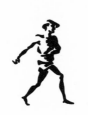

# THE COMPLETE

# MEDICAL GUIDE

by BENJAMIN F. MILLER, M.D.

with Lawrence Galton

---

## 4th Edition—Revised and Updated

---

ILLUSTRATED BY R. PAUL LARKIN

---

SIMON AND SCHUSTER · NEW YORK

PUBLISHED BY SIMON AND SCHUSTER
A DIVISION OF GULF & WESTERN CORPORATION
SIMON & SCHUSTER BUILDING
ROCKEFELLER CENTER
1230 AVENUE OF THE AMERICAS
NEW YORK, NEW YORK 10020
FOURTH REVISED EDITION

MANUFACTURED IN THE UNITED STATES OF AMERICA

1  2  3  4  5  6  7  8  9  10

LIBRARY OF CONGRESS CATALOGING IN PUBLICATION DATA

MILLER, BENJAMIN FRANK, 1907–1971.
    THE COMPLETE MEDICAL GUIDE.

    INCLUDES INDEX.
     1. MEDICINE, POPULAR.   I. GALTON, LAWRENCE.
II. TITLE.
RC81.M66   1978   610'.24   78–9574

ISBN 0-671-24107-9

The 8-page color insert following page 32 is used by permission of the W. B. Saunders Company. It appeared in *Good Health—Personal and Community* by Miller and Burt, 2nd edition, published in 1966.

TO

CHESTER M. JONES, M.D.

> *who taught me so much at medical school, and then in later years generously and skillfully guided me back to health during a long illness.*

# CONTENTS

---

# INTRODUCTION

This is a book written for all adults. I believe it will serve the health information needs of the mother and father in the home, as well as those of unmarried men and women. I hope, too, that older people—our senior citizens—will find sound advice in it to make their golden years even richer.

Because of the many sections dealing with purely adult matters I do not recommend the book for children or adolescents. However, any person old enough to contemplate marriage, or mature enough to be working for a livelihood, is surely old enough to be concerned with the intimate matters of health and sexual hygiene that are contained in some chapters.

The book has several purposes. I have written it as a *guide* to the complex world of health and medical matters. I believe people will be healthier and happier if they read and follow the advice on nutrition, alcohol, posture, mental health, first aid, and the many other matters which play a part in everybody's life. Other chapters dealing with job hazards, marital problems, housing, pregnancy, child care, home nursing, etc., contain information that is of special interest and value to different members of the family.

Another chief purpose of the book is to serve as a *reference work.* Every major disease such as cancer and diabetes has been described, as well as many of the less common ones. The "nuisance" ailments from dandruff to hemorrhoids have been given space. All this information is at your disposal by reference to the chapter headings and to the Index, which has been made as comprehensive as possible.

Third, the book provides a dictionary and glossary of medical terms. Today, an educated person must be conversant with such technical matters as the electrocardiogram, basal metabolism, antibiotics, Papanicolaou smears for cancer detection, and hundreds of other terms. To help in this sometimes bewildering area, I have prepared the glossary with both definitions and pronunciations of the terms you are most likely to encounter in daily life.

Finally this book is designed as *an integral part of the doctor-patient relationship.* I view my book as an extension of your personal physician, not as a replacement for him. Doctors who have read this book agree with me. They point out that no physician can take complete responsibility for the health of his patient. Your doctor has to assume that you will read and educate yourself regarding matters as vital as balanced diets, prevention of accidents, mental hygiene, and the dozens of other subjects covered in this book. It would take several days if he sat down with you and gave you even a digest of the health information contained in a comprehensive health manual such as this. No doctor can afford the time to do that.

Your doctor will welcome the fact that I stress (1) prevention of illness, (2) detection of sickness in its earliest stages if it is not a preventable type, and (3) recognition of the danger of self-treatment in potentially serious conditions. Thus, this book helps your doctor do his important job better.

Physicians in particular may wonder how one person has "dared" write a comprehensive health book alone, especially in this day of specialization. I wanted this book to convey a unified point of view, with a consistent approach to the many problems concerning the prevention of sickness and the achievement of ideal health. I also felt the need of a book in which one style of writing was maintained, so that the reader would become well acquainted with the author, instead of having to adapt to a new personality with each chapter. Therefore, I determined to write the book myself. However, I wanted the book to have the advantages made possible by specialization, and so experts in various fields were consulted, particularly in areas outside my special training or experience. The chapters dealing with these subjects have been carefully checked by them. I owe a tremendous debt to the following specialists for their expert advice and suggestions: Frances Bowen, R.N., Leslie Falk, M.D., David Goodfriend, D.D.S., Harriet L. Hardy, M.D., David Harris, M.D., Ralph J. Kahana, M.D., Maxwell P. Lewitus, D.M.D., Richard J. Manley, Ph.D., M. M. Osborne, M.D., Leon Resnik, M.D., Melvin H. Rosen, D.M.D., Arthur J. Schramm, M.D., Kenneth Sterling, M.D., and John Vester, M.D.

## ADDITIONAL ACKNOWLEDGMENTS

I started this book a number of years ago, and have been thinking about it and planning it for a long time. Then, for the revisions, everything I had done had to be brought up to date because medical knowledge fortunately is always moving ahead. During all these years I have been discussing the book with physicians and nurses and nonmedical people—in fact, anyone who would listen to my obsession about writing a comprehensive, understandable health book. I doubt that I can remember everyone who has offered suggestions and criticisms. If I have omitted someone, I beg his or her forgiveness.

There are some persons who have worked actively with me in a research or editorial capacity during various phases of the writing of this book. I want particularly to thank my wife, Judith, who has been an invaluable helper and critic. Also, Rhoda Truax, who helped in the preparation of the first edition, and Edward B. Rosenberg, who helped with the third edition. To Philip James I owe much gratitude for his careful reading and rereading of the manuscript of the third revised edition and now of this new edition.

I am indebted to the following for permission to reprint or adapt material from their books: Dr. Maurice Levine, from his *Psychotherapy in Medical Practice,* and to the publisher, The Macmillan Company, for their permission; to St. Martin's Press Incorporated, New York, and The Macmillan Company of Canada, Ltd., for the quotation written by A. J. Amor in *Medicine,* edited by Hugh G. Garland, 1953; Harcourt, Brace and Company, Inc., for the passage from Carl Sandburg's *The People, Yes,* 1936; Alfred A. Knopf, Inc., for the quotation from *The Happy Family* by Levy and Monroe, 1938; The Metropolitan Life Insurance Company for the table on "Desirable Weights for Men and Women."

The illustrator, R. Paul Larkin, has been a joy to work with because he conveyed to me so much enthusiasm for the book along with his artistic skill.

In the preparation of this fourth, revised edition, Lawrence Galton has served as research and editorial associate.

B. F. M.

# PART ONE

## You and Your Body

# 1
# GENERAL CARE OF THE BODY

If you bought your body as you do an automobile, a piece of furniture or a garment, you would undoubtedly receive instructions with it telling you how to take *reasonable care* of your purchase. I am sure you would read them carefully. You would want to avoid fussing or worrying about things needlessly and yet be sufficiently careful so that your purchase would remain in good condition as long as possible.

This chapter covers the subject of reasonable care of the precious human body. Here, I shall deal with matters involving the entire body, such as fresh air, cleanliness, sleep, posture, exercise, smoking, and alcohol. The food you eat belongs in this category, but the subject is so large I devote all of Chapter 2 to it. Chapter 6 tells you how to take care of the individual parts—the various organs and tissues—of the body.

Books on health were limited to these subjects in the past, and this tradition continued even after doctors came to realize that they were only one (although an essential) part of your total health program. Many of these books would tell you exactly how long you should sleep, how far open the windows should be, how cold a shower you should take, and what setting-up exercises you should do. They failed to take into account such matters as differences in individual life-styles—where and how people live, their work, housing circumstances, physical activities and more—as well as varying individual needs and preferences. There may still be a few doctors inclined to believe that what is best or customary for them and the majority of their patients is essential for everyone. It is possible, for example, that you might find

a small-town European doctor who, if asked how often people should take baths, might say, "Once or twice a week," and perhaps an American physician who might answer automatically, "Every day." But more and more doctors now take a more relaxed position and suggest that while a daily bath or shower is a good idea in hot weather, two or three times a week may be enough otherwise, especially for a person who is not very physically active. Actually this, like many other things, depends on your situation, needs, and personal preference.

## THE AIR YOU BREATHE

"Fresh air" is a frequently misunderstood term. It doesn't mean that our bodies need air blowing through a room all the time. Unless a room is completely sealed up, enough air comes in around doors and windows to provide oxygen for breathing. Whether more air should be circulated through the room depends on your own comfort and desires.

These vary a great deal. A few generations ago air in itself was considered dangerous, especially night air, which was supposed to carry disease-laden vapors (called miasmas) and drafts, which doctors blamed for any number of illnesses. The result was that many of our ancestors accustomed themselves to wearing several layers of underclothing in all seasons, and to sleeping with their windows tightly closed. They even had draperies hanging from canopies over their beds for added protection, and babies were wrapped up like mummies. (See pages 264-65 concerning air and clothing for infants.)

With such discoveries as the fact that malaria was caused by mosquitoes and not by night air, the pendulum began to swing in the opposite direction. One of the results of this was the "fresh-air fiend" who went around flinging windows open to the discomfort of his associates. A former patient of mine, a middle-aged woman from a well-to-do New York City family, told me that her parents were so sold on the virtues of fresh air that they insisted on her being out of doors regardless of the temperature. As she was not a very active child, she was cold most of the time, even suffering from frostbitten fingers and toes. In some countries and among some groups, drafts are still carefully avoided, while other folks enjoy rooms that resemble the great open spaces.

There is no evidence to prove that one situation is more healthful than another. Some people feel definitely better with windows open while others feel uncomfortable—even sick—when exposed to drafts of cold air. *Each person needs to find the condition to which he reacts best.*

## Dangerous Heating Appliances

When coal, wood, or gas is burned in fireplaces, stoves, or radiators, it consumes oxygen. Oxygen is essential for life. When such heating methods are used, make certain that air is entering the room. If the doors and windows fit snugly (so that you don't feel any air coming in when you place your hand near the sills), be sure to open one of them a little. Always be careful to protect a gas flame from drafts that might blow it out, leaving the gas pouring into the room. This has been the cause of many serious accidents (see page 322). Electric heaters and electric stoves *do not* use up the oxygen in the air. They warm the air around them by various means, but they do not themselves interact chemically with the oxygen in the atmosphere.

## Temperature of Rooms

There is, of course, a problem when it comes to getting along with people whose standards of comfort differ from your own. The average person seems to prefer a room temperature between 70°

and 75° F. If you like to be warmer or colder than your associates, try to take care of this by the clothing you wear; there is a big difference between the warmth provided by various suits, or between a sweater and a thin blouse. Garments should be loose enough not to restrict the body in any way and should permit the absorption or evaporation of perspiration. They should be chosen for comfort rather than simply for style.

AIR CONDITIONING. Air conditioning is becoming so common in the United States that few of us could avoid it even if we wanted to. Not only in stores and offices but in apartments, houses, theaters, trains, buses, and automobiles, the air is cooled, sometimes uncomfortably so.

Air conditioning is certainly an aid to comfort, but it sometimes is a problem, especially if the control is fixed. If at all possible, you should have the temperature adjusted to your own comfort and health requirements. Many people are exposed to an air-conditioned environment so much of the time that they rarely have the advantage of breathing outdoor air during the summer. Going from an air-conditioned apartment, in an air-conditioned car, to an air-conditioned office, and back again at the end of the day means that the body has had little opportunity to make the healthy adjustment to varying climatic conditions that is so important to maintaining a sturdy constitution.

On the other hand, air conditioning can be a lifesaver. Hot, humid weather places added strain on the circulatory system. For persons suffering from some heart disease, this added strain may be intolerable. Living in an air-conditioned environment may be advised by your physician if you have a coronary condition. (Heart diseases are discussed beginning on page 416.)

## Humidity and Comfort

Besides the freshness and temperature of air, its moisture content (humidity) may influence health. Again, each individual must find his own prescription. Some people feel well in cold winter climates where the *indoor* air is extremely dry. Other people notice that this dry atmosphere causes irritation of the nose and throat. They react very much better after they humidify the air by putting pans of water around the house, especially on or near the radiators. Some people are relatively comfortable when the air is warm and moist in summer. Others are so oppressed by it that they need a fan or an air conditioner. Because perspiration evaporates more readily in dry air, thus cooling the body, most people mind the heat less when it is not combined with dampness.

A number of room humidifiers and dehumidifiers have come on the market in recent years. Many of them are useless, but some have limited value. Before you spend the considerable amount any such device costs, examine it carefully. Best of all, consult a reliable consumer rating service.

It is best not to expose the body directly to a fan, especially at night, because the chilling may predispose to an attack of neuralgia, bursitis, or even pneumonia. Air conditioners should have thermostats so that they will not cool rooms to uncomfortable temperatures.

## REST AND SLEEP

The number of hours of sleep required for good health varies tremendously from person to person. Eight hours each night appears to be average, but we have all heard about people like the famous inventor Thomas A. Edison, who got along very well on five hours, and others who require more than eight hours a night. The essential test is whether you feel rested in the morning and have sufficient energy to carry through the day's activities. If you don't, chronic fatigue may accumulate and contribute to what can be a serious illness. Many men and women find they really can get along on fewer than eight hours sleep a night as they grow older. If you are concerned about having trouble sleeping, it is possible that you are getting less sleep because you need less sleep. Insomnia, or the inability to sleep, is discussed under Nuisance Diseases, page 494.

We all know about the need for a good night's sleep, but too few of us recognize the need for *rest during the day*. Businessmen, professional people, executives, and many others, who not only work hard but are under heavy stress, could live more comfortably and probably longer if they managed to rest during the day. Even a brief period of relaxation would be healthful. I suggest that you place a couch, or at least a reclining chair, in your office. If this is impossible, you could relax by having lunch in a quiet restaurant, instead of in a crowded, noisy one. Or you might bring lunch from home and eat it in a park.

I have always found it refreshing to rest at home for a half hour at the end of the day instead of rushing right to the dinner table. It is really sad that this time of day, which could be a peaceful meeting time for the family, can become a time of short tempers and unpleasantness, just because you, and perhaps your wife too, are tired. An eight-hour workday, plus another hour or two for commuting, is too long for many people. If you can't do anything about your hours of work, try to relax at other times.

Periods of *relaxation* which are found in *pleasant recreation* are necessary to most people at least once a week. More and more it is being recognized that a yearly *vacation* helps to safeguard good health. (See Chapter 9 on vacations.) Church affairs and social activities with friends and one's family provide excellent relaxation. So do *hobbies* and *exercise*, or sports, which are discussed below.

## HOBBIES

Hobbies provide relaxation and help to maintain your zest for living, which we doctors have come to realize is immensely important to your health. Like most physicians, I have observed this frequently. People who have developed hobbies tend to be healthier as well as happier, especially in their later years, than those who lack outside interests.

Ideally, each of us should have an indoor and an outdoor hobby that gives us genuine, long-range satisfaction. Some energetic folks change their hobbies every year or two, keeping a direct relationship between the indoor and outdoor activity. For example, one year the outdoor hobby will be archery and the indoor diversion Indian art; the next year the combination may be sailing and ship models. I prefer to be more casual, letting the hobby grow with time. I enjoy photography, which lends itself to both indoors and outdoors; piano playing and fishing or swimming have also served well for me.

Hobbies need not be expensive. Some of them, like gardening and refinishing old furniture, can more than pay for themselves. Be sure to find something you enjoy. Don't be like a patient of mine who came to me some time ago when his own physician retired. A businessman in his fifties, he had been collecting stamps for years; it was only after I got to know him fairly well that he admitted it had always bored him. He had taken it up because his doctor recommended a hobby, and it was the only one he could think of! While he was telling me this, he doodled on a pad lying on the desk; and in reply to a comment of mine he remarked that he had always liked to draw but had never thought of it as a suitable hobby for a man in his position. Now he belongs to the ever growing group of amateur "Sunday artists."

There are several things to consider when you choose a hobby, most of which this man ignored when he chose his. The hobby should be something *you* want to do. Never mind what anyone else thinks. It should give you both satisfaction and relaxation. Your hobby should be worth doing. If it is a mere time-filler with no built-in value, you will soon become bored. Being worthwhile, it will sooner or later be productive, most likely in terms of inner satisfaction but possibly even financially. Many women who started sewing or embroidering for fun, and many men who turned to cabinetmaking for relaxation, later found their skills and services in demand, at a profit. Finally, don't wait to begin until you are retired. How you develop your interests and activities as a young person, then in middle age, will largely determine how enjoyably you will spend your later years.

Adult education is becoming more and more popular. The motives range from completing degree requirements, to acquiring new knowledge or skill for its own sake, to developing a hobby. Whatever the reasons, the newspapers and magazines are full of advertisements and notices of adult education courses in colleges and universities everywhere. Your local public school board may also offer adult courses at night. The Adult Education Association of the U.S.A., 1225 14th Street, NW, Washington, D.C., will tell you about the opportunities in your vicinity. These courses usually include everything from the arts and crafts to languages, current events, and such subjects as science, philosophy, and psychology. One of them is almost certain to appeal to you.

## EXERCISE AND SPORTS

Although a reasonable level of physical activity is important in maintaining health and even in warding off some diseases, most of us today have less and less routine opportunity for activity in our daily lives unless we deliberately seek it out.

You can almost certainly expect to derive a long list of benefits by giving proper attention to exercise and other physical activity. Muscles will, of course, be strengthened. So, too, will be the heart, lungs, and circulatory system. Along with increased strength, you will find that endurance, coordination, and joint flexibility will be increased, and there may well be a reduction of minor aches and pains.

There is increasing evidence that physical activity is of value in helping to overcome or prevent emotional tension and in helping to prevent many critical diseases such as heart disease, stroke, and peripheral vascular disorders which affect circulation in the extremities.

### Do You Need More Activity?

If you need specific indications that you can benefit from more activity, here are some: hard breathing or pounding of your heart after relatively slight exertion; a long period before your heartbeat returns to normal after heavy exertion (you can measure the heart rate by the wrist pulse); stiffening of legs and thighs after climbing stairs; waking up from sleep as tired as before; frequent restlessness.

I suggest that you discuss the matter of activity with your physician. He will be glad to determine with you—on the basis of your specific present condition, daily activities, and other personal factors—whether you need more exercise, how much time you need to devote to it, and what kinds of activity would be best suited for you.

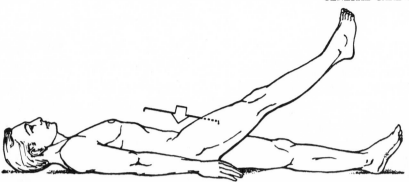

*Figure 1–1. Exercise for Muscles of Lower Abdomen.* Exhale; raise leg slowly without bending; hold it up while counting to ten (about ten seconds); lower it slowly; inhale. Do the same with the other leg. To strengthen the muscles without straining them, begin by repeating the exercise two or three times, and increase gradually until you can do them about twenty times without straining.

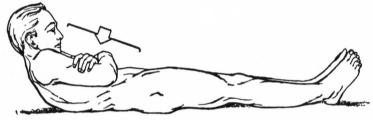

*Figure 1–2. Exercise for Muscles of Upper Abdomen.* Exhale; with arms folded over chest, raise head slowly, keeping legs on the floor; hold for about ten seconds; relax and inhale. Repeat two or three times. As muscles grow stronger, increase gradually to about twenty times.

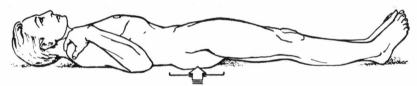

*Figure 1–3. Exercise for Muscles of Buttocks.* While lying flat, tighten the buttocks as much as possible, and hold for about ten seconds before relaxing. Repeat two or three times. Increase gradually to about twenty times.

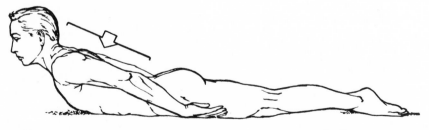

*Figure 1–4. Exercise for Muscles of Back.* Keeping arms at side and legs on the floor, slowly raise chest and shoulders; hold for about ten seconds; lower slowly. Increase gradually from two or three times to about twenty times.

## Choice of Sports and Athletics

I always suggest that patients get their exercise as much as possible from games they enjoy. A game stimulates interest so that exercise becomes positively pleasurable. However, too many young people, especially young men, become proficient only in those sports which cannot be carried into later life. Some of these, such as boxing, carry the continual threat of body injury. Highly competitive sports including football, baseball, basketball, crew; and track do not serve a useful purpose in the individual health program in later life. Either they are too strenuous, or they require too many participants. A busy adult with job and family responsibilities can rarely get up a neighborhood baseball game.

It is wise for the athletically inclined to take advantage of their high school and college facilities to become proficient in one or two of the following sports. I have selected some that can be carried into middle and even late life, to the benefit of body and muscle health, strength, and good posture:

| | |
|---|---|
| Swimming | Hiking |
| Golf | Badminton |
| Tennis | Squash rackets |
| Handball | Horseback riding |
| Canoeing | |

These are desirable because they require only one or two people. They lend themselves to weekend relaxation. Married couples can enjoy them together, later participating in them with their children.

Hiking and swimming are good sports for people of all ages, especially those who enjoy the outdoors. Many communities have indoor pools so that it is possible to swim regardless of the season. Neither of these sports need be expensive.

## A Balanced Program

Your activity program should be balanced, just as diet should be. You need one or more activities to exercise the heart and lungs and to build endurance. Brisk walking, jogging, and swimming relatively long distances are good for this. Other parts of the program should be aimed at improving strength, agility, flexibility, and muscle tone.

Your physician may have suggestions for a program to achieve these objectives. Suggestions also can be found in such publications as these:

*Adult Physical Fitness*, President's Council on Physical Fitness, Superintendent of Documents, U.S. Government Printing Office, Washington, D.C. 20402

*Physical Fitness*, Department of Health Education, American Medical Association, 535 N. Dearborn, Chicago, Illinois 60610

*Seven Paths to Fitness*, Department of Health Education, American Medical Association, 535 N. Dearborn, Chicago, Illinois 60610

Whatever activities you engage in, start slowly. There should be no sudden demand on your body for a burst of tremendous effort. Start easily and then gradually begin to work a little harder—just slightly beyond the first feeling of tiredness but still within your limits of tolerance. Your body has more capacity than it is routinely called upon to use. Give it a bit more load than usual and it can handle it. Progressively, it will become able to handle more.

If, for example, you should choose jogging as an activity, at first you might jog for fifty yards, walk for fifty yards, keep alternating, and cover about a mile. As you continue to work out, you will find you can increase the distance, jog more and walk less, jog faster, perhaps even interspersing some sprints, running as fast as you can for fifty yards, then dropping back to a jog or walk. Over a period of months, you may progress until you can cover as much as three miles at a good pace, walking very little of the time.

Physical activity should become part of your daily routine. This means setting aside a period —perhaps thirty minutes to an hour a day—about five times a week. It should be considered as essential a part of your life as eating, sleeping, and bathing. Pick a time most suitable for you. If it is convenient for you to carry out much or all of your activity in one period each day, fine; divided periods of activity can also serve the purpose. Never perform any exercise sooner than one hour after a meal.

## What to Do About the Sagging Waistline

Few people are lucky enough to get much beyond the age of thirty-five or forty without some extra fat or muscle sag around the waistline. By combining the reducing diet, or "hold your weight" advice, that I give on pages 44 to 56, with a daily period of the exercises on page 17, you should restore your waistline to normal within a few months.

## The "Middle-Aged Spread"

Women in their forties and fifties usually develop flabby muscles and extra fat around the hips (really around the thighs, buttocks, and lower abdomen). This combination of fat and poor muscle tone gives the so-called middle-aged spread. The following measures are helpful: (a) weight control or reduction of weight as described on page 49, (b) use of special exercises, (c) some discretion in the selection of clothes, with the realization that at forty a woman can no longer wear the styles that are becoming to a twenty-year-old (especially true of slacks and dungarees!), (d) a philosophic approach to middle life with some sense of humor about the exaggerated importance placed on a trim figure in our society. By forty or fifty, a woman's beauty should reflect her sense of accomplishment as a human being, whether wife, mother, teacher, nurse, etc.—and not merely as a glamorized "clothes horse."

Look at almost any man past the age of thirty. His arms aren't fat and his legs are probably in good shape. But his waistline is getting out of control! For the specific problem of a flabby middle, the exercises I have illustrated will be helpful.

## The Pleasures of Walking

If you don't especially care for sports or games, just a brisk regular walk will do a lot for your muscle tone, circulation, and general health. Instead of driving all the way to work, you might try parking a mile or so from your office and getting in your walk at the beginning and end of your workday. My system, in part, is to park at the end of the very large lot near my hospital and walk to the entrance of the building. This is only a modest amount of exercise, but it makes me feel good, and it gives me a chance to relax a little before and after the pressures of the day.

# POSTURE

Good posture is usually an expression of good health rather than a major factor in producing good health. A healthy person will as a rule automatically find a comfortable, attractive posture. Pride and poise will do away with slight slouches or round shoulders. You'll be surprised by the feeling of well-being that comes with good posture.

If your posture is not easy to correct, there is probably some medical reason for it, unless you are being influenced by some foolish fashion such as the debutante slouch of the 1920's or the sloppy Joe pose of more recent years. It is far wiser to invest in an examination by your doctor or at a hospital clinic than to spend money on a course in posture building. Your doctor can establish the cause, and if special exercises or braces are needed, he will prescribe what is right for you. Foot troubles caused by badly fitting shoes can be responsible for poor posture (see page 115).

There are a few posture rules worth putting into practice every day. At work, at school, or at home, your chair should feel comfortable and should give sufficient support so that your back rests against its back. The chair should be strong and solid enough to take your weight comfortably, and not sag or rock when you sit in it. This is particularly true of the soft chairs found in so many homes, which tempt us to curl up or slump until we are practically "sitting on the back of the neck." Difficult as it may be to believe, people would be far more comfortable, especially over a long period of time, if they sat in relatively hard chairs with sturdy, fairly straight back supports. The choice of a well-designed chair is especially important for people who sit for long periods at their work—for example, typists and office workers.

They should sit squarely, with their feet placed on the floor a short distance in front of their chairs, avoiding bad habits such as wrapping one leg around the leg of the chair.

A patient of mine, a six-footer who travels a great deal by car, told me that he always pulls the seat as far forward as possible when he is driving. In this way he sits quite straight, his back sup- ported, and is able to press down on the accelera- tor instead of having to stretch out his leg to reach it at an angle; this is far easier on the muscles of the back as well as of the leg.

*Posture for the standing position* is important if your work requires you to be on your feet for long hours at a time. Study the illustrations which show good and bad posture. When correcting your

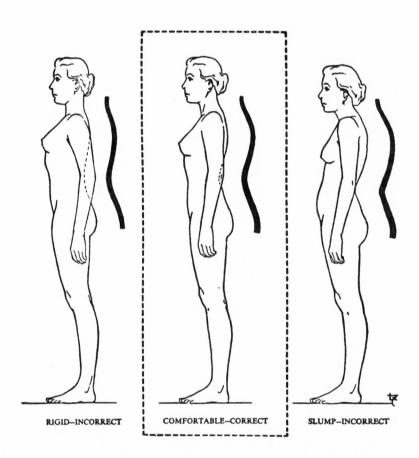

RIGID—INCORRECT     COMFORTABLE—CORRECT     SLUMP—INCORRECT

*Figure 1-5. Standing Posture.* LEFT: *Incorrect. Standing in this rigid, military position, with the chin pulled in and the backbone unnaturally straight, causes tension and strain, especially on the knees and the back muscles.* CENTER: *Correct. A minimum of fatigue results when standing in this easy, comfortable manner, with the chest slightly raised and the buttocks "tucked in." It is also important because it permits organs such as the lungs and stomach to be in their proper positions.* RIGHT: *Incorrect. Slumping in this too-relaxed manner, with the chin thrust forward, the chest sunken, and the stomach protruding, can cause a number of ailments, including "round shoulders" and backache.*

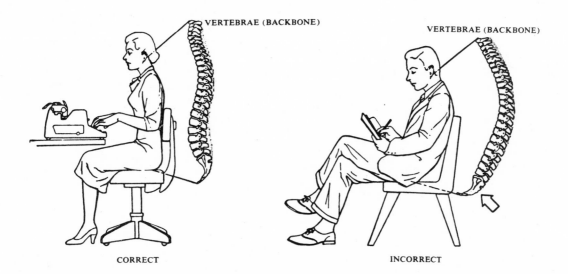

VERTEBRAE (BACKBONE)

VERTEBRAE (BACKBONE)

CORRECT

INCORRECT

*Figure 1–6. Posture When Seated.* LEFT: *Correct. The backbone is in its normal position, with its burden equally distributed. The feet rest on the floor. The chair is adjustable, so that the work surface is at the proper height.* RIGHT: *Incorrect. Slouching puts too much of the weight on the end of the spine (indicated by arrow). The shoulders are rounded, the internal organs compressed, and the legs twisted, straining the muscles and interfering with the circulation.*

posture, find a relaxed, attractive stance that feels restful. Do not try to stand as erect as a soldier at a military parade.

If your posture does not satisfy you, try to improve it by a period of exercises. Also, be sure your weight is correct as judged by the information I give in Chapter 3, page 45. Develop skill in one of the sports I have suggested, or take long walks. If after several months you are still troubled by a faulty standing position, or rounded shoulders, or protruding abdomen, see your doctor for a checkup and advice.

## Posture During and After Pregnancy

Many women lose their fine carriage and figure during pregnancy, and never regain their former good posture and muscle tone. There is no need for this. During pregnancy, the pull on the abdominal and back muscles can be reduced by the use of maternity corsets, which your doctor will prescribe if they are necessary.

After the baby has been born, the mother should carry through the series of exercises given on page 257. These will help bring back the strength of the abdominal muscles. Many women have borne a half-dozen children and have retained youthful, trim body outlines.

## Posture for Children and Adolescents

Correct posture for children and adolescents is discussed on pages 302.

# USE OF ALCOHOL, TOBACCO, DRUGS

Before I take up these subjects individually, I want to remind you that I am speaking as a physician. I feel it would be presumptuous of me to discuss the purely moral or religious aspects of these matters. For example, even the most moderate use of tobacco or alcoholic beverages is forbidden by some religious denominations. Nothing I say should influence you regarding matters that each of us must decide in accordance with his or her own conscience and with the help of spiritual advisers. I am limiting myself to telling you what medical science has, to date, discovered about the effect of stimulants upon your body.

## ALCOHOL

Although usually considered a stimulant, alcohol is actually a depressant. It *appears* to lessen fatigue and make you peppy because it, in effect, takes the brake off certain processes. For example, even a fairly small amount of alcohol lessens the cerebral inhibitions which we normally exert in order to "behave properly," and this makes us feel relieved and free.

Alcohol is useful in certain diseases and harmful in others. People who consider a drink of whiskey as the initial step in all first-aid treatment can do a lot of damage. (It is definitely harmful, for instance, in cases of heatstroke and snakebite.) People with some diseases may have a certain amount of alcohol prescribed for them; in other illnesses it is forbidden. If you or anyone in your family is suffering from any ailment, be sure to discuss the matter with your doctor before taking or offering drinks.

## Alcohol for the Normal, Healthy Individual

There is no evidence to prove that moderate drinking will *cause* any disease, or injure the general health, or shorten the life of the healthy adult. What do I mean by moderate drinking? This is not easy to define exactly, since the amount which different people can tolerate varies considerably. Most of us doctors would describe the moderate drinker as one who takes one or two drinks a day, e.g., a couple of highballs containing one and a half ounces each of whiskey, or a quart of beer during the course of several hours. The moderate drinker takes his alcoholic beverages for relaxation, never as a constant necessity. He does not become intoxicated. Taken in this way, there is no physical harm in the use of liquor. It can be a source of great pleasure. Yet even under these circumstances there may be some impairment of judgment or coordination; there are people who ought not to drive a car after drinking even one small glass of sherry.

## Excessive Drinking

Again, this does not depend solely upon the amount of alcohol consumed. Some people—the French, for example—drink as much as a pint of wine with every dinner but are not excessive drinkers. By excessive drinking I mean getting intoxicated or drinking to the point where it interferes with one's job, one's family life, and one's relation to society. The person who drinks excessively is practically a criminal when he is behind the wheel of a car or otherwise assumes responsibilities he is not capable of fulfilling. He or she often has hangovers. Excessive drinkers often fail to eat properly and otherwise neglect to observe the rules of good health, thereby suffering from a number of illnesses as a direct consequence of drinking. There is some recent evidence, although it is not conclusive, that in addition to all the other physical problems created by excessive drinking, cancer of the mouth is more likely to afflict the heavy drinker than the person who drinks moderately or not at all.

## The Chronic Alcoholic

We doctors distinguish between the excessive drinker and the chronic alcoholic, although the former may become the latter without realizing it. The excessive drinker uses alcohol on occasion to escape from unpleasant situations, but the alcoholic wants to escape from life, or from himself,

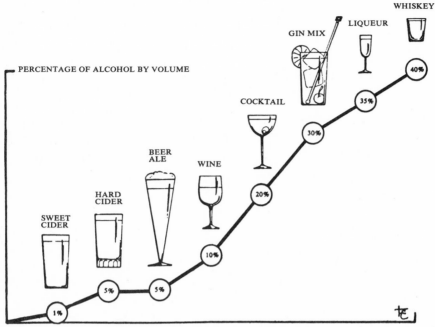

PERCENTAGE OF ALCOHOL BY VOLUME

*Figure 1–7. Alcoholic Content of Beverages.*

completely. No matter how bad a hangover he may have, the alcoholic craves a drink again, often in the morning before (or instead of) breakfast. One of the surest signs of the chronic alcoholic is that he cannot take one drink without wanting more; "one drink is too many, a hundred not enough."

Sooner or later, the alcoholic cares for nothing but drinking. His health suffers for a number of reasons, one of the main ones being his failure to eat properly. Alcohol provides him with calories enough to keep him from feeling hungry, but alcoholic beverages lack vitamins, minerals, and other requirements. Deficiency diseases (see page 471) result; eventually, a number of afflictions may involve the brain, the nerves, and the liver. Some of these illnesses are fatal, and all are relatively disabling.

## Chronic Alcoholism Is an Illness

I discuss this fully in the chapter on disabling diseases, page 470. The one fact which you should always bear in mind, if you or someone close to you suffers from or is threatened by this condition, is that your doctor recognizes it as a serious *medical* problem. Unlike some of your neighbors, he will not condemn or joke or sermonize or dismiss you with some pious words of sympathy. Don't try patented "cures." Be sure to consult a physician or go to a hospital clinic for proper advice and treatment. You may say an alcoholic can't be helped unless he wants to be cured, but this does not mean alcoholism is not an illness. There are many diseases which doctors cannot help without the cooperation of the patient—for example, diabetes can't be handled unless the patient is willing to take his insulin and observe his diet. A doctor will know how best to get cooperation from an alcoholic, which ones will be benefited by joining the well-known organization called Alcoholics Anonymous, and which will respond better in a hospital or sanatorium where new and excellent treatments for alcoholism have been worked out.

## TOBACCO

Enough is known about the direct relationship between smoking and several extremely serious diseases to make me, like many other doctors, say, "If you don't smoke, don't start. If you do smoke, stop. If you can't stop, then at least cut down." This is now my advice to *everyone*.

Smoking is a direct cause of lung cancer. The death rate from lung cancer for cigarette smokers is more than ten times higher than for nonsmokers. Air pollution also is considered a factor, but scientists and physicians are convinced that smoking is far more significant. Smoking also has been blamed for cancer of the larynx (upper throat or voicebox) and several serious respiratory ailments, including bronchitis and emphysema of the lungs. The effect of tobacco smoke inside the body is to slow down or stop the natural cleansing processes of the bronchial tubes leading to the lungs, leaving those organs more susceptible to the irritants of the smoke itself and of other substances in the air. Some of these substances can bring about cancer.

A significant association has also been made between smoking and heart disease, now the most common cause of death in the United States. The death rate from coronary heart disease is much higher among smokers than nonsmokers, and higher among men than women, especially men in their forties and fifties.

Smoking also contributes to other diseases, including peptic ulcer and cancer of the bladder. The vital thing to remember is that the risk of incurring any of these diseases grows with the number of cigarettes smoked daily, the length of each cigarette consumed, and the length of time the smoking habit has lasted. It is a fact that heavy smokers as a group die younger than nonsmokers.

You may wonder why I don't just tell everyone to stop smoking, without even suggesting they cut down. One reason is that my experience as a doctor tells me most people won't listen to such a flat ban. Habits are hard to break, even habits that injure our health. But I do emphasize two things —if you have children, do everything you can to persuade them never to start smoking. For yourself, if you can't stop, cut down on your smoking until it becomes a *low-risk activity*. Personally, I found it impossible just to stop doing something I had been in the habit of doing for some thirty-five years. Now, instead of chain-smoking two or three packs of cigarettes daily, I smoke nothing but a pipeful of mild tobacco, and even that only occasionally during the day. There is no reason to panic at the knowledge of how smoking damages the body, but it certainly makes sense to indulge in low-risk, not high-risk, smoking, if you can't break the habit.

## For the Determined— How to Stop Smoking

It would be a mistake to believe that if you have tried to give up smoking in the past and have failed, you are doomed to go on smoking. If you have failed before, that in itself is no indication of hopeless weak will. Along with determination, you also need insight, a plan, a constructive attitude.

A most important factor in quitting is to view the process positively. If you regard it as simply giving up something of value, you may feel sorry for yourself. Rather, you must view the process as one of teaching yourself a more rewarding behavior pattern, one that will represent a huge gain.

Many methods have been suggested for quitting, and the American Cancer Society has compiled expert recommendations. To begin with, set a date when you plan to quit. Call it Q day—for complete quitting day. You may want to allow yourself as much as a month to get ready for that day. And getting ready can involve a gradual reduction in the number of cigarettes you smoke day by day.

A good system is to determine that you will smoke only once an hour or that you will not smoke between the hours of 9 and 10, or 12 and 1, or 3 and 4, for example. And then extend the nonsmoking time by half an hour, an hour, and more. You may find it helpful, too, to smoke just half of each cigarette.

Make it a deliberate effort to light a cigarette. If you habitually carry a pack in a certain pocket, start using another pocket so you have to do some fumbling for a smoke. If you habitually use your right hand to bring a cigarette to your mouth, determine to use the left hand.

Wrap your pack in several sheets of paper so it becomes an involved process to get at a cigarette. Shift from your usual brand to one you don't like.

Each time before lighting up, make it a point to ask yourself a direct question: Do I really want this cigarette right now or am I just lighting up out of habit? For whatever else it is, cigarette smoking is a habit, and anything you can do to put even small crimps in the automation involved can help.

Along with determination to break the habit, you need deep motivation. Think carefully and then write out a list of reasons why you smoke, and another list of reasons why you should give up cigarettes.

THE LAST WEEK. In the week before Q day, go over your reasons for not smoking: the disease risk, the cost, the cough, the bad breath, the bad taste, etc. Each evening, before falling asleep, concentrate on one dire result of smoking: repeat and repeat that fact, and another the next night, etc.

Remind yourself all during the week of some established facts: that if you continue smoking, you risk losing six and a half years of life; that if you smoke heavily, you have twice the chance of a nonsmoker of dying between twenty-five and sixty-five. Are the six minutes of pleasure, if such they really be, in a cigarette worth six fewer minutes of life? Consider that 100,000 American physicians have quit smoking cigarettes.

Q DAY. On Q day you get up—and don't smoke. You may find it helpful to drink water often; to nibble fruit, celery, carrots; to suck candy mints or chew gum. You may resort—and good if it helps —to chewing bits of fresh ginger or biting a clove when you start reaching for a cigarette.

Exercise. Physical activity, if your physician says you are up to it, can help work off irritation from not having a cigarette in your mouth. Even mild calisthenics, stretching exercises, and walks can help relax you. Breathe deeply from time to time; deep breathing can have a calming effect.

After-meal times can be difficult. Instead of a cigarette, try a mouthwash. Change habit patterns that have gone with after-meal smoking. Immediately after eating, if you are used to relaxing in one chair, use another; if you are accustomed to reading a newspaper, read a magazine or book instead, or try a puzzle.

Reward yourself. Have your favorite meal on Q day. Treat yourself to things you like best— except cigarettes. After saving some money from not smoking, reward yourself with a present: a new record, book, trinket.

Will this method work for you? It has worked for many. It is worth trying.

CAUTION: WATCH YOUR WEIGHT. People who give up smoking usually gain weight. After the first week or so, or when you no longer crave a smoke, start taking the precautions about diet I suggest on page 52.

## USE OF COFFEE AND TEA

Both coffee and tea contain caffeine, which is a stimulating compound. Coffee and tea in moderate amounts are not harmful. The use of more than three to four cups of coffee or tea per day may lead to restlessness, overactivity, nervousness, insomnia, and excessive urination. Each person needs to find the correct amount for his own particular system and habits of life. Some people can take coffee or tea shortly before going to bed without any interference with sleep; others find that the caffeine in these beverages keeps them awake for several hours or more.

The coffee habit can become a very serious one. A patient once came to me complaining of severe attacks of dizziness which almost reached the fainting stage. She was greatly worried for fear that she had high blood pressure or some serious illness. It turned out that she had become addicted to coffee, always had a pot boiling on the stove, and was consuming twenty to twenty-five cups of strong coffee each day! Her symptoms disappeared as soon as she reduced her consumption of coffee to a few cups daily.

Nor is she a rare exception. Recent studies have indicated that excessive caffeine intake can produce symptoms much like those of a psychiatric disorder—chronic anxiety. The symptoms include restlessness, irritability, insomnia, headaches, muscle twitching, and sometimes vomiting and diarrhea. The studies also suggest that some patients may be treated unsuccessfully with tranquilizers and other drugs when they need no new drugs but to cut the intake of the responsible drug, caffeine.

Coffee and tea should not be given to children. Even when so much water is added that there is practically no caffeine present in a cup of these beverages, they should not be substituted for nutritious drinks like milk and fruit juices which growing children and adolescents need even more than adults. (The caffeine in cocoa is negligible.)

### Cola Drinks

Most cola drinks contain caffeine—approximately the same amount as is in a cup of coffee. Obviously, the cola-drink habit can be as serious as the coffee habit I discussed above. In fact, it can be more serious, since many people do not realize that there is caffeine in these drinks and consume quantities of them, or let their children have a number of them a day, spoiling their appetites for essential foods.

Always think of cola drinks as though they were coffee. Your children are better off without them; and you yourself should set a daily quota which does not make you suffer from any of the symptoms caused by too much coffee.

## HOW MUCH WATER SHOULD WE DRINK?

The amount of water drunk each day is usually correctly adjusted by your sense of thirst. The body loses each day about a quart of water in the invisible perspiration from the skin, and as water vapor expired in the air from the lungs. This loss of water plus the quart or more of water contained in the daily urine must be supplied chiefly by:

1. *Water in solid foods,* e.g., vegetables and fruits are high in water content.
2. *Water in fluids* such as milk, soups and beverages.
3. *Water* taken as such. This will balance any difference between the above intake and the output.

In hot weather, or when you work in a hot area, your body requires more water to compensate for the loss of sweat (the *visible* perspiration may amount to many quarts a day). Because the sweat contains salt, too, it is necessary to replace the salt also (see page 40).

### Is Extra Water Necessary for Good Health?

There is an old belief among some people that it is necessary to drink very large amounts of water and other fluids to remain healthy. Some people have an almost mystical belief that this large amount of water washes poisons out of the system, especially through the kidneys. Medical research has shown that this is not true and that the ordinary amounts of fluid that are taken in are sufficient to remove all the waste products through the kidneys. Only in exceptional cases, such as I list below, is it necessary to take larger amounts of water and fluid than are mentioned above.

### Is It Dangerous to Drink Water?

On the other hand, there are people, including some large national groups, who have the suspicion that water is harmful to health. This idea very likely arose during times when sanitation was so poor that typhoid fever, dysentery, and many other diseases were spread through impure drinking water. (See page 136 for a discussion of diseases transmitted through impure water, and how to prevent them.) When water is pure, it is perfectly healthful. There is no need to substitute wine or beer or other drinks with the idea that they will aid your health. In hot weather there is a tendency for some people to take in huge quan-

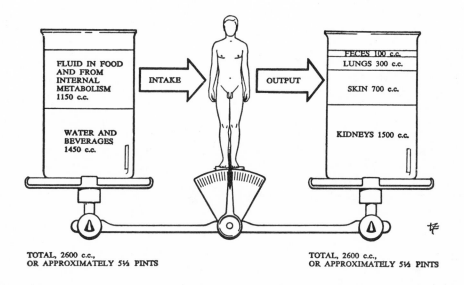

FLUID IN FOOD
AND FROM
INTERNAL
METABOLISM
1150 c.c.

INTAKE

OUTPUT

FECES 100 c.c.
LUNGS 300 c.c.

SKIN 700 c.c.

WATER AND
BEVERAGES
1450 c.c.

KIDNEYS 1500 c.c.

TOTAL, 2600 c.c.,
OR APPROXIMATELY 5½ PINTS

TOTAL, 2600 c.c.,
OR APPROXIMATELY 5½ PINTS

*Figure 1–8. Fluid Balance of the Body. This diagram shows the sources and the quantity of fluids required by the average, moderately active man, and how they are eliminated.*

tities of extremely cold, iced water. This may overload the stomach with too much cold fluid. It is best to take iced water and other iced drinks in small quantities.

## When Is Extra Water Required?

In certain illnesses it is necessary to take extra water as part of the treatment and for prevention of complications. This is particularly true for people who have a tendency to form *kidney stones.* The stones form more readily when the urine is concentrated. Therefore, doctors prescribe extra fluids to keep the urine dilute during both the day and the night. Sometimes it is even necessary to take an extra glass of water during the night to make sure the urine doesn't become too concentrated during the night hours. In infections of the kidneys such as *pyelitis* and *pyelonephritis,* or in infections of the urinary bladder, such as *cystitis,* extra water may be useful to help wash out the infection. In *gout* there is a tendency for the extra uric acid to precipitate in the urine. Therefore, doc-

tors advise extra water to keep the uric acid in solution. (See page 457 for a discussion of gout.) There is a disease in which the body cannot retain water in a normal manner, and amounts of urine up to such huge quantities as thirty quarts a day are passed. This sickness is called *diabetes insipidus.* Whenever there is excessive thirst, you should tell your doctor about it because it may be a warning that some ailment has set in.

## When Is It Necessary to Restrict Water Intake?

In some diseases, particularly where there is a tendency toward *edema* (see page 417), part of the treatment may consist of restricting the intake of fluid. This may be true in *heart disease* (see page 417), *cirrhosis of the liver* (see page 445), and the edematous stages of *Bright's disease* (see page 423). Actually, the *salt* in fluids other than water is more important in causing edema than the water itself.

# USE OF MEDICINES, DRUGS, AND NARCOTICS

In the 1950's and 1960's, a revolution took place in the field of medicine. It meant that the public could be protected against and cured of many ailments that had been disabling or fatal or had taken tedious weeks or months for recovery in the past. But there have been some bad effects. A new category of disease has arisen, called *iatrogenic disease*, meaning those caused by the administration of medicines and drugs. More than 250 such ailments have been recognized.

More than ever, it is necessary to use only those medicines your doctor recommends for you, and to use them exactly as he directs. Your doctor knows of the dangerous side effects of many drugs. He will use only carefully prescribed amounts of whatever you need for your condition. The habit of using an old medicine months or years later, when apparently similar symptoms occur, or worse, taking a drug prescribed for a friend who "had the same thing," is worse than foolish. It can be extremely dangerous.

I want to warn pregnant women especially to stay away from all medicines, except those ordered by their own doctor. Even a seemingly innocent preparation may harm the woman or her growing baby. A particularly shocking example occurred in the early 1960's, when the drug *thalidomide* was used by thousands of women. It was created to bring about a deep and restful sleep, and in some countries, particularly Germany, it was sold without prescription. Its effect was soon apparent. Newborn babies had deformed or rudimentary arms, sometimes little more than flippers. Thousands of such deformed infants were born in Germany, England, France, Belgium, Australia, and Canada. American women were spared this horror only through the caution exercised by Dr. Frances Kelsey, a medical officer of the Food and Drug Administration, who refused to license thalidomide for sale in this country because she believed it had not been properly tested.

It isn't only the new prescription drugs that can cause trouble. Even Vitamin D has been fatal when taken in an extremely high dosage over a long time.

Most people are not harmed by *aspirin*, although it *can* be harmful—for example, aspirin may cause peptic ulcers to bleed. However, I want to caution you against using it indiscriminately, as some people do. They carry a box of tablets with them at all times, swallowing a couple of pills at the first real or fancied sign of discomfort. *Bicarbonate of soda* and other remedies for indigestion, "sour stomach," should not be taken continually, either. While there is no need to fear medicines, they should never be taken regularly unless your doctor tells you to. Pain, indigestion, and other symptoms may be nature's warning signals of disease and should not be obscured by self-medication.

*Sleeping tablets* should be taken only upon a doctor's prescription. They cannot be obtained without one. This is a wise provision, as they can be extremely dangerous. (Sleeping pills are discussed under Insomnia, page 494.)

Pills containing *caffeine* or *Benzedrine* to keep you from getting sleepy or to pep you up can also be very harmful.

Pain-killers like *codeine, Darvon,* and *Demerol* are habit-forming. Only a physician knows how the more powerful narcotics such as *morphine, cocaine,* and *heroin* can safely be used to relieve intolerable pain. *There is no such thing as a safe, small dose of any of these narcotics except when a doctor administers them.* Otherwise, even the most high-minded individual runs a very grave risk of becoming a "dope addict," with resulting deterioration of body and mind. For example: some years ago a group of young scientists became addicted to cocaine as a result of repeatedly experimenting on themselves in their search for a local anesthetic; only one of them, after undergoing terrible agony, was able to conquer the habit and complete the work, eventually becoming the outstanding surgeon of his day.

If you feel a desire to use these drugs, or do use them, or have used them in the past, you should talk over the matter very frankly with your doctor. He will pass no moral judgment on you, but will advise you how to prevent or to overcome the habit before it is too late. The U.S. Public Health Service runs free hospitals which treat severe cases of drug addiction. You or your doctor can obtain information about them by communicating with the U.S. Public Health Service, Washington, D.C. 20201.

## "ONLY ONE TO A CUSTOMER"

Your body is the one "machine" which is "unconditionally guaranteed to last a lifetime."

How long and good a lifetime this will be depends a great deal on you, on whether you neglect and abuse your body out of carelessness or ignorance, or whether you treat it with the respect so wonderful an organism deserves.

# 2

# THE FOOD YOU EAT

---

Getting enough to eat is less of a problem in America than in most of the world, or than it has been at any other period in history. Throughout the ages the vast majority of the population seldom if ever knew what it was like not to be hungry; and in many parts of the modern world, people are little if any better off.

Yet there is more to food than the simple matter of satisfying one's hunger pangs. Some people enjoy food so much that they practically "live in order to eat." Others care little about it, and simply "eat in order to live." I have seen patients from *both* these groups whose diets are inadequate, sometimes even incompatible with good health. I am not talking about patients who are too fat or too thin—a subject I discuss fully in the next chapter—but about the people who fail to get the proper nourishment because they are not eating right. This chapter is devoted to information about good diets and eating habits for everyone.

## WHEN TO EAT

We doctors advise "three square meals a day," with or without additional snacks. The latter depend on you—your weight, whether or not they spoil your appetite for the food you should have, and how much you want them. Some people are miserable when deprived of their coffee break or afternoon tea or a bedtime raid on the icebox. On the other hand, some people are undernourished because they drink countless cups of tea or coffee instead of eating regular meals, or spend restless nights because they indulge in sandwiches before going to bed.

Why *three* meals? Why not just eat when you feel like it? Mainly because it is more practical in our present civilization. (And, incidentally, some primitive people eat a morning, noon, and late evening meal.) Energy-producing foods can be spaced better when one has three meals a day; if you eat one huge meal you are apt to feel like a hibernating python when you're finished! Adhering to the custom of three meals a day makes it easier to plan an adequate diet and make sure you are getting it.

The proportionate size of the meals is up to you—whether, for example, you eat your largest meal in the middle or at the end of the day. The only point I stress is: if you have your dinner at noon, allow time enough for it. The average lunch hour isn't long enough for the trip to your home or a good restaurant, with a few stops on the way to attend to errands, *and* a hearty dinner. We doctors no longer advise people to chew each mouthful of food a specific number of times; but we do urge you not to bolt it. Chewing mixes it with saliva and gets your digestion off to a good start; and having time enough to relax encourages the whole digestive process considerably. Besides, many women would be better cooks if their families didn't gulp down their best efforts like seals being thrown a piece of fish—as a housewife complained to me recently.

When I write about three meals a day, I am thinking of the man or woman in reasonably good health. Persons with certain illnesses, like coronary artery disease, may be better off eating four or five smaller meals a day. In this way, they cut down the work their bodies must do at any one time. (Heart diseases are discussed beginning on page 416.)

## How About Breakfast?

Many a patient has said to me, "I know it would be good for me, but honestly, Doctor, I just can't eat much breakfast!" She (it's usually a woman) may be right. Some people awaken slowly and painfully, and anything more than orange juice, black coffee, and a few bites of toast doesn't appeal to them. However, many people *think* they don't like breakfast simply because they've never given themselves a chance to enjoy one. Because a good high-protein breakfast makes one feel better and have more energy during the morning, I usually ask people who say they can't eat much in the morning to make the following experiment for a month. If you belong to this group, why don't you try it?

If you awaken slowly, set the alarm ahead by ten or fifteen minutes. Spend *at least* fifteen minutes every morning eating breakfast, or just sitting at the breakfast table. Try adding various things that appeal to you such as a bit of crisp bacon, a small dish of cereal, an extra piece of buttered toast, a small portion of egg, some milk.

Usually by the end of a week or two people find they are enjoying a larger breakfast. If not, I tell them to forget it; it is better to get one's extra energy from a midmorning snack than it is to force one's self to eat or to worry about not eating a good breakfast.

If you have succeeded in eating a larger breakfast, then try to convert to a high-protein breakfast. It has been observed by medical scientists that a high-protein diet provides energy at a more uniform level throughout the morning than do other types of breakfast. The sugar in the blood doesn't fluctuate nearly as much as it does after a high-starch type of breakfast. These changes in sugar level affect your appetite and energy capacity. Also, because the appetite is satisfied for a long time thereafter by the high-protein breakfast, the actual calorie intake later in the day is reduced —thus keeping total body weight down.

For the high-protein breakfast, concentrate on *eggs; cereals and milk;* meats such as crisp bacon, ham, crisp sausages; and *milk* (use skimmed, fat-free milk if you have a tendency to overweight [p. 44]). Reduce the amounts of sugary and starchy foods to a minimum, e.g., toast, jelly, marmalade, pancakes, waffles.

If you can't eat a good-sized breakfast, or if you don't eat sufficient protein, then by midmorning you may possibly feel the effect of a low blood sugar—by hunger and even sensations of dizziness and faintness. Try before this time arrives to take some solid foods and a glass of orange juice.

## ATTRACTIVE MEALS

No one should have to force himself, or be forced, to eat at any meal. But it is not "forcing" to encourage your appetite or that of some member of your family, by giving time and thought to meals. This means not only preparing them well but serving them in a pleasant atmosphere and making them look attractive. If that isn't enough to make an individual like food, a doctor should be consulted.

## WHAT TO EAT

Foods can properly be classified into seven groups. If the meals you and your family eat during the course of a day include at least one food from each of these groups, they will be well-balanced, nutritious meals containing what is needed for health.

The groups are

1. Milk and milk products
2. Meat, fish, poultry, eggs, nuts, dried beans, and peas
3. Green, yellow, and leafy vegetables
4. Citrus fruits, tomatoes, raw cabbage, and salad greens
5. Noncitrus fruits, potatoes, and other vegetables not included in group 3
6. Bread, cereals, and pasta
7. Butter, margarine, or vegetable oil

Milk or milk products include cottage cheese, yogurt, cheeses, and ice cream, and provide vitamins A, $B_2$, and $B_{12}$, calcium and many other minerals (but not iron), and protein. Instead of whole milk, you can use low-fat milk.

Meat, fish, poultry, and the other foods of group 2 contribute large quantities of protein. Fish and poultry have less fats than most meats. Eggs contain virtually all vitamins and minerals but large amounts of cholesterol. Liver is rich in iron and vitamin A but also in cholesterol.

Green, yellow, and leafy vegetables, which are excellent sources of minerals and A, B, and E vitamins, include spinach, kale, Swiss chard, watercress, collard, mustard and turnip (the greens), and carrots, pumpkin, squash of various types, and yams (the yellows).

Citrus fruits, tomatoes, raw cabbage, and salad greens contribute vitamin C. Lettuce, cabbage, and salad greens provide somewhat less of the vitamin than do tomatoes, oranges, grapefruit, tangerines, and other citrus fruits.

Potatoes and other vegetables and fruits—including broccoli, Brussels sprouts, green peppers, cauliflower, berries, cherries, melons, and peaches—contribute vitamin C, minerals, some protein, and energy.

Bread, cereals, and pasta provide protein, iron, and B vitamins as well as carbohydrates. They help meet energy needs. Enriched flour and cornmeal offer vitamins $B_1$ and $B_2$, niacin, and iron. And whole-grain flour, bread, and brown rice contain other B vitamins, minerals, and desirable dietary fiber.

Butter, fortified margarine, and vegetable oil provide vitamin A as well as calories.

If you and your family not only get at least one food from each of the seven groups each day but also get varied choices from each group, the likelihood of your getting everything needed in adequate and well-proportioned amounts will be increased.

Your family may not like many of the items listed; and you have found that it isn't easy to change people's eating habits. I realize that, too. I have had many a patient tell me he won't eat vegetables and that salads are rabbit food. Many a woman who lives alone doesn't want to bother with anything but tea and toast, while business girls may eat practically nothing but sandwiches, coffee, and sodas. Don't try to change eating habits—your own or those of others—in a tactless manner. Use ingenuity: if someone won't drink milk, see that he or she gets the required amount in puddings, soups, cheese, and the many other foods that can contain milk products.

Tastes vary according to national and regional customs. Some people of Italian descent eat spaghetti almost every day, while in parts of the United States dinner consists of meat and potatoes, bread and butter, and pie. Every group has some justification for thinking its dishes are the best in the world. Many of them are, indeed, excellent, and all customs need not be changed. I wouldn't think of saying that rye bread, which Slavic people prefer, is a better source of cereal carbohydrate than spaghetti, or vice versa.

However, it is important to realize that many groups ate certain foods almost exclusively (rice, for example) because they couldn't get anything else. Here in the United States we need not limit ourselves. A tremendous number of foods are easy to obtain here. The many national groups that have contributed to the melting pot of American cookery have made it possible to enjoy the best and most varied dishes in the world. A restaurant in the United States may serve French onion soup or Russian borscht, lamb cooked with vegetables in the Greek, Armenian, or Turkish manner, American corn-on-the-cob, Chinese chop suey, East Indian curried rice, or Hungarian goulash.

Tastes in eating grow and develop. But again —be tactful in your approach if you want to encourage change. Don't try something "too queer," like Japanese-style raw fish. Introduce something new as a side dish rather than as the main course. A little experimenting with some of the slightly Americanized versions of inexpensive national or regional specialties may help to broaden the eating habits of your family.

If you still aren't able to include the required items in your diet, it is probably because of lack of money. In that case, the first thing to do is to go over your budget carefully. Clothes, entertainment, and the car often demand too large a portion of the family income. Soft drinks, candy, and

# I: THE HUMAN BODY

## HIGHLIGHTS of STRUCTURE and FUNCTION

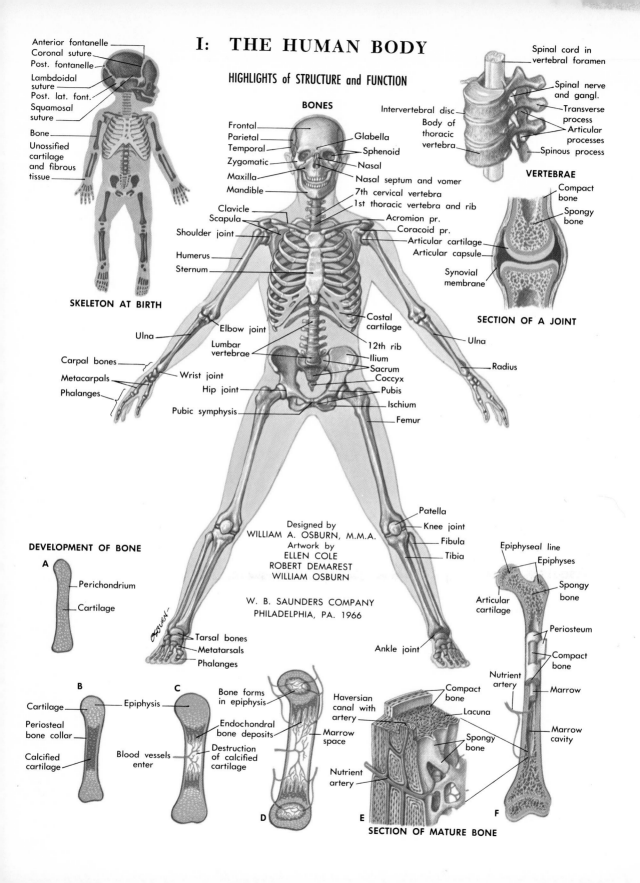

**SKELETON AT BIRTH**

- Anterior fontanelle
- Coronal suture
- Post. fontanelle
- Lambdoidal suture
- Post. lat. font.
- Squamosal suture
- Bone
- Unossified cartilage and fibrous tissue

**BONES**

- Frontal
- Parietal
- Temporal
- Zygomatic
- Maxilla
- Mandible
- Glabella
- Sphenoid
- Nasal
- Nasal septum and vomer
- 7th cervical vertebra
- 1st thoracic vertebra and rib
- Clavicle
- Scapula
- Shoulder joint
- Humerus
- Sternum
- Acromion pr.
- Coracoid pr.
- Articular cartilage
- Articular capsule
- Elbow joint
- Ulna
- Lumbar vertebrae
- Carpal bones
- Metacarpals
- Phalanges
- Wrist joint
- Hip joint
- Pubic symphysis
- Costal cartilage
- 12th rib
- Ilium
- Sacrum
- Coccyx
- Pubis
- Ischium
- Femur
- Ulna
- Radius
- Patella
- Knee joint
- Fibula
- Tibia
- Tarsal bones
- Metatarsals
- Phalanges
- Ankle joint

**VERTEBRAE**

- Spinal cord in vertebral foramen
- Spinal nerve and gangl.
- Transverse process
- Articular processes
- Spinous process
- Intervertebral disc
- Body of thoracic vertebra

**SECTION OF A JOINT**

- Compact bone
- Spongy bone
- Synovial membrane

Designed by
WILLIAM A. OSBURN, M.M.A.
Artwork by
ELLEN COLE
ROBERT DEMAREST
WILLIAM OSBURN

W. B. SAUNDERS COMPANY
PHILADELPHIA, PA. 1966

**DEVELOPMENT OF BONE**

A
- Perichondrium
- Cartilage

B
- Cartilage
- Periosteal bone collar
- Calcified cartilage
- Epiphysis
- Blood vessels enter

C
- Endochondral bone deposits
- Destruction of calcified cartilage

D
- Bone forms in epiphysis
- Marrow space

E
- Haversian canal with artery
- Compact bone
- Lacuna
- Spongy bone
- Nutrient artery

**SECTION OF MATURE BONE**

F
- Epiphyseal line
- Epiphyses
- Spongy bone
- Articular cartilage
- Periosteum
- Compact bone
- Nutrient artery
- Marrow
- Marrow cavity

# II: SKELETAL MUSCLES

**HOW A MUSCLE ATTACHES TO BONE**

Penetrating fibers
Periosteum
Muscle fiber
Int. perimysium
Ext. perimysium
Muscle fasciculus
Tendon

The connective tissue which surrounds the muscle fibers and bundles may (1) form a tendon which fuses with the periosteum, or (2) may fuse directly with the periosteum without forming a tendon.

Biceps
Biceps
Triceps
Triceps
Triceps
Elbow joint

**FLEXION:**
Biceps contracts;
triceps relaxes

**EXTENSION:**
Triceps contracts;
biceps relaxes

Frontalis
Temporalis
Orbicularis oculi
Masseter
Sternocleido-mastoid
Trapezius
Deltoid
Pectoralis major
Biceps brachii
Latissimus dorsi
Flexor carpi radialis
Pronator teres
Palmaris longus
Tensor fascia lata
Rectus abdominis (beneath rectus sheath)
Iliotibial band
Vastus lateralis
Patella
Peroneus longus
Tibialis anterior
Extensor digitorum longus
Lateral malleolus (fibula)
Extensor digitorum tendons

Orbicularis oris
Clavicle
Sternum
Triceps brachii
Serratus anterior
Brachialis
Brachioradialis
Ext. oblique
Extensor carpi radialis longus
Crest of iliac bone
Inguinal ligament
Iliopsoas
Pectineus
Adductor longus
Rectus femoris
Vastus lateralis
Tendon of quadriceps femoris muscle group
Patella
Patellar ligament
Soleus
Sup. extensor retinaculum
Inf. extensor retinaculum
Extensor hallucis longus tendon

Gracilis
Sartorius
Vastus medialis
Gastrocnemius
Soleus
Tibia
Medial malleolus (tibia)

**HOW A MUSCLE CONTRACTS**

Epimysium (muscle fascia)
Ext. perimysium
Blood vessels
FIBER
FIBRILS
FASCICULUS
Z A Z
Sarcomere
SECTION OF A MUSCLE
MYOFIBRIL

Thick myofilament
Thin myofilament
A
I
Z
Z
Myofilaments relaxed
Z
Z
Myofilaments contracted

# III: THE ORGANS OF DIGESTION

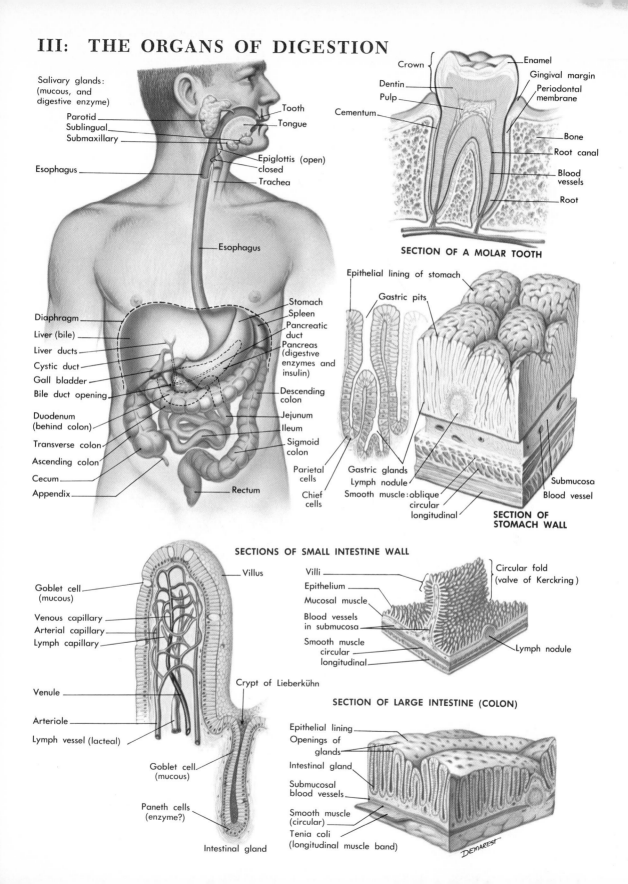

Salivary glands:
(mucous, and
digestive enzyme)

Parotid
Sublingual
Submaxillary

Esophagus

Tooth
Tongue

Epiglottis (open)
closed
Trachea

Esophagus

Diaphragm
Liver (bile)
Liver ducts
Cystic duct
Gall bladder
Bile duct opening
Duodenum
(behind colon)
Transverse colon
Ascending colon
Cecum
Appendix

Stomach
Spleen
Pancreatic
duct
Pancreas
(digestive
enzymes and
insulin)
Descending
colon
Jejunum
Ileum
Sigmoid
colon

Rectum

## SECTION OF A MOLAR TOOTH

Crown
Dentin
Pulp
Cementum

Enamel
Gingival margin
Periodontal
membrane

Bone
Root canal
Blood
vessels
Root

## SECTION OF STOMACH WALL

Epithelial lining of stomach
Gastric pits

Parietal
cells
Chief
cells

Gastric glands
Lymph nodule
Smooth muscle: oblique
circular
longitudinal

Submucosa
Blood vessel

## SECTIONS OF SMALL INTESTINE WALL

Villus

Goblet cell
(mucous)
Venous capillary
Arterial capillary
Lymph capillary

Venule

Arteriole

Lymph vessel (lacteal)

Crypt of Lieberkühn

Goblet cell
(mucous)

Paneth cells
(enzyme?)

Intestinal gland

Villi
Epithelium
Mucosal muscle
Blood vessels
in submucosa
Smooth muscle
circular
longitudinal

Circular fold
(valve of Kerckring)

Lymph nodule

## SECTION OF LARGE INTESTINE (COLON)

Epithelial lining
Openings of
glands
Intestinal gland
Submucosal
blood vessels
Smooth muscle
(circular)
Tenia coli
(longitudinal muscle band)

DEMAREST

# IV: THE ORGANS OF RESPIRATION AND THE HEART

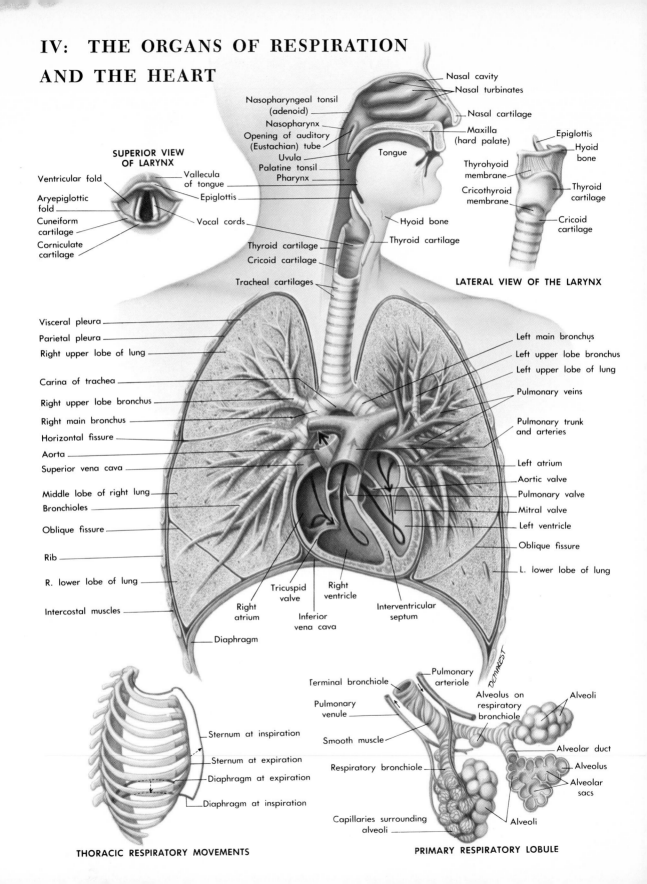

SUPERIOR VIEW OF LARYNX

Ventricular fold
Aryepiglottic fold
Cuneiform cartilage
Corniculate cartilage
Vallecula of tongue
Epiglottis
Vocal cords

Nasopharyngeal tonsil (adenoid)
Nasopharynx
Opening of auditory (Eustachian) tube
Uvula
Palatine tonsil
Pharynx
Tongue

Nasal cavity
Nasal turbinates
Nasal cartilage
Maxilla (hard palate)

Epiglottis
Hyoid bone
Thyrohyoid membrane
Cricothyroid membrane
Thyroid cartilage
Cricoid cartilage

LATERAL VIEW OF THE LARYNX

Hyoid bone
Thyroid cartilage
Thyroid cartilage
Cricoid cartilage
Tracheal cartilages

Visceral pleura
Parietal pleura
Right upper lobe of lung
Carina of trachea
Right upper lobe bronchus
Right main bronchus
Horizontal fissure
Aorta
Superior vena cava
Middle lobe of right lung
Bronchioles
Oblique fissure
Rib
R. lower lobe of lung
Intercostal muscles
Diaphragm

Left main bronchus
Left upper lobe bronchus
Left upper lobe of lung
Pulmonary veins
Pulmonary trunk and arteries
Left atrium
Aortic valve
Pulmonary valve
Mitral valve
Left ventricle
Oblique fissure
L. lower lobe of lung

Tricuspid valve
Right atrium
Right ventricle
Inferior vena cava
Interventricular septum

Sternum at inspiration
Sternum at expiration
Diaphragm at expiration
Diaphragm at inspiration

Terminal bronchiole
Pulmonary venule
Smooth muscle
Respiratory bronchiole
Capillaries surrounding alveoli
Pulmonary arteriole
Alveolus on respiratory bronchiole
Alveoli
Alveolar duct
Alveolus
Alveolar sacs
Alveoli

DEMAREST

THORACIC RESPIRATORY MOVEMENTS

PRIMARY RESPIRATORY LOBULE

# V: THE MAJOR BLOOD VESSELS

## A VEIN

Tunica intima:
Endothelium

Tunica media:
Circular smooth muscle and elastic tissue

Tunica adventitia:
White fibrous connective tissue

Valve open

Muscle contracted

Valve closed

Muscle relaxed

Valve open

Venule

## VEINS

Int. jugular
Ext. jugular
Sup. vena cava
Subclavian
Intercostal
Basilic
Brachial
Cephalic
Hepatic
Median cubital
Portal
Renal
Sup. mesen.
Inf. mes.
Inf. vena cava
Ext. iliac
Femoral
Greater saphenous
Popliteal
Peroneal
Post. tibial
Ant. tibial
Dorsal venous arch of foot

## ARTERIES

Int. carotid
Ext. carotid
Arch of aorta
Subclavian
Pulmonary
Axillary
Heart
Intercostal
Internal thoracic
Brachial
Deep brachial
Aorta
Splenic
Radial
Ulnar
Sup. mesen.
Com. iliac
Int. iliac
Ext. iliac
Obturator
Deep femoral
Femoral
Popliteal
Ant. tibial
Peroneal
Post. tibial
Dorsal arterial arch of foot

## A LARGE ARTERY

Tunica intima:
Endothelium
Loose connective tissue
Internal elastic membrane

Tunica media:
Circular smooth muscle and elastic tissue
External elastic membrane

Tunica adventitia:
White fibrous connective tissue

### ARTERIOLES

Tunica intima:
Endothelium
Circular internal elastic fibers

Tunica media:
Sparse transverse smooth muscle

Tunica adventitia:
Loose fibers

**RELAXED**

Tunica intima:
Endothelium constricted
Int. elastic fibers

Tunica media:
Smooth muscle contracted

Tunica adventitia:
Loose fibers

**CONSTRICTED**

Valve
Lymph vessel

Tissue fluids:
extracellular
intracellular

Lymphatic capillaries

Arteriole

Tissue cells
Venous capillaries
Arterial capillaries

Cole + OSBURN

## A CAPILLARY BED

# VI: THE BRAIN AND SPINAL NERVES

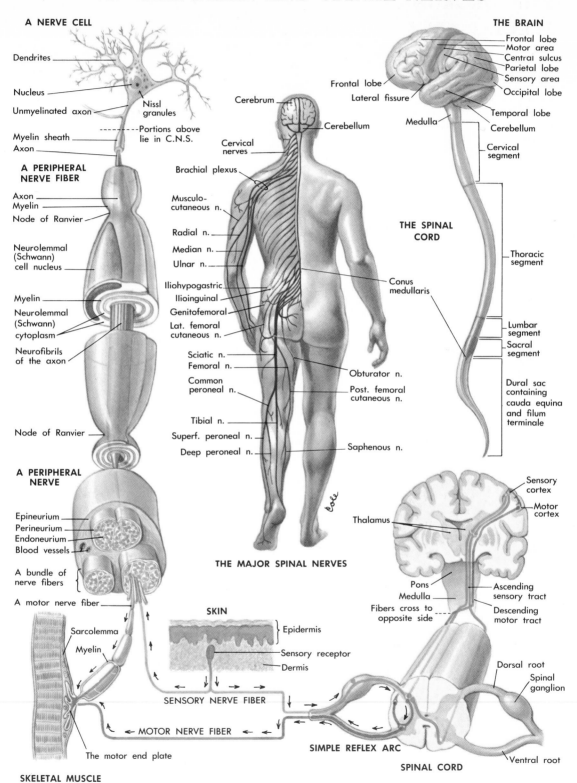

### A NERVE CELL

Dendrites

Nucleus

Unmyelinated axon

Nissl granules

Portions above lie in C.N.S.

Myelin sheath

Axon

### A PERIPHERAL NERVE FIBER

Axon

Myelin

Node of Ranvier

Neurolemmal (Schwann) cell nucleus

Myelin

Neurolemmal (Schwann) cytoplasm

Neurofibrils of the axon

Node of Ranvier

### A PERIPHERAL NERVE

Epineurium

Perineurium

Endoneurium

Blood vessels

A bundle of nerve fibers

A motor nerve fiber

Sarcolemma

Myelin

The motor end plate

**SKELETAL MUSCLE**

Cerebrum

Cerebellum

Cervical nerves

Brachial plexus

Musculo-cutaneous n.

Radial n.

Median n.

Ulnar n.

Iliohypogastric

Ilioinguinal

Genitofemoral

Lat. femoral cutaneous n.

Sciatic n.

Femoral n.

Common peroneal n.

Tibial n.

Superf. peroneal n.

Deep peroneal n.

Conus medullaris

Obturator n.

Post. femoral cutaneous n.

Saphenous n.

**THE MAJOR SPINAL NERVES**

### THE BRAIN

Frontal lobe

Motor area

Central sulcus

Parietal lobe

Sensory area

Occipital lobe

Temporal lobe

Cerebellum

Frontal lobe

Lateral fissure

Medulla

Cervical segment

### THE SPINAL CORD

Thoracic segment

Lumbar segment

Sacral segment

Dural sac containing cauda equina and filum terminale

Sensory cortex

Motor cortex

Thalamus

Pons

Medulla

Fibers cross to opposite side

Ascending sensory tract

Descending motor tract

**SKIN**

Epidermis

Sensory receptor

Dermis

SENSORY NERVE FIBER

◄ MOTOR NERVE FIBER ◄

**SIMPLE REFLEX ARC**

Dorsal root

Spinal ganglion

Ventral root

**SPINAL CORD**

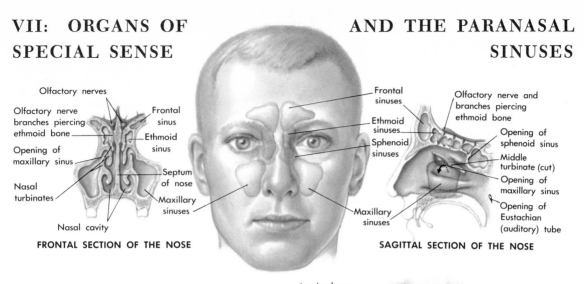

**Olfactory nerves**
**Olfactory nerve branches piercing ethmoid bone**
**Opening of maxillary sinus**
**Nasal turbinates**
**Frontal sinus**
**Ethmoid sinus**
**Septum of nose**
**Maxillary sinuses**
**Nasal cavity**

**FRONTAL SECTION OF THE NOSE**

**Frontal sinuses**
**Ethmoid sinuses**
**Sphenoid sinuses**
**Maxillary sinuses**

**Olfactory nerve and branches piercing ethmoid bone**
**Opening of sphenoid sinus**
**Middle turbinate (cut)**
**Opening of maxillary sinus**
**Opening of Eustachian (auditory) tube**

**SAGITTAL SECTION OF THE NOSE**

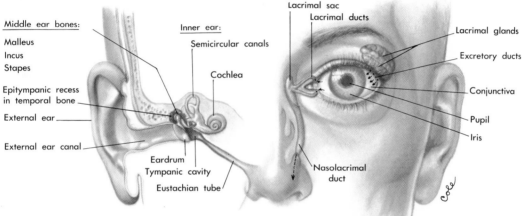

**Middle ear bones:**
Malleus
Incus
Stapes
**Epitympanic recess in temporal bone**
**External ear**
**External ear canal**

**Inner ear:**
**Semicircular canals**
**Cochlea**

**Eardrum**
**Tympanic cavity**
**Eustachian tube**

**THE ORGAN OF HEARING**

**Lacrimal sac**
**Lacrimal ducts**
**Lacrimal glands**
**Excretory ducts**
**Conjunctiva**
**Pupil**
**Iris**
**Nasolacrimal duct**

**THE LACRIMAL APPARATUS AND THE EYE**

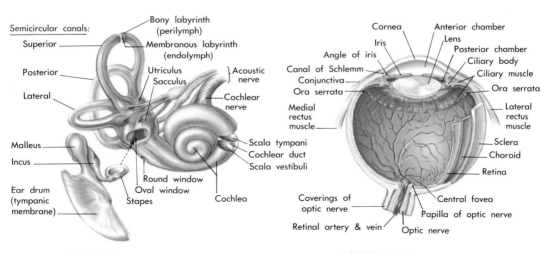

**Semicircular canals:**
Superior
Posterior
Lateral

**Bony labyrinth (perilymph)**
**Membranous labyrinth (endolymph)**
**Utriculus**
**Sacculus**
**Acoustic nerve**
**Cochlear nerve**

Malleus
Incus

**Ear drum (tympanic membrane)**

**Round window**
**Oval window**
**Stapes**
**Scala tympani**
**Cochlear duct**
**Scala vestibuli**
**Cochlea**

**THE MIDDLE EAR AND INNER EAR**

**Cornea**
**Iris**
**Angle of iris**
**Canal of Schlemm**
**Conjunctiva**
**Ora serrata**
**Medial rectus muscle**

**Anterior chamber**
**Lens**
**Posterior chamber**
**Ciliary body**
**Ciliary muscle**
**Ora serrata**
**Lateral rectus muscle**
**Sclera**
**Choroid**
**Retina**

**Coverings of optic nerve**
**Retinal artery & vein**
**Central fovea**
**Papilla of optic nerve**
**Optic nerve**

**HORIZONTAL SECTION OF THE EYE**

# VIII: THE AUTONOMIC NERVES

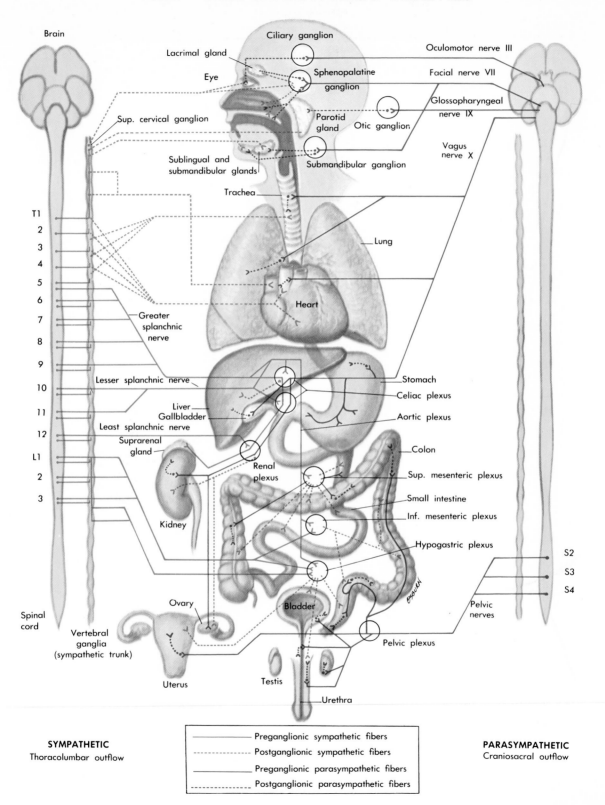

Brain

Ciliary ganglion

Lacrimal gland

Oculomotor nerve III

Eye

Sphenopalatine ganglion

Facial nerve VII

Sup. cervical ganglion

Glossopharyngeal nerve IX

Parotid gland

Otic ganglion

Sublingual and submandibular glands

Vagus nerve X

Submandibular ganglion

Trachea

T1
2
3
4
5
6
7
8
9
10
11
12
L1
2
3

Lung

Heart

Greater splanchnic nerve

Lesser splanchnic nerve

Liver
Gallbladder

Least splanchnic nerve

Suprarenal gland

Renal plexus

Kidney

Stomach

Celiac plexus

Aortic plexus

Colon

Sup. mesenteric plexus

Small intestine

Inf. mesenteric plexus

Hypogastric plexus

S2
S3
S4

Ovary

Bladder

Pelvic nerves

Spinal cord

Vertebral ganglia (sympathetic trunk)

Pelvic plexus

Uterus

Testis

Urethra

**SYMPATHETIC**
Thoracolumbar outflow

**PARASYMPATHETIC**
Craniosacral outflow

| | |
|---|---|
| Preganglionic sympathetic fibers | |
| Postganglionic sympathetic fibers | |
| Preganglionic parasympathetic fibers | |
| Postganglionic parasympathetic fibers | |

sodas do not give you their money's worth in food value if substituted for protein foods.

You may also be able to learn some new tricks for stretching your food dollar. If, after trying the suggestions in the following section, your diet still doesn't come up to the recommended ones, you need outside assistance. Ask your local health department or your community services headquarters whether they can refer you to an agency or a trained social worker who can go over your problem with you and make certain you are providing the best that can be managed on your income. The U.S. Department of Agriculture, Agricultural Research Service, Beltsville, Maryland 20705, will send you up-to-date pamphlets on family food plans, for budgets of different sizes. This agency will also give you accurate information about food values and up-to-the-minute cost information. It's all free. All you need is an envelope and a stamp for your request.

If you still can't purchase the things on the recommended diet, you need financial help from your community. *Don't be reluctant to ask for it.* It is far better to accept some assistance now than to injure your health and that of your family so that you will need greater assistance later. *No one should be exposed to the slow starvation which results from a substandard diet.*

## HOW TO MAKE THE MOST OF YOUR FOOD DOLLARS

### Don't Waste Food

Many foreigners insist they could live on the food which we Americans throw into our garbage cans! Stop and think before you empty anything into yours. Don't pour the liquid from canned vegetables down the sink; it is rich in minerals and vitamins. Boil it down as rapidly as possible to one-half or one-quarter of its original volume, then add the vegetables and heat for serving. Or use the liquid to make valuable soups. The best stews are often made from leftovers. Don't pare away the best part of your vegetables and potatoes; leave the skins on or scrape away the outer surface (a pot cleaner is good for this).

Don't let food spoil. It is cheaper to buy nonperishable foods in bulk if your storage space permits, but it isn't economical to buy a bargain-lot of perishable foods and then throw most of them away.

PERISHABLE FOODS. Meat, fish, cheese, etc., must be kept cool. Fruits and vegetables lose some of their vitamin content as well as their palatability if allowed to become stale. The wise housewife plans her menus for several days ahead and buys just enough of the perishable items for immediate use. Even food in cans will eventually deteriorate if exposed to high temperatures, that is, near hot pipes or radiators or directly under noninsulated roofing.

Moist or liquid foods spoil most rapidly. Bacteria, yeasts, and molds from the air can contaminate them. This process goes like wildfire if the liquid or moist food is slightly warm, the temperature which most microbes like best. Since bacteria do not thrive in cooler temperatures, these foods should be kept cooled or refrigerated. Milk must be guarded more carefully than almost any other food. It should be cool when it is delivered to the home or taken from the store, and it should not be allowed to sit around on porches or in halls for several hours getting warmed up before it is put into the cooler or refrigerator. It spoils if left in the sun, and may even be dangerous to use because of the increased number of bacteria in it. Exposure to light also destroys some of its precious vitamin B.

It is perfectly safe to keep canned foods in the icebox after they have been opened. Many people still believe that canned goods must be put into a dish or discarded in order not to risk getting "ptomaine poisoning." Modern cans are perfectly safe; food may be left in them in the refrigerator. Some foods such as tomatoes and pineapple take on a slightly metallic taste after a few days in an open can, but they may be eaten without harm. So many housewives worry about this that the U.S. Department of Agriculture published a news release entitled, "Oh, Sure! You Can Keep It in a Can." These experts said, "It is just as safe to keep canned food in the can it comes in—if the can is cool and covered—as it is to empty the food into another container." The important thing is to remember to keep the unused portion of canned food covered and in the refrigerator.

## Other Dollar Stretchers

Gardening, and the home canning of fruits and vegetables purchased when they are at their cheapest, will help make your food budget cover your needs. It takes very little space to grow a few tomato plants, and even a window box will do for chives and herbs that can transform dull, inexpensive dishes into tasty ones. You can learn how to utilize inexpensive cuts of meat which are just as good for you as expensive ones (see Table 2-1). Cheese is a good, inexpensive meat substitute, and so are baked beans and lentils. Canned or powdered milk can be used instead of fresh, and margarine, which is "fortified" with vitamins, is as good as butter.

### TABLE 2–1

SOME LESS EXPENSIVE SOURCES OF PROTEIN FOODS

| MEATS | FISH IN SEASON |
|---|---|
| Short ribs of beef | |
| Lamb and beef stew meat | FOWL |
| Beef chuck roast | DRIED PEAS AND BEANS |
| Livers | |
| Hearts | LENTILS |
| Tongues | |
| Kidneys | SOY BEANS |
| Brains | POWDERED MILK |

Perhaps you are spending too much of your food money on tea or coffee. These beverages are pleasant, and although they contain a stimulant, caffeine, they are usually harmless to adults, in moderation (see page 25). However, these beverages are expensive and they are *not actually food*.

The following pamphlets contain valuable money-saving information. Send for them.

Human Nutrition Research Branch
Agricultural Research Service
U.S. Department of Agriculture
Beltsville, Maryland 20705
*Family Food Plans and Food Costs*

*Food for Fitness*
*Home Canning of Meat*
*Home Freezing of Fruits and Vegetables*
*Nutritive Value of Foods*
*Storing Perishable Foods in the Home*

National Canners Association
1133 Twentieth Street, N.W.
Washington, D.C. 20036
*Focus on Canned Foods*

American Meat Institute
59 East Van Buren Street
Chicago, Illinois 60605
*Buying Guide to the Thriftier Cuts of Meat*

## FOOD POISONING

We used to hear a great deal about "ptomaine poisoning," a diagnosis made on the incorrect theory that mysterious poisons were created by the digestion of certain foods. However, certain kinds of *food poisoning* do occur. They can be caused by the contamination of food at its source, as, for example, milk from a diseased cow, oysters from a polluted bed, or vegetables fertilized by human manure; by food that has spoiled, lobsters, for example; or by the contamination of food during its preparation. Dysentery and typhoid fever have been spread in the last manner, perhaps by a cook who was suffering from the disease or who happened to be a carrier—that is, one of the rare individuals who can harbor and pass on a certain germ without being made ill by it himself. A baker with a sore on his hand might introduce bacteria from it into food—perhaps cream puffs or custard pies, which make excellent breeding spots for such microbes, especially in hot weather.

People who eat such foods are apt to get sick; but if the condition is treated in time the mortality is very low. Therefore it is important to see the doctor immediately if you suspect food poisoning. Fortunately, our public health officials do an excellent job of inspecting our water, milk, and food supplies to make certain they are safe. You can do your share by not buying food that has spoiled, particularly meat, fish, and shellfish, or by not serving it if it "goes bad" after being purchased. If you can't be certain from its appearance whether or not food is safe to eat, smell it; usually "your nose knows." Be sure that you and anyone else who handles the food you eat observe the obvious rules of cleanliness. Don't let food stand around all day on the back of the warm stove where any germs that fall on it will flourish. If food should cook a long time, let it *cook*—heat destroys germs —and not just sit. Home canning must be carried out properly to avoid botulism.

Poisoning by *inedible berries, toadstools,* etc., is discussed on page 159. It can easily be avoided by purchasing your food at the store, or *really* knowing what you are about. (Your experiences in Scout camp do not, for example, enable you to pick "mushrooms" for dinner!)

## SPECIAL DIETS

### Diet for Children

The formula for infants should be prescribed by your doctor or hospital clinic, who will tell you when to supplement it with cereal, vegetables, egg, and so on, and how much cod-liver oil, orange juice, or vitamin concentrates to give (see chapter on child care, page 271).

From the time the doctor says your child can eat everything, his diet can be much the same as that of the adult given in the preceding pages, except that (1) the child needs a quart of milk a day, and (2) he may need "pick-me-ups" between meals to supply extra energy. Bread or crackers covered with cheese, butter, or jam; ice cream; cocoa and chocolate milk are good for this purpose. (However, read my remarks on sweets and tendency toward tooth decay, page 67.)

### Diet for the Adolescent

During their rapid growth in adolescence, boys and girls need extra milk, proteins, and vitamins. It is essential that they eat the balanced diet listed at the beginning of this chapter. They need extra food and milk drinks between meals to add poundage to the lengthening body. Good dietary habits are especially important at this age as explained in my chapter on adolescence, page 310.

### Diet During Pregnancy

The pregnant woman must supply her own body with proper food, and at the same time eat foods to build the baby's bones and tissues. This means that extra minerals, proteins, and vitamins are needed. The diet during pregnancy should be regulated by a physician, which is one of the reasons why every pregnant woman should be under the care of a doctor. (See chapter on pregnancy, page 234.)

### Diets for the Later Years of Life

The elderly person needs the well-balanced, basic diet I have described (pages 31-32). Many doctors feel that older people benefit from additional vitamins. These can be obtained from natural sources by taking a glassful of orange or tomato juice *each day* and a daily teaspoonful of cod-liver oil. A serving of liver and a pork chop *each week* will add the vitamin B group. These extra vitamins can also be taken in capsule or concentrated form. Let your doctor decide what is best for you. He will probably caution you against gaining weight, and you will undoubtedly want to read my next chapter on overweight and underweight. You will also want to read the chapter on aging, page 530.

## WHY YOU NEED A BALANCED DIET

So far, this chapter has consisted almost entirely of "what to do" and has said almost nothing of "why to do it." This is because I want to provide workable rules and ready facts about foods for the many people who "aren't interested in proteins, vitamins, calories, and so on," but do want to eat the proper foods. The following section of this chapter is written for those of you who would like to know *why* a diet must be scientifically balanced.

Food provides the body with four essentials:

1. Energy
2. Repair materials

3. Growth materials (from infancy through the period of active growth)
4. Vitamins and other special substances

The largest solid parts of the body are the muscles and bones. This framework must be built out of food, mostly from proteins and minerals. The muscles, heart, liver, kidney, and other organs are composed chiefly of proteins. The child and the growing adolescent need plenty of proteins to build up the muscles and vital organs. Meat, fish, milk, and eggs are among the main sources of protein in our diet. Even after the period of growth is over, the body tissues, which are continually being worn out, must be replaced with new materials. That is why adults, as well as children, must have ample protein in their diets. Lacking protein, the body becomes weakened and exhausted, with lowered resistance especially to infections. Certain other conditions can result from "protein starvation." I shall never forget one such case I saw because the patient was a nurse who certainly should have known better! She was working very hard in a doctor's office, and foolishly existed on jelly sandwiches, soft drinks, and black coffee—which caused her to develop *starvation edema!*

In addition to the organs and muscles, the body must build its solid framework of bones. They are composed chiefly of the mineral substances calcium and phosphorus. The best source of these two minerals is milk, either fresh or canned, dried, skimmed, or whole. Milk is a splendid, all-round food because it is rich in both minerals and proteins. Other good sources of calcium are American and Swiss cheese, molasses, turnip tops, dandelion greens.

Other good sources of phosphorus are cereals, meat, and fish.

Minerals and proteins build the bones and flesh. But what supplies the energy? An automobile cannot go without gasoline, no matter how good an engine it has, nor can a stove or furnace operate without fuel. The fuel of life—which the body burns for energy—is glucose (sugar). Carbohydrates, which include both sugar and starches, provide the fuel most readily, for in the body starches are quickly converted to glucose.

Children need extra carbohydrates between meals to keep them supplied with fuel for the tremendous amount of activity they indulge in. Anyone doing hard physical labor requires plenty of energy-giving foods such as bread, pancakes, syrup, jelly, honey, and sugar. (Scientific tests indicate that boys of thirteen or so can use up as much food as a lumberjack does—which will come as no surprise to most mothers!)

Fat and protein can also be used to provide energy, and these the body can store up to use as reserves. For that reason Eskimos and others who eat proteins and fats almost exclusively at certain seasons of the year do not have "stalled engines" during these periods. However, starches and sugars act more promptly in providing energy than do proteins and fats.

Usually your appetite will tell you just how much food your body needs. This indicator is so sensitive that some people go for years at almost precisely the same weight. If more food is taken in than is needed for fuel, building, and repair, the body stores it as fat. If too little food is consumed, the body burns its reserves of fat and protein. Neither of these conditions is desirable, and I explain how to avoid or correct them in the next chapter.

## CALORIES

A calorie is a *unit of measurement* of the energy value of food. It represents the energy for heat and physical work which can be obtained from a certain weight of food. A pound of fat in butter or meat equals 4,000 calories. If—to cite an extreme case—a person consumed 4,000 more calories a day than he needed, the body would have to dispose of them. It could do so by laying down a pound of fat in the abdominal wall and elsewhere! On the other hand, if the food consumed each day were not enough to furnish heat and energy, the individual would have to "burn up" a part of his own body fat or tissues.

The caloric intake per day needed by one person is not necessarily the same as for another. The range can be all the way from under 2,000 calories a day to well over 4,000. It is evident that a lumberjack will burn up more calories than an office worker.

A caloric intake that keeps an individual at proper weight, feeling able to accomplish all he or she wants to accomplish, can be considered ideal. And what that ideal is can be found in some general guidelines.

Some years ago, the Food and Nutrition Board (FNB) of the National Research Council drew up tables of Recommended Dietary Allowances, setting caloric intake levels at 2,900 for men and 2,100 for women. But with further study, it had to make modifications.

In 1963, the FNB advocated a somewhat lower intake. Basing its figures on a "reference" man and woman, each 22 years of age, the man weighing 154 pounds and the woman 127, both living in a mean temperature of 68 degrees Fahrenheit and engaging in light physical activity, the FNB recommended 2,800 calories for men and 2,000 for women.

But in 1968, it made further modifications. It recommended that since weight gain after the age of 22 no longer involves gain associated with growth but is all a matter of fatty tissue, desirable weight (defined as the average weight of individuals of a given sex and height at age 22) should be maintained throughout the rest of life.

That means adjusting caloric intake according to age, for it has been found that the metabolic rate at rest—the calories burned up when you are resting—falls off about 2 percent per decade of adult life. Moreover, physical activity, too, is likely to decrease after early adulthood.

So, starting from the base caloric intake at age 22—2,800 for men and 2,000 for women—the FNB proposed these reductions: 5 percent between ages 22 and 35; 3 more percent for each decade between ages 35 and 55; 5 additional percent for each decade between 55 and 75; and 7 percent more for age 75 and beyond.

That means 1,900 calories a day for a woman of 30; 1,843 at age 40; 1,788 at age 50; 1,697 at age 60; 1,602 at age 70; and 1,490 at age 80.

And for a man, it means 2,660 calories at age 30; 2,580 at age 40; 2,503 at age 50; 2,378 at age 60; 2,160 at age 70; and 2,009 at age 80.

At any age, from very young to very old, even as caloric requirements differ, there remains the need for all of the basic nutrients and food values.

It is possible to consume a great many calories without getting the benefit of body-building food values. Alcohol and soft drinks contain many "empty calories." Among the problems associated with drinking alcoholic beverages are these: A few drinks, in addition to adding calories, can stimulate the appetite so that you might eat too much. Excessive drinking, to the point of alcoholism, can ruin the appetite. In using alcohol instead of food, the drinker is taking in a great many calories, but none of the essential bone- and tissue-building nutrients.

All this information about protein foods for tissues and muscles, minerals as bone builders, and carbohydrates for fuel seems complicated enough. Yet we have to go still further.

## VITAMINS

Vitamins are food substances that are essential for growth, health, and life itself. You need them only in tiny quantities, but you cannot get along without them. Vitamins help change the food we eat into bones, skin, muscles, nerves, and other parts of our bodies. A basic, balanced diet, such as I describe in this chapter, provides all the vitamins and minerals you need. About a billion and a half dollars are spent for vitamins every year. Much of that money is spent by perfectly healthy people who have been convinced by high-powered advertisements that they need extra vitamins. Your doctor will certainly tell you if you need a supplement to the vitamins present in your normal diet.

If your diet is not balanced, the accompanying lack of vitamins may produce what we doctors call *deficiency diseases*.

Some of these diseases have been recognized for centuries. The disease known as *scurvy* was a familiar one to seafaring people for hundreds of years before they suspected it had anything to do with the diet on which sailors had to exist when they went on long voyages. Scurvy made them weak, caused their gums to bleed and their teeth to fall out, made their muscles ache, and eventually ended in death. About two hundred years ago, Dr. Joseph Lind, a British naval surgeon, found that the juice of citrus fruits would cure or prevent scurvy. Lime juice was subsequently carried on British ships so that sailors could have some every day, with the result that scurvy was eliminated—and British sailors came to be known as "limeys." Now we know that the value of the juice was in the *vitamin C* which citrus fruits contain.

Lack of *vitamin A* causes poor vision in dim light (called "night blindness"). Without *vitamin D* the bones fail to harden properly, causing *rickets,* one result of which we could see in bow-legs, from which so many children used to suffer. Lack of *B vitamins* causes several diseases such as beriberi and pellagra. Victims of this latter deficiency disease are weakened to the point of helplessness, their minds frequently being affected. *Pellagra* is widespread in certain poverty-stricken areas where the people have to exist on a monotonous diet: for example, the sharecropper in the South. However, it is not limited to any group. Some years ago the son of a well-to-do family was referred to the hospital with which I was associated; his poor school record had led his teachers to believe he was mentally retarded. Fortunately he was given a complete checkup which revealed —perhaps the last thing a doctor would have suspected—that he was suffering from pellagra. It was then discovered that his father, who had undergone several stomach operations and had been limited to a diet consisting of soups and gruel, had decided this diet would be good for his son if it was good for him, and had limited the boy to the same fare!

In addition to these striking deficiency diseases, lack of vitamins can cause milder disturbances that are more difficult to detect. Both the mild and the severe cases can be prevented by a balanced diet which contains all of the vitamins.

It is necessary for us to get our vitamins from foods because the human body cannot manufacture them—with the exception of *vitamin D.* Our bodies can make this when sunlight falls on the skin. However, we seldom can manufacture enough *vitamin D* all through the year, especially those of us who work indoors or live in the North. So we·must obtain *vitamin D,* too, in our food.

The following table shows some good sources of each of the principal vitamins:

### VITAMIN A

Vegetable greens, e.g., beet, kale, chard, mustard, spinach, turnip
Yellow vegetables, e.g., carrots, yellow squash, sweet potato
Beef liver
Cod-liver oil; halibut-liver oil

### VITAMIN B

(The vitamin B family consists of several vitamins, including thiamine, niacin, etc.)
Liver, pork, beef, salmon
Whole-wheat bread, enriched bread, cereals, e.g., oatmeal
Peanut butter, peanuts

### VITAMIN C

Citrus fruits—oranges, lemons, grapefruits, limes
Tomato juice (fresh or canned)
Strawberries, raspberries, gooseberries, currants

### VITAMIN D

Halibut-liver oil and other refined fish-oil preparations
Vitamin D milk
Exposure to sunlight (not sufficient alone, especially for dark-skinned people. Sunlight through glass will not make vitamin D).
(Concentrates of vitamin D are frequently prescribed by doctors for children.)

"But why should I bother with this chart?" you may ask. "Why shouldn't I just buy my vitamins at the drugstore?"

In the first place, it is more expensive. No one should spend money to purchase only vitamins if it is needed to buy foods which contain other essentials in addition to the vitamins in them. In the second place, there is still no guarantee that all the purified vitamins known at present to medical science are as good as those which nature provides. So don't buy vitamin pills, capsules, or other products unless your doctor says you need some concentrated supplements.

# OTHER DIETARY REQUIREMENTS

In addition to vitamins, the body needs small amounts of other valuable materials. Only a fraction of an ounce of iron is required, but without this the body develops a form of anemia. The blood's rich redness is produced by hemoglobin containing iron and protein. Foods rich in iron include kidney and navy beans; liver and other meats; turnip tops, beet greens, and spinach; whole-meal bread. A trace of iodine is necessary to prevent goiter; this can easily and safely be obtained by always using iodized salt.

Small quantities of still other materials are essential. The need for some has been discovered only in very recent years. Zinc, for example, is now known to be valuable for growth, sexual maturation, wound healing, and even for taste and smell. Copper is a part of many enzymes in the body. Chromium, manganese, magnesium, selenium, cobalt, and still other substances play important roles. Nature provides them in balanced and varied diets.

FIBER. Until recent times, man ate much fiber. It's the indigestible part of plant cell walls, present in many fruits and vegetables, and present naturally in large amounts in grains and cereals.

But about the turn of the century, the invention of modern roller mills made it possible economically to remove the outer husk of cereal grain kernels, and with it the fiber, to produce refined white flour. Ever since, fiber intake has decreased sharply. Today, cereal fiber intake in the United States and most Western countries is one tenth of what it was.

And as the fiber intake has gone down, the incidence of many diseases has shot up. Appendicitis, for example, became common only in this century. Constipation has become extremely common. Diverticular disease—abnormal outpouchings of the colon that can cause severe pain and may require surgery—is present in over one third of Americans and other Westerners over age forty.

Yet there has been nothing comparable among rural Africans living on native unrefined diets. They get infections; they sometimes go hungry; but eating unrefined cereal as a staple, getting about 25 grams (almost an ounce) of fiber a day—

many times as much as the average American or other Westerner—they rarely experience many common chronic Western diseases.

Fibrous foods add bulk. Once in the intestinal tract, the fiber absorbs water and swells. That makes stools soft and large, helping to prevent constipation with its characteristically small, hard, pebbly stools.

Constipation, rare in rural Africans, is more than a nuisance, since it leads to straining which, in turn, may provoke a series of problems. Straining raises pressure in the colon, and the increased pressure may cause the outpouching of diverticular disease. With straining, intra-abdominal pressure also is raised and may tend to push the stomach up through the diaphragm, some research suggests, producing hiatus hernia with its heartburn, regurgitation of stomach acid back up into the esophagus, and burning pain in back of the breastbone.

Some investigators now believe that raised pressure in the abdomen also can be transmitted elsewhere—to the leg veins, dilating them so they become varicose veins, and to veins in the anal region, causing hemorrhoids, which also are varicose or unnaturally swollen veins.

In recent studies, fiber-rich foods not only have overcome constipation problems but also have benefited diverticular disease patients. Many hemorrhoid sufferers have been relieved as stools have softened and straining has been eliminated.

The irritable bowel syndrome—also called spastic colon and mucous colitis—is a very common problem causing abdominal distention, cramps or dull deep pain, and sometimes, too, heartburn, excessive belching, nausea, weakness, headaches, or faintness. Irritable colon has responded gratifyingly to a high-fiber diet.

A diet with a full complement of fiber also may have value for combating obesity for several reasons. Fiber, providing no calories, displaces other nutrients that do. It also requires chewing, which slows intake. And there is evidence that fiber cuts down on body absorption of other foods. Some studies indicate that whereas 97 percent of total dietary calories are absorbed on a low-fiber diet, only 92.5 percent are absorbed on a high-fiber diet.

You can make certain you and your family are

getting enough fiber in several ways. One is to use bran, the fiber-rich material removed when flour is milled. It's available in breakfast cereals with "bran" in their name—and also in unprocessed brans, obtainable from health food stores and perhaps other stores. You can sprinkle unprocessed bran on cereals or mix it with soup or with flour in baking.

You can use naturally fiber-rich cereals such as oatmeal (the old-fashioned, slow-cooking kind, not the "instant"), a whole-grain wheat cereal designed to be cooked, or shredded wheat. And if you look for them, you can now find commercial whole-meal breads, rich in fiber, and whole-meal flour you can use at home to make your own bread, rolls, muffins, pancakes, and other items.

A study of more than twenty fruits and vegetables indicates them to be valuable for fiber content in this order: mango, carrot, apple, Brussels sprouts, eggplant, spring cabbage, orange, pear, green beans, lettuce, winter cabbage, pea, onion, celery, cucumber, banana, rhubarb, old potato, new potato, turnip. As much as possible, eat fruit skins for their fiber content.

SALT. Salt, of course, is sodium chloride. The body requires it. In addition to salt we add at table, some sodium occurs naturally in fresh vegetables such as artichokes, beets and beet greens, carrots, kale, dandelion and mustard greens, spinach, and Swiss chard. It is present in milk, eggs, cheeses, and meats. Canned vegetables are rich in it. It is in baking powder and soda, in the flavor intensifier monosodium glutamate, and in the preservative sodium benzoate.

Although only 1 gram or less of salt intake daily may be needed, we commonly take in as much as 15 grams a day. Too much? There is evidence that excessive salt may play a role in high blood pressure, an extremely common problem affecting upward of 23 million Americans. It would seem to be wise to moderate salt intake under normal circumstances.

There are circumstances under which more salt than usual may be needed. Salt is lost in perspiration, so during very hot days, especially with vigorous physical activity, extra salt may be needed to replenish what is lost. Salt then can be added to tomato juice and various foods. If

necessary, one-fourth teaspoonful can be added to each glass of water.

SUGAR. We consume an amazing amount—even a worrisome amount—of sugar in this country. Our average consumption per person runs to 140 to 150 pounds per year, more than 2 pounds per week. Of the 525 pounds of food consumed in the United States and in many other Western nations per person yearly on a dry basis, sugar makes up about one fourth.

The huge consumption has long been of concern —largely, at first, in connection with dental disease. That sugar plays a significant role in dental decay—feeding the bacteria that attack tooth enamel—has long been established. More recently, evidence has been accumulating that sugar may be a factor in producing periodontal, or gum, disease.

Sugar has come in for indictment as an important factor in the obesity problem. An "empty-calorie" food containing no proteins, vitamins, or minerals, it provides only energy—calories. With most of us leading relatively inactive lives, there is less and less reason to have something in the diet that provides only calories.

It could well be that many people could avoid excess weight or lose it by restricting sugar. If, for example, you take just one spoon of sugar in each cup of coffee or tea and drink only five cups daily, you could drop more than ten pounds a year by eliminating the sugar in your coffee or tea.

Some recent studies suggest that excessive sugar intake may also contribute to diabetes.

If yours is a sugar-loving family, what can you do to manage well with less? If, for example, there must be a sweet dessert, try fruit with a little liqueur. Instead of cakes, try fruit and cheese or crackers and cheese. For baking, use half the sugar recommended in some recipes and give yourself and your family an opportunity to like things that taste less sweet.

CHOLESTEROL. Cholesterol has become a household word because of evidence indicating that excesses of it in the blood are associated with coronary atherosclerosis, the narrowing of the coronary arteries which may lead to heart attacks.

Actually, the soft, waxy, yellowish substance is

essential in the body, needed in every body cell, and the body itself is equipped to produce a supply.

It is not cholesterol per se but an excess of it in the blood that is the problem. To some extent, an excess can be traced to a diet heavy in foods rich in cholesterol itself. In addition, a diet containing large amounts of fats may raise blood cholesterol levels abnormally, apparently because increased deposits of fat in the liver provide an increased source of material for liver manufacture of cholesterol.

Moreover, it is the nature of the fat in the diet that is significant. Some fats, called saturated, increase blood cholesterol levels. Others, called unsaturated and polyunsaturated, do not and may, in fact, tend to slightly decrease cholesterol levels.

The difference between the saturated and unsaturated fats is a matter of hydrogen atoms, in technical terms. In everyday terms, the primary saturated fats are milk fat, meat fat, coconut oil, and cocoa fat. Milk fat includes the fat in butter, most cheeses, and ice cream as well as whole milk. Meat fat means primarily the fat of beef, pork, and lamb; veal has less fat, and chicken and turkey are low in fat and the fat they contain is less saturated. Polyunsaturated fats are the liquid vegetable oils such as safflower, soybean, corn, and cottonseed.

A definitive answer to whether lowering cholesterol levels will reduce heart attacks will require long-term studies with large numbers of people. But there is enough evidence at hand, many authorities agree, to make it seem wise to encourage changes in the typical American diet, which tends to include excessive amounts of cholesterol and fats.

If your blood cholesterol level, as shown by a blood test, is high, your doctor may well prescribe a diet to help bring it down. If it is not yet high, he may suggest dietary changes to help prevent a future rise.

The average daily American diet contains about 600 milligrams of cholesterol, and authorities recommend that this be cut to 300. The ideal quantity of fat needed in the diet is not known, but an intake of less than the 40 percent of calories now common in the American diet is considered desirable. And of this total, polyunsaturated fats probably should compose two thirds.

Following these recommendations, you can control cholesterol intake by eating no more than three egg yolks a week, including eggs used in cooking. You will also need to limit your use of shellfish and organ meats.

To control the amounts and types of fats, authorities recommend that you

1. Use fish, chicken, turkey, and veal in most meals, limiting beef, lamb, pork, and ham to five moderate-sized portions a week.
2. Choose the leanest possible cuts of meat, trimming any visible fat, and discarding any fat that cooks out.
3. Avoid deep-fat frying, using instead such cooking methods as baking, broiling, boiling, roasting, and stewing, which help to remove fats.
4. Restrict use of fatty "luncheon" and "variety" meats such as sausages and salami.
5. Make use of liquid vegetable oils and margarines rich in polyunsaturated fats, and use less butter and other cooking fats that are solid or completely hydrogenated.
6. Use more skimmed milk and skimmed milk cheeses, less whole milk and cheeses made from whole milk and cream.

# FOOD FADS

## Vegetarian Diets

There are three types of "vegetarian" diets: (a) the strictest, which excludes all animal products in addition to the flesh and organs of all animate creatures; (b) the intermediate, which permits the eating of such animal products as milk, cheese, eggs, etc.; (c) the mildest, which permits the eating of fish and shellfish in addition to dairy products.

We doctors have been unable to find any virtue in vegetarian diets, except for the fact that people who adhere to them are apt to be lean, which is usually a good thing. For every vegetarianist who attributes his healthy old age to his diet, we have seen an even older person who gives credit to something else, perhaps the fact that he eats beef every day.

Vegetarian diets, particularly of type (a), can be harmful because they lack sufficient protein, which, as I explained on page 34, is essential for adults as well as children.

## Diets as Cures

We constantly hear about diets which will "prevent acid or alkaline stomach," cure skin disease, cancer, high blood pressure and tooth decay, or "increase virility and guarantee long life." Some of these systems are advocated by quacks; some by reputable physicians who become unduly optimistic and fail to test their theories sufficiently. (Dr. Elie Metchnikoff, one of the great pioneers in bacteriology, was convinced that drinking sour goats' milk would tremendously extend the span of human life. Thousands of people followed his advice, to no avail.)

Some diets are sound. For example, a special diet is essential in certain diseases such as diabetes. Other diets may be helpful in celiac disease, some allergic states, anemias, acne, and so on.

Nevertheless, I wouldn't think of saying that everyone with a poor complexion should cut out sugars, starches, and fats, or that people with a low hemoglobin count should eat additional portions of liver. Before I recommended such diets, I would find out what was causing the condition: the anemia could be due to the constant loss of blood from hemorrhoids (piles), and the poor complexion might be an allergic reaction to some scented soap. I wouldn't tell an adolescent who was underweight to eliminate fats and carbohydrates from his diet. Cutting out meat in order to reduce high blood pressure may result in an insufficient protein intake or in the substitution of fattening foods with weight gain that may be harmful.

I have mentioned just a few of the many examples I might give, in order to show you why it isn't safe for you to adopt a special diet on your own. (High blood pressure is discussed fully on page 421, constipation on page 504, dyspepsia [indigestion] on page 492, allergies on page 498, and anemias on page 477.)

If you need a special diet, your doctor will tell you so, making certain it is good for *you* and not just for a possibly imaginary symptom. Don't try a special diet without consulting your physician, even though a doctor may have prescribed it for some friends of yours for whom it has done miracles. Remember that the diet prescribed for the man I mentioned earlier caused his young son to suffer from pellagra. The old saying "one man's meat is another's poison" has some truth to it.

# SOME MISCELLANEOUS FOOD FACTS

Don't worry about "mixing" foods. There is no truth to the old superstition that something terrible will happen when "acid" and "alkaline" foods get together in your stomach, or that you are bound to get sick if you have lobster and milk at the same meal, or ice cream and cherries. I can find no scientific basis for the Orthodox Jewish interdiction of the simultaneous use of meat and dairy foods. On the other hand the Mosaic Law was very sound in the attitude toward pork, the washing of hands before eating, and the killing of animals intended for human consumption.

You may react violently to certain foods because you are allergic to them (see page 501). However, some foods may "disagree" with you because of an association; for example, one patient of mine says he is always nauseated by orange juice because his parents used to give him foul-tasting castor oil in it, while another can't eat shrimp salad because her attack of acute appendicitis followed a luncheon at which that was the main dish. You yourself know best whether to try to overcome the aversion or to avoid the food.

Seasonings don't injure foods. The danger from highly seasoned foods in the past came from the fact that the seasonings were often added to hide the fact that the food had spoiled. The new meat tenderizers and flavor enhancers apparently do not injure the foods in any way.

There is no basis for such superstitions as that eating oysters will increase virility, or that fish is "brain food." Garlic will not "purify the blood," and carrots will never make your hair curl.

You don't need to cut down on the quantity of food you eat in the summer, unless, of course, you cut down on your activity and don't want to gain weight. But foods won't "thicken" or "heat" the blood.

## WHAT DOCTORS DON'T KNOW ABOUT FOOD

Despite all that has been discovered about food, there is still a great deal to be learned. Scientists are constantly investigating the relationship between what we eat and our general physical and mental health. A new vitamin might be discovered at any time, or the special value of some humble food item. Because we doctors don't know everything about food, I urge you to make certain you are getting the basic requirements given at the beginning of the chapter, and also to branch out as much as you can with seafoods, etc., so you will be apt to include all foods which may happen to be particularly valuable.

## EAT RIGHT AND LIKE IT

As a physician who happens to enjoy food, I want everyone to get pleasure as well as nourishment from eating. Good meals needn't cost more or take longer to prepare than poor ones. Combining two different kinds of canned soups, for example, is no more trouble than serving your family two cans of the same variety. Herbs and seasoning help tremendously at the cost of very little time and money. Why not start collecting recipes so that the food you eat will be good—as well as good for you?

# 3
# UNDERWEIGHT AND OVERWEIGHT

Sooner or later almost everyone is faced with the problem of losing or gaining weight—or, at the least, wonders whether he or she ought to diet. Medical statistics show that 2,500,000 individuals in the United States actually consulted doctors during one year recently to ask for help in reducing. Scientific estimates indicate that in this country one fifth of the people over thirty years of age, and undoubtedly a large number of younger people, are overweight.

## WEIGHT DOES MAKE A DIFFERENCE

Anyone who is markedly underweight or overweight is suffering from a kind of illness; at any rate, he has received a danger signal. By definition, an obese person weighs 30 percent or more over what he should. Even if you are not that seriously overweight, you should be alert to the potential troubles that may lie ahead. *The obese person may suffer from one or more of the following:* (1) an overworked heart and circulation, (2) shortness of breath, (3) a tendency to high blood pressure, (4) a tendency to diabetes, (5) poor adjustment to hot weather and changes of temperature, (6) increased strain on joints and ligaments, often leading to chronic back and joint pains, (7) reduced capacity for physical exertion and sometimes for mental work, (8) increased susceptibility to infectious disease, and (9) personality problems due to poor appearance.

Surely such a person cannot be enjoying good health. And the final proof comes from incontestable medical evidence which shows that *overweight shortens the span of life itself*. For example, the mortality from circulatory conditions is 44 percent higher in males who are 5 to 15 percent overweight than it is in men whose weight is what it ought to be. "The larger the waistline, the shorter the lifeline."

I know people who have taken this so seriously that dieting is practically the most important thing in their lives—sometimes when their weight is perfectly compatible with health. On the other hand, I've had patients dismiss it as nonsense, informing me that it is natural for them to be fat or thin, and they don't think it makes any difference anyway. Of course, I tell them they are mistaken.

We should regard obesity as a potentially serious type of illness, not as a matter for jokes and ridicule.

People who are markedly *underweight* are in less danger, provided, of course, that their condition is not due to illness. However, they often lack energy, endurance, and resistance to infection, being more susceptible to illnesses such as tuberculosis, especially when they are young. To be "skinny" is not funny, either.

Obviously, people in these two groups don't look as well as they would if their weight were normal. Appearances, as well as health, contribute to happiness and success.

## DOES THIS MEAN YOU?

Your doctor can answer this question better than anyone else. Usually your mirror has provided you with a pretty good clue. Consult Table 3-1 and Figure 3-2 to determine whether or not your eyes have been deceiving you.

---

**TABLE 3-1**

DESIRABLE WEIGHTS FOR MEN AND WOMEN*

Weight in Pounds According to Frame
(as ordinarily dressed, including shoes)

MEN

| *Height* (with shoes on) Ft. In. | *Small Frame* | *Medium Frame* | *Large Frame* |
|---|---|---|---|
| 5  2 | 116–125 | 124–133 | 131–142 |
| 5  3 | 119–128 | 127–136 | 133–144 |
| 5  4 | 122–132 | 130–140 | 137–149 |
| 5  5 | 126–136 | 134–144 | 141–153 |
| 5  6 | 129–139 | 137–147 | 145–157 |
| 5  7 | 133–143 | 141–151 | 149–162 |
| 5  8 | 136–147 | 145–160 | 153–166 |
| 5  9 | 140–151 | 149–160 | 157–170 |
| 5  10 | 144–155 | 153–164 | 161–175 |
| 5  11 | 148–164 | 157–168 | 165–180 |
| 6  0 | 152–164 | 161–173 | 169–185 |
| 6  1 | 157–169 | 166–178 | 174–190 |
| 6  2 | 163–175 | 171–184 | 179–196 |
| 6  3 | 168–180 | 176–189 | 184–202 |

WOMEN

| Ft. In. | *Small Frame* | *Medium Frame* | *Large Frame* |
|---|---|---|---|
| 4  11 | 104–111 | 110–118 | 117–127 |
| 5  0 | 105–113 | 112–120 | 119–129 |
| 5  1 | 107–115 | 114–122 | 121–131 |
| 5  2 | 110–118 | 117–125 | 124–135 |
| 5  3 | 113–121 | 120–128 | 127–138 |
| 5  4 | 116–125 | 124–132 | 131–142 |
| 5  5 | 119–128 | 127–135 | 133–145 |
| 5  6 | 123–132 | 130–140 | 138–150 |
| 5  7 | 126–136 | 134–144 | 142–154 |
| 5  8 | 129–139 | 137–147 | 145–158 |
| 5  9 | 133–143 | 141–151 | 149–162 |
| 5  10 | 136–147 | 145–155 | 152–166 |
| 5  11 | 139–150 | 148–158 | 155–169 |

* From "Overweight and Underweight," Metropolitan Life Insurance Company.

Unlike some tables, this one does not give *average* weights but, rather, the *desirable* weight for you. The average person tends to become fat with the passing of the years, and this is most undesirable.

You will notice that there is an allowance of about ten pounds in each ideal weight group. If you have dropped or risen a few pounds above or below these limits, discuss the matter with your doctor at your next visit. If you vary *fifteen* or more pounds from the given limits, *make an appointment for an immediate checkup*. The older you are, the more important it is for you not to be overweight. The younger you are, the more dangerous it is to be underweight.

## CAN SOMETHING BE DONE ABOUT YOUR WEIGHT?

*Practically everybody can achieve and maintain an ideal weight.* Don't delude yourself with the excuse that you have inherited your fat or your thinness; don't pay any attention to the stories you have heard about glandular or metabolic disturbances. We doctors find that most of these stories are untrue.

A large proportion of the men and women with whom I discuss the problem of dieting assure me that there must be something wrong with them, hoping to have it confirmed by a metabolism test (see page 82). They are often incredulous and sometimes indignant when I tell them that the only thing wrong about them is the amount or kinds of food they eat.

It is true that a few diseases can be responsible for overweight or underweight. Certain glandular disturbances can affect the appetite or influence the *distribution* of fat. But a healthy individual gains or loses weight in direct relation to the *amount and kind of food eaten* and the *amount of energy expended* in his physical activity.

## FOOD AND WEIGHT

The body burns food to provide heat and energy (in addition to using it for the growth, building, repairing, protecting, and regulating of the body, as described in the previous chapter). The harder we work, the more food we require, just as an automobile consumes more gasoline when going fast or going uphill, and a stove has to be stoked more often on a cold day than on a warm one. The work or energy which can be obtained from food is measured in *calories*. A lumberjack may expend as many as 6,000 calories a day when he is working; a stenographer or other sedentary worker, only 2,000. If the stenographer ate as much as the lumberjack, she would take in a great deal of food which the body would store as fat; if the lumberjack limited himself to the stenographer's diet, he would shrink away to skin and bones.

However, quality as well as quantity counts. Some foods contain far more calories than others, as you will see by consulting Table 3-2.

Some starchy vegetables have a high-calorie value. They include baked and canned beans, green and canned corn, fresh peas, lima beans, potatoes, and rice. Also, fruits prepared with *added sugar* may be high-calorie.

The following vegetables are intermediate between the low- and high-calorie ones: beets, carrots, canned green peas, okra, onions, parsnips, pumpkin, squash, and turnips.

Among fruits, too, there are those which are high-calorie, e.g., canned apricots, bananas, cherries, huckleberries, nectarines, pears, and plums; the following ones are especially fattening: dates, figs, raisins, dried peaches, prunes, and apricots. The intermediate fruits include apples, blackberries, fresh grapes, fresh pears, and raspberries.

Not everyone can gain or lose weight simply by substituting some high-calorie for some low-calorie foods or *vice versa*. You may be eating *so much* or *so little* that this would make almost no impression on your total calorie intake.

## WHY DO PEOPLE EAT TOO MUCH OR TOO LITTLE?

If I had to answer that question in one word, I would say "habit." Many fortunate individuals

**TABLE 3–2**

CALORIE CONTENT OF FOODS AND BEVERAGES

| FOODS | AMOUNT | CALORIES |
|---|---|---|
| *Soup* | | |
| Bouillon or consomme | 1 cup | 30 |
| Cream soups | 1 cup | 150 |
| Split-pea soup | 1 cup | 200 |
| Vegetable-beef or chicken | 1 cup | 70 |
| Tomato | 1 cup | 90 |
| Chicken noodle | 1 cup | 65 |
| Clam chowder | 1 cup | 85 |
| | | |
| *Meat and Fish* | | |
| Beef steak | 4″ x 2¼″ x 1″, 3 oz. | 300 |
| Roast beef | average portion, 3 oz. | 300 |
| Ground beef | 1 patty, 3 oz. | 245 |
| Roast leg of lamb | average portion, 3 oz. | 250 |
| Rib lamb chop | 1 medium | 130 |
| Loin pork chop | 1 medium | 235 |
| Ham, smoked or boiled | 2 slices | 240 |
| Bacon | 2 strips | 100 |
| Frankfurter | 5½″ x ¾″ | 125 |
| Tongue, kidney | average portion | 150 |
| Chicken | average breast, 6 oz. | 190 |
| Turkey | 3 slices or 3½ oz. | 200 |
| Salami | 2 slices or 2 oz. | 260 |
| Bologna | 4 slices 4½″ x ⅛″ or 4 oz. | 260 |
| Veal cutlet (without breading) | 1 piece, 4″ x 2½″ x ½″, 3 oz. | 185 |
| Hamburger patty (regular ground beef) | 5 patties per pound of ground meat, 3 oz. | 245 |
| Beef liver, fried | 1 thick piece, 3″ x 2½″, 2 oz. | 130 |
| Bluefish, baked | 1 piece, 3½″ x 2″ x ½″, 3 oz. | 135 |
| Fish sticks, breaded (including fat for frying) | 5 fish sticks, 4 oz. | 200 |
| Tuna fish, canned, drained | ⅔ cup | 170 |
| Salmon, drained | ⅔ cup | 140 |
| Sardines, drained | 10 sardines or 4 oz. | 260 |
| Shrimp, canned | 4 to 6 | 65 |
| Trout | average portion | 250 |

| FOODS | AMOUNT | CALORIES |
|---|---|---|
| Fish (cod, haddock, mackerel, halibut, white fish), broiled or baked | average portion | 190 |
| Whole lobster | 1 lb. | 145 |

*Vegetables*

| | | |
|---|---|---|
| Asparagus | 6-7 stalks | 20 |
| Beans, green | ½ cup | 15 |
| kidney | ½ cup | 335 |
| lima | ½ cup | 80 |
| Beets | ½ cup | 30 |
| Broccoli | 1 large stalk | 30 |
| Cabbage, raw | ½ cup | 12 |
| cooked | ½ cup | 20 |
| Carrots | 1 medium or ½ cup | 25 |
| Cauliflower | ½ cup | 15 |
| Celery | 1 large stalk | 5 |
| Corn | 5″ ear or ½ cup | 70 |
| Cucumber | ½ medium | 5 |
| Eggplant | 2 slices or ½ cup | 25 |
| Green pepper | 1 pepper | 20 |
| Lettuce | 3 small leaves | 3 |
| Peas | ½ cup | 55 |
| Potato, sweet | 1 medium | 200 |
| white | 1 medium | 100 |
| Potato chips | 10 chips | 100 |
| Radishes | 2 small | 4 |
| Spinach | ½ cup | 25 |
| Squash, summer | ½ cup | 15 |
| winter | ¼ cup | 45 |
| Tomatoes, raw | 1 medium | 30 |
| canned or cooked | ½ cup | 25 |

*Fruits*

| | | |
|---|---|---|
| Apple | 1 medium | 75 |
| Applesauce, unsweetened | ½ cup | 50 |
| sweetened | ½ cup | 95 |
| Apricots, raw | 2 to 3 | 50 |
| canned or dried | halves, 4 to 6 | 85 |
| Avocado | ½ small | 250 |
| Banana | 1 medium | 85 |
| Cantaloupe | ⅓ medium | 35 |
| Cherries, fresh | 15 large | 60 |
| canned, syrup | ½ cup | 100 |
| Cranberry sauce | ½ cup | 250 |

| FOODS | AMOUNT | CALORIES |
|---|---|---|
| Fruit cocktail, canned | ½ cup | 90 |
| Grapefruit | ½ medium (4¼″ diameter) | 55 |
| Olives | 1 large | 8 |
| Orange | 1 medium | 70 |
| Peach, fresh | 1 medium | 45 |
| canned, syrup | 2 halves, 1 tbsp. juice | 70 |
| Pear, fresh | 1 medium | 80 |
| canned, syrup | 2 halves, 1 tbsp. juice | 70 |
| Pineapple, canned (with syrup) | 1 slice | 90 |
| Plums, fresh | 2 medium | 50 |
| canned, syrup | 2 medium | 75 |
| Prunes, cooked with sugar | 5 large | 135 |
| Raisins, dried | ½ cup | 200 |
| Tangerine | 1 large | 45 |

*Cereal, Bread, and Crackers*

| | | |
|---|---|---|
| Puffed wheat | 1 cup | 45 |
| Other dry cereal | average portion | 100 |
| Farina, cooked | ¾ cup | 100 |
| Oatmeal, cooked | 1 cup | 135 |
| Rice, cooked | 1 cup | 200 |
| Macaroni or spaghetti, cooked | 1 cup | 200 |
| Egg noodles, cooked | 1 cup | 100 |
| Flour | 1 cup | 400 |
| Bread, white, rye, or whole wheat | 1 slice | 70 |
| Ry-Krisp | 1 double square | 20 |
| Saltine | 1 cracker 2″ sq. | 15 |
| Ritz cracker | 1 cracker | 15 |
| Biscuit | 1 biscuit, 2″ diameter | 110 |
| Hard roll | 1 average | 95 |
| Pancakes | 2 medium | 130 |
| Waffle | 1 medium | 230 |
| Bun—cinnamon with raisins | 1 average | 185 |
| Danish pastry | 1 small | 140 |
| Muffin | 1 medium | 130 |

*Dairy Products*

| | | |
|---|---|---|
| Whole milk | 1 cup | 160 |
| Evaporated milk | ½ cup | 170 |
| Skim milk | 1 cup | 90 |
| Buttermilk (from skim milk) | 1 cup | 90 |

| FOODS | AMOUNT | CALORIES |
|---|---|---|
| Light cream, sweet or sour | 1 tbsp. | 30 |
| Heavy cream | 1 tbsp. | 50 |
| Yoghurt | 1 cup | 120 |
| Whipped cream | 1 tbsp. | 50 |
| Ice cream | 1/8 qt. | 200 |
| Cottage cheese | 1/2 cup | 100 |
| Cheese | 1 oz. or 1 slice | 100 |
| Butter | 1 tbsp. | 100 |
| | 1 pat | 60 |
| Egg, plain | | 80 |
| fried or scrambled | | 110 |

### Cake and Other Desserts

| | | |
|---|---|---|
| Chocolate layer cake | 1/12 cake | 350 |
| Angel cake | 1/12 cake | 115 |
| Sponge cake | 2" x 2¾" x ½" | 100 |
| Fruit pie | 1/6 pie | 375 |
| Cream pie | 1/6 pie | 200 |
| Lemon meringue pie | 1/6 pie | 280 |
| Chocolate pudding | 1/2 cup | 220 |
| Jello | 1 serving (1/5 package) | 65 |
| Fruit ice | 1/2 cup | 145 |
| Doughnut, plain | 1 doughnut | 130 |
| Brownie | 2" sq. | 140 |
| Cookie, plain | 3" in diameter | 75 |

### Miscellaneous

| | | |
|---|---|---|
| Sugar | 1 level tbsp. or 3 level tsp. | 50 |
| Jam or jelly | 1 level tbsp. | 60 |
| Peanut butter | 1 tbsp. | 100 |
| Catsup or chili sauce | 2 tbsp. | 35 |
| White sauce, medium | 1/4 cup | 100 |
| Brown gravy | 1/2 cup | 80 |
| Boiled dressing (cooked) | 1 tbsp. | 30 |
| Mayonnaise | 1 tbsp. | 100 |
| French dressing | 1 tbsp. | 60 |
| Salad oil, olive oil, etc. | 1 tbsp. | 125 |
| Margarine | 1 tbsp. | 100 |
| Herbs and spices | | 0 |
| Chocolate sauce | 2 tbsp. | 90 |
| Cheese sauce | 2 tbsp. | 65 |
| Butterscotch sauce | 2 tbsp. | 200 |

### Beverages

| | | |
|---|---|---|
| Ice-cream soda | 1 regular | 250 |

| FOODS | AMOUNT | CALORIES |
|---|---|---|
| Chocolate malted | 8-oz. glass | 300 |
| Chocolate milk | 8-oz. glass | 185 |
| Cocoa made with milk | 1 cup | 175 |
| Tea or coffee, plain | | 0 |
| Apple juice or cider | 1/2 cup | 65 |
| Grape juice | 1/2 cup | 90 |
| Cola drink | 8 oz. | 95 |
| Ginger ale | 8 oz. | 70 |
| Grapefruit juice, unsweetened | 1/2 cup | 40 |
| Pineapple juice | 1/2 cup | 55 |
| Prune juice | 1/2 cup | 85 |
| Tomato juice | 1/2 cup | 25 |

The person who "eats nothing and gains weight" is undoubtedly concentrating on fattening foods. Some of these high-calorie foods are:

Butter, oleomargarine, and cream
Oils and salad dressings
Lards and all foods fried in deep fat
Candy, sugar, jelly, jam, etc.
Ice cream, malted milk, sodas
Carbonated drinks
Bread, crackers, cookies, cakes, pastries, rice, noodles, macaroni, and spaghetti
Fat meats and gravies
Potatoes
Corn, peas, beans (except string beans), figs, dates, and other dried fruits
Nuts and olives
Chocolate and cocoa

On the other hand, the person who "eats all the time and doesn't gain weight" is apt to be selecting the less fattening, low-calorie foods. Some of these are:

Lean meats, eggs
Skimmed milk, cottage cheese (most other cheeses are not low in calories)
Vegetables: e.g., asparagus, string and wax beans, Brussels sprouts, cabbage, cauliflower, celery, cucumber, eggplant, endive, lettuce, mushrooms, pickles, radishes, sauerkraut, spinach, Swiss chard, tomatoes
Fresh fruits: e.g., blackberries, cranberries, currants, gooseberries, grapefruit, muskmelon, oranges, fresh peaches, fresh pineapple, strawberries, watermelon

never want to eat more or less than they need to maintain their ideal weight. When they exercise a great deal they eat more heartily than when they spend a quiet day at home; and if they have a huge Thanksgiving dinner at noon, they just aren't hungry for their next meal. Their appetites are regulated by their requirements, and they seldom develop bad eating habits.

Dr. Norman Jolliffe, in his excellent book *Reduce and Stay Reduced,* has coined the term "appestat" for the mechanism that regulates the appetite. People who don't go above or below their normal weights usually have appestats that are set exactly right.

In many people, however, the appestat is easily influenced or conditioned by habit. A patient of mine who had been visiting relatives and eating the huge meals they set before her, in order to be polite, came home two months later and told me her appetite had increased until she wasn't satisfied with less. On the other hand, people who don't get enough to eat for some time may develop poor appetites. Children coming from families that love food and make a happy event out of each meal, often grow up to be adults whose appestats are set too high, while those from homes where mealtimes are unpleasant, the food skimpy and poorly prepared, may have low appestats. I have frequently had patients who observe this themselves, although they usually express it by saying their stomachs "stretch" or "shrink."

*Emotional factors can play an important part in overeating or undereating.* People who feel lonely and unwanted often eat a great deal because it is one of their few pleasures. Women with small children have frequently told me they eat simply in order to have something to do, being bored by having to stay home so much, or because it makes them feel calmer and better able to cope with the children. On the other hand, worry and tension can also keep people from eating, together with such psychological quirks as the desire for attention and sympathy. Deep psychological problems naturally call for the help of a specialist. However, I have found that many of my patients who have fallen into bad eating habits can break them by will power and the type of knowledge given in this chapter.

# IF YOU NEED TO REDUCE

Too many sincere but misguided friends and relatives give incorrect and even dangerous advice about reducing and reducing diets. Let's take up a few of the things you may have heard or want to know about.

## Should One Take Drugs and Medicines in Order to Reduce?

Without a doctor's supervision and prescription, *never.* If you are under a doctor's care while you are reducing, take the medicine he selects exactly as prescribed; however, most doctors prefer to persuade a patient to rely on good judgment and self-control rather than on drugs. At one time, most medicines for weight reduction were based on Benzedrine, which so stimulated patients that physicians were reluctant to use such drugs. Now, a number of antiappetite agents are available, free of the side effect of overstimulation. Some of these medicines, which are apparently safe, include Preludin, Pre-Sate, and Tenuate, all available only through a doctor's order. The over-the-counter, so-called reducing drugs have become big business. An estimated $100 million was recently spent for these preparations in one year. At best, the money was foolishly spent; at worst, it was a risky expenditure, because of the possibility of side effects. The problem with even the safe reducing drugs is that they are only a shortcut, a prop that helps only temporarily. It is far more sensible to regulate your diet by a change in your eating habits, a change that must be permanent to be effective. A built-in adjustment of your appestat is the most effective insurance against obesity.

## Can Exercise Reduce Weight?

For many years, the role of exercise in weight control was disregarded, if not openly minimized. But regular exercise is now considered highly important, not only for the maintenance of good health but as an adjunct to a carefully regulated diet. Regular and moderate exercise (as discussed on pages 16 and 18) does burn up a measurable

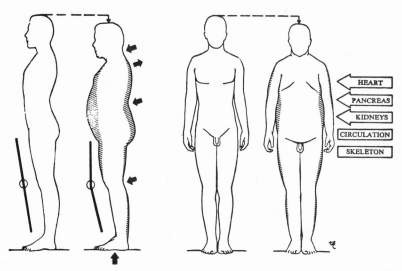

*Figure 3-1. Obesity. Note the decrease in height due to increased weight. LEFT: The black arrows indicate the location of the most severe skeletal strain. RIGHT: The organs most severely affected.*

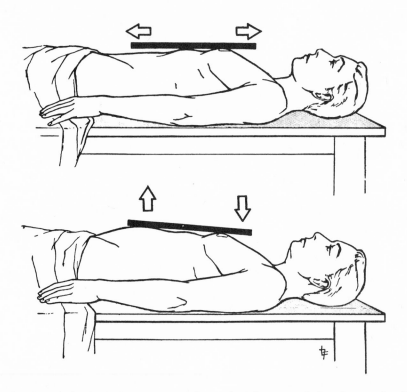

*Figure 3-2. Indication of Obesity in Men. UPPER: The board is level, indicating normal weight. LOWER: The board is raised by the man's abdomen, indicating obesity.*

number of calories. Besides, it has a beneficial effect on the cholesterol level and helps prevent heart disease.

The combination of diet and exercise, if the goal is substantial weight loss, should be carried out under a doctor's supervision.

## Can Unsightly Fat Be Removed Surgically?

Operations have been performed to trim layers of fat from the ankles, abdomen, or some other area. This is a very difficult and by no means always effective method, which is very rarely undertaken only to improve appearance. But if obesity has made a woman's breasts pendulous and quite painful, for example, a plastic surgeon would probably consider removing some of the fatty tissues.

## Can Massage Reduce Weight?

No. Massage may tone up the skin and muscles and may help the body to adjust to its new, slimmer contours. Your doctor knows when to prescribe massage.

## Can Sweating or Hot Baths Reduce Weight?

Only temporarily. They remove water, which is almost immediately regained. Not only do these methods accomplish nothing permanent, but they may put a dangerous strain on the heart and circulation. The recently fashionable *sauna baths* are a good example. In a sauna, the body is exposed to high temperatures to induce violent perspiration. This is a shock to the body, in which the pulse rate may double. It can be as much of a jolt as sudden and violent exercise. True, they have been popular in Finland for a long time, but keep two things in mind: the Finns subject themselves to saunas over a lifetime, instead of suddenly beginning in flabby middle age, and they dash water on heated stones, producing a much more humid and more tolerable heat than the new American saunas, which are electrically heated and produce a very hot and dry air.

## How About the New Reducing Diets?

So many new diets appear and disappear that it is impossible to discuss them all. Some of them are based on sensible calorie control, with a harmless "gimmick" added (perhaps in the form of a catchy title) to make them popular. The main danger I see in many of these diets is that they tend to encourage people to reduce at a rate that is too rapid for safety. Some diets are too expensive or difficult to be practical, while others are based on theories that have not yet been scientifically proved. From time to time a patient has shown me the current diet craze, saying she could stick to it far more easily than she could follow any general instructions. "Everything's written down," she explains. "I don't have to count calories or consult charts; and best of all, I don't have to make any decisions." If you feel the way she does, take any diet that appeals to you to your doctor, and let him approve or modify it, or write you out one of his own.

## Is a Doctor Necessary for Supervision of Loss of Weight?

Reduction of weight calls for the special knowledge of a physician; he will make certain that you don't lose your health while you lose your excess weight. He will see to it that you don't reduce too rapidly and thereby put a strain on your heart and circulation. He will prescribe the correct amount of minerals, proteins, and vitamins to prevent weakening of your bones and organs, and also to maintain your resistance to disease. For example, if you use a "no calorie" salad dressing made of mineral oil, your doctor may want you to take some vitamin pills, because mineral oil prevents the absorption of some of the vitamins your diet would ordinarily provide.

Your doctor has learned many helpful things by studying various people who have been on reducing diets. Individual preferences vary tremendously, and it helps a great deal if you can have your diet adjusted to your taste. Some people are miserable if they are deprived of a bedtime snack;

some want a substantial dinner at night and are willing to cut down on lunch in order to have it. Patients are occasionally reconciled to dieting when I tell them they may have hot or cold consomme and celery whenever they want it, or a cup of slightly sweetened tea to control hunger pangs. (I'll go into the matter of personal preferences more fully a little later in this chapter.)

Faddists and quacks who advocate reducing diets do not follow correct, medically exact rules for dieting. Stay away from them.

## Can You Ever Reduce "On Your Own"?

Although I see no reason why you shouldn't at least mention it to your physician, it isn't actually necessary to visit him in order to lose five or ten pounds over a period of a few months. However, report to him immediately if you notice any untoward symptoms such as constipation or diarrhea.

Let's assume that you were in excellent condition at your last checkup, just before going on your vacation, and that, in spite of all your resolutions, you put on another five pounds. If you're sensible, you can get rid of them without danger. *Be sure to maintain an adequate diet as described on page 31 in the previous chapter.* Get rid of your excess weight at the rate of one-half to one pound a week by exercising self-control. Cut out eating between meals, except for practically no-calorie foods. Eliminate desserts except for low-calorie fruits. Go easy on high-calorie foods at mealtime, substituting low-calorie ones whenever possible; avoid alcoholic beverages and soft drinks, and resign yourself to getting up from the table without feeling really full (see page 53 for sample menus of reducing diets). In a month or two your appestat will be back where it belongs. Of course this takes self-control.

## Is It Worth It?

Decidedly! Don't wait until you are actually obese before you do something about your weight. *Prevention is important.* It is much easier to prevent overweight than to correct it, easier to lose a few pounds than to readjust your appestat to a more healthful point after years of indulgence.

Watch your weight. If you can't control it, see a doctor.

You may say you don't care, that anything is better than bothering with scales and calories. Occasionally I hear someone, usually an elderly person, who means it when he or she says, "Eating is practically my only remaining pleasure. I'd rather eat myself into my grave than restrain myself and live a little longer." If you feel that way —go ahead. I mean it seriously. But be sure *you really mean it*. You might be surprised at how much satisfaction you can get from eating even while reducing if you follow a carefully supervised diet.

## HELP FOR THE PROBLEM DIETER

Almost everyone with whom I've discussed dieting has told me, usually in an apologetic manner, "It's particularly hard for me to diet, Doctor, because . . ." Then, as a rule, he or she gives one or several of the following reasons:

"It's so expensive."

"I have to cook for nondieters."

"I eat most of my meals in restaurants."

"I get cross and tired and my work (or my family) suffers."

"I often have to be a guest, and I can't be rude."

"I love good food."

Some books and articles on dieting dismiss these things as excuses. It is true that some people use them as excuses; but I, having been faced with several of them myself, know that they are real problems. There is no doubt in my mind that

Low-calorie foods *tend* to be more expensive than high ones. It is cheaper to fill up on baked beans, rice, or macaroni than it is on lobster or steak.

A housewife can't think only of her own diet when she is cooking for a husband who does hard physical work and for several teenagers who need to gain weight.

It is not easy to count calories in a restaurant when you don't even know what is in some of the dishes, and when the price includes dessert and unlimited bread and butter.

Very few bosses or families will make allowances for the fact that you're cross and tired because you're hungry.

You simply cannot tell certain hostesses that you are dieting, or ignore the creamed chicken and French fries on your plate at a business luncheon.

Being deprived of good food is certainly very hard on some people. Yes, dieting would be ever so much simpler if it weren't for the problems of money, family, work, society, and tastes. But then, so would life itself! Since these are problems almost all of us have to face, I've purposely put off giving samples of reducing diets until this section, so that I can combine them with suggestions which I hope will help you solve some of these problems. Read them all, paying especial attention to the ones that apply to you.

First of all, look at the examples of reducing diets for one day (given in Tables 3-3, 3-4, 3-5). They are for 1,000 calories a day. This is probably lower than the diet you require, so you have a certain amount of leeway. Consult Table 3-2 (page 46) and add the extra calories to which you are entitled in any way you like: a few at each meal or all of them at your most important meal, or in the form of between-meal snacks.

---

**TABLE 3–3**

### 1,000 CALORIE MENU A

*Breakfast*

| | |
|---|---:|
| Orange juice (½ cup) | 85 |
| Soft-boiled egg | 75 |
| Toast, 1 slice | 75 |
| Butter (1 tsp.) | 30 |
| Coffee | 0 |
|    with cream (1 tbsp.) | 30 |
| | 295 |

*Luncheon*

| | |
|---|---:|
| Consommé (1 cup) | 25 |
| 1 Lamb chop | 130 |
| Broccoli (1 large stalk) | 40 |
| Carrots (½ cup) | 25 |
| Pineapple slice | 50 |
| Coffee or tea | 0 |
|    with cream | 30 |
| | 300 |

*Dinner*

| | |
|---|---:|
| Crabmeat (3 oz.) | 90 |
| Green peas (½ cup) | 55 |
| Cole slaw | 15 |
|    with vinegar | 0 |
| Apple | 75 |
| 1 Cookie | 75 |
| Skim milk | 90 |
| | 400 |

TOTAL 995

---

**TABLE 3–4**

### 1,000 CALORIE MENU B

*Breakfast*

| | |
|---|---:|
| Grapefruit, ½ | 70 |
| Poached egg | 75 |
| Hard roll | 95 |
| Butter (1 tsp. or half a pat) | 30 |
| Skim milk | 90 |
| | 360 |

*Luncheon*

| | |
|---|---:|
| Bouillon | 25 |
| Beef tongue (3 thin slices) | 160 |
| Asparagus (6-7 stalks) | 20 |
| Summer squash (½ cup) | 15 |
| Canned peaches (2 halves) | 100 |
| Coffee | 0 |
|    with skim milk | 10 |
| | 330 |

*Dinner*

| | |
|---|---:|
| Clear tomato soup (¾ cup) | 75 |
| Slice of chicken | 100 |
| Green beans (1 cup) | 30 |
| Eggplant (4 slices) | 50 |
| Cantaloupe, ½ | 50 |
| Tea with lemon | 0 |
| | 305 |

TOTAL 995

**TABLE 3–5**

## Some Dieting Suggestions

1,000 CALORIE MENU C

### Breakfast

| | |
|---|---:|
| Cantaloupe, ⅓ | 35 |
| Boiled egg | 75 |
| Black coffee or tea | 0 |
| | 110 |

### Luncheon

| | |
|---|---:|
| Casserole of eggplant, ground lean meat, tomatoes, egg, and buttermilk | 250 |
| Cole slaw with vinegar | 12 |
| Fresh peach | 50 |
| Skim milk | 90 |
| | 402 |

### Dinner

| | |
|---|---:|
| Bouillon | 25 |
| Shish kabob (broiled, skewered lamb) | 340 |
| Lettuce salad (¼ head) | 10 |
| with boiled dressing | 30 |
| Asparagus (6 spears) | 20 |
| Small slice sponge cake | 100 |
| Black coffee | 0 |
| | 525 |

TOTAL 1037

To add extra calories one may add sugar and cream to the coffee or add a moderate amount of snacks such as:

| | |
|---|---:|
| Carbonated beverage or cider (1 glass) | 180 |
| Ritz crackers | 15 each |
| Peach or tangerine | 50 |
| Raw carrot | 25 |

Menu A is an average diet; Menu B provides a bulky intestinal residue for those who need it; Menu C is for those people who want special dishes.

FATS. Use skim milk or powdered milk; or take the cream off whole milk and use the fat-free milk for your beverages (hot skimmed milk is good in breakfast coffee) and in cooking soups, mashed potatoes, gravies, etc. Powdered milk is excellent for gravies. You can remove your portion and then add the cream or butter or margarine for the rest of your family. The cream you save can be used to convert *your* low-calorie gelatin or fruit desserts into high-calorie ones for the rest of your family. Use cottage cheese instead of butter or margarine. It is especially good with chives, or onion or celery salt, on thin dry (Melba) toast. Cook finely chopped spinach and other greens in very little water to which a bouillon cube has been added, and you won't miss the butter. Avoid fried foods, especially those that are French fried. It is difficult to tell exactly how many calories these dishes contain as they absorb varying amounts of fat—but it is always a great deal. Boil or poach eggs; you won't mind unbuttered toast if you serve your egg on it. Try cooking eggs on a griddle or the type of pan that doesn't require greasing. Cook stews ahead of time, let them cool, and remove the hardened fat, at least from your portion. (Stews are even better when warmed up again.) Trim the fat from your meat. Omit the rich gravy.

SWEETS. If you serve fruit stewed in sugar, give the syrup to someone who needs the calories. Sponge and angel cake aren't very high in calories if you remove your portion before icing them for the family or before adding jam or fruit syrup. Take very small portions of any dessert. Avoid soft drinks, unless you use those that contain a no-calorie type of sweetener.

STARCHES. Eat leafy green vegetables to provide the bulk you are accustomed to getting from starches. Don't munch on bread and butter, especially in restaurants. Ask the waiter not to bring it until he serves the main course. In some parts of the country salads are served first. This is a good idea because salads take the edge off your hunger before you get to the higher-calorie foods. Use wine vinegar with herbs or lemon juice on yours, while serving mayonnaise for the others.

Good gravies can be made without flour—powdered milk is one way; vegetables, either dried ones or fresh ones cooked down, and herbs such as filé will thicken stews.

Chinese restaurants serve bulky, low-calorie dishes—if you avoid the rice. You can buy many Chinese vegetables in stores.

Avoid restaurants that enforce the "no substitute" rule. Many restaurants will give you an extra vegetable or an extra serving of the one on your dinner, or a salad, in place of potatoes.

When serving soups such as minestrone, chowder, etc., take mainly the clear part for yourself, leaving most of the macaroni, potatoes, and so on, for the others. Restaurants will usually do this if you ask.

## Other Suggestions

Don't taste while cooking. This may spoil some appetites, but probably not yours! Don't lick the bowl when you've finished cooking. It has been jokingly estimated that half the overweight housewives in this country have tasted or licked themselves fat.

SNACKS add a great deal in calories. Are they worth it? If you're a "snacker," study the snack chart (Table 3-6) carefully so you will know whether it is worth it. A cup of tea or coffee, without cream, with one teaspoonful of sugar is only 16 calories; it may satisfy your hunger and provide the quick energy you need. A chocolate sundae will run between 300 and 400 calories, while half a brick of plain ice cream is 200 ("low-calorie" ice cream is 100). Nibbling between meals helps some people to diet by decreasing their appetite at mealtime. If you try this, keep careful count of calories so you'll know whether or not it's really helping you. Nibbling may be suggested by a doctor for a patient suffering from a certain type of heart condition, in which the body can manage five or six very small meals daily better than the customary three, one or two of which may be fairly heavy.

Helping your children by sampling their dinners or finishing their portions, a common form of nibbling, really helps neither them nor you. I don't know why so many parents do this. Maybe they think they're encouraging the children to clean their plates. It is, of course, only one more way to add calories. This is a very fattening habit, since any parent who does it never stops to think of the extra calories he is putting away.

EATING BINGES. Just as some people can take a drink without becoming alcoholics, so some dieters are able to go off their diets occasionally without ill effect. Their morale may even benefit from knowing they can do this every month, which is better than constant "cheating." But remember, your appestat is probably easily conditioned, or you wouldn't be dieting in the first place, so be very careful.

TALKING ABOUT YOUR DIET. This may make people shun you as a bore. Some people will try to get you to break your diet, while others will help you to keep it. You have to know which kind you are with before you start discussing your diet. Sometimes it will save embarrassment for you to say that the doctor has told you not to eat certain foods. As a general rule, the best social technique is to avoid attracting attention to yourself and your problem. Simply eat very little of fattening foods that are placed before you.

BREAKFAST. For reasons explained previously, a hearty, *high-protein* meal in the morning usually keeps people from being hungry in the mid-morning and from eating too much at noon.

ALCOHOLIC BEVERAGES. Consult the calorie chart in Table 3-7, and you will see that these are high in calories; they don't satisfy your hunger except, sometimes, when taken in excess. Usually they make you forget you're on a diet. For example, three glasses of beer, at 120 calories per 8-ounce glass, will supply as many calories as a fairly substantial breakfast. A party evening of cocktails will ensure you almost as many calories as a full day's reducing diet. Even more serious is the fact that alcohol supplies "empty calories," or energy without any of the other necessary food values, such as proteins or minerals (see page 36).

MODERATION. This should be your key word. Remember, it took a long time for you to put on this fat you want to lose, so be moderate about reducing, too. Fat lost at the rate of one-half pound to a pound a week stays off much better than that lost in a hurry—and a pound a week adds up to 52 pounds a year! When you lose weight slowly, your skin adjusts itself and you don't get that deflated-balloon look.

## TABLE 3–6

### CALORIE CONTENT OF SNACK FOODS

| FOOD | AMOUNT | CALORIES |
|---|---|---|
| Chocolate bar | 1 small bar | 155 |
| Chocolate creams | 1 average size | 50 |
| Cookies | 1 medium size | 75 |
| Doughnut | 1 plain | 135 |
| Banana | 1 large | 100 |
| Peach | 1 medium size | 50 |
| Apple | 1 medium size | 75 |
| Raisins | ½ cup | 200 |
| Popcorn | 1 cup popped | 55 |
| Potato chips | 8-10 or ½ cup | 100 |
| Peanuts or pistachio nuts | 1 | 5 |
| Walnuts, pecans, filberts, or cashews | 4 whole or 1 tbsp. chopped | 40 |
| Brazil nuts | 1 | 50 |
| Butternuts | 1 | 25 |
| Peanut butter | 1 tbsp. | 100 |
| Pickles | 1 large sour | 10 |
| | 1 average sweet | 15 |
| Olives | 1 | 10 |
| Ice cream | ½ cup | 200 |
| Chocolate-nut sundae | | 270 |
| Ice cream soda | | 255 |
| Chocolate malted milk | 1 glass | 450 |
| Eggnog (without liquor) | 1 glass | 235 |
| Carbonated beverages | 6 oz. or 1 bottle | 80 |

## TABLE 3–7

| ALCOHOLIC BEVERAGES | | CALORIES |
|---|---|---|
| Beer | 8 oz. glass | 120 |
| Wine | 1 wine glass | 75 |
| Gin | 1 jigger | 115 |
| Rum | 1 jigger | 125 |
| Whiskey | 1 jigger | 120 |
| Brandy | 1 brandy glass | 80 |
| Cocktail | 1 cocktail glass | 150 |

# IF YOU NEED TO GAIN WEIGHT

If you are markedly underweight or are losing weight, you, even more than the overweight person, should consult a doctor.

A chronic underweight condition or a sudden loss of weight is an indication of poor health. It may indicate the onset or presence of a disease; chronic undernutrition is very apt to make one more susceptible to sickness. In either case, it is a signal for action to protect one's health.

Loss of weight or undernutrition may be warnings that diabetes has set in, or that the thyroid gland is overactive; tuberculosis may be the cause, although, contrary to popular opinion, it frequently does not produce loss of weight. Intestinal worms, especially in children, may be responsible.

These are just a few of the causes. All kinds of chronic infections and many other illnesses can result in loss of weight. Finding the cause is your doctor's concern. It is your responsibility only to watch your weight and that of your children. If you notice a definite loss of weight, report it to your doctor or to a hospital clinic. They, and not you, will be able to track down the cause and prescribe the treatment.

## How to Tell If You Are Underweight

Usually you need the help of a doctor, even more than the overweight person does, in deciding whether or not you are actually underweight. If you are ten to fifteen pounds below the figures given on page 45, and if the bones stick out all over your body, or the muscles don't cover the back, thighs, and buttocks with resilient protection, or your face is thin and drawn, you are very likely underweight. But the figures in this table can't always answer your question. You may be the long, lean type whose weight normally runs below those given. Your doctor, by considering the results of your physical examination, including observations of the size and bony framework of your body, can decide fairly accurately whether you are underweight. Too many people worry over an underweight condition that does not actually exist, because they have accepted the "diagnosis" of well-intentioned friends or relatives—often individuals whose age or background leads them to believe "it is healthy to be stout." Let your doctor decide whether you are truly underweight in the sense of needing special treatment for it.

## What to Do About It

If your extreme thinness is not due to ill health, it is due to a failure to eat enough of the right food. A good diet provides (a) flesh-building proteins, (b) minerals for the bones and teeth, (c) vitamins, iron, iodine, etc., and (d) carbohydrates to provide a reservoir of energy. If the diet is too low in protein, the muscles are thin; unless sufficient carbohydrates are consumed, the body obtains its energy from fats; if these, too, are lacking, it draws on the muscles and some of the organs which start to shrink. The Eskimos eat little carbohydrate, getting their energy and keeping up their weight with fats and protein. Americans usually prefer a diet with less fat and protein, and depend on carbohydrates to provide energy.

Having decided your diet is inadequate, your doctor will try to discover whether you have a psychological resistance to eating. Although such attitudes may be deep-seated, I have had quite a few patients whose appestats were low because they had been told it was wrong, or greedy, or wasteful to eat unless they were really hungry, or that it was fashionable to look excessively thin.

Just as your doctor worked out ways for your obese friend to consume fewer calories, he will help you to take in additional ones. Gaining weight is not a simple matter of eating more. Your problems, too, will have to be solved. The doctor can help a great deal, but you will have to cooperate wholeheartedly. You must remind yourself that (1) you *can* eat even though you aren't hungry, (2) you *can* get in the habit of substituting high-calorie foods for the low-calorie ones you prefer.

Your doctor will probably recommend a high-calorie diet, medication, appetite-stimulating exercises, or a combination of these measures. To be safe, follow his instructions.

## Gaining Weight without Medical Supervision

As in the case of the moderately obese, people who are somewhat underweight can gain on their own if they have been given a clean bill of health by their physicians. Perhaps your doctor has cautioned you against losing weight by neglecting to eat three good meals a day, and you know you have been getting careless. Or perhaps he has said he would like you to gain five to ten pounds, but since he also said you were in good condition, you've ignored his advice until today, when something injured your vanity. You can gain weight on your own, but be sure to consult your doctor if, for example, cutting down on bulky low-calorie vegetables should make you constipated. Don't take laxatives or mineral oil, which may deprive you of some of the vitamins you need (see Constipation, page 504).

## ADVICE TO THE PROBLEM EATER

### Time

It takes time to eat proper meals and learn to enjoy them instead of getting through with the task of swallowing your food as fast as possible. Pleasant, relaxing company may help you to prolong your mealtime so you can eat more without feeling stuffed. Some people who eat alone find it helps to listen to the radio, particularly to musical selections, or even to read to keep from being bored. Some find large portions discourage them from eating, while others who "can't take seconds" do better with big servings. Meals that look attractive usually encourage appetite. As a rule, people eat more at "family style" meals, at which the food is all placed on the table and they help themselves, than they do when they have it passed to them formally. It takes thought and attention for you to find out what is best for you.

You also should take time to relax before meals. It is difficult to eat when you are tired. And you should set aside plenty of time for a good night's rest, to avoid fatigue at breakfast time.

## Eat More

You can do it. Another piece of bread and butter, a second helping, soon become matters of habit.

## Using High-Calorie Foods

Higher-calorie vegetables such as peas, potatoes, and lima beans provide more carbohydrates than the leafy vegetables you may have been eating. Use them but continue to use salads, which help to provide bulk.

If your doctor approves after a check into any cholesterol problem, you can use such high-calorie foods as cream soups, chowders, cereals with cream, mayonnaise, sauces made with butter or margarine or thickened with flour, and rich desserts.

## Snacks

You can learn to enjoy them, finding ones that don't spoil your appetite. For example, an eggnog with some crackers can add plenty of calories and may even make you sleep better. Try it and see whether it does, cutting it out if insomnia or restless sleep results, in which case you may be able to add snacks between meals. (See Table 3-6 for the high-calorie snacks.)

Although candy and other foods such as jellies, pastry, cake, and ice cream are concentrated energy sources, they may satiate hunger for more valuable foods and increase tooth decay. Other snacks such as peanut butter, eggnog, and fruit are valuable because, beyond calories, they provide essential nutrients.

## Consult the Suggestions for Problem Dieters (page 52)

Some of these may be useful to you *in reverse*. But remember, you are different from the person with a tendency to overweight. Tasting is apt to spoil your appetite. *Don't* eat a light breakfast in the hope of being hungrier at noon. You need a good, high-protein breakfast to get you off to a good start every day. Remember, your long-range goal is to reset your appestat at a favorable point, so that you will have a natural desire to eat enough to keep your weight at a healthful level.

## Smoking

There is no doubt that smoking, particularly chain or any excessive smoking, tends to keep people from eating and interferes with the enjoyment of good food. However, some people become so nervous when they give up smoking that I would scarcely make so drastic a suggestion to everyone who wants to gain. Try it, but also try cutting down. At least, avoid cigarettes just before meals and at mealtimes. As discussed on pages 427 and 434, heavy smoking is such a health hazard in so many other ways that your weight problem is only *one* good reason for cutting down.

## Alcoholic Beverages

This, too, is a matter for each individual to decide. Many people find that an apéritif such as a glass of sherry sipped in a leisurely manner before dinner helps them to relax and stimulates the appetite. But don't substitute alcohol for food.

Consult the sample *high-calorie diets* in Tables 3-8, 3-9, and 3-10. Take your dieting seriously; it is important to your health. Menu D and Menu E contain rich, concentrated, high-calorie foods. They are less bulky than Menu F, which gets its large number of calories from employing large quantities of lower-calorie materials. Try these high-calorie diets until you find the type which you like—and which helps add the pounds.

# UNDERWEIGHT AND OVERWEIGHT IN CHILDREN

The proper diet for infants, children, and adolescents is described on pages 268, 271, and 310-11. *All cases of underweight or overweight should be discussed with your doctor.* If you are in any doubt, let him decide.

Parents can do great harm by trying to make children eat more or less because someone—perhaps a relative or neighbor—has decided they are

## TABLE 3–8

### 3,500 CALORIE MENU D

#### Breakfast

| | |
|---|---|
| 1 Banana sliced | 100 |
| with cream (½ cup) | 120 |
| 2 Griddle cakes | 200 |
| with syrup and | 50 |
| butter (1 tbsp.) | 100 |
| 2 Sausages | 350 |
| Black coffee | 0 |
| | 920 |

#### Luncheon

| | |
|---|---|
| Cup of cream of potato soup | 250 |
| Macaroni and cheese (1 cup) | 300 |
| Apple and nut salad | 150 |
| Pie a la mode | 400 |
| Cocoa | 210 |
| | 1,310 |

#### Dinner

| | |
|---|---|
| Fruit cocktail | 90 |
| Duck (4 oz.) | 350 |
| gravy | 20 |
| Baked potato | 90 |
| with butter | 100 |
| Green peas | 55 |
| Avocado pear salad | 250 |
| with mayonnaise | 100 |
| Chocolate pudding | 200 |
| Tea or coffee | 0 |
| | 1,255 |

DAILY TOTAL 3,485

## TABLE 3–9

### 3,500 CALORIE MENU E

#### Breakfast

| | |
|---|---|
| Dry cereal | 100 |
| with cream and sugar and | 140 |
| ½ banana, sliced | 50 |
| Toast | 75 |
| with butter (1 tbsp.) and | 100 |
| jelly | 100 |
| Coffee or tea | 0 |
| with 1 tsp. sugar and | 20 |
| 2 tbsp. cream | 60 |
| | 645 |

#### Luncheon

| | |
|---|---|
| Cup of cream of tomato soup | 250 |
| 3 Saltines | 45 |
| Ham and cheese sandwich | 350 |
| 2 Celery stalks | 15 |
| filled with mayonnaise | 100 |
| Milk (half cream) or cocoa | 210 |
| Chocolate layer cake | 400 |
| | 1,370 |

#### Dinner

| | |
|---|---|
| Pineapple juice (4 oz. glass) | 55 |
| 1 Pork chop or veal chop | 235 |
| gravy | 20 |
| Mashed potatoes (1 potato) | 100 |
| Creamed broccoli | 140 |
| Bread and butter | 100 |
| Sweetened applesauce (½ cup) | 100 |
| Ice cream sundae or | |
| lemon meringue pie | 335 |
| Milk (8 oz. glass) | 170 |
| | 1,255 |

#### Bedtime

| | |
|---|---|
| Eggnog | 230 |

DAILY TOTAL 3,485

TABLE 3–10

3,500 CALORIE MENU F

### Breakfast

| | |
|---|---|
| 5 large prunes | 135 |
| Dry cereal | 100 |
| with sugar and cream | 140 |
| Scrambled eggs (1) | 100 |
| 2 strips bacon | 100 |
| Toast | 75 |
| and butter | 100 |
| Coffee | 0 |
| with sugar and cream | 80 |
| | 830 |

### Luncheon

| | |
|---|---|
| Split pea soup | 200 |
| with croutons | 40 |
| Baked ham or veal cutlet | 240 |
| Potato | 90 |
| Carrots | 25 |
| Cottage cheese salad | 50 |
| with peach | 100 |
| Bread | 75 |
| and butter | 100 |
| Jello | 90 |
| with whipped cream | 60 |
| Tea with lemon | 0 |
| | 1,070 |

### Dinner

| | |
|---|---|
| Tomato juice | 25 |
| Pork and beans (1 cup) | 500 |
| 2 Frankfurters | 300 |
| Tossed green salad | 25 |
| with French dressing | 60 |
| Large roll | 95 |
| and butter | 100 |
| Ice cream | 200 |
| Brownie | 140 |
| Milk | 170 |
| | 1,615 |

DAILY TOTAL 3,515

too thin or too fat. They can also do great harm by dismissing the subject with, "Oh, Johnny will grow out of it!"

Underweight and overweight in young people can be serious; only a doctor can determine this and decide how it should be dealt with according to the cause, the age of the child, and the entire situation. The only thing parents should do on their own is to provide proper meals and a proper attitude toward them.

Don't use food as a reward or withhold it as a punishment. Make meals pleasant and relaxed without overemphasizing them. In this way you will help to develop well-functioning appestats in your children, for which they will be grateful all their lives.

I discuss punishments as a method of maintaining discipline in children on page 279. The problem of *underweight and overweight in adolescence* is described on page 311.

Ideal weights for adolescent boys and girls are given on page 312.

# 4
# CARE OF THE TEETH AND GUMS

Tooth decay—which your dentist calls *dental caries*—is the most common disease in the country. It is the chief cause of toothache and of your fillings and inlays; it is the major source of pulp and root abscesses, and a very common reason why teeth have to be extracted and artificial ones substituted for them.

Another important disease, which involves the gums and tooth sockets, is periodontal disease or, as it is better known, pyorrhea. This is a progressive disease, which starts with gingivitis, in which the gums become inflamed, swollen, and tender. Left uncontrolled, the inflammation advances and the gums begin to stand away from the teeth so that pockets are formed which harbor bacteria and pus; this is pyorrhea. As pyorrhea progresses, fibers holding the teeth in their sockets weaken and gradually the bone supporting the teeth is destroyed, and the teeth become loose and are lost.

Aside from caries and periodontal disease, there are other tooth troubles, such as impacted teeth, accident cases, and problems resulting from poor alignment of teeth. When teeth are not correctly aligned the bite doesn't work properly, and our chewing is inadequate or difficult; or the teeth overlap and stick out in an unattractive manner. The correction of this condition is called *orthodontia*, and is slow, difficult work, usually handled by specialists. These dentists are called *orthodontists*. You have seen some of their work in children who wear braces to correct the alignment of their teeth.

An alternative to dentures is the *reconstruction* of teeth. A specialist in this field of dentistry can grind your teeth and cap them with natural-looking materials. This process can involve a few teeth only or the entire mouth. The effect of reconstruction is that the combination of your teeth and caps becomes permanent. In the process, the dental specialist also may adjust the alignment of your teeth. Discuss reconstruction in detail with your dentist; it is a slow, tedious, and expensive undertaking.

By now you may be asking, "Wouldn't it be simpler to have all my teeth pulled before caries and/or pyorrhea ruin them—and get some artificial ones right away?" At one time people used to do just that: they would have a tooth extracted as soon as it started to ache, or even before. Fortunately, no reputable dentist would do such a thing today. Dentists now try to save every tooth they can. Dentures involve time, trouble, and expense, and they seldom do as good a job of chewing as one's own teeth can do—and the proper chewing of food is of great value to digestion. However, modern dentures are remarkable, and many of my patients who have artificial teeth tell me that they look much better than they expected. The new dentures are also far more comfortable than the older models.

## PAINLESS DENTISTRY

Today dentists are able to save many teeth which formerly they would have extracted. The main reason for this lies in the advances dentistry has made, especially in the direction of painless dentistry. New instruments and improved techniques make it possible for the dentist to work faster, more gently, and less painfully. Fear of pain probably is the main reason people postpone visits to the dentist. The heat and vibration of slow-running dental instruments do cause pain, but newer types of drills now can eliminate most of the discomfort—sometimes, all of it.

Water-cooled air drills avoid creating pain-producing heat. Ultrasonic (faster than sound) devices and extremely high-speed rotary drills (they may run as fast as 400,000 revolutions a minute) are other recent developments. It is worthwhile to check with your dentist for his view on painless dentistry and his equipment for making it possible.

Years ago dentists used anesthetics only when extracting teeth. Today most dentists use them for almost all painful procedures, including preparing teeth for fillings, with children as well as adults. The most popular methods are the injections of procaine, Novocain, etc., into the nerves or gums, or the inhalation of nitrous oxide gas. Some dentists use the "light nitrous oxide analgesia method" (analgesia means insensibility to pain). The patient inhales a mixture of nitrous oxide and oxygen through a nosepiece. Although he remains conscious and is aware of the drilling, his sensations are dulled so that it does not hurt him. Some patients actually enjoy taking nitrous oxide in this way, and most children prefer it to an injection of Novocain. Of course, the gas must be administered by a skilled dentist; and there are people who should not take it because they are suffering from certain diseases.

A type of mild analgesia which I recommend for nervous or sensitive patients is a pain-killing medicine such as ordinary aspirin (or stronger pain-relievers such as codeine or Demerol). The tablets taken an hour *before* your appointment can make a real difference. If you are apprehensive about having work done on your teeth, ask your doctor or dentist about this. Sometimes a sedative such as phenobarbital will be very helpful, especially for children. Don't be ashamed to ask for something for relief of your pain or to enable you to get a good night's sleep after a long, difficult session. Some people are surprised when I suggest such things, and even more so when I tell them that I am certainly not above taking a pain-reliever before a session with the dentist. Be-

cause some people don't mind dental work, doctors and dentists may fail to take the time to discuss this with you unless you ask about it. Always remember that your doctor and dentist don't want you to suffer needlessly.

## YOUR TEETH

Nature provides two sets of teeth in one's lifetime: the twenty deciduous (first, baby, or milk) teeth, and the thirty-two permanent (second) teeth. This is not extravagant of nature, for the jaws of an infant aren't large enough for the teeth he will get in later life. But don't make the mistake of assuming that the first teeth are not important because they are expendable. If these teeth become badly decayed and have to be pulled, the permanent teeth may not come into place properly. Those thirty-two teeth are all that nature will ever give you. There is no case on record of anyone ever having developed a third set of natural teeth.

The first teeth start to appear (erupt) when the infant is about six months old, and continue to erupt until he is about thirty months old. Shedding

TABLE 4–1

AGES AT WHICH INDIVIDUAL TEETH APPEAR

| Tooth | Baby Teeth* (Age in Months) | Permanent Teeth (Age in Years) | |
|---|---|---|---|
| | | Upper Teeth | Lower Teeth |
| Central incisor | 5–8 | 7–8 | 6–7 |
| Lateral incisor | 7–11 | 8–9 | 7–8 |
| Cuspid | 16–20 | 11–12 | 9–10 |
| First bicuspid | | 10–11 | 10–12 |
| Second bicuspid | 10–16 | 10–12 | 11–12 |
| First molar | 20–30 | 6–7 | 6–7 |
| Second molar | | 12–13 | 11–13 |
| Third molar | | 17–21 | 17–21 |

* The baby teeth referred to as the second bicuspid and the first molar are also called the first molar and the second molar.

usually begins when the child is six or seven years old. At that age the first permanent teeth, the first molars (six-year molars), also usually appear. Table 4-1 is a rough guide to when the different teeth erupt.

I say "rough guide" because these ages vary according to the individual. However, be sure to consult your dentist or physician if your child's teeth don't appear at about the time they should. He can then start searching for the reason.

Proper nourishment is essential to the development of both the first and the permanent teeth (see page 36). Cleanliness and dental care are also necessary, so start taking your child to the dentist early. Various ages are recommended by different authorities. Personally, I think it is a good idea to begin soon after the twenty first teeth have appeared (at two and a half to three years). The chances are that no treatment will be needed then, so the child's first (and very important) experience with the dentist will be a pleasant one, especially if you take a little trouble to prepare him for it. Play "going to the dentist" with your child and mark the occasion by the gift of some simple toy such as a balloon.

Give your child a small, soft-bristle toothbrush for his own. Let him brush his teeth at the same time as one of his parents. Children are great im-

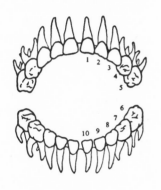

*BABY TEETH*

1. *central incisor—7½ mos.*
2. *lateral incisor—9 mos.*
3. *cuspid—18 mos.*
4. *first molar—14 mos.*
5. *second molar—24 mos.*
6. *second molar—20 mos.*
7. *first molar—15 mos.*
8. *cuspid—16 mos.*
9. *lateral incisor—7 mos.*
10. *central incisor—6 mos.*

*PERMANENT TEETH*

1. *central incisor—7-8 yrs.*
2. *lateral incisor—8-9 yrs.*
3. *cuspid—11-12 yrs.*
4. *first bicuspid—10-11 yrs.*
5. *second bicuspid—10-12 yrs.*
6. *first molar—6-7 yrs.*
7. *second molar—12-13 yrs.*
8. *third molar—17-21 yrs.*
9. *third molar—17-21 yrs.*
10. *second molar—11-13 yrs.*
11. *first molar—6-7 yrs.*
12. *second bicuspid—11-12 yrs.*
13. *first bicuspid—10-12 yrs.*
14. *cuspid—9-10 yrs.*
15. *lateral incisor—7-8 yrs.*
16. *central incisor—6-7 yrs.*

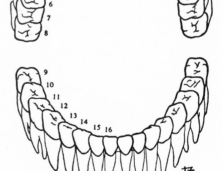

*Figure 4–1. Baby Teeth and Permanent Teeth. Approximate time of their appearance.*

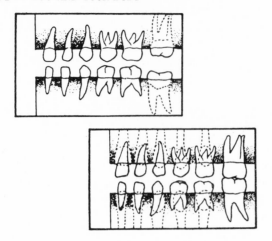

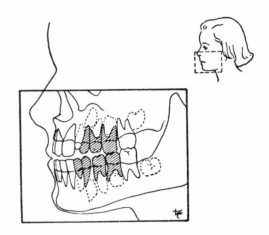

*Figure 4–2. Replacement of Baby Teeth by Permanent Teeth.* UPPER LEFT: *One side of the jaw at about 6 years of age, showing the milk teeth, in diagrammatic form. The first permanent molars are appearing.* LOWER LEFT: *At about 8 years of age. The first permanent molars have appeared, and other permanent teeth are appearing.* RIGHT: *At about 9½ years of age. Some baby teeth (shaded) are still in; some permanent teeth have fully appeared (solid outline); and some permanent teeth are about to appear (dotted lines).*

itators. Encourage the child to use a small amount of dentifrice. Praise his performance even though his efforts for some time will appear clumsy and poorly coordinated.

## CHOOSE YOUR DENTIST CAREFULLY

Every family needs a competent dentist. Also, the decisive factor in your child's attitude toward dental work will depend on your dentist. As in medicine, there are tremendous differences among the men in the dental profession—only now you have your doctor or your pediatrician to help you make your choice. Your local dental school, dental society, or health officer will also help you to find a dentist or, if you can't afford a private one, will direct you to the nearest good clinic. But remember that however well qualified a dentist may be, his skill and personality can make all the difference in the world to you. I add "personality" because a good deal of our suffering in the dentist's chair comes from fear and tension, and a sympathetic dentist, willing to take time and trouble, can spare you most of it. It is worth your time

and trouble to find such a dentist, especially for your children. It may be worthwhile for you to travel to a dental center or clinic in order to find a person especially trained and suited to working with children.

## IMPACTED TEETH

Look at the chart again. You've heard about impacted teeth. This means a tooth which, although formed, does not come through the gums, or pushes only partway through. This happens most frequently in the case of the third molars (wisdom teeth). If a tooth fails to come through, causing pain or swelling, consult your dentist. Only he, with the help of his x-ray, will be able to tell you what, if anything, should be done. The surgery necessary to remedy this condition can quite well be performed in the dentist's office, but sometimes this procedure may be so complicated and long that it is better done in a hospital operating room. This is to the patient's benefit, for a surgical operation on the gums is no less serious than on other parts of the body.

## ALIGNMENT OF TEETH

Everyone has seen teeth that are irregular, or which overlap, or stick out in odd directions. Sometimes the upper and lower teeth do not meet (occlude) properly. This may be due to the fact that the first teeth were lost too soon because of decay or accident—a good reason for taking your child to the dentist early. It may also be due to the fact that the teeth failed to fall out when they should. Some dentists believe that excessive thumb or finger sucking at the time the second teeth are coming in may be responsible. (Since the happy child has usually given up sucking his thumb by the time he is six, it is advisable to discuss this habit with your doctor if it persists.) Another important cause of irregular tooth alignment and a faulty bite is insufficient chewing, because the diet is overloaded with soft foods.

### Correcting Irregular Teeth

Poorly aligned teeth are apt to give trouble because the food collects behind them and the gums become irritated. Because only a few of the teeth meet in chewing, the force of the bite falls entirely upon them, and loosens them. Perhaps equally important, they detract from the individual's appearance. Many people would be happier if they didn't have "buck teeth" or a "weak" receding chin. Your dentist can tell you whether your child's bite is so poor he can't chew his food properly; he will suggest that you see an orthodontist, and help you to find a qualified one.

You may be so anxious to do the right thing by your child that you fail to realize what a financial burden the prolonged treatment is going to be. It may result in only a slight improvement. Also, some people suggest having teeth straightened for purposes of appearance when actually an irregular tooth or two may not really be disfiguring. Be sure to discuss this matter frankly with your dentist, and you and he can undoubtedly arrive at a suitable decision together. As for payment, your dentist may be willing to spread out the payment of his bills. If your child really needs orthodontic braces and you can't afford them, don't hesitate to investigate dental clinics, as suggested on page 408. I have had patients whose expenditures for a child's tooth braces resulted in their using money they should have spent on more vital matters. People frequently spend the entire sum they have allocated to health on dental bills, and then fail to go to the doctor because they can't afford it. *Medical and dental care should be two separate items in your budget.*

## DENTAL CARIES

Look at the picture of the tooth on page 66. You will see that the part of it (called the crown) that

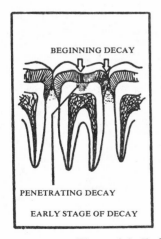 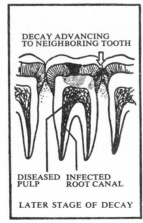 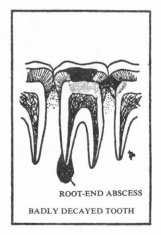

*Figure 4–3. Early and Late Stages of Dental Caries (Decay).*

lies above the surface of the gum is covered with a coating of enamel; fortunately this is thickest on the "grinding surface" where it wears down from use. The part of the tooth (called the root) that lies within the jaw is covered with a thin bonelike layer (cementum). Beneath the enamel lies the resilient, leathery dentin, with a chamber, called the pulp chamber, and the root canal. They contain the blood vessels and nerve fibers which nourish the tooth and maintain its life and sensations.

It is important to realize, first of all, that *dental caries is a disease,* not a vague, mysterious "rotting" of the teeth which must be accepted fatalistically. Dental caries *always* starts on the outside of the teeth, in the enamel. If we focus a microscope on a section of enamel where the tiniest new cavity is developing, we see a pinhead-sized collection of bacteria and food adhering to the smooth surface of the tooth, similar to barnacles gathering on the smooth hull of a ship. The dentists call this collection *plaque.*

It is generally believed that a good proportion of these bacteria are the kind that thrive best on starchy and sugary foods, which they change into *lactic acid.* Although tooth enamel is the strongest material in the body, able to withstand repeatedly enormous biting pressures in pounds per square inch, lactic acid quickly and permanently dissolves it. Eating minute pits and furrows in the surface of the tooth, the acid opens up new territory for the bacteria. Soon they reach the softer, richer dentin, where they grow faster and spread rapidly. They proceed into the root canal, attacking the nerves and causing great pain. (For temporary, partial relief from toothache, see page 340.) Infected pulps or decaying teeth make excellent breeding places for bacteria; they can cause localized abscesses, and may even enter the blood stream to spread their poison to various parts of the body.

## Filling Teeth

Enamel that has been destroyed by acid won't grow and come together again; neither will the dentin of the tooth destroyed by bacteria. Unless the decay has gone too far, the dentist can save the tooth by removing the diseased portion and filling the cavity. The dentist drills out the decayed area, treats it with an antiseptic, and puts in a perfectly fitting filling.

When decay has entered the pulp and root canal, the tooth may begin to ache. The nerve dies and the infection spreads around the ends of the roots in the jawbone. This may cause infections elsewhere even though the tooth may not ache at all. The dentist tries to save most of the tooth by cleaning out the decay and residue of the pulp and nerve. He sterilizes the root canals with antibiotics and antiseptics, then fills the root canals and the cavity to seal them and keep them sterile. Thereafter, such a tooth must be examined regularly by x-ray. If the infection continues or recurs, the tooth should be extracted.

## Why Do YOU Get So Many Cavities?

Some people seem to have teeth that are particularly prone to decay. Others seem to be immune to caries. We may have an immunity at certain times and not at others; the same patient may have many cavities one year and none the following year. Such types of immunity, which are not understood, usually occur from about

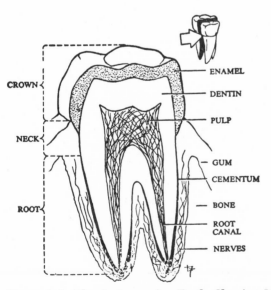

CROWN
NECK
ROOT

ENAMEL
DENTIN
PULP
GUM
CEMENTUM
BONE
ROOT CANAL
NERVES

*Figure 4-4. The Anatomy of a Tooth. Showing Its Construction and Placement in the Jaw.*

twenty-five to forty-five years of age.

In some communities the residents are practically free from tooth decay: some Alaskan Eskimos, natives of parts of the Hebrides Islands off the coast of Scotland, several South African Zulu tribes, and a few others. In some areas, there is partial immunity. Resistance to decay in such areas in the United States appears to be directly related to the fluoride content of the water.

## Fluoridation

The role of fluoride in minimizing or preventing decay has come in for intensive study. Research, which began following the discovery that there is a markedly lesser incidence of decay in communities in which fluoride is present naturally in drinking water, indicates that fluoride can combine with tooth enamel to make it more acid-resistant.

The addition of small amounts of fluoride to community water supplies in areas where water was lacking in it began in 1945. Since then, it has been recommended as an effective measure by the American Dental and Medical Associations, the U.S. Public Health Service, and other bodies concerned with health. Currently, more than 100 million Americans in 10,000 communities drink fluoridated water. There is still opposition to fluoridation, and some communities have been influenced to vote against it. Although reasons for opposition range from political to religious, fluoridation is dangerous only if the concentration in the water is too great. A safe and effective proportion is one and a half parts of flourine to one million parts of water. Many dentists in non-fluoridated areas prescribe fluoride tablets or vitamins with added fluoride for children.

Additionally, applications of fluoride directly to the teeth by dentists and use of toothpastes containing fluoride have been found to aid further in reducing decay.

## A Plastic Sealant

Recently, a promising transparent plastic sealant has been developed to protect the biting surfaces of the teeth against decay. The biting surfaces contain pits and fissures—narrow crevices and indentations. Fluorides have proved to be less effective here than on the smooth surfaces of teeth.

Application of the sealant—a clear, plastic liquid—by a dentist is painless. It is painted on the biting surfaces. Then a gunlike device is used to direct rays of ultraviolet light onto the coating to harden it and form a transparent film. Studies indicate that the sealant is effective in helping to minimize chewing surface decay.

## Can Anything Else Be Done to Prevent Dental Caries?

A great deal. Many dental scientists are investigating ways to directly attack the bacteria that dissolve enamel by producing acid. Efforts are being made to develop a vaccine for the purpose, and work has advanced to the point where such a vaccine, which may even take the form of a simple pill, appears to be a good possibility within a few years.

Meanwhile, other weapons are available. One of the best ways of conquering an enemy is to starve him. This is an excellent weapon against tooth decay. *All cavities start from the outside.* The bacteria on the tooth surfaces demand carbohydrates (sugars) for food. Therefore, if you deprive them of carbohydrates, these bacteria will have nothing to convert to acid, and so the enamel will not be penetrated.

"But that's impossible," you will tell me. "All balanced diets contain starches and sugars."

You are quite right. Nevertheless, we can go a long way toward starving these bacteria without cutting down on our sugar intake too much. Reduction or elimination of rich, concentrated sticky sugars from the diet almost always diminishes the number of new cavities and the spread of existing ones. The worst enemies of the teeth are the all-day suckers, the chewy candies, and the sweetened chewing gums. Sweetened, carbonated beverages contain concentrated sugars. Also, pastries and pies and cookies should be limited, especially in those children with a strong tendency toward tooth decay. *A sweet tooth can ruin all the teeth!*

And yet most children love candy. It, and other sweets, are a symbol of love to a little child, and so we don't like to remove them entirely from his diet. I meet this problem in my family by restricting candy to a special treat once a day, but *not* just before bedtime, because children (and many adults) do not remove all candy and cake from the teeth when they brush. It is better to regulate the eating of candy so that it is followed by other foods, like apples or carrots that cleanse the teeth rather than stick to them.

## EFFECTIVE HOME MOUTH CARE

Gum, or periodontal, disease has come in for hard study recently. And effective methods to help prevent it have been developed; these very same methods provide for even further improvement in reducing decay, also.

There is now evidence that, just as in tooth decay, bacteria are involved in gum disease. Clinging to the teeth and producing acid from food particles, bacteria also produce a plaque, or film, that covers them over, allowing them to work undisturbed.

Plaque not only furthers decay but triggers formation of tartar, or calculus. And calculus, spreading down below the gumline, irritates the gums, starts up inflammation and gingivitis, and opens the way for pyorrhea and gum disease progression.

Against both decay and periodontal disease, effective home care to prevent plaque formation is a prime weapon. Many prevention-oriented dentists now take time to educate patients in proper home-care methods—exactly how to break up and clean away plaque with toothbrushing methods different from those most of us have used; how to use dental floss, not as most of us have used it, merely to dislodge food particles from between the teeth, but also to get plaque off the sides of the teeth. Often, they send patients home with a supply of special "disclosing wafers" and a little dental mirror to be used for self-checking on home cleaning. Plaque on the teeth is invisible. But a disclosing wafer contains a harmless vegetable dye. When the wafer is chewed up, it stains teeth temporarily, but only where any plaque is.

Ideally, the mouth should be cleansed immediately after a meal or snack. Practically, that is difficult for many people. Many dentists now emphasize that, because it takes twenty-four hours or more for plaque to reform once it is removed thoroughly, even a single thorough cleansing of the mouth at night before retiring can go a long way toward minimizing decay and gum disease.

Among the prevention-minded dentists today are periodontists, specialists in gum diseases, who have referred to them only the worst cases—so far advanced that surgery to eliminate the deep gum pockets is necessary. But, typically, many now will not operate until the patient is shown how to care for his mouth at home and goes on a home-prevention program for several weeks or even months. In virtually every case, these periodontists report, they are able to demonstrate that the patient himself or herself, with proper home care, can bring even the most advanced periodontal disease under control so that, once surgical repairs are made, there will be no recurrence.

## A Guide for Effective Home Mouth Care

TOOLS. A toothbrush, preferably soft-bristled, never hard, since it will be used at the gumline as well as on the teeth. Dental floss. *Also helpful:* an irrigator, or water spray, attachable to the bathroom faucet (your dentist may recommend one); a small, inexpensive plastic-handled mouth mirror, available from your dentist or drugstore; disclosing wafers, available from your dentist or drugstore (if not immediately available, the store may order them for you from the maker: Amurol Products, Box 300, Naperville, Illinois 60540; they are called Xpose).

HOW TO BRUSH. Properly used, a toothbrush can clean three of the five surfaces of the teeth—chewing surface, cheek side, and tongue side. *Note:* An often-missed but critical area is the last one-sixteenth inch of the tooth at the gum margin; plaque and bacteria near the gum as well as on the rest of the tooth must be removed.

Direct the brush bristles gently into the crevice between gum and teeth. Mildly vibrate the brush handle so bristles do not travel and skip about but can dislodge material in this area. Next, move the brush, applying gentle but firm pressure, so the bristles travel over the surface of the tooth. Brush the upper teeth with a downward motion; the lower, with an upward motion. Brush the surfaces on the tongue side and the surfaces next to the cheek. Then clean the chewing surfaces, brushing across the tops of the teeth. Brush at least half a dozen strokes in each area.

How to Floss. Plaque must be cleaned away from the other two surfaces of the teeth—the sides between the teeth, or the interdental surfaces. Floss can accomplish this.

Cut off a piece of floss 18 to 24 inches long. Wrap the ends around the forefinger and middle finger of each hand, leaving the thumb free. To floss between the upper teeth, use the thumbs as a guide; hold the thumbs about 1 inch apart, keeping the floss taut. For the lower teeth, use the forefingers as a guide, keeping them 1 inch apart.

Slip the floss between each pair of teeth. Do not try to snap the floss through a tight area; work it gently back and forth until it passes through. Carry the floss to the base of one tooth, stopping when it is just under the edge of the gum. Scrape the floss up and down against the side of the tooth until you get a rough or squeaky feeling, which indicates you have broken through the plaque and are actually touching the tooth.

After cleaning the side of one tooth, clean the side of the adjoining tooth. Move to the next pair of teeth, and the next, until all interdental surfaces are cleaned.

How to Rinse. After brushing and flossing, vigorous rinsing will remove dislodged food particles, plaque, and bacteria. Your dentist may suggest an irrigating spray which also helps clean under any bridges or braces and in gum pockets where brush and floss cannot reach. Place the spray tip in the mouth pointing toward the tongue, and adjust the water flow until pressure and temperature feel good. Move the tip so warm water washes spaces between teeth and between gums and teeth. The spray should not be painful at any time.

Checking. Disclosing wafers with their harmless red dye can help you make certain you are doing a good cleaning job. For the first week, you can use one before and another after each nightly cleaning. In the second week, clean first, then use a wafer to check on whether any areas have been missed. Once proper cleaning habits are established, use a wafer about once a month for checking.

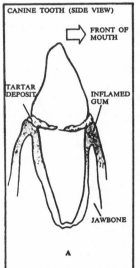
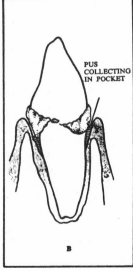
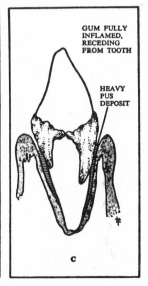

*Figure 4–5. Early and Advanced Periodontal Disease.*

Place a wafer in the mouth, chew slowly to help it dissolve, then swish around as if it were a mouth rinse. You may then swallow it. Any bright red stains you see on the teeth (use the mouth mirror to help view the tongue side of the teeth) indicate areas of plaque and bacteria; pay particular attention to brushing and flossing these areas. The dye, which will color tongue and lips, can be removed readily from lips with a wet cloth. Brush it from the tongue and you will simultaneously remove bacteria that grow on the tongue's furry surface and may contribute to bad breath. As the bacteria are brushed off, much of the dye color goes with them; the rest is gone, dissolved in mouth fluids, by morning.

## RESTORING KNOCKED-OUT TEETH

Often now, a knocked-out tooth, child's or adult's, can be reimplanted if certain conditions are met.

Timing is crucial. If a tooth can be set back in place within half an hour, it very often can be saved. Beyond that, for periods of up to six hours there is a fair chance that interior pulp and outer periodontal tissues may survive and allow successful reimplantation.

Dental authorities emphasize that keeping the tooth moist until the patient can reach a dentist also is crucial. They urge that you wrap a knocked-out tooth in a cloth wetted in water to which a little salt has been added and get to a dentist as fast as possible. If there is going to be a delay, try placing the tooth in the socket yourself, or if that can't be done, put it in a container of water until help can be obtained.

## TEETH AS FOCI (CENTERS) OF INFECTION

Not long ago some doctors were inclined to blame infected teeth for many diseases, especially arthritis, and very frequently recommended the extraction of "bad" teeth. Now we feel that infected teeth are apt to be an accessory factor rather than the primary cause. The decision to have your teeth pulled is a big one; as in the case of any operation, you should feel free to tell your dentist you want a consultation with your physician or a specialist before having it done. *Be sure to get your doctor's advice before having even one tooth pulled* if you are suffering from potentially dangerous diseases such as chronic heart trouble, rheumatic fever, high blood pressure, diabetes, or nephritis.

## REMOTE SYMPTOMS RELATED TO A FAULTY BITE

The way your teeth meet as you chew and swallow food may cause or aggravate certain symptoms far from your teeth. A faulty bite can displace the joints just in front of your ears, where your jaws meet (the *temporomandibular joints*). Displacement of these joints can cause pain in the face or head, noise or blocking of the ears, and dizziness with or without nausea and vomiting. Patients usually seek their doctor's advice for such conditions, but your doctor may advise you that your bite may be the cause of such distress.

## HALITOSIS (BAD BREATH)

This condition almost always accompanies pyorrhea. It can also be caused by teeth and gums which are not clean or in good condition. However, it may be due to inflamed tonsils, infections in or behind the nose, and conditions of the stomach or intestines. Also, certain foods cause odoriferous breath. Some diseases such as uremia produce foul breath. It is hard to tell whether or not one has halitosis, but there is no need to worry about it or spend time and money on "remedies," since your dentist or physician will tell you —and help you to find its cause and cure.

## ARTIFICIAL TEETH

Dentures should be removed and cleaned and the mouth rinsed after every meal, if possible. Don't use hot water, as it may warp or crack them. Putting them in a glass of water overnight helps to keep them clean. Of course, artificial teeth should be checked regularly to make certain that they have not warped out of shape and that a change in your mouth or gums hasn't made them fit badly.

## PERIODIC DENTAL CHECKUPS

How often should you see your dentist? *As often as necessary*. Let him decide. If dental decay is on a rampage or you are fighting off a threatened case of pyorrhea, you may have to see him every month. At other times, a visit a year may suffice. The only definite piece of advice I can safely give you is to *make an appointment now*—because the chances are, if you are like the rest of us, you are probably overdue for a visit.

The dentist can save you time, money, and suffering. He can fill small cavities quickly and almost painlessly; he will take x-rays to discover tiny and easily repaired cavities; he will remove tartar before it irritates the gums.

Regular visits to the dentist will not only save you time, money, and suffering, but they will SAVE YOUR TEETH!

# 5
# ENDOCRINE GLANDS

The term *gland* is given to any part of the body that develops a secretion. There are two types of glands, the *exocrine* and the *endocrine*. *Lymph glands*, which I discuss on page 115, are more aptly described by the term *lymph nodes*, and belong in a different category.

Exocrine glands are usually called glands of external secretion. Among them are the *salivary glands* which pour saliva into the mouth, and the breast or *mammary glands* which produce milk. Glands of this type also secrete the digestive juices of the stomach and bile.

While the glands of external secretion send their products through a duct or tube, the secretions which endocrine glands produce go directly into the blood stream. That is why they are called *endocrine glands—endo* means within—and why they are also referred to as ductless glands.

The existence of many of these glands has been recognized for ages, but their functions were, in the main, shrouded in mystery. Centuries ago, a connection was noted between the sex glands, the testes and ovaries, and what are called the secondary sexual characteristics such as the beard in men and the breast in women. It was quite apparent, for example, that a boy whose testes had been destroyed failed to develop masculine characteristics. Now we know a great deal about the reasons for this, and about the other endocrine glands as well. We know that the substances (*hormones*) these glands create are chemical in nature. The exact chemical composition of most of them has been discovered by scientists, who can even create a few of them in the laboratory.

They can be extracted in pure form from the gland, which is a great advantage in using them medically.

We have found out a great deal about what the various hormones do and about what happens to the body when a certain gland fails to function properly, creating too much or too little of its secretion. Although our knowledge of this subject is still incomplete, some of the most remarkable and dramatic treatments in medicine are possible because of advances in endocrinology.

## SOME WONDERFUL RESULTS

Not very long ago a woman brought her baby to our hospital—a pathetic little boy with a strangely old face, dull eyes, and a tongue so thick it protruded from his mouth. Examination showed that the infant was a *cretin* (see Figure 5-1).

When I was young, one of the families living in our neighborhood had a child of this type. My mother always insisted we must be kind to the poor, dwarfed imbecile, saying, "To have such a child is the greatest tragedy that can happen to a woman."

Remembering this as I looked at the infant in the hospital, I thought how fortunate I was to be a doctor of medicine today rather than several generations ago. Then the mother would have been told that nothing could be done. Now, tablets containing an extract prepared from the thy-

72

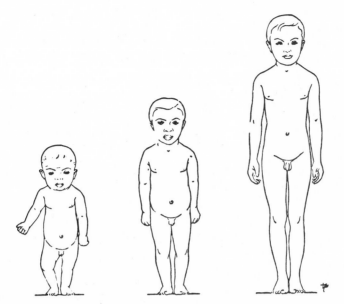

*Figure 5–1. Treated and Untreated Cretinism.* LEFT: *A typical cretin about a year old. Height approximately normal; puffiness about eyes; nose broadened; tongue thick and protruding; difficulty in sitting and standing.* CENTER: *Untreated cretin about 10 years old. Height, 40 inches, far below normal; physically undeveloped;* *mentally deficient.* RIGHT: *Child about 10 years old, treated for cretinism regularly from the time symptoms were first observed. Height 55 inches, almost normal; physical development almost normal; mentally somewhat retarded.*

roid glands of sheep will enable this baby to develop normally because the treatment can be started early enough.

Or take the case of a patient suffering from a malady called *Addison's disease,* which is destroying his adrenal glands. He is weak and emaciated, with a faint pulse, a low blood pressure, and discolored, darkened skin. Not too many years ago any doctor would have said he was doomed to die very soon. Today, watching the change taking place in him after the administration of the proper hormones from the adrenal cortex, one is inclined to think of the miracle of Lazarus rising from the dead.

Almost equally miraculous is the change that has taken place in regions which used to be referred to as the *"goiter belts"*—areas such as those in the Swiss Alps and around our own Great Lakes. Within our lifetime, visitors to such places had been shocked by the number of people they saw, including children, who were disfigured by

these swellings of the thyroid gland, at the base of the throat, sometimes so large as to interfere with breathing. Now, merely because of the use of table salt to which a tiny amount of *iodine* has been added, simple goiter no longer characterizes the residents of these areas.

Stories about these and other remarkable cures spread rapidly. To them were added tall tales of imaginary cures. A wave of hysteria spread, carrying away even some of our scientists. People cried out that glands, wonderful glands, could do anything! The fountain of eternal youth was supposed to be just around the corner, in the form of transplanted monkey glands. Articles, books, and even plays were written dealing with this new way of staying young and virile forever.

These claims soon proved to be unfounded, and the monkey-gland craze went the way of other crazes. Yet even now aging men and women will ask whether they can't be rejuvenated by means of some gland or hormone. Many such people are victimized by quacks who can't do them any good, and frequently cause great harm. However, the problems of aging are being scientifically studied by a number of able doctors who are making valuable discoveries. (See chapter on the later years, page 530.)

While many glandular disturbances can be cured, it is always dangerous to attempt treatment except under a doctor's direction. It is even risky to use a "hormone face cream" to beautify the complexion, because if this actually does contain a hormone, it may disturb the delicate balance of endocrine functioning.

## THE FAMILY OF ENDOCRINE GLANDS

The endocrine glands and their location in the body are shown in Figure 5-2. These glands include:

The *pituitary,* which consists of three parts
The *thyroid*
The *parathyroids,* which are actually four small glands quite different from, but attached to, the thyroid
The *islets of Langerhans,* tiny cells forming "islands" in the pancreas
The *adrenal glands,* one on each side above each kidney; each gland consists of two different parts
The *gonads,* or *sex glands,* consisting of the testes in men and the ovaries in women

In addition, there are the *pineal* gland in the upper, back part of the brain, and the *thymus* gland, which is found below the thyroid in young people and later atrophies (withers away). Very little is known as yet about the pineal gland, nor have the functions of the thymus been fully determined. The latter is believed to play a role in the body's immune system, which defends against foreign invaders.

The hormones that the endocrine glands send through the blood to the various parts of the body act like messengers. (The word *hormone* comes from the Greek word meaning to excite or to stir up.) They don't actually create processes, but rather tell certain processes to speed up or to slow

down, encouraging or discouraging them. They exert their influence on such fundamental processes as growth, reproduction, and sex. How great a part they play in our mental and emotional states is not yet fully understood. However, it is known that some glandular disturbances cause mental conditions or personality changes, and that these disappear with treatment.

The endocrine glands form an *interdependent* system. In that respect they are like a family: what happens to one can affect them all. Again, we don't know exactly *how* this happens, but it has been shown that the removal of one gland often alters the functioning of them all. Similarly, an increase in the functioning of one will change the others. That is one reason why *it is extremely dangerous to dose oneself with hormones, glandular tissue or extract,* or whatever it may be called, for the purpose of reducing, getting rid of excess hair, developing the breasts, becoming more virile, or for any other reason.

The table on page 76 lists a number of the hormones produced by the endocrine glands, and some of the diseases resulting when a gland functions too actively or too little.

## THE ISLETS OF LANGERHANS IN THE PANCREAS

DIABETES is the most familiar of the diseases caused by an endocrine gland disorder. There are ten million diabetics in the United States. Diabetes (or, to give it its full name, diabetes mellitus) was once a major cause of early death in children and young adults and a seriously disabling condition in many older people. It is now often controllable. A major advance against the disease was made possible in the early 1920's by the discoveries of a young Canadian doctor, Frederick G. Banting, assisted by Dr. Charles H. Best.

Many years ago, a scientist named Langerhans studied small clusters of cells that formed what he called "islets" scattered throughout the *pancreas.* The pancreas is the flat organ situated below and behind the stomach. Although the masses of cells which are now called the islets (or islands) of Langerhans lie within the pancreas, their func-

*Figure 5–2. Location of the Endocrine Glands.*

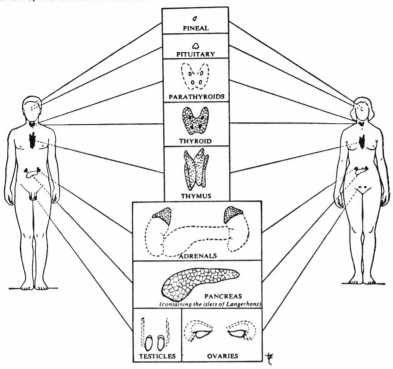

PINEAL

PITUITARY

PARATHYROIDS

THYROID

THYMUS

ADRENALS

PANCREAS
*(containing the islets of Langerhans)*

TESTICLES   OVARIES

tion is entirely different from the functions of the rest of the organ. The main part of the pancreas produces juices which play a major part in the digestion of proteins and fats, while the islets control the use of sugar by the body.

## Cause of Diabetes

Diabetes is not a contagious or infectious disease. It is caused by the failure of the body to provide or properly utilize something that it needs.

The islets of Langerhans secrete the hormone called *insulin*. This hormone enables the body to use (or "burn") sugar and starch after they have been converted into glucose by the digestive juices. The body has to utilize this glucose (sugar) in order to provide heat and energy and to help in the utilization of other foods. Any sugar the normal body does not immediately need is stored in the tissues, to be drawn on later—like money in the bank.

When there is a disturbance in the insulin mechanism, nourishment is seriously disturbed. No matter how much food is eaten, glucose is not utilized. The sugar accumulates in the blood and even spills over into and is eliminated in the urine. The quantity of urine eliminated increases, causing the diabetic to be thirsty and drink more fluid, which in turn is quickly eliminated.

One factor leading to disturbance in the insulin mechanism and onset of diabetes is insufficient production of insulin by the islets of Langerhans. Diabetes also may be the result of an increase in the insulin requirement, or there may be a decrease in the effectiveness of insulin.

We do not know all the reasons why these factors arise. Heredity is an important influence, as evidenced by the frequent occurrence of diabetes in the same family. Diabetes also is more frequent in people who are overweight. The disease occurs more often in women than in men, and its incidence increases with age.

Two types of diabetes are generally recognized:

the juvenile-onset and the adult-onset. Although there are exceptions, the juvenile-onset, occurring in children and young adults, tends to be more serious than diabetes appearing in later life.

## Untreated Diabetes

Without insulin and its ability to utilize sugars, the body is deprived of an essential food. No matter how much the diabetic eats—and he is apt to eat a great deal—he is unable to utilize the food he eats, and so he is always hungry. He is also, as I have said, always thirsty. The word *diabetes,* which comes from a Greek word meaning *fountain,* was used to describe this disease because of the excessive urination which is one of its main symptoms.

Sugar piles up in the blood faster than the body can get rid of it in the urine. This makes the individual less capable of coping with infections of any kind. If large amounts of sugar accumulate in the blood, the patient will become tired, weak, and nauseated; these are the signs of *diabetic acidosis* which precedes *diabetic coma,* which, if untreated, usually results in death within about twenty-four hours.

In a prolonged severe diabetic condition, damage to blood vessels and to tissues and organs containing blood vessels may occur. The consequent poor blood circulation may be a factor leading to

| Gland | Hormone | Disease Caused by | |
| --- | --- | --- | --- |
| | | Overactivity | Underactivity |
| Thyroid | Thyroxin | Exophthalmic goiter (also called Graves' disease or hyper-thyroidism) | Myxedema Cretinism (in infants) |
| Parathyroid | Parathormone | Hyperparathyroidism (osteitis fibrosa cystica) | Parathyroid tetany |
| Islets of Langerhans (in the pancreas) | Insulin | Hyperinsulinism | Diabetes mellitus |
| Adrenal (a) Cortex | Cortin Cortisone, etc. | Cushing's syndrome Adrenal hypercorticism Adrenal virilism | Addison's disease |
| (b) Medulla | Adrenaline | Hyperadrenalism Pheochromocytoma | May contribute to symptoms of Addison's disease |
| Gonads Female (ovary) | Estrogen (estrin) | Menstrual irregularities | Menopause |
| —or— Male (testis) | Androgen (testosterone) | Excessive virilism | Eunuchism |
| Pituitary (a) Anterior lobe | Corticotropin Thyrotropin Gonadotropins Lactogenic hormone, prolactin | Cushing's syndrome (hyperadrenalism) Gigantism ( acromegaly ) | Dwarfism Simmonds' disease |
| (b) Posterior lobe | Vasopressin (Oxytocin) | | Diabetes insipidus |

other complications, such as gangrene of the feet or hands. The heart or kidneys may suffer damage, difficulty with vision may develop, or the nervous system may be affected.

## Symptoms of Diabetes

Everyone should be alert for the following symptoms of diabetes:

Excessive thirst and urination (in children, bed-wetting may be a sign)

Loss of weight (especially where there is an increased consumption of food)

Weakness, listlessness, fatigue

Decreased resistance to infection—often manifested in frequent boils or carbuncles; or, especially in elderly people, in gangrenous conditions particularly in the feet

Itching of the genitals

Indications of approaching diabetic acidosis and coma (I describe these more fully on page 78.)

Even when the disease is in an early and mild stage, it can be detected by tests of the urine and the blood for sugar. A complete medical examination should include an analysis of the urine and the blood after a test meal of sugar. Good clinics provide low-cost tests for sugar in the urine and the blood. The American Diabetic Association conducts frequent drives for detection of this disease. In some cities, it sets up diabetes detection centers, which you should visit, possibly to your advantage. It's so easy to find out whether you have a tendency to diabetes, which usually can be handled easily if recognized early!

## Treatment of Diabetes by Diet

Until about 1923, when insulin was introduced, the only thing that could be done for diabetics was to eliminate, as nearly as possible, sugars and starches from their diet. The small amount of insulin manufactured in all but the most severe cases might be enough to handle the decreased amount of work it was called upon to do.

*This treatment is still the best and simplest one for mild, borderline cases of diabetes in adults.* The doctor prescribes a diet which the patient follows exactly, testing the urine to discover how much starch and sugar he can utilize without having any excess sugar spill over into the urine. If he sticks to such a diet, testing his urine regularly, the borderline diabetic can keep his disease under control. Sometimes, especially in obese individuals who lose weight on their diets, the condition may clear up; the rested islets of Langerhans may once more take up the task that had been too much for them!

*Never attempt to treat even the mildest form of diabetes yourself.* The diet must be exact, and only a doctor is capable of working out its details with you. To be successful, treatment by diet requires a capable physician *plus* a cooperating patient.

Diet alone can never control severe diabetes or diabetes in children. Too little insulin is provided by the body in such cases to take care of even the small amount of starch and sugar in any diet. The body *has* to have a small amount of sugar; larger quantities are essential to the growth and development of children. In the past, children with diabetes, and adults with severe cases, were doomed to waste away or die in a coma.

## Insulin Treatment

Today, because insulin can be obtained, even the most severe types of diabetes can be controlled. Diabetic children can grow to healthy adulthood. Diabetics can live as normally and actively as anyone else. The individual who cannot manufacture his own insulin can substitute for it the identical hormone extracted from animal glands.

This insulin must be injected under the skin. It is useless if taken· by mouth. It is a natural hormone, not in any sense a "drug" or form of "dope"; it is never habit-forming, as are narcotics.

The doctor can teach the average individual how to inject insulin into himself or into a member of the family not capable of doing so. He can also show the diabetic how to make the simple test to determine whether or not there is sugar in his urine—the test involves only a specially treated slip of paper, to be supplied by your physician. This is absolutely essential, as the amount of insulin required by his body may decrease, or it may increase, owing to, for example, *an infection.*

Even with injections of insulin, the diabetic must learn to regulate his diet. This may scarcely vary from the diet of the normal person. The same kinds of food are eaten; nothing is eliminated. The only difference lies in the fact that the day's menu must be planned, because the same amount of sugar must be eaten every day. By keeping the daily quantity of sugar constant, the doctor can tell how much insulin the patient needs in his daily dose. It is almost impossible, from a practical point of view, for a diabetic to vary the amount of insulin he takes because he wants to eat more or less sugar than his regular amount. He cannot take extra insulin "to be on the safe side" because this is far from safe. An *insulin reaction* will probably result.

If too much insulin is taken (or too little food eaten to utilize the amount of insulin injected), the blood sugar becomes low and the urine contains no sugar instead of the small amount usually present. The result is shaky tremors, cold sweats, and an extreme feeling of hunger. In severe cases, *insulin shock* results. An insulin reaction calls for emergency treatment, since coma may follow. Eat a few lumps of sugar or drink a glass of orange juice with sugar added. No insulin should be taken until the reaction has completely passed. Diabetics who take insulin should carry a few lumps of sugar with them so that, in case they are forced to miss a meal or two, and feel a reaction coming on, they can prevent the condition from becoming serious.

*Diabetic acidosis* is just the opposite of an insulin reaction. People sometimes have difficulty in distinguishing between the two, especially since, in extreme cases of either condition, coma may result. Diabetic acidosis is caused by *too much* sugar (and not enough insulin). This may happen if injections are neglected or too much food is eaten. The symptoms are deep breathing, tremendous thirst, dryness of the skin and tongue, and often pains in the back and stomach as well as nausea and vomiting. In diabetic acidosis the urine always contains a large amount of sugar; in an insulin reaction the urine is always free of sugar. Diabetic acidosis is worse than ordinary untreated diabetes: that is, the disease is far out of control and has become extreme and dangerous.

## What to Do for Diabetic Acidosis

*Call your doctor.* Until he arrives, do the following: Go to bed and keep quiet and warm. Drink a cup of warm fluid—soup or broth—every hour.

Change to an emergency diet consisting of milk and crackers and either poached eggs on toast and cocoa, or any bland vegetables you can tolerate. These feedings should be taken about every two hours. The purpose is to make certain you get enough nourishment, in spite of nausea and vomiting.

*Take insulin.* Get the required dosage from the doctor over the phone. If he cannot be reached, take 20 units of regular insulin at once and 10 to 15 units every six hours until the urine is clear or shows only traces of sugar.

If improvement doesn't set in fast, and your doctor cannot be reached, go by taxi, ambulance —or if by your own automobile, have *someone helping you*—to the nearest good hospital.

In neglected cases, diabetic coma may result. Unconsciousness sets in. This is an emergency calling for immediate medical attention. A person in a coma should be rushed to the hospital.

One of the main causes of this condition is overeating or neglecting to take insulin. Like most of the problems facing the diabetic, this is usually the result of negligence. The diabetic person must learn to be strong-willed enough to avoid going on food sprees, and must never neglect his insulin injections. (Similarly, he must not skip meals, thus running the risk of an insulin reaction.) Diabetes is no longer a dangerous, disabling disease, *provided* the diabetic has enough self-control and good sense to adhere strictly to his diet and the few rules his physician has given him.

Diabetic acidosis or coma can also be caused by infections or by surgery and dental extractions performed without adequate preparation. If any operations or dental extractions are needed, the diabetic should make certain his condition is known to the dentist or doctor who will then be able to take the proper precautions.

Diabetics make a note of their conditions on their identification cards, just as perfectly healthy persons carry the address of a relative to be notified in case of accident. It is even a better idea to carry a separate card for this purpose, something like the one illustrated.

The diabetic should also be careful not to catch colds and should avoid people with infectious diseases. He should get plenty of rest and sleep. An infection diminishes the efficacy of insulin and may bring on acidosis. One way to avoid infections of the skin is to be clean. Sensible diabetics are among the cleanest people in the world.

## Oral Medications for Diabetes

In place of insulin, which must be injected into the body, some diabetics now may be treated with oral medications. (Some doctors may prescribe *both* insulin and the newer oral drugs.) These are called *hypoglycemic agents* because they reduce the sugar content of the blood. They also act on the liver to reduce its output of glucose. Only certain kinds of diabetics can safely and successfully take medication by mouth. Some of these preparations are Orinase, Diabinese, and Dymelor. Diabetics being treated with these drugs still must watch their diets scrupulously.

## Care of Feet

A great deal of emphasis is placed on foot care because there is danger of gangrene (a condition in which tissues actually die) if the feet are neglected. This is because diabetes often brings about poor circulation, especially in the feet and legs. The feet are exposed to many possible avenues of infection such as corns, calluses, blisters, cuts, and ingrown toenails. Any of these may result in gangrene.

The older the diabetic person, the more attention his feet require. Diabetics over forty-five should be particularly careful about carrying out the following measures:

Wash the feet daily with soap and water, then dry thoroughly.

Massage daily with lanolin, rubbing from the toes to the knees.

Raise yourself on your toes twenty times, twice a day.

Treat ingrown toenails by the method described on page 117.

Have toenails cut carefully by someone other than yourself, preferably a chiropodist who must be told that you are diabetic.

Wear shoes that are comfortable, and wide enough not to rub against the feet.

Stockings should be washed daily, and should be free of imperfections that may irritate the skin.

## Try to Avoid Diabetes— or Learn to Live with It

Although the tendency toward diabetes may be inherited, you can help to avoid the disease by keeping slim. Overweight people, especially

---

**I AM A DIABETIC**

Name_____ Telephone_____

Address_____

City_____ State_____

If ill, call a **DOCTOR** or send me to a **HOSPITAL.**

My Doctor: Name_____

City_____ Telephone_____

Also, please notify_____

City_____ Telephone_____

(see other side)

---

**DIABETIC IDENTIFICATION**

If ill, call a **DOCTOR** or send me to a **HOSPITAL.**

I am a diabetic. My behavior during reactions to therapy may resemble that of an intoxicated person.

I have been taking_____
INDICATE DOSAGE OF INSULIN

_____
OR NAME AND DOSAGE OF ORAL ANTIDIABETIC DRUG.

(see other side)

women in their forties, seem to be more susceptible to diabetes than underweight ones. One of the many good reasons not to put on fat as you get older!

You can have a good, active life even if you have diabetes. Even though you cannot be cured, you can get along very well with your diabetes once you make up your mind to it. Keep in touch with your doctor. Stick to your diet. Take your medication regularly. And most important of all, exercise your will power. You will probably discover there is a great deal of truth to the saying "the best way to lead a long, healthy life is to have an incurable disease and take care of it."

Always remember, diabetes is a lifetime condition. It cannot be ignored, for it will neither go away nor be cured. More than any other chronic condition, its progress is affected by the patient's daily activity. A carefully worked out combination of diet, weight control, exercise, regular urine testing, and foot care is necessary to keep the disease under control. The reward for patience and care is the greatest possible—a virtually normal life, for as many years as a nondiabetic might expect to live.

This has been a long section on one disease, but diabetes affects millions of people in the United States, half of whom are unaware of their illness. To sum up, the diabetic patient should:

See the doctor regularly.

Have a complete medical checkup periodically.

Follow the prescribed course of diet, medication, urine testing, and exercise, exactly.

Get adequate rest and sleep.

Take good care of his feet, as discussed on page 79.

Have his eyes checked regularly.

Carry a special identification card, as shown on page 79.

For further information, write to the American Diabetes Association, Inc., 1 West 48th Street, New York, N.Y. 10017.

## Hypoglycemia

Hypoglycemia, an abnormally low level of sugar (glucose) in the blood, has a number of possible causes and may produce many diverse symptoms.

Among the common symptoms when the blood sugar level remains low for a prolonged period are weakness, dizziness, palpitation, shaking, sweating, headache, and blurred vision. Sometimes, difficulty in concentration, anxiety, mental confusion, bizarre behavior, and blackout spells may occur. With severe hypoglycemia, convulsions and eventually deep coma may develop as the nervous system is deprived of the glucose needed for its normal functioning.

CAUSES OF HYPOGLYCEMIA. One cause of low blood sugar is an excess of insulin. This may be the result of an uncommon insulin-secreting tumor of the pancreas. It also may follow an overdose of insulin or oral hypoglycemic medication by a diabetic.

Because the liver is the source of most of the glucose entering the blood between meals, disease of the liver interfering with glucose release may lead to hypoglycemia.

In addition to insulin, hormones from the adrenal glands are involved in the regulation of blood sugar levels, and hypoglycemia may develop when there is adrenal insufficiency.

Occasionally, hypoglycemia may be caused by a sensitivity to fructose (a sugar present in large amounts in fruits) or galactose (a carbohydrate in milk).

The most common type of hypoglycemia, often called reactive, occurs several hours after meals rich in carbohydrates, without apparent reason.

Some symptoms similar to those of hypoglycemia can be produced by other conditions, including anxiety states. Hypoglycemia, however, can be diagnosed by measuring the blood glucose level after a high carbohydrate intake, commonly a drink of glucose solution.

Once hypoglycemia is established, it is important to try to find the cause if possible.

TREATMENT FOR HYPOGLYCEMIA. When an organic cause can be determined, treatment is directed at correcting it. If the problem lies with a tumor of the pancreas, its removal by surgery can provide a cure. If adrenal insufficiency is the source, adrenal hormone replacement treatment is usually adequate. If it is a matter of sensitivity to fructose or galactose, avoidance is required. If the problem lies with excessive dosages of insulin or oral hypoglycemic drugs, reduced dosages must be used.

Patients with reactive hypoglycemia can usually be greatly helped by frequent feedings of a high-protein, high-fat, low-carbohydrate diet. Commonly, for an adult, a satisfactory diet consists of 120 to 140 grams of protein and 80 to 100 grams of carbohydrate daily, with enough fat to maintain ideal body weight.

## THE THYROID GLAND

The thyroid, a small, butterfly-shaped gland located in front of the throat, below the Adam's apple and just above the breastbone, weighs less than an ounce. Yet it is impossible to overemphasize its importance.

It is the thyroid that controls the rate of metabolism—the process by which food is converted to energy and many essential chemical changes take place. Minute thyroid secretions, less than a spoonful in a year, are responsible for much of the body's heat production. They help maintain the blood circulation system, are necessary for muscle health, heighten the sensitivity of nerves, and affect every organ and tissue.

HYPOTHYROIDISM. Severe hypothyroidism, or underfunctioning of the thyroid, can have devastating effects. A cretin child (that is, one who is born with a grossly defective thyroid gland) will remain a dwarf and become an idiot unless given thyroid hormone to make up for the gland's total or almost-total failure to produce secretions.

A severely hypothyroid adult, whose gland produces grossly inadequate amounts of secretions, may have coarse features, a "moon-shaped" face, thick nostrils, slow and thick speech, and suffer from weakness and listlessness. Here, too, regular use of thyroid hormone usually brings marked improvement.

Extreme hypothyroidism (also known as myxedema) is rare. But mild to moderate underfunctioning of the gland is not uncommon. Although the lesser degrees of hypothyroidism do not pro-

duce the gross changes of features seen in the extreme form, they may produce varied symptoms, including fatigue, menstrual disturbances, repeated infections, memory disturbances, concentration difficulties, weight gain, dry hair, and hair loss. When the presence of thyroid gland underfunctioning is established by blood or other tests, regular treatment with thyroid hormone extract or synthetic thyroid substitutes can eliminate all these symptoms.

SIMPLE GOITER. The thyroid gland needs iodine in order to function normally. Without sufficient iodine, the gland cannot manufacture the normal quantity of its hormone (called *thyroxin*). In an effort to make up for this, the gland becomes enlarged. As the swelling continues, a noticeable lump appears in the throat. This swelling, or goiter, may be large enough to interfere with breathing or swallowing.

The hormone of the thyroid gland contains about 65 percent iodine, but the amount of iodine needed in food to avoid goiter is very small. The amount of *iodized* table salt we use in meals is sufficient, even in areas where the soil is completely lacking in natural iodine. Too much iodine may lead to a skin eruption. Although consuming iodine does not cure a simple goiter, it will prevent one or will stop an existing goiter from getting larger. Anyone with even a small goiter should consult a doctor.

It is especially important for expectant mothers who live in regions such as the Rocky Mountain states, the Great Lakes Basin, or the upper Mississippi River Valley, where the soil is lacking in iodine, to follow the doctor's orders about the amount of iodine they need. Insufficient iodine in the diet may cause a pregnant woman to produce a child with thyroid deficiency. However, all expectant mothers develop a slight enlargement of the thyroid, and this should not cause them to worry unduly. Children whose diets lack iodine may show signs of goiter when they reach adolescence. Girls and women are more susceptible than are boys and men.

HYPERTHYROIDISM. A more serious type of goiter develops when the thyroid manufactures too much hormone. *Hyper* means too much; hence the disorder is called hyperthyroidism. People with hyperthyroidism are nervous and irritable and suffer from insomnia. Heat makes them extremely uncomfortable, so that they frequently sleep with the covers thrown off, even in cool weather. The excess secretion also produces an overactive heart, manifesting itself in palpitation (which people frequently mistake for a true cardiac condition).

Another symptom of this disease is loss of weight—as much as twenty pounds or even more —in spite of increased hunger. (This unusual combination is also a symptom of diabetes, as I have just explained on page 77.)

Other names for hyperthyroidism are thyrotoxicosis and Graves' disease. Hyperthyroidism is sometimes called *exophthalmic goiter* because many patients have protruding eyes, causing them to look continually startled. This is a fairly common symptom (Figure 5-3).

For many years the only treatment was surgery; about 90% of the gland was removed, and most patients were cured. Today, radioactive iodine is employed to cut down the gland's activity. Like ordinary iodine, radioactive iodine is taken up by the thyroid. The radiation given off within the gland suppresses its functioning. A medicine called propylthiouracil is sometimes used in treatment, either by itself or in preparation for surgery. (Operations on the thyroid may be dangerous, and should be performed by specialists: see page 399.)

Any enlargement or lump in the throat should be examined by a physician. Do not make the diagnosis yourself and decide you have thyroid trouble, and what kind it is. The tests for glandular disturbances of any kind are not simple. Many laboratory studies and examinations may be necessary before your doctor can determine the nature of the illness. One of the tests employed is the *basal metabolism* test, which records the amount of oxygen you use. In hyperthyroidism this amount is increased, and in myxedema the absorption of oxygen during breathing decreases. One of the laboratory tests for thyroid disorders utilizes radioactive iodine as a *tracer*. The severity of the disease can be determined by the amount of radioactive iodine taken up by the thyroid gland: an overactive gland will use up more of the tracer iodine; an underactive one will con-

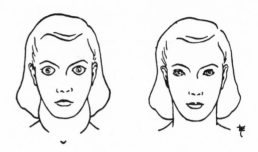

*Figure 5–3. Exophthalmic Goiter.* LEFT: *Characteristic staring eyes and enlarged area in the neck.* RIGHT: *A healthy girl.*

sume less. Another test is the protein-bound iodine (PBI) test. This is an examination of the blood taken from a vein to determine whether the amount of PBI normally produced in the body is elevated, as in hyperthyroidism, or low, as in the opposite condition.

TUMORS of the thyroid are a separate condition from most other ailments involving this gland. That is, they are distinct from the problem of overproduction or underproduction of the hormone. Most of these tumors turn out to be benign, or harmless, but some are malignant. Surgery is the usual procedure in cases of cancer of the thyroid gland, but radiation is also sometimes used, particularly if the malignancy has begun to spread.

## THE PARATHYROID GLANDS

These tiny glands, about the size of a very small pea, and usually found in clusters of four, are embedded near the base of the thyroid. They control the excretion in urine of calcium and phosphorus, which make the bones hard.

The parathyroid glands are so much smaller than the thyroid that before doctors were certain of their presence they were sometimes removed with the thyroid when it had to be taken out surgically. The significance and location of the parathyroids is well known today, and there is little danger of their accidental removal.

In *parathyroid deficiency* the calcium regulation is disturbed and the muscles become subjected to spasms (*tetany*). In severe cases convulsions and death may result. The administration of the parathyroid hormone, or certain synthetically manufactured compounds with similar actions, or a potent vitamin D preparation, will keep the calcium output normal and stop the spasms. Feeding calcium is extremely helpful in such cases.

*Parathyroid tumors* cause *hyperparathyroidism* with generalized depletion of calcium, sometimes kidney stones, and in some cases a cystic degeneration of the bones. Hyperparathyroidism is a rare disease and curable if diagnosed early.

# THE SEX GLANDS (GONADS)

The gonads (from the Greek word *gonē*, meaning *seed*) consist of the *testes* in men and the *ovaries* in women. Besides producing *sperm* and *ova*, the sex glands make the hormones which are responsible for the special characteristics of the male and female.

Human beings have always been aware of the outward physical differences between men and women, but understanding the cause of these differences has been a slow process. The discovery and understanding of the gonads and their hormones have gradually removed much of the mystery from sexual differentiation.

## The Male Sex Glands

The male sex glands consist of two testes which lie enclosed in the scrotal sac of skin, just below the penis. They secrete semen containing the male element of reproduction, the sperm, and also the very important male sex hormone, *testosterone.*

Testosterone was one of the earliest known of the endocrine hormones. This followed logically from the fact that the most easily observed effect of glandular deficiency was that following removal of the testes. It has been known for centuries that if the testes of a boy were removed or destroyed *before puberty,* he would not develop masculine characteristics. He would have a gentle personality and a soft, often high-pitched voice. His chest would be narrow and flat, his muscles undeveloped, with excess fat on the hips, abdomen, and breasts. He would lack hair on the face, armpits, and pubic region. His penis would be small or underdeveloped, and he would fail to develop sexual desire, or lose what he did have; he would be impotent. In the past, especially in the Orient and Middle East, it was customary to castrate (remove the testes from) a number of boys so that they could be trusted to take care of the women of the household. They were called eunuchs, from the Greek word *eunouchos,* meaning guarding the couch. Boys were also castrated to keep their voices from changing, and thus provide sopranos for male choirs. Castration is still practiced on animals to make them easier to manage or so that their flesh will be plump and tender.

In addition to affecting the male sex organs and secondary sexual characteristics, testosterone stimulates muscular and bone development, and helps maintain the strength of muscles.

If testosterone is injected into a female animal, certain masculine characteristics develop, and the female hormonal function is inhibited. This is only temporary; the female functioning is restored when testosterone injections are terminated.

If testosterone is injected into a eunuch or a man with an underactive secretion, the size of the sexual organ increases, the secondary sexual characteristics develop, and there is an increase in sexual desire and potency. The effect of injected testosterone is transitory. People suffering from a lack of this hormone must be treated medically for their entire lives. (The growth of the testes is also stimulated by pituitary hormones, described on page **86.**)

"I thought you said it was impossible to increase or restore virility, and this seems to be a way to do it!" you may be saying. It is true that *certain injections are beneficial in cases of hormone deficiency.* It has also been found that implanting sex glands in male animals may lead to a temporary surge of sexual activity. However, injections of testosterone not only are unsatisfactory and ineffectual as far as "rejuvenation" is concerned, but may be dangerous, leading to tumors of the *prostate* (see page **434**). Let me repeat: the process of aging is not confined to the sexual function, and cannot be halted by a single hormone or any combination of hormones so far discovered.

Actually, many men can reproduce at the age of seventy or older. The feeling of decline which some elderly men experience is more apt to be due to other factors than to the sex glands—either some other physical ailment or a psychological difficulty. A thorough medical checkup is advisable rather than costly and dangerous injections.

IMPOTENCE IN MEN. The problem of impotence, or the inability to have sexual relations, is very difficult and complicated. It can occur if the testicles are removed, and it may result from a disease of the testes or the pituitary gland. Some maladies of the nervous system cause impotence. Most frequently, however, impotence is due to *psychological factors which inhibit sexual ability*. In a great majority of cases of impotence, the testes are present and normal, as is the entire endocrine system. Such impotent individuals suffer from emotional troubles or psychoneuroses, as explained further in Chapter 12. Proper treatment of these conditions often restores the sexual function. Anyone suffering from impotence should have a complete examination by a doctor who is qualified to understand emotional factors. A competent family doctor or internist should study the problem first and, if necessary, refer the patient for psychotherapy or endocrine treatment.

STERILITY IN MEN. Sterility means the inability to have children; it occurs in some men who are by no means impotent. It may be due to the failure (for a number of causes) to produce sperm that are sufficiently strong or numerous to reach and fertilize the female cell. Only one healthy sperm is necessary for that, and the male usually provides from 300 million to 400 million sperm in each sexual act. However, the journey these cells must take to reach the female cell is so hazardous for them that a great many lively ones are needed to ensure there being a survivor in the proper place at the proper time. Ways have been found to help this to take place, and I discuss them, and the problem of sterility in general, on page 232.

## The Female Sex Glands

The female sex glands are called the *ovaries*. Like the testes, there are two of them. Besides producing ova, the eggs, the ovaries secrete hormones necessary both for the feminine characteristics and for reproduction.

The plum-sized ovaries lie in the front portion of the abdomen, below the navel. Each ovary is connected with the womb by a tube called the *fallopian tube*. These tubes are hollow and open out into the womb, or uterus, which is a pear-shaped organ meant to house the unborn child. In the diagram on page 106, the womb, tubes, and ovaries look like the head of an animal with two horns.

The hormones produced by the ovaries are called *estrogen* and *progesterone*. There is very little secretion of them before puberty and after the menopause. They are produced abundantly, however, during a woman's childbearing years, which start around the age of twelve to fourteen and usually end between the ages of forty and fifty. During that period, a woman has her regular monthly cycles.

MENSTRUATION AND OVULATION. Menstruation is the discharge from the body of the extra blood and tissue which have been built up in preparation for a baby and have not been used. Menstrual cycles vary, the time from one menstrual period to the next usually being about 28 days. Differences in the length of this cycle are not unusual, nor are they necessarily to be considered abnormal. The 28-day cycle is merely an average one, rather than being indicative of good health.

Doctors customarily start counting the first day of menstruation as Day 1. During the first 14 days of this cycle, the ovary contains a follicle—a small hollow ball the size of a pinhead. Within it lies an egg. This follicle grows during these 14 days until it is several times its original size, becoming as large as a pea. While it is growing, the follicle makes the hormone *estrogen*. The menstrual cycle in general and the growth of the follicle are under the control of the pituitary gland. On about Day 14, stimulated by the pituitary gland, the follicle

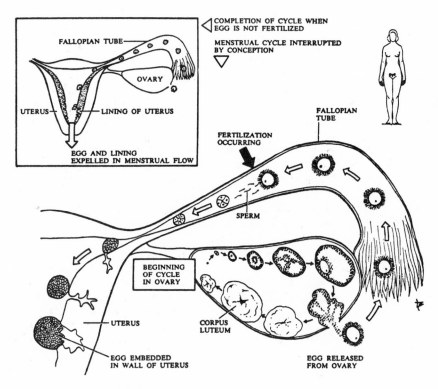

*Figure 5–4. Diagram of the Menstrual Cycle.*

bursts and the egg is discharged from the ovary. The discharged egg enters the tube on its way down to the uterus. If any sperm are present in the fallopian tubes at that time, fertilization may take place in the tube. The fertilized egg continues its journey to the uterus. Once there, it plants itself in the wall of the uterus. Meanwhile, the ruptured follicle from which the egg was discharged is transformed into a yellowish, solid ball now called the *corpus luteum* (Latin: yellow body). The corpus luteum produces a second hormone, *progesterone.*

Scientists have learned how to make synthetic hormones in the laboratory, so that the process of ovulation can be controlled at will. The contraceptive pill "imitates" the natural body processes in preventing ovulation. I discuss this and other birth-control methods in Chapter 16, The Strategy of Becoming Good Parents.

Estrogen and progesterone play two important roles in the female body. They are greatly responsible for feminine characteristics, and they help build up the lining of the uterus for receiving and nourishing the fertilized egg. The lining becomes thicker and develops a rich blood supply to feed the unborn baby.

During the last 14 days of the cycle, the two hormones are produced by the corpus luteum to stimulate the manufacture of the tissues and blood supply in the uterus. The fertilized egg in turn secretes its own hormone. This hormone helps the corpus luteum to persist and continue making estrogen and progesterone. In other words, this is like a chain reaction, with one hormone prodding the other two hormones to keep going. The hormone from the fertilized egg is necessary because at the end of the 28-day cycle the pituitary "resigns" and will no longer maintain the corpus luteum. So the fertilized egg has to take over the job.

If pregnancy has not occurred, the corpus luteum degenerates and its secretions stop abruptly. With the stopping of the hormones, the rich supply built up in the lining of the uterus sloughs off and leaves the body. This bleeding is called menstruation. (I discuss menstruation and menstrual difficulties in detail on page 514.)

MENOPAUSE. The menopause, or change of life, is as natural for women as is menstruation or the bearing of children. I want to do everything I can to dispel the dread which many women feel regarding this change in their reproductive systems. I discuss this fully on page 517. Nothing more disastrous occurs than the tapering off and stopping of the monthly cycle!

True, certain natural changes do take place. Estrogen secretion is reduced. The follicles no longer release an egg each month. Menstruation ceases. It may end suddenly, or gradually—skipping a few months, or stopping and then returning for several months. After the menopause has been well established for about a year, there should be no more bleeding. (Be sure to consult a doctor *immediately* if bleeding or "spotting" should occur. This may be a danger signal of cancer or some other disorder requiring prompt medical attention. See page 432.)

Unfounded fears concerning the menopause are largely responsible for the emotional disturbances some women experience during this period. Certain physical symptoms may be present because of the glandular changes taking place. If they become troublesome, they can be relieved by hormonal injections or tablets—*but never without a doctor's prescription*. I discuss menopausal symptoms, both physical and emotional, on page 517.

## THE ADRENAL GLANDS

These glands fit like small cups on the top of each of the two kidneys (Figure 5-2, p. 75). Each adrenal gland is divided into two parts: the *cortex* or outer portion, and the *medulla*, the central section. The cortex and the medulla produce hormones of different natures. The cortex, absolutely essential to life, secretes about thirty hormones

and regulates many of our metabolic processes.

The medulla of the adrenal gland produces the hormone *epinephrine*, more commonly called *adrenaline*. The output of this hormone is immediately stepped up when you become angry, fearful, or excited. This makes the heart beat faster and produces chemical changes that prepare the body for action. You have undoubtedly observed the effects of adrenaline, when you were angry or alarmed, for it makes you feel tense and on edge; or perhaps you have said, "I was so scared (or angry) that I did things I couldn't possibly have been able to do normally."

The two main functions of the adrenal *cortex* hormones are

1. To control the salt and water content of the body.
2. To control the sugar and protein metabolism, acting exactly opposite to insulin. In some tumors of the adrenal cortex, with a condition called *Cushing's syndrome*, diabetes occurs.

The cortex appears also to secrete a hormone similar to that put out by the testes. In certain tumors of the cortex, females develop marked masculine characteristics such as a deep voice and hair on the face; menstruation may slow down or cease. In men with such tumors the secondary sex characteristics may become more pronounced.

Atrophy or underfunction of the adrenal cortex produces a rare disease called *Addison's disease*, which is discussed on page 73. The recently developed adrenal preparations make it possible to control Addison's disease and enable the afflicted person to lead a normal life.

## THE PITUITARY GLAND

This gland is located at the base of the brain. Imagine a line drawn through your head from ear to ear and another line going backward from between your eyes. The pituitary gland lies at the spot where these two lines cross. It is about the size of a pea. It consists of an anterior lobe, an intermediate part, and a posterior lobe.

The most important function of the pituitary is the part it plays in stimulating, regulating, and coordinating the functions of the other endocrine glands. For this reason it is called the "master gland." Research is constantly revealing new facts about the pituitary gland and the relationship between the various glands of the endocrine family. Scientists are also delving into the secrets of the thymus gland and the pineal gland, about which little is now known. When these problems are solved, we shall probably be able to cure or prevent many more diseases and also to gain deeper insights into the questions of health versus disease and of normal aging versus senile degeneration.

One hormone of the pituitary gland has a powerful effect on growth of the body in general. Another hormone regulates the thyroid. Pituitary hormones stimulate the development of the ovaries and the testes, making sexual development and reproduction possible. Still another hormone stimulates the milk production of the breasts. The pituitary hormone which controls the adrenal glands, the adrenocorticotropic hormone, is popularly known as ACTH.

## Diseases of the Pituitary Gland

These diseases are fortunately quite rare. Too little pituitary secretion will cause certain types of *dwarfism,* while too much stimulates the body to grow to gigantic proportions. Pituitary tumors may press on the optic nerves and cause some loss of vision and headaches. *Acromegaly,* in which the bones increase in size, particularly those of the face and hands and feet, is caused by an overactive pituitary gland (see Figure 5-5). *Cushing's disease* is also sometimes caused in this way. Underactivity of the front section of this complex gland leads to a thin, malnourished condition called *Simmonds' disease.* Underactivity, or pituitary insufficiency, can cause children to be excessively fat. In some cases a condition called *Fröhlich's syndrome* results; these children are excessively fat, underdeveloped sexually, and mentally bright although unusual. If given an extract of pituitary gland in time, they will become normal and be spared unhappy lives. If the pituitary secretion decreases after puberty, fat may accumulate around certain portions of the body, particularly the hips. When the back portion of the pituitary fails to function properly, excessive urination results—as much as 30 quarts a day. This rare malady is called *diabetes insipidus,* and should not be confused with "ordinary" diabetes.

There is no effective replacement for every pituitary hormone, but treatment of the parts of the body affected by overproduction or underproduction of the pituitary is often possible and often successful. Cortisone and similar preparations, and thyroid and sex hormones are frequently used for patients suffering from pituitary diseases. For persons suffering from dwarfism, human growth hormone has become available, but it is useful with only a relatively few persons. It is effective only if administered before the normal period of growth has ended.

## OTHER HORMONES

In recent years it has become evident that hormones produced by tissues other than the endocrine glands play vital roles in the body.

*Figure 5-5. Acromegaly.* LEFT: *A typical case. The lower jaw and the bones of the hand are enlarged; the nose and the ridges above the eyes are thickened.* RIGHT: *A normal man of the same size.*

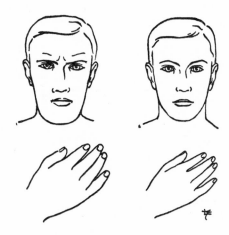

For example, gastrin, a hormone produced by small glands in the stomach lining, serves to stimulate the flow of gastric juices needed for digestion. Secretin, a hormone produced by cells in the wall of the small intestine, stimulates the secretion of digestive juices from the pancreas and bile from the liver and gallbladder, both essential to normal digestion, with the bile serving to aid in the handling of fats.

# 6

# CARE OF THE INDIVIDUAL PARTS OF THE BODY

Our total health is the summation of the workings of individual parts of the body and the efficiency with which they work together in complex ways. If these parts, such as the heart, lungs, and liver, work at maximum efficiency and are aided by a mind free from excess nervous tensions, then there is given us the basis for full enjoyment of the wonderful human body.

This chapter deals with most of the *individual parts* of the body. Some, such as the teeth and gums and the endocrine glands, have chapters to themselves, and I devote an entire part of this book to the mind, beginning on page 169. Here, I describe what the various organs of the body do, and what you should do to care for them, without, however, discussing every illness that can involve each part.

This section is also written to counteract such misinformation as "a chronic pain in the back means you have kidney trouble," or "you should take pills to stimulate your liver," and use "eyedrops to relieve eyestrain." It will answer questions you have undoubtedly asked, from whether you should do something to protect your heart and lungs, to whether you could throw away your eyeglasses if you took eye exercises.

We can do things in our everyday living to protect the various parts of the body. To check more directly yourself on my proposition, read at least the next few sections on the brain, heart, lungs, and blood. (Many readers have surprised me by the statement that they have read this whole, long chapter at one time. One reader told me, "I never realized what fascinating parts and organs make up our bodies; I guess I was always squeamish when it came to learning about such organs as the heart, lungs, and liver.")

## BRAIN

The brain is the master organ of our bodies, and the nervous system is the intricate network through which it controls our body functions and feelings. With the brain we carry out functions possible only to human beings: complex thought, creative work in the arts and sciences, and the control of speech. This wonderful organ contains fifteen billion nerve units which permit the storage of millions of memory images and all the other learning that we accumulate. In addition to the memory cells, the brain has huge numbers of connections which control the more than six hundred muscles in our bodies. Other connections into the brain from the eye, ear, and the nerves in the skin permit us to record and remember what our eyes see, our ears hear, and our skin feels.

It is not surprising that nature had to evolve a system of defenses to guard this amazing three-pound structure against injuries. Thus the bony skull protects the brain. The scalp is a tough wrapping outside the skull that can absorb blows. Inside the skull, a tough membrane called the *dura mater* protects the brain. Also, the brain has

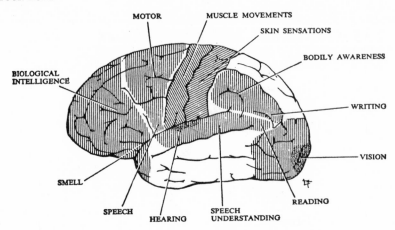

Figure 6–1. The Brain, Viewed from the Left Side, Indicating the Areas Involved in Various Functions.

an additional, wonderful protective device against blows and falls: it is encased in fluid and "floats" in liquid which helps absorb traumatic shocks. (See Figure 6–2, which shows you how this layer of spinal and brain fluid bathes the brain.) But nature can't provide infinite protection for the brain. The automobile and other modern devices can deal terrific blows against which even the admirable natural defenses we enjoy cannot shield us.

We can help nature by protecting our brains against severe trauma. *Young people* should know the hazards of boxing, football, diving, and other sports, and act to avoid skull injuries. Employ recognized safeguards learned from your athletic coach. Using safety measures doesn't make you a "sissy"; it stamps you as a resourceful, rather than a reckless, human being. *Automobile drivers* should remember the terrible consequences of brain injuries when indulging in reckless speeding or other hazards. *Workers* must learn the physical as well as the chemical hazards on the job to prevent brain and nerve injuries (see fuller comments in the chapter on your job and your health, page 141). *Alcoholics* should realize that excessive drinking can injure the brain (page 471).

Suppose you are now alerted to protection of your brain against injuries from blows and accidents: what other protection can you give it in your daily life? You can let it operate at maximum efficiency by providing sleep (page 15) which rests and revitalizes the brain. And you can help the brain by not overstimulating or depressing it with too much caffeine from coffee, soft drinks, and tea, or by too frequent use of sedatives such as barbiturates or bromides. And never go in for "pep pills" such as Benzedrine without the advice of your doctor.

The brain works best when it is free from anxieties, fears, and other mental conflicts. The part of this book entitled You and Your Mind gives detailed advice on how to keep your psyche (the functional part of your brain) in the best possible daily condition (see page 168).

Do you need special "brain foods" and tonics to keep your brain in good condition? *No.* The well-balanced diet described in the chapter on the food you eat will provide the brain with all the vitamins and nourishment it requires (p. 32). Fish is not any better for the brain than other protein foods.

Can the effects of aging on the brain be prevented? Some of the harmful effects of hardening of the arteries can be prevented or diminished by following the suggestions given in the section on obesity (p. 44), high blood pressure (p. 421), and other conditions that weaken the arteries of the brain.

Remember, too, that the mind and emotions react quickly to diseases in other parts of the body.

Headaches, dizziness, fainting, impaired memory, and other brain symptoms can be due to conditions in and around the brain, e.g., sinus trouble or a tumor; or these symptoms could be the result of poisons because damaged kidneys are not removing toxic materials from the blood. In other words, brain symptoms call for a complete medical checkup by your doctor.

And always be on the optimistic side about your brain and its future. I think of Michelangelo, producing some of the greatest art of all times when he was more than eighty; of Toscanini at eighty-seven, directing a hundred-piece symphony orchestra without referring to any musical score; and the many other people we meet in everyday life, who continue to have active, useful brains long beyond the traditional "three score and ten years." (See Chapter 37, The Later Years, page 530.)

## NERVES

If we compare the brain to a control center, we can think of the nervous system as a communications network that directly or indirectly associates all our activities with that center. Messages from both the outside world and from within our own bodies come to the brain via the nerve network, for a decision on what is to be done. In addition to the fifteen billion nerve units in the brain, there are billions of receiving points, called *receptors*, all over the body. These are for vision, hearing, pain, pressure, and other functions and feelings.

The network of nerves is divided into two groups: the central nervous system and the autonomic nervous system. The brain itself and the spinal cord make up the central nervous system. There are twelve sets of nerves running directly from the brain to the sensory organs, the heart, and other major internal organs. From the spine, another set of thirty-one nerves reaches out to muscles, controlling both feeling and the ability to move. The autonomic system controls the smooth muscles of the internal organs. This whole system is ordinarily beyond our conscious control. It takes charge of narrowing or dilating the blood vessels, adjusting the pupil of the eye to light, regulating the digestive process, and, in general, masterminding our body.

Like any other part of the body, the nervous system is subject to many ailments. These may be organic, in which the nerve structure is affected. They may be functional, which means that a part of the body or mind is in trouble but that no change in the nerve structure is apparent. I dis-

*Figure 6–2. How the Brain Is Protected. Note the number of outer coverings which provide excellent protec-* tion for the brain, and the fluid which helps to absorb shocks.

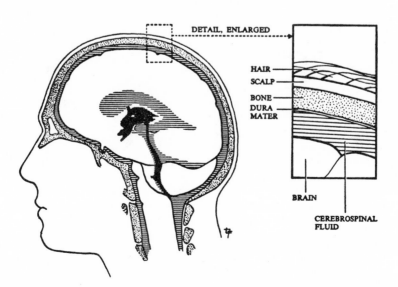

DETAIL, ENLARGED

HAIR
SCALP
BONE
DURA MATER
BRAIN
CEREBROSPINAL FLUID

cuss some of the more common nerve ailments, such as neuritis, beginning on page 467. For information on some of the functional ailments, such as neuroses and psychoses, see Chapter 12, The Partially Sick Mind, and Chapter 13, The Sick Mind.

A neurologist is a medical specialist who deals with ailments of the nervous system. Psychiatrists and psychoanalysts specialize in the functional aspects of nervous disorders and with the problems of the troubled mind and personality.

Many people blame their "nerves" when they have some vague ailment or complaint. Most likely, there is nothing wrong with their nerves at all, but they are foolish to try to diagnose themselves. So-called nuisance symptoms, if they persist, should always be discussed with a doctor.

## HEART

The heart is a muscular, pear-shaped organ, slightly bigger than your fist, composed of four chambers with valves in them. Enclosed by a protecting sac (the *pericardium*), it is located in the left front portion of the chest. It is a pump, sending blood to all parts of the body through the *arteries* which divide and subdivide, eventually

merging with tiny vessels called *capillaries* which, in turn, merge with *veins* that carry the blood back to the heart.

Your heart beats automatically at the rate of about 70 to 80 times a minute—or about 40,000,000 times a year, every year of your life. Its pace increases when the body is active, decreases when it is at rest. Most people cannot consciously influence its speed. However, if your heart beats at a slower rate, that doesn't mean there is anything wrong with it. It may also beat somewhat faster than 80 times a minute and still be perfectly normal.

Since the heart is so essential an organ, it is fortunate that it is a tough one. Although you may have heard that it is "delicate," the heart has been handled by surgeons who have successfully sewn up wounds in it and have even repaired the valves and corrected malformations. Protected by the tough and resilient ribs, the heart is rarely damaged by a blow.

Guarding the health of your heart does not mean that you should spend most of your life in bed! Quite the contrary. Like any healthy muscle, a healthy heart is not injured by regular exercise and, indeed, benefits from it. Sudden, vigorous overexertion by someone who has led a sedentary life—shoveling snow or engaging, without adequate preparation, in a demanding sport, for ex-

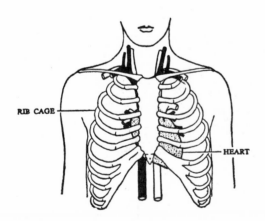

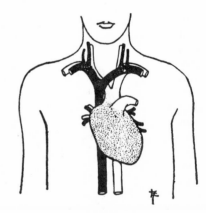

*Figure 6–3. Location of the Heart.* Left: *the protective bony structure.* Right: *the blood vessels from the* body *(in black) and to the body (in white).*

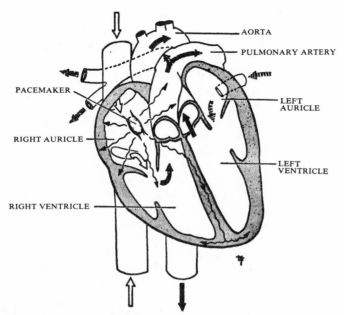

AORTA

PULMONARY ARTERY

PACEMAKER

LEFT AURICLE

RIGHT AURICLE

LEFT VENTRICLE

RIGHT VENTRICLE

*Figure 6–4. Course of Blood Through the Heart. The blood flows from the body (white arrows) into the right side of the heart; from there (stippled arrows) it goes to the lungs; it returns (striped arrows) to the left side of the heart, and is sent through the body (black arrows).*

ample—can put dangerous strain on the heart. But sensible regular exercise may well be protective for the heart; in fact, lack of such exercise in our modern society is blamed by many distinguished researchers as a factor in our high incidence of heart disease.

Exercise can be beneficial to the heart in another way. It helps to relax and counter the effects of stress and tension.

Guard your heart, too, by avoiding obesity. Excess weight taxes the heart and has been linked with a higher incidence of heart disease and of other diseases as well.

Smoking, as we have already indicated (p. 24), is dangerous to the heart as well as to the lungs and other organs. By all means, don't smoke if you don't have the habit. If you're a habitual smoker, make every effort to stop. If you must smoke, use cigarettes in moderation, or preferably, switch to an occasional pipe or mild cigar.

A good diet helps to keep the heart working at its best. In addition to the information in Chapter 2 on diet, we will have more to say about diet in connection with the heart later in our discussion of hardening of the arteries (p. 427).

Keep your work and social life under control so you are not chronically fatigued. If you are so tense and driven in our competitive world that you may be prone to high blood pressure or heart pains (angina pectoris), ask your doctor for his suggestions about counteracting stress and possibly about the advisability of a talk with a psychotherapist. You may be able to reduce the nervous tension to the point where you may avoid trouble with your heart in later life.

The great enemies of your heart are the following diseases. Read the detailed accounts of them in this book so that you will be alerted to their dangers, and know what medical science has learned about their prevention or mitigation: hyperthyroidism page 81; high blood pressure (hypertension), page 421; rheumatic fever, page 292 (not rheumatism or arthritis, which do not affect the heart); hardening of the arteries (coronary artery disease), page 419; diabetes, page 74; nephritis (Bright's disease), page 423; syphilis, page 447.

## LUNGS

The two lungs, which like the heart are completely encased by the ribs of the *thorax* (chest cavity), lie on each side of the heart. They supply the body with oxygen. The blood picks up, from the lung capillaries, the oxygen which the tissues must have, and carries it in its red cells throughout the body. Carbon dioxide, which the tissues give off as a waste product, is carried back to the lungs and expelled.

The air goes to the lungs via the *trachea* (windpipe), which divides into smaller tubes called the *bronchi*. The lungs are subdivided into lobes. Hence, *bronchopneumonia* means infection of the bronchial tubes, whereas *lobar pneumonia* refers to infection of one of the large portions of the lungs. Asthma is properly called *bronchial asthma* because it affects the air tubes.

The lungs act like bellows, sucking in air through the trachea when the chest cavity gets bigger, and expelling it when the cavity contracts. The *diaphragm* and other muscles expand the chest during respiration. This process goes on at the rate of about sixteen times a minute, increasing in speed when more oxygen is needed, as when the body is active. It is an automatic process, although we can deliberately take in a breath and keep from expelling it for a while. It is possible to work the "bellows" by artificial respiration or by means of an iron lung, if they cannot function by themselves.

What common sense precautions should you take to care for your lungs? First of all, especially in view of what we know about the effects of smoking on the lungs, you should give up smoking or cut down from high-risk cigarettes to the lower-risk mild cigar or pipe. I discuss this in detail in the sections on tobacco, beginning on page 24, and on cancer, page 429. Chapter 38, The Calculated Risk in Health, is also pertinent.

Next if you are a worker in any industry where dust, gases, and smoke are inhaled, you must learn the risks involved *now*, because industrial materials such as silica will have produced their irreversible damage to the lungs by the time symptoms

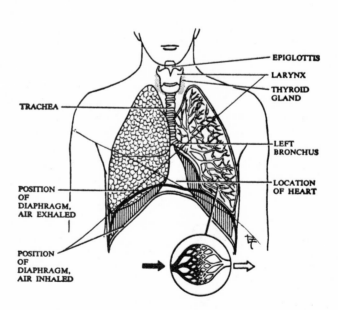

*Figure 6–5. The Lungs.* LEFT: *Outer surface of the lung.* RIGHT: *Internal structure of the lung.* INSET: *Network of blood vessels in a microscopic section of the lung, showing (in black) the blood before picking up oxygen, and (in white) the blood containing oxygen.*

appear. Read the section on your job and your health if you work in an industrial job (p. 140).

You can do a great deal to protect your lungs against infections from pneumonia and tuberculosis if you acquaint yourself with the information given elsewhere about these diseases (see Index). I have also discussed the question of climate and lung disease in my chapter on climate and illness, page 163.

And with advances in the treatment of diseases such as pneumonia, tuberculosis, and even cancer of the lungs, you can enjoy the wonderful pair of lungs nature has furnished—provided you equip yourself with adequate knowledge about these diseases, so that if they did occur you would recognize them in the early, *curable* stages.

## BLOOD

Blood is the "elixir of life." Nourishment (including oxygen) is carried in the blood by the *red cells* to the organs and tissues; waste materials go from the tissues into the blood. It carries essential products made by various organs (for example, the liver) to other organs which need these products. It helps keep the temperature equal throughout the body. Its *white cells* devour germs. Other parts of the blood, including its fluid portion (*plasma*), carry other germ-killing materials. Proteins in the plasma play a vital role in the reaction. The blood also contains substances, including the *platelets*, that make it coagulate—that is, turn solid so that serious bleeding won't result from a cut or wound.

Right here I want to mention one thing sometimes attributed to the blood that it does *not* do. It has no connection with the good or evil in human nature; people don't become criminals because there is "bad blood in the family." Similarly, it has no connection with so-called racial characteristics; our skin is not brown or yellow or white because of anything in the blood. The blood *types*, which are important where transfusions of whole blood (but *not* of plasma) are concerned, have to do with the dangerous tendency of blood cells to *agglutinate* (clump) under certain circumstances. But these blood types are not arranged according to race. The blood of a Negro or a Chinese may match that of a Scandinavian, for instance, while that of his brother might not match his and could, if it were transfused into him, cause serious trouble.

In addition to the four blood types, there is another factor, the *Rh (rhesus) factor,* which can cause incompatibility in case of a transfusion. Only about 15 percent of all people do not have this factor in their blood; they are called Rh negatives and should have transfusions of whole blood only from others like themselves. The baby of an Rh-negative mother and an Rh-positive father may (in about 5 percent of such cases) suffer from a blood disorder which was often fatal in the past but now can be counteracted by transfusions of blood from an Rh-negative person. More recently, it has become possible to immunize Rh-negative mothers and thus prevent Rh incompatibility reactions. I discuss this fully when I deal with pregnancy (p. 234).

Your blood does not need to be "purified," so don't waste money on tonics that could not possibly purify it anyway. It doesn't get thicker in cold weather and thinner in hot weather, so avoid medicines that promise to remedy anything of the sort. It will take your doctor only a minute to examine a drop of your blood and find out whether or not it contains sufficient red blood cells, so don't waste money on "iron pills" or tonics which you may not need, and which may upset your digestion. The kidneys remove most of the toxic materials in the blood and thus purify it. The lungs breathe out the carbon dioxide that accumulates in it. Nature regulates so perfectly the acid and alkaline states of the blood and tissues that you don't need to do anything about that, either. *Acidosis* or *acid blood* does not arise from eating citrus fruits or anything else, contrary to some ideas. It results only from serious illnesses such as untreated diabetes (p. 76).

All that a healthy person needs to do for the blood is to maintain an adequate diet, avoid poisonous substances, and keep germs out of the blood stream by preventing infections.

*Disorders of the blood* can affect the white cells, the red cells, or the ability of the blood to clot. *Leukemia* is a kind of cancer in which the number of white cells is tremendously increased (p.

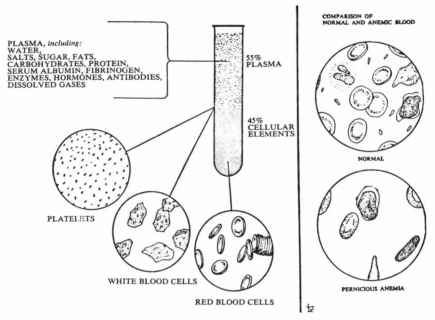

PLASMA, *including:*
WATER,
SALTS, SUGAR, FATS,
CARBOHYDRATES, PROTEIN,
SERUM ALBUMIN, FIBRINOGEN,
ENZYMES, HORMONES, ANTIBODIES,
DISSOLVED GASES

55% PLASMA

45% CELLULAR ELEMENTS

COMPARISON OF NORMAL AND ANEMIC BLOOD

NORMAL

PERNICIOUS ANEMIA

PLATELETS

WHITE BLOOD CELLS

RED BLOOD CELLS

*Figure 6–6. Composition of the Blood.*

431). In *pernicious anemia* (p. 479), which is entirely different from ordinary anemia (p. 478), the number of red cells is seriously diminished. Treatment can eliminate the danger from this disease, which was once usually fatal. In ordinary *anemia*, the low number of red cells is usually due to a loss by bleeding or to an incorrect diet. This anemia, too, can be corrected, but don't take "blood tonics" because only a doctor can determine the cause of anemia and eliminate it, in addition to giving you the proper medicine.

*Hemophilia* (p. 231) is a rare hereditary disease in which the blood fails to clot, so that its victims may bleed to death from a slight injury. It is found only in men, who inherit it from their mothers; thus it always skips a generation. *Purpura hemorrhagica*, in which bleeding takes place inside the body, is caused by a shortage of blood platelets. Although all of its causes are not known, it can result from the action of a poison such as benzol (p. 147). The cause of *polycythemia*, which means an abnormally large number of red blood cells, is usually not known. *Blood poisoning* is due to getting germs into the bloodstream (also called *septicemia*).

## BONES

The bones form the basic framework or chassis of the human body. There are 206 bones in the body. Some of these, such as the skull, which encloses the brain, the eyes, the inner ear, have chiefly a protective function. Others are mainly supporting structures, such as the vertebral column with its 24 individual bones. This encases the vital spinal cord and also helps support the back. Other bones are concerned chiefly with movements, for example, those of the fingers. The various types of bones are shown in Figure 6-7.

Bones contain a hard, stony chemical structure which gives them the tremendous strength required of them. Yet they are so marvelously constructed that they are resilient and light enough to permit the wonderful feats of strength and agility of which the human being is capable. The basic chemical of bones is calcium phosphate, found so plentifully in milk. That is why milk is such a basic item in the diet of growing infants and children (p. 36) and is also very important for the pregnant and nursing mother (p. 244).

Vitamins, especially vitamin D, are required in the proper manufacture of the bones, as described more fully in the section on the vitamins, page 37, and on page 271, in which I discuss the feeding of infants.

As people grow older their bones may become more brittle and heal less readily. That is why physicians fear certain fractures in elderly people much more than in children and younger adults.

The bones have another quite different function in addition to protection, support, and movement. They are vital elements in the manufacture of the blood cells. The bone marrow carries on this important work. After the red and white blood cells are manufactured in the marrow of the various bones, these cells enter the blood to carry on the functions described in the section on blood.

The bone marrow requires nutrient foods and vitamins different from those needed by the hard outer calcified part of the bones. The red blood cells must have iron and proteins to build hemoglobin, their important oxygen-carrying pigment. Other vitamins in the vitamin B family are required to nourish the bone marrow.

What everyday care do I recommend for the bones? If you follow the good diets prescribed in this book (p. 32), and utilize the precautions against accidents described in Chapter 22 (p. 321), you will give your bones the care they need.

There are a number of diseases of the bone and the bone marrow, which are described on pages 458 and 480.

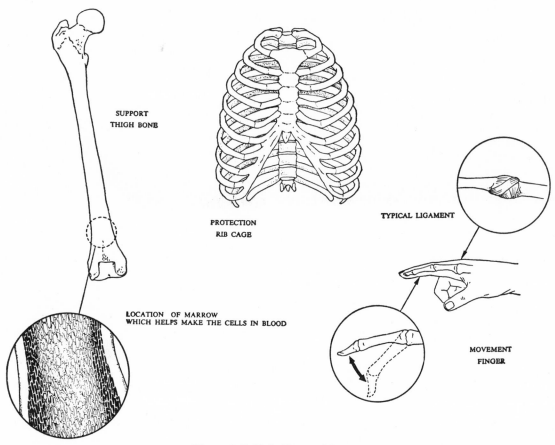

SUPPORT
THIGH BONE

PROTECTION
RIB CAGE

TYPICAL LIGAMENT

LOCATION OF MARROW
WHICH HELPS MAKE THE CELLS IN BLOOD

MOVEMENT
FINGER

*Figure 6–7. Main Types of Bones.*

# JOINTS, LIGAMENTS, AND BURSAS

Joints and ligaments connect the bones to each other. The joints provide the smooth, gliding surfaces at the ends of the bones so that movements can be carried out easily and painlessly. As shown in Figure 23-6 (p. 339), the joint consists of a fibrous sheath that is attached to the smooth end of the bones. Nature provides for the ends of the bones concerned in our bodily movements a special material, called *cartilage*. This material has special resiliency and smoothness so that fingers, arms, and legs can move thousands of times daily without our being actually conscious of their activities.

To bind bones together, or to strengthen joints, nature uses special tough bands of tissue called *ligaments*. These are attached to the bones so well that only exceptional strains will tear them away. A similar type of strong tissue called *tendons* connects bones to muscles. Tendons are so durable they are seldom torn, even when an injury is severe enough to break a bone or tear a muscle.

A final element in the wonderful, smooth, and effective movement of our joints is the *bursa*. The bursa is a sac or bag with smooth surfaces, containing a small amount of lubricating material. The bursa permits the smoother functioning of the joints. The location of a typical bursa is shown in Figure 34-3 (p. 461).

The everyday care of the joints, ligaments, and bursas is extremely important to you. An injured joint, a torn ligament, or an inflamed bursa can interfere seriously with your enjoyment of life—or incapacitate you from work. It is of primary importance that you work with—not against—nature so that there will be no extra stresses on joints, ligaments, and bursas. That means keeping a normal weight; if you are greatly overweight you are overloading the joints of the knees and feet every time you stand or walk. Good posture also keeps the joints in their best condition because weight is distributed as nature intended. Good physical condition prevents the joints from being strained by lifting and strenuous sports.

I suggest that you read the previous chapter on the general care of the body, especially those sections dealing with posture and exercises (pp. 19-21). Also, if you are overweight, consult Chapter 3. Everyone, whether a man lifting heavy objects at work, or a housewife moving the furniture at home, should know the proper techniques for lifting, as explained in the illustration on page 527. Older people are subject to the wear-and-tear type of arthritis described on page 456; they should have their joints checked at their regular medical checkups (see Chapter 27). Also, workers in the many occupations that require constant use of certain joints are subject to joint and bursa trouble. "Housemaid's knee" is a form of chronic bursitis; typists and pianists may develop aches in the finger joints, or the wrist, elbow, or shoulder; coal miners are subject to backstrains as are farmers and workers in many other jobs requiring hard physical labor. (See the chapter Your Job and Your Health, page 141, for precautions at work.)

There are many injuries and diseases which can affect the joints, ligaments, and bursas. I discuss these later, e.g., rheumatism and arthritis, page 456; bursitis, page 461; sprains, page 338; backache, page 458.

# MUSCLES

There are over six hundred muscles of voluntary movement in the human body. These give us the power to carry out the enormous variety of movements we are capable of. I described the bones, joints, ligaments, and bursas first so that you would understand the basic bony framework or skeleton of the body, and how the bones are connected for motion at the joints. But there could be no action unless there were muscles capable of moving the bones. The muscles of movement are called voluntary, skeletal, striped, or striated muscles. These synonyms refer to muscles such as the biceps which is the powerful one in the front of your upper arm, which lifts the forearm. You can feel the powerful tendon in the elbow where the biceps muscle is attached to the bone.

These voluntary muscles are quick-acting, and are under control of the conscious part of our brains. There is another group of muscles in the body which carries on activities over which we have little or no control. These muscles propel the food along the intestines; they contract the heart; they control the pupil of the eye. Therefore, they are called *involuntary muscles.*

The voluntary muscles are the only ones that require your everyday care. Muscles remain in good condition only when they are exercised properly. Healthy muscles are important to a sense of well-being, and to good posture, graceful walking, and other movements. Also, strong muscles protect the bones, joints, and contents of the abdomen against injury. Read my section on keeping muscles in good condition by pleasurable forms of exercise and sports (pages 16-18) if you are not in ideal "muscular" condition. Almost every older person, or many others who do light work, needs to strengthen the abdominal and back muscles by the exercises described in the illustrations on page 17.

Muscles are composed chiefly of protein. A good diet containing the sources of protein, described on page 36, will help you build good muscles.

Almost everyone has experienced a *"charley horse."* This results from too violent use of a muscle or group of muscles, e.g., at the start of a new job, or shoveling the first snow, or, very frequently, during vacation when there is a natural tendency to go "all out" for strenuous sports. The muscles "protest" against the too violent use by soreness, stiffness, and pain. The "charley horse" will clear up with rest of the sore muscles. Warm baths will help. A tablet or two of aspirin by mouth will also be useful in relieving the painful feeling. *Muscle twitchings* result from various causes, usually minor ones like temporary fatigue, overwork of a group of muscles, or nervousness or insomnia. If muscle twitches become frequent or painful, or if they involve the face, producing unpleasant grimaces, then you should discuss them without delay with your doctor. The same is true of *muscle cramps,* especially the ones that occur at night which sometimes wake people from their sleep because of intense pain in the calf of the leg or in other muscles.

Muscles are affected by a great variety of diseases. There are the intrinsic ailments of the muscles such as *muscular dystrophy,* described in the section on muscle diseases (p. 474). Muscles waste away if the nerves that connect them to the brain

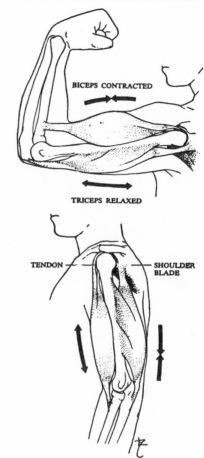

*Figure 6–8. Voluntary Muscular Action.*

are damaged. This happens in polio and other afflictions of the nerves and spinal cord (see page 464). Also, if a stroke damages a section of the brain which controls an arm or leg, then the muscles of the limb may atrophy, as explained on page 428. Similarly, in severe disease of the joints or bones, there may be inability to move a limb which then causes "secondary" wasting of the muscles.

## STOMACH, INTESTINES, AND COLON

The *stomach,* which is located in the abdominal cavity, resembles a bag approximately a foot long and six inches wide. The narrow small intestines are about twenty feet long, and the *colon,* or large intestine, is about five feet long. A tube called the *esophagus* connects the throat to the stomach. The place where the stomach ends and the small intestine begins is called the *duodenum.* It is very important because the main tubes from the *pancreas,* the *liver* and the *gallbladder* discharge juices and bile into it. Ulcers are frequently located in the duodenum.

Food is churned up, acted upon by juices, and digested in the stomach and intestines, the residue being eliminated through the opening known as the *rectum* and *anus.* Actually, the mouth itself, in which the food is chewed and mixed with saliva, is a part of the *digestive system,* or *gastrointestinal system* as it is also called.

The delicate and sensitive lining of the stomach and intestines is actually a busy chemical factory, making juices and enzymes for the digestion and absorption of food. The stomach and intestines,

which are controlled by a network of nerves, are constantly in motion, pushing the food along. It takes about twenty-four hours for the food you eat to move through and to the end of the digestive tract.

Disorders of the gastrointestinal system are among the most common illnesses we doctors encounter. Almost everyone has had some degree of difficulty at one time or another.

These disorders can be functional. Because of the extensive nerve connections involved in the digestive system, fear, anger, and other nervous upsets set off attacks of nausea, cramps, diarrhea, and other symptoms. Organic diseases such as ulcer and cancer can affect these organs, as do contagious ones such as typhoid fever and virus infections, as well as food poisoning, constipation, dyspepsia, allergies—and a list almost as long as the digestive tract itself!

You can protect your digestive system by taking precautions against infectious diseases (p. 136);

*Figure 6–9. The Gastrointestinal (Digestive) Tract.* LEFT: *Shaded areas indicate the location of the organs associated with digestion.* RIGHT: *As food passes through the mouth, stomach, and small and large in-* *testines, it is worked upon by juices manufactured in these and other organs (such as the liver and pancreas). The food is then absorbed, mainly through the intestinal walls. The residue is excreted through the rectum.*

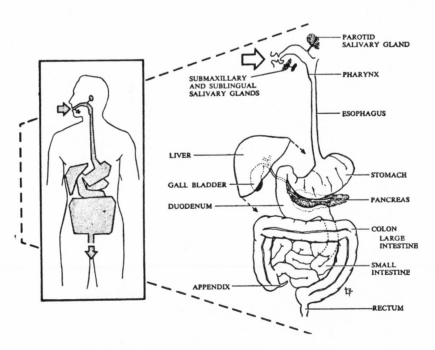

by being sensible about the food you eat and the way you eat it; by avoiding poisonous and irritating substances (including excessive amounts of alcohol); and by maintaining mental health in order to prevent "nervous stomach" and other psychosomatic digestive diseases.

Perhaps even more important, you can guard the health of your stomach and intestines by *leaving them alone.* Don't take enemas to "clean out the colon and get rid of germs." Nature intended them to be there, and a great many people would have better digestions if they had never heard the term *autointoxication.* I wish you would remove it from your vocabulary, and also the words *acid stomach* and *alkaline stomach.* You can't "cure" these nonexistent diseases by taking stomach "sweeteners," or "aids" to digestion, which can do real harm.

It is unfortunate that there are so many "simple remedies" for indigestion on the market, when this is by no means a simple disease. In fact, it isn't a disease at all, but a condition or group of symptoms which can be caused by any number of diseases, from *migraine headaches* (p. 493) to *heart disease* (p. 416), *gallbladder trouble* (p. 445), the fact that you are coming down with the flu—or simply to the fact that you bolted your dinner when you were tense and tired!

Even a skilled physician often finds it a long and difficult task to determine the cause—and hence the treatment—of indigestion. Don't object if your doctor asks you to have a complete set of x-rays, after having you drink some barium compound, so that he can find out whether the indigestion is caused by a tumor or an ulcer, or if he wants to examine your stomach with a prism-equipped instrument called a *gastroscope.* These tests are well worth while. Almost every disturbance of the gastrointestinal system which makes itself known by the symptoms of indigestion can be helped *if* it is identified in time.

On the other hand, a disease can progress to a serious, even fatal, stage while you are engaged in "treating" your indigestion—for example, if you took a cathartic for indigestion and it happened to be caused by *appendicitis* (p. 449). Let the doctor decide whether or not you should take any medicine.

I know that everybody isn't going to the doctor each time he has a *mildly upset stomach.* If that's really all you are suffering from, I recommend one of the following remedies:

A level teaspoonful of bicarbonate of soda in something, such as fruit juice, that appeals to the individual.

Ten to 20 drops of essence of peppermint taken on a lump of sugar, or in a teaspoonful of sugar, and chewed slowly.

A teaspoonful or two of *creme de menthe,* or other liqueur or brandy, sipped slowly; or a little wine such as sherry.

For *nausea* or *cramping,* tincture of belladonna is helpful. Adults require from 10 to 20 drops in water. Each person must find his proper dosage. Usually, an effective amount will cause some dryness of the mouth or a slight blurring of vision. The dosage can be repeated in 4 to 6 hours.

For more *intense abdominal cramps,* one to two teaspoonfuls of *paregoric* will be helpful (see page 449 on appendicitis).

A persistent *"nervous stomach"* can be helped by mild sedatives such as phenobarbital, especially if given in combination with tincture of belladonna. However, this medication should be prescribed only by a physician.

Aspirin, taken for a headache, cold, or rheumatism, sometimes causes stomach distress. This may be alleviated by a teaspoonful of bicarbonate of soda or by using a buffered aspirin. Alternatively, an aspirin substitute, acetaminophen (available under various trade names), can be used.

If you are *occasionally* (*not* habitually) constipated, it is safe for you to take mild *laxatives* such as a tablespoonful or two of *milk of magnesia,* as I suggest in the section on *constipation* (p. 504). Avoid dosing yourself regularly with any laxative or cathartic.

Be sure to consult a doctor if you suffer persistently or repeatedly from any of the following symptoms: nausea, vomiting, excessive belching, fullness or burning sensations in the abdomen, cramps, constipation, or diarrhea. Be sure to see him *immediately* if you pass stools that are blood-streaked, blackish, colorless, or very foul smelling.

## The Appendix

At the juncture of the small intestine and the large intestine is a little wormlike appendage called the *vermiform appendix* (see Figure 33-5, on page 449). No one knows why nature placed it there. Unfortunately, this apparently useless structure can be the source of serious or even fatal illness. No age group is immune to it. It may surprise you to learn that it is a more serious threat to children than it is to adults. Be sure to read the section in which I tell you the details about appendicitis (p. 449); and always remember this fact: the one thing you can do for your appendix is to realize that, if it is inflamed by appendicitis, you may cause it to rupture by taking a laxative or by applying a hot-water bottle over it.

Can appendicitis be prevented? Unfortunately, there is no way known at present to prevent this potentially serious illness. However, its prompt diagnosis can lead to effective removal of the inflamed organ before serious complications set in. The operation when performed early by a competent surgeon is a comparatively simple and safe one.

## LIVER

If you place your left hand over the lowermost ribs on the right side of your chest, it will cover the liver, which is the largest internal organ in the body (see Figure 6-9, page 100). It has at least five hundred functions which are concerned with the processes of digestion, nutrition, and with the development of the red blood cells. It produces *bile,* which flows out through a channel into the small intestine. It helps detoxify harmful substances in the blood.

The liver in a healthy body requires no particular care or concern. It certainly does *not* need to be "stimulated" by medicines such as those which claim to "increase the flow of bile."

However, there are a few things you can do to prevent damage to your liver. Protect it from the harm which can result from excessive drinking of alcoholic beverages, and from poisons such as *carbon tetrachloride* to which you may be exposed at work (p. 147) or during some hobbies that require solvents. Obesity also damages the liver. A good, balanced diet (p. 31) and normal weight (p. 45) are necessary to help keep your liver healthy.

Hepatitis, a viral disease of the liver, can manifest itself by jaundice (p. 444), in which the skin and whites of the eyes become yellow. If you notice such a condition, report it immediately to your doctor. Hepatitis can be transmitted by transfusions of contaminated blood and by improperly sterilized needles or syringes. Do not use one—for example, in giving insulin—that has been employed by another person. Alcohol and ordinary boiling do not kill the virus; the high temperature of an autoclave type of sterilizer is required. We doctors are now using individually sterilized disposable needles to draw off even a drop of blood, because of the danger of transmitting the hepatitis virus. Hepatitis can also be spread by contaminated food or water. (A discussion of several liver diseases begins on page 444.)

## GALLBLADDER

The gallbladder is a "side pocket" in the channel through which the bile flows from the liver into the intestine; it acts as a storage place for the bile (see Figure 33-4, page 446). Infection may cause an acute or chronic inflammation of the gallbladder (p. 444). Gallstones (p. 444) sometimes cause a great deal of pain, or they may block the flow of bile, causing jaundice and an inflammation in the liver and gallbladder. Fortunately, the gallbladder can be surgically removed; the body can get along without it.

There is nothing you need to do about the everyday care of your gallbladder except to keep your weight normal. Obesity probably increases the tendency toward gallbladder disease. Women who have had more than one or two children are somewhat more likely to suffer gallstones, and in general, after the fortieth birthday, about twice as many women have this problem as do men. Once stones have formed, they do not dissolve; sometimes they pass spontaneously into the intestines (p. 446). However, your doctor has ways

CARE OF THE INDIVIDUAL PARTS OF THE BODY — 103

of stimulating the flow of bile and of decreasing the inflammation in the gallbladder; these measures may conceivably reduce the formation of additional stones. Now under study is a chemical which, in the trial stage, is showing promise of dissolving some stones.

## KIDNEYS

The kidneys are two organs located deep in the abdomen at about the level of the lowest ("floating") ribs. By means of more than two million tiny, separate filters, they filter out, and remove from the blood, the urea and other useless material it contains. This they excrete in the urine. The kidneys "know" how to hold back the valuable vitamins and minerals the body needs. They also regulate the volume of fluid in the body: when a person drinks a large amount of fluid, the kidneys excrete the excess, but in hot weather, when extra fluid is lost via the sweat, the kidneys excrete smaller amounts of urine.

Your kidneys do *not* need to be "flushed" or "stimulated" or any of the things that patented medicines falsely claim to do. Trouble in the kidneys can cause pain in the lower back, and this symptom, together with changes in the urine, should always be reported immediately to a doctor. However, contrary to the claims made for certain "kidney medicines," they can't cure *chronic pain in the back,* which is *seldom* caused by kidney trouble. Don't take *any* medicines for your kidneys except on a doctor's orders.

Some of the causes of kidney stones (renal calculi) are beyond our control, but preventing or curing infections will help to keep them from forming (p. 27). Another thing you can do to prevent the formation of stones is to see to it that you always have *an adequate flow of urine.* This should amount to at least a quart or slightly more a day. When the urine becomes highly concentrated during hot weather or as a result of excessive sweating at work, there is an increased tendency toward the formation of stones and the occurrence of infections. This can be avoided by drinking sufficient water if you are perspiring a great deal.

A floating (or movable) kidney is usually not se-rious, although it may cause discomfort. *Nephritis* (also called Bright's disease) is a *potentially serious illness* (p. 422). Whenever the urine appears bloody, wine-colored, smoky, or at all unusual, it may be a sign of kidney disease. Always see your doctor *immediately* if you notice any of the above conditions in your urine. You should also see him immediately or go to a hospital if your urine looks cloudy or full of pus. If treated early, many kidney disorders can be completely cured. However, if not cured, diseases of the kidneys can slowly destroy these vital organs, leading years later to *uremic poisoning* (p. 426) and high blood pressure (p. 421). Fortunately, many patients with kidney failure now can be helped by dialysis, a process in which blood is filtered by a machine to remove toxic materials. Kidney transplants also are proving successful.

## URINARY BLADDER

The urinary bladder and the tubes leading to and from it form, together with the kidneys, the *urinary system.* The tubes called the *ureters* carry waste products, including urea, from the kidneys to the bladder. After a sufficient quantity has collected there, it is eliminated by urination, through the tube called the *urethra.* The external opening of the urethra is called the *meatus* (see Figure 6-10). No everyday care is required for the bladder.

Infections and inflammations are fairly common, especially in the bladder (*cystitis* is the name for infections of the bladder) (p. 246). They usually yield to treatment with antibiotic medicines, but these *must* be given under the supervision of a doctor. Never use a "bladder purifier" or other home remedy. Infections can be the cause of *incontinence*—the inability to control urination. This is natural in young children; in older ones it may take the form of *bed-wetting,* and is frequently due to emotional tension, although it can have a physical cause. Frequency of urination can be a symptom of a disease such as *diabetes* (p. 74). Difficult urination can be caused by a *urethral stricture.* Always consult a doctor if you experience *frequent, difficult, or painful urination.* Don't attempt to treat these conditions yourself. They are often due to an easily cured inflammation, but they can be caused by a disease; for example, in men by an enlargement of the *prostate gland* (p. 481). *Stones* can also form in the urinary bladder. Never take any "home remedies" to "dissolve" them. If necessary, stones can be removed by a surgeon.

## SPLEEN

This pulpy organ is tucked away under the ribs in the upper left-hand corner of the abdomen. It performs important functions associated with the blood, particularly the red blood cells, especially in breaking down worn-out red cells. Enlargement of the spleen often occurs in diseases such as mononucleosis, cirrhosis of the liver, rheumatoid arthritis, and some anemias. The internal bleeding you may have heard mentioned in connection with some accident might very well have come from a broken or ruptured spleen. Yet it's only relatively rarely that the spleen causes trouble, and there is nothing you need do about the organ. Fortunately, the body can get along without the spleen so it can be removed if injury or disease should require it.

## PANCREAS

The pancreas lies high up in the abdomen, deep behind the stomach. It produces important digestive juices which flow into the small intestine. Equally important are the islets of Langerhans which are contained in the pancreas and which produce insulin. A lack of insulin causes *diabetes* (p. 74). The best thing you can do for your pancreas is to avoid overweight (p. 44), which predisposes people to diabetes.

## GENITALS (MALE)

Look at the diagram showing the structure of the male genital system.

Before a male baby is born, his *testes* lie within the abdominal cavity; at the time he is born, they descend through the *inguinal canal* into the *scrotum*. (Testes that do not descend can usually be surgically placed in their proper spot.) It is because of this passageway that *rupture* (hernia, page 483) occurs so much more frequently in men than in women. Always consult your doctor if you notice a bulge in the groin toward the upper part of the scrotum or in the lowest part of the abdomen just above the tight cord that separates it from the thigh. Don't listen to people who tell you to wear a truss. Only a doctor is capable of deciding between the relative merit of an operation and a truss in case of a hernia (see discussion of hernia, page 483).

IS CIRCUMCISION NECESSARY? This operation is the removal of the fold of skin called the *foreskin* or *prepuce*. It is performed if this fold covers the entire end of the penis (the *glans*) and obstructs the passage of urine, or is so tight that irritation results. Otherwise, circumcision is a personal matter. It has been customary among certain groups for centuries; the Egyptians practiced it before the Hebrews made it a part of their religious customs. The practice is safe and simple when performed in accordance with the principles of modern aseptic surgery. Although circumcision can be performed later in life, it is best to circumcise a boy when he is seven or eight days old and will experience no physical or emotional discomfort from it (see also page 261). Talk the matter over with your family doctor or pediatrician.

CLEANSING THE GENITALS. The genitals should be kept clean and free from infection. Uncircumcised males should pull back the foreskin and wash off any secretions with soap and water as frequently as required to keep the penis clean. The genitals should be protected from blows and other injuries during football and other strenuous sports. Masturbation causes no organic harm (p. 315). However, because of the feelings of guilt often associated with this practice, conflicts, tensions, and other emotional problems frequently arise.

VENERAL DISEASE. The penis can be affected by *venereal diseases* (referred to as VD). *Syphilis*

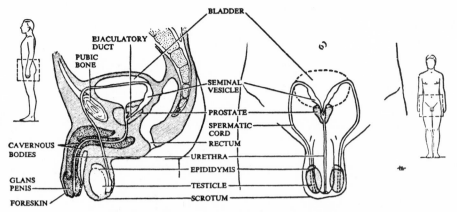

*Figure 6–10. The Male Genitalia. The bladder is shown by dotted lines, in order not to obscure the organs in back of it.*

(p. 447) is the most serious of these. I can't remind you too often that this disease can be cured completely; I urge you to read the section on this disease so that you won't fail to seek medical advice if you have any reason to suspect that you have contracted syphilis. No one except a competent physician is capable of treating it. The fact that this disease can be cured completely is no reason for carelessness. The number of syphilis cases in the United States and in many other countries has risen alarmingly fast. One reason seems to be that many people take it for granted that they have nothing to worry about. However, syphilis is serious, and precautions against it should always be taken.

Another common venereal disease is *gonorrhea* (p. 485). Before the development of drugs such as penicillin, it was a very serious illness. Now it can usually be cured with one injection of penicillin. Every person, female as well as male, should read the section on gonorrhea. Even children are susceptible, and it can be transmitted in ways other than sexual contact. If you learn the facts, you will know how to prevent gonorrhea.

The other venereal diseases are less common and less important. They are chancroid, lymphogranuloma inguinale, and venereal warts (p. 486). They will be made evident, in men, by sores on the penis or enlarged glands in the groin, and respond to treatment provided a doctor is consulted while they are in their early stages.

CAN VENEREAL DISEASE BE PREVENTED IN THE MALE? The simplest, most effective prophylactic is the condom (rubber sheath, "safety"). Some males seem to think that it diminishes the pleasure of intercourse; others feel it isn't "manly" to wear one. However, all I can say, as a doctor who has seen some of the really severe cases of gonorrhea or syphilis, is this—if a male must expose himself to the dangers of venereal disease, he can well afford to reduce the physical pleasure a slight amount in return for the mental relief he will obtain after the act by not having to worry about syphilis and other types of VD. And, too, the condom prevents conception, a very important factor in providing emotional relaxation.

As I think back on some patients who have had venereal disease, I believe the most pathetic males have been those who indulged in sexual relations during heavy alcoholic sprees—and couldn't even remember the event or the person who had given them a serious disease.

Other methods of prophylaxis toward venereal disease are described elsewhere in this book (p. 448).

Nature has been kinder with respect to cancer. It rarely involves the penis.

The *testicles* are not often affected by illness. They can be involved, in adults, as a result of a disease such as mumps (p. 296), undulant fever (p. 486), or gonorrhea (p. 485). The cord which supports them may be invaded by an extension of a hernia, or there may be enlarged veins. The *epididymis* may become diseased. If you notice a swelling, lump, or congestion of the scrotum or testicles, be sure to see your doctor as soon as possible. It may be an early cancer or some other illness; almost all of these conditions are completely curable if treated early. The skin in and around the *scrotum* may be infected by *ringworm fungus* (p. 133), causing the so-called jockstrap itch. Keeping these areas clean and dry (a simple drying powder, such as that used for babies, is useful) will help prevent these fungus infections.

The *prostate gland*, which plays a part in the process of reproduction (it creates *prostatic fluid*, which helps to make up the *semen*), can be affected by cancer and infections. In men of about fifty years of age or older, it frequently enlarges for reasons which are not yet fully understood. This is called benign hypertrophy of the prostate gland (p. 481).

## GENITALS (FEMALE)

The anatomy of the female sex organs is illustrated below. I devote an entire chapter to pregnancy and childbirth (p. 234). Sterility is discussed on page 232. Chapters 21 and 36 contain sections devoted to menstruation and to the menopause (see pages 313, 514, and 517).

HYGIENE. *Feminine hygiene* does not require the taking of douches. Nature has provided for the cleansing of the internal passages. Altogether too many women have been persuaded to take frequent douches with antiseptic solutions because of advertisements which imply that no woman can be dainty or clean without them. They *can* be the cause of irritation. If you wish to take an occasional douche, it should be of the mildest type, imitating nature's own secretions. Use what is called a *physiological salt solution,* by adding two level teaspoonfuls of table salt to a quart of moderately warm water. The douche should be given under gentle pressure.

Should external or internal pads be used during the menstrual period? This depends on individual choice. Some women prefer the external sanitary pad, while others like an internal absorptive pad (*tampon*). Either is safe. Each woman should decide for herself, dependent upon the amount of flow and other factors, which type she prefers. An unmarried woman can wear a tampon if her hymen happens to be well perforated; contrary to some opinion, this may be the case even though she has never had sexual relations. Certain kinds of exercise may cause the hymen of a virgin to rupture. (The structure of the hymen is illustrated on page 213).

If the hymen is completely lacking in perforations (an *imperforate hymen*), menstruation may be interfered with, and a minor surgical operation may be necessary.

An irregularity in menstruation, after it has been well established, should be reported to a doctor.

*Figure 6–11. The Female Genitalia. The bladder is shown by dotted lines, in order not to obscure the organs in back of it.*

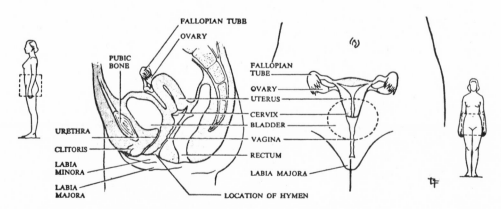

FALLOPIAN TUBE
OVARY
PUBIC BONE
FALLOPIAN TUBE
OVARY
UTERUS
CERVIX
BLADDER
VAGINA
URETHRA
RECTUM
CLITORIS
LABIA MINORA
LABIA MAJORA
LABIA MAJORA
LOCATION OF HYMEN

INFECTIONS, including venereal ones (syphilis and gonorrhea), can seriously damage the female genitals. A sudden, profuse, odorous, colored, or painful discharge may indicate a potentially serious infection that may not only affect the vaginal passage but could spread into the uterus (womb) and the tubes and ovaries. If such a discharge is accompanied by chills and fever, real trouble may be developing. Such infections can usually be healed by penicillin or other medicines, provided you give a competent M.D. or hospital clinic the opportunity to help you. Keep away from quacks, advertising doctors, and neighbors and friends who like to dispense advice about feminine hygiene. *These infections, if not treated promptly, can cause sterility.* If they advance far enough, they may cause a condition that requires surgery, possibly the removal of one of the reproductive organs. Remember that *gonorrheal vulvovaginitis* in young girls can be contracted without sexual intercourse, so be sure not to neglect any discharge in your young daughters.

*What can the adult female do to prevent venereal infection?* This is frequently considered too delicate a subject even for a health book. However, please remember that physicians are pledged to treat and prevent disease in everyone, regardless of his or her moral status. For those women who are for any reason exposed to the dangerous fire of venereal disease, I can recommend only one safe preventive measure: that is, to insist that the male employ a condom during *the entire time* of the sexual act. Obviously, if the sheath is applied only to prevent conception at the time just before the male orgasm, there will not be protection from syphilis if the male organ has a syphilitic sore on it; nor will protection result if the male is infected with gonorrhea and his germs are present in the lubricating secretions that are produced at the earliest moments of the male erection.

Of course a vaginal discharge, *leukorrhea,* is not always serious. A certain amount of fluid is normally produced to keep the tissues moist. It is practically odorless and colorless and is not irritating. Congestion, tension, and minor inflammations can increase this discharge. Germs far less dangerous than those causing syphilis and gonorrhea can cause infections which may become troublesome unless they are cleared up. Your doctor must find the cause of the infection before he can prescribe the right treatment. That is why you should not use an antiseptic or germicidal solution as a douche unless you are under a doctor's orders; you may be "curing" the wrong infection! (See page 519.)

The female organs are subject to tumors and cancers, and should be examined regularly at your medical checkup. At that time, your doctor may decide to take a "Pap smear," a painless and simple procedure that can give him much useful information about the health of your uterus. This is a test for a cancerous, or precancerous, condition. Thousands of women owe their lives to the fact that their physician included this test as part of a routine checkup. (See page 435.) Any unexpected bleeding or discharge, especially after the menopause, and any change in menstruation, should be immediately reported to your doctor. Even if these symptoms are due to a cancer, the percentage of cures is *very* high if the growth is detected in its early stages (Cancer, p. 429).

* * *

We now go to the external organs of the body. Because they are located externally they are subject to more frequent accidents and require more attention by you than many of the internal organs. Everyone of us has been faced with the problem of a cinder in the eye or a cut in the skin, but most of us will go through life without a foreign body in the brain or heart or a cut in the lungs or other vital internal organ.

Even though these sections on the skin and eyes are long, I truly believe you will obtain a rich reward by reading them carefully.

## EYES

The eye is like a camera (see Figure 6-12). The front part consists of the *cornea,* the transparent area in the center, which is surrounded by the *sclera,* as the white of the eye is called. Behind the cornea is the colored part, in the middle of which is the *pupil,* which grows larger or smaller to control the amount of light let into the "camera." The clear, transparent *lens,* located slightly in back of the front surface, focuses the image on the *retina,* which is about three quarters of an inch behind it. The *optic nerve* carries the picture from the retina to the brain. The eye also contains muscles to do this work and fluid to keep the parts in working condition.

If I asked you whether you would mind being blind, you would call it a ridiculous question. Most people consider blindness the worst thing that could happen to them. But you'd never guess it from the way they treat their eyes!

Probably some of you who are reading this have to squint to do so, or hold the book close to your nose, or wish your arms were longer so you could hold it farther away. You know you *should* have your eyes examined—but you put it off because it can wait, or because you don't want to be told you have to wear glasses. Even some serious eye conditions have been neglected, with tragic consequences, for these foolish reasons.

One such condition is *glaucoma.* In this disease, increased pressure within the eyeball seriously injures the vision. In the acute type of glaucoma, dimming of the vision may be sudden: the eyeball becomes painful, and the affected person feels quite ill. However, the insidious type of glaucoma doesn't cause pain, and injures the vision very slowly. Sometimes it may make itself known by the appearance of colored rings and halos about bright objects, or by the fact that the vision in front remains good while that on the sides becomes dim. About half of the blindness occurring in adults in this country is due to glaucoma, which occurs most frequently in people over forty. There is a great deal that can be done to preserve the vision in most cases, provided the disease is caught in time. It is easily recognized by a doctor specializing in the eyes (an *ophthalmologist*). Isn't it foolhardy not to have your eyes examined once a year after you have reached the age of forty? Once every three years is sufficient if you are between twenty-five and forty.

*Cataracts* impair the vision of many elderly people and some younger ones. These are opaque spots which form on the lens. Why put off going to the doctor if you suspect you have cataracts? They can be removed surgically at any time and practically at any age. It isn't necessary to wait for the cataract to become complete, or "ripe," as was believed in the past. Depending on the condition of the lens, the retina, and other considerations, some cataracts can be treated successfully without surgery.

INFECTIONS OF THE EYE can be serious. Today, even the chronic eye infection called *trachoma,* and other diseases that used to cause blindness such as tuberculosis, gonorrhea, and pneumonia, can be cured by the "wonder drugs." Don't decide for yourself that an eye infection is nothing to worry about.

Of course there are minor eye infections, the most common of which is *conjunctivitis,* or *pink eye.* In this disease, the eyes become red, the lids swell and are usually stuck together in the morning. Symptoms of conjunctivitis resemble those of other eye infections, so let a doctor make the diagnosis and provide suitable treatment.

It is safe for you to treat an *occasional stye* (an infection resembling a pimple in the tiny glands of the eyelid) at home. Apply hot compresses every 2 hours for 15 minutes at a time. If the stye doesn't open and drain, and heal in a few days, be sure to see a doctor. See him, too, if you have styes repeatedly.

CLEANING THE EYES. If your eyelids become irritated by wind or dust, you can relieve them by washing them out, using an eyedropper or an eyecup, as you prefer, with a warm solution of pure table salt—a level teaspoonful to a pint of warm water, being sure that the utensils you use have been thoroughly cleaned and scalded. It is *not* necessary to wash your eyes as a routine measure. Nature has provided for that through the tear glands. So *don't* use any kind of eyedrops or wash your eyes every day with any solution. Incidentally, *boric acid* does not warrant its reputation as an antiseptic for the eyes. All you should do to keep your eyes clean is to wash the skin around them. Always use a clean washcloth, your own, not one someone else has used. Be careful not to rub your eyes with your fingers.

EYE INJURY. Of course, you can't be too careful in guarding your eyes against accidents at home or at work. Always see a doctor *immediately* if you have hurt an eye. Delay can mean blindness,

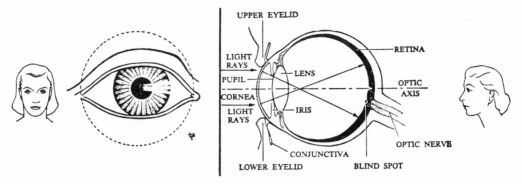

*Figure 6–12. The Eye.* LEFT: *Front view. The approximate orbit of the eye is indicated by dotted lines.*

RIGHT: Side view, showing the light rays passing through the lens.

plus possibly the loss of an eye. Dirt, cinders, and other bits of foreign material are so apt to get into the eyes that everyone should read the section (under First Aid, page 326) in which I tell you what to do and what *not* to do when this happens to you or someone in your family.

EYESTRAIN can best be treated by putting an end to the conditions that are causing it. *Improper lighting,* especially when reading or using your eyes for other close work, is a frequent cause of eyestrain. Don't face the light; it should come from in back of you and from the side so you won't be in your own shadow. Be sure the light bulbs are strong enough (75 to 100 watts) and are not dusty. Hold your book or paper about 16 or 18 inches away from you and a little lower than eye level. Reading when you're lying on your back in bed or propped up on an elbow will strain your eyes, and so will reading for a long time in a vibrating train or subway. Rest your eyes from time to time by looking off into the distance—which is easier said than done, I know, in some places. Avoid glare.

NIGHT BLINDNESS (*nyctalopia*) is an impairment in vision that makes a person unable to see well, if at all, in dim light. It can mean something is wrong not only with the eyes but with the entire system. Night blindness is a threat to safety, particularly on the highway, because a driver may have 20/20 vision and not realize that he has night blindness. This condition also causes no observable changes in the tissues of the eyes, so it can't be

diagnosed unless the patient tells his eye doctor that he can't read road signs at night or has trouble picking out objects on a dimly lighted street. It is not normal to have trouble seeing in dim light after a two- or three-minute period of adjustment. If you do detect such a condition in your vision, discuss it with an eye specialist. It can be treated temporarily by the addition of special vitamins to your diet.

If you are in the *bright sun,* dark glasses can protect your eyes—*good* sunglasses, that is. Poor ones can add to your troubles, especially if you wear them for a long time, and so can glasses that fit so badly you see the rims. Don't wear glasses with irregularities or scratches in them: plastic lenses scratch very easily. Some glasses are too lightly tinted to do any good. Unfortunately, good sunglasses are expensive. Don't look directly into the sun even though you are wearing glasses, and don't wear them indoors and at night—even though some Hollywood stars consider it smart! If you wear glasses, it is worthwhile to have a pair of sunglasses ground to your prescription, rather than clip a pair of possibly inferior sunglasses over your carefully made regular glasses.

*Movies* can cause eyestrain if the lighting is poor, the film flickery, or you sit too far to the side—or if you're such an addict that you go practically every day. It is easy to become addicted to *television* without realizing it, and this, too, can cause eyestrain. Television won't bother your eyes unless you have a room totally dark, sit too close or at an angle, or watch too steadily for a long time. I think it is wise to be arbitrary about children watching television, and set the limit at an hour, with a good long rest period before the next program. It is best, too, to mark a spot about six feet away from the set, because children are apt to sit practically next to the screen.

EYEGLASSES. A most important source of eyestrain is in our eyes themselves. A large number of us are *nearsighted, farsighted,* or *astigmatic.* These conditions are caused by the shape of the eyeball. It may be formed in such a way that the lens focuses well on nearby objects but not on those at a distance, or vice versa; or it may be "squeezed" out of shape so that things look slightly distorted to the astigmatic eye no matter how hard the focusing muscles work. *Strabismus* (also called cross-eyes and squint) is caused by an imbalance of the muscles of the eyes. Babies are apt to be cross-eyed, but they should begin to lose this tendency by the time they are three months old. Don't put off consulting a doctor if your child is cross-eyed. His vision may be impaired unless he is treated. Sometimes a fairly simple surgical operation is necessary.

Fortunately, nearsightedness, farsightedness, and astigmatism are readily corrected by wearing the proper eyeglasses. It is essential for these conditions to be corrected, not only to prevent eyestrain but to keep them from getting worse. If, for example, one eye is normal and the other is not, the good one will do all the work, which is bad for the one that is not being used. Even if your eyes have always been perfect, they tend to change as you get older, and they are then unable to adjust to anything close at hand. That is why you should have your eyes examined as soon as you find yourself holding things off at a distance in order to see them, or notice that you cannot see as well as you used to in a poor light. Always have an eye doctor examine your eyes and prescribe the proper lenses. In some places you can still buy eyeglasses over the counter. Think about how much your eyes mean to you, and resist this temptation to economize!

I must confess it is difficult for me to understand why so many people object to wearing glasses. It is true that they are an expense and a bit of a nuisance, but what a joy it is to see properly. Fortunately, glasses have become so "glamorized" that resistance to them is disappearing.

For actresses and others in special occupations who would find ordinary glasses a real handicap, contact lenses which fit directly over the eyeball are a boon. However, they are expensive, are not always easy to insert, and can usually be tolerated for only limited periods. These new types of "invisible eyeglasses" are constantly being improved. Your eye doctor can advise about their suitability for *you.*

It is most unwise to try to avoid wearing glasses by spending hours on various systems of exercises which have not as yet been scientifically proved effective. Exercising the eyes can help under some circumstances; and in themselves, the exercises usually don't do any harm. Their main danger lies in the fact that they may be used when poor vision is due to some eye disease such as glaucoma, or in the fact that people who use the exercises fail to go to an ophthalmologist who might, in his examination, discover some illness that first reveals itself in the eyes. "Pop-eyes" for example—that is, eyes that are prominent and staring—may mean an overactive thyroid gland which, unless corrected, may lead to serious damage of the heart. Isn't it wise to see an eye specialist who has spent four years at medical school and five more in postgraduate training? The specialist will *really* know if you need corrective exercises or glasses.

## EARS

The ear is made up of three parts, the *outer ear,* the *middle ear,* and the *inner ear* (see Figure 6-13). The part you see, that is, the *lobe* and the *ear canal,* make up the outer ear. The canal leads to the *eardrum* and the middle ear in which lie the "bones of hearing," called the *hammer, anvil,* and *stirrup* because of their resemblance to these objects. The middle ear is connected to the upper rear part of the throat by the *eustachian tube,* and to the *mastoid cells* inside the skullbone just behind the outer ear. The inner ear contains the *semicircular canals* (or *labyrinth*), which are essential to our sense of balance, and the *cochlea,* in which nerves analyze the sounds from the outer world and carry them to the brain.

INFECTIONS. *Middle ear infections* do not usually come from outside, as some people believe, but from the nose and throat through the eustachian tube. That is why inflamed tonsils and adenoids, a severe cold, sore throat, or sinusitis are usually accompanied by a sense of pressure or pain in the ears. Infection may spread up the eustachian tube into the middle ear, especially in children. Your doctor can prevent this, which is one of the reasons for calling him whenever you or a member of your family has a sore throat, a severe cold, or sinusitis.

*If the middle ear becomes seriously infected, hearing may be impaired.* The infection may spread, causing rupture and destruction of the eardrum. It may continue into the mastoid cells and, unless checked there, can enter the nearby brain and its covering. Children are very susceptible to middle ear infections. Before the development of the "wonder drugs," *mastoiditis* was a common, and rightly dreaded, disease, especially in children. Now, if a doctor is called in early, he can control these infections successfully. Operations for infected middle ears and mastoids, which were so common until recently, are fortunately seldom necessary today.

*Infections of the outer ear,* involving the lining of the auditory canal, are common. They may be caused by fungi or by germs, resulting in boils of the canal. Eczema also frequently affects this area. If these exterior infections are ignored, they may travel inward and involve the eardrum and the middle ear.

Infections which injure hearing can also be caused by *foreign objects,* such as beads or pencil erasers, which very young children sometimes push into the ear canal. *Such objects should be kept away from them.* Adults can cause similar trouble by "cleaning" their ears with hairpins, matchsticks, or other long objects. There's a lot of sense in the old saying, "Never put anything smaller than your elbow into your ear." Follow this rule for *cleaning the ear canal:* what you cannot remove with your little finger, which has previously been thoroughly cleaned with soap and water, should be removed by a doctor or nurse or at an ear clinic. If wax is deeply embedded, a doctor can wash it out with an ear syringe; ask him to show you how to do this if wax tends to accumulate frequently in your ear canal. Never try to clean out a child's ear unless a doctor or nurse has given you instructions. Ordinary washing of the external portions with soap and water is all that is necessary in most cases.

Some people believe that a *chronic running ear* cannot be cured. This is completely false. It is possible to cure almost every case of chronically infected ears. Sometimes it may be necessary to go to an ear specialist or to a hospital many miles away, but it is always worthwhile to clear up a

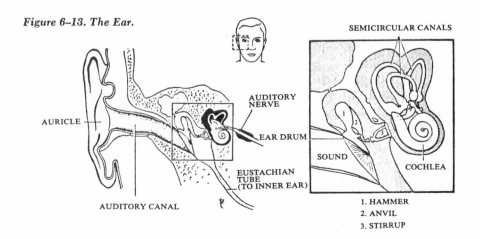

*Figure 6–13. The Ear.*

AURICLE

AUDITORY NERVE

EAR DRUM

EUSTACHIAN TUBE (TO INNER EAR)

AUDITORY CANAL

SEMICIRCULAR CANALS

SOUND

COCHLEA

1. HAMMER
2. ANVIL
3. STIRRUP

condition which may ruin your hearing or that of your child.

*Swimming* rarely causes any trouble to the ears unless there is an infection in the nose, sinuses, or throat. Learning how to breathe *in* through the mouth and *out* through the nose when you are swimming will help prevent this. Of course, the situation is different with a *perforated eardrum*. In that case, you *must* have your doctor's permission and advice before you go swimming. Once in a great while the eardrum can be perforated by the pressure of high diving. Pain and sometimes bleeding will result. If you see a doctor immediately afterward, there will probably be no permanent harm from such an accident.

DEAFNESS. Infections are not the only cause of *deafness*. The changes of old age may gradually bring on deafness, which in many cases can be somewhat relieved by a doctor. Another type of deafness, called *otosclerosis*, may start in earlier years. It involves bone changes within the ear that impair the transmission of sound vibrations. A special operation can relieve this type of deafness. Your doctor will probably need the help of an ear specialist (*otologist*) to decide whether this type of hearing loss can be helped in this way.

Many types of deafness can be greatly helped by *hearing aids*. It is tragic to think of all the people whose lives have been seriously handicapped because, as I have so often heard a deaf person say, "People will make fun of me if I wear such a thing." Personally, I can't see anything funny in today's well-designed hearing aids. I wish everyone who needs one would forget the ancient and seedy jokes on the subject, and think of hearing aids in the same way we are learning to think of eyeglasses. Since all types of deafness are not alike, these instruments vary, and it is important to find the right one. An ear specialist, not a salesman, can give you the right advice. Hearing aids for the elderly are discussed on page 536.

The most important thing you can do to prevent deafness is to have your hearing, and especially that of your children, tested and to see a doctor the minute you or your child feels any pain, has a discharge from the ear, notices any unusual buzzing, ringing or pressure in the ears, or experiences any loss of hearing.

## NOSE

The nose, with its bones, cartilage, nerves, and mucous membranes (which contain glands secreting a watery fluid) is the organ of smell; and more important, it is the means by which we take air into our bodies. We can—and some people do —get along by breathing through the mouth. While this is not dangerous, as some people believe, it is by no means satisfactory. The nose is a far better ventilator. It filters out dust, provides moisture, and acts as an air conditioner by warming the air we take in.

The most common disease of the nose—in fact, the most common disease in the world—is the *common cold*, which involves the mucous membrane of the upper part of the nose. You'll certainly want to read the section I devote to prevention and treatment of the cold (p. 495).

In addition to colds, the following diseases cause *congestion of the nose*: hay fever and other allergies (p. 498), chronic infections, nasal polyps, sinusitis (p. 498), and a deviated or crooked septum. Adenoids may also be the cause in children (p. 290). Your doctor, or a specialist in ear, nose, and throat (usually referred to as an ENT specialist) can help all these conditions.

*Ozena* is a disease characterized by crusting in the nose and unpleasant odor. However, a persistent, foul-smelling discharge in children is usually caused by the fact that some *foreign object* such as a bean or pencil eraser is lodged deep in the nasal passage. Always have a doctor take care of this.

How to stop a *nosebleed* is an essential part of the first aid information everyone should have (p. 340). It may simply mean that a small blood vessel in the nose needs to be cauterized, which your doctor can attend to in a few minutes. On the other hand, nosebleeds are sometimes a sign of rheumatic fever, typhoid fever, or other diseases. If your nose bleeds frequently without any obvious cause, it requires your doctor's attention.

Should an *unsightly nose* be changed by *plastic surgery*? This is a problem you should talk over with your doctor. If he advises an operation he will refer you to a surgeon who specializes in this type of surgery. Beware of the many quacks who advertise themselves as plastic surgeons. "Nose-shapers," from the time-honored clothespin to patented gadgets, don't do any good.

CLEANSING THE NOSE. Your nose needs little regular care. Don't use nose drops, sprays, or "sniffers" unless your doctor tells you to. Continued use can cause irritation or injury. They won't cure chronic sinusitis or catarrh (*postnasal drip* is one of the current terms for this condition). The chances are that you don't have chronic sinusitis; this condition is quite rare and can only be diagnosed by a physician (see the discussion of sinusitis, p. 498). Catarrh simply means an inflammation of the mucous membranes with increased secretions of their glands. It can be caused by a great many things, such as an allergy, a vitamin deficiency, or by spending most of your time in dry rooms filled with cigarette smoke. Nose drops and sprays won't help under any of these circumstances. They will just add to your troubles if your catarrh is due, as it often is, to the fact that your membranes happen to be overly sensitive. I know that a postnasal drip is unpleasant, and it can cause irritation in the throat; but if you won't go to a doctor, the next best thing you can do for it is to leave it alone! I can at least assure you that the

mucus which accumulates is *not*, as you may have been told, "full of dangerous germs and will poison you or ruin your digestion if you swallow it." It's quite harmless.

## LIPS, TONGUE, AND MOUTH

Most diseases and sores of the lips, tongue, and mouth are either very minor or very serious. The slight cracks from dried-out lips heal readily, and the irritating lumpy spots in the mouth called *cankers* disappear quickly. But other whitish spots, lumps, or sores may indicate early stages of cancer, or they may be signs of syphilis or some other serious disease. You can usually tell the mild from the serious conditions by the rapidity with which they heal. *Any canker, cold sore, or lump that does not heal readily should be seen by a doctor or a dentist* (it may be due to a rough spot on a tooth which is irritating the lining of the mouth). Even some serious conditions can be corrected if they are discovered early enough, so never delay.

*Vincent's angina* (trench mouth) is a common infection characterized by sores and ulcers on the lining of the cheeks, the gums, and the back of the throat. Some people, particularly young ones, conceal the fact that they have trench mouth because they have heard that it is "a disease of filth" or "it can only be caught by kissing." Both ideas are false. Never neglect trench mouth. Your doctor or dentist can usually cure it quickly in its early stages, and even later it responds well to penicillin.

The *parotid* and *submaxillary glands* in the mouth can be affected, most commonly by mumps, and rarely by tumors or stones that block their passages.

Most lipsticks are harmless unless you happen to be allergic to something in them. They have no value except for their appearance. Cracked chapped lips, from which you may suffer during cold or dry, hot weather, will usually get better if you apply a soothing ointment such as boric acid ointment, petroleum jelly, or cold cream.

Your mouth does not need, and may actually be harmed by, "medication" that claims to cure

*Figure 6–14. The Nose. Side view. Note the opening of the eustachian tube which runs from the middle ear.*

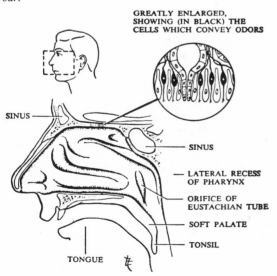

GREATLY ENLARGED, SHOWING (IN BLACK) THE CELLS WHICH CONVEY ODORS

SINUS

SINUS

LATERAL RECESS OF PHARYNX

ORIFICE OF EUSTACHIAN TUBE

SOFT PALATE

TONSIL

TONGUE

*halitosis* (p. 70) and other conditions. Mouth washes, antiseptic lozenges, and gargles come in contact with only the surface of the mouth, and do not reach the germs which are more deeply located when infection is present. They may provide a pleasant taste.

## THROAT AND TONSILS

The throat cavity, or *pharynx,* is separated from the mouth by the *soft palate* and the *uvula,* and leads into the *esophagus* (the gullet). The *tonsils* lie on each side of the back of the mouth. Like the *adenoids,* which are located in back of the throat, near the nasal passages at the eustachian tubes, the tonsils are masses of *lymphoid tissue* which play a part in dealing with germs that enter the throat.

Like your nose and mouth, your throat does not need sprays, gargles, or lozenges to keep it healthy. Avoid them because their regular use may cause irritation.

*Sore throats* are almost as common as colds, for a certain amount of inflammation in the throat usually results from the cold itself. They may even be due to irritation caused by excessive smoking. If cutting down on your smoking and gargling every two to three hours (I suggest a third of a glassful of warm water containing two crushed aspirin tablets) do not bring relief in a few days, visit your doctor or a hospital clinic. Serious conditions may begin with a sore throat (see page 290).

*Cancer* of the lip, mouth, and throat are definitely connected with smoking, especially heavy smoking. This does not mean that everyone who smokes must live in fear of cancer, but that smokers should be alert to any sores of the lip, mouth, or throat, and have any stubborn irritation checked by a doctor quickly.

Any *acutely sore throat* accompanied by fever in either an adult or a child may mean trouble. It may indicate the early stages of *diphtheria* (p. 297), *scarlet fever* (p. 291), a *septic sore throat* (an acute streptococcal infection) (p. 290), or a *serious infection of the tonsils* (tonsillitis) (p. 290). Be sure to call a doctor or go to a hospital immediately. If these conditions are treated promptly, they can quickly be cured. You may wonder why your doctor gives you an injection or some pills to swallow instead of applying something directly to the infected throat area. He does this because local applications do not reach the germs which are below the surface, whereas medication taken internally attacks the germs through the bloodstream. *Penicillin* works wonders in most throat infections. However, if a doctor is available, don't take it in any form, not even penicillin lozenges, unless he says you should. Always be very careful to avoid getting fatigued or chilled while you are recovering from a sore throat. These simple precautions will help prevent you from getting a serious illness such as *pneumonia* (p. 443) or Bright's disease (p. 422).

REMOVAL OF TONSILS. Should your child's tonsils (and adenoids) or your own be removed? Certainly not as a routine measure. If they are chronically diseased, that is, so full of germs that they can't possibly act as a protection but become a source of infection themselves, they should be taken out. The fact that they are large is not, in itself, cause for removal. Only a doctor—not a friend or neighbor—is qualified to decide whether or not tonsils should be removed. He will take into consideration not only the tonsils themselves, but the condition of the individual and the time of the year, avoiding seasons when polio (infantile paralysis) and certain other diseases are prevalent (see polio, page 464).

## LARYNX, TRACHEA, AND NECK

The *larynx,* which projects itself on the outside of the body as the Adam's apple, is part of the breathing apparatus. Its main function, however, is to act as a voice box in producing sounds.

Hoarseness is a sign that something may be wrong with your larynx. Naturally, if you have been shouting and cheering at a football game the day before, the reason is obvious. But if hoarseness or a change in your voice comes on without apparent cause, and lasts longer than a few days, it may indicate a tumor or some other potentially serious condition of the larynx. Immediate attention is essential. See your doctor or the throat specialist he recommends, without delay.

The *trachea* is the windpipe through which air enters and leaves the lungs. (See Figure 6-5, page 94.) It is connected with the throat by way of the larynx. Although it is protected by a lid (the *epiglottis*), food particles sometimes get into it; most of us have, on some occasion, "swallowed something the wrong way." People, particularly children, have choked to death because an object large enough to block the trachea completely has entered it or has lodged in the throat and shut off the passage of air. This is one of the situations in which a knowledge of first aid can mean the difference between life and death (see page 336 for emergency treatment). One reason I have cautioned you against using nose or throat drops and sprays lies in the fact that they (especially if they have an oily base) may be inhaled through the windpipe and irritate it, the bronchi, or the lungs.

The neck contains the *thyroid gland* (p. 81), an endocrine gland which is subject to several disorders that respond readily to treatment if it is started early. Simple goiter (p. 81), now quite rare, reveals itself in an enlargement of this gland, which is located below the Adam's apple and slightly above the notch of the breastbone. A more serious type of goiter is caused by an overactive thyroid gland; this is called hyperthyroidism, Graves' disease, and exophthalmic goiter (p. 82).

You are probably familiar with a fairly common condition of the neck usually called *swollen glands.* This is an enlargement of the *lymph nodes,* usually called the *lymph glands.* If these glands are painful, it means that there is an infection somewhere in the head. It may be in the scalp, for example, and be caused by nits or cuts and sores; or it may be due to sore throat, tonsillitis, sinusitis, and other types of infection. Relatively painless swollen glands may be caused by potentially serious illnesses such as tuberculosis (p. 441) and Hodgkin's disease (p. 431).

Make it a rule to see a doctor immediately whenever a swelling occurs in *any* of the glands of the throat. Let him know if you notice unusual lumps of any kind. They may not mean anything serious, but the cause *must* be satisfactorily established.

A stiff neck commonly is the result of a muscle cramp precipitated by a chill, sleeping in a cramped position, tonsillitis, unaccustomed exercise, or sudden twisting of the neck. This type usually yields to hot wet packs, hot showers, massage, and aspirin. Other kinds of stiff neck, such as those caused by arthritis or a spinal disc problem, need professional help. A form of stiff neck that is difficult to treat is *spasmodic torticollis,* in which the head becomes abnormally twisted to the side. Sometimes, injection of a local anesthetic into tender muscle areas (trigger points) helps.

## FEET

I am going to tell you a good deal about how to care for your feet because many of the troubles involving this part of the body are due solely to improper care, neglect, or downright abuse. I am inclined to believe that the feet cause a big percentage of *avoidable* man (and woman) hours of suffering in the world. Seven out of ten people have some foot trouble. I don't know why they

*Figure 6–15. A Normal Foot. Note the correct angle (indicated by dotted lines), the "bridge," and the footprint.*

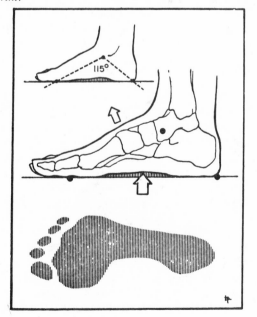

endure this type of pain stoically, when a far smaller amount of suffering in any other part of the body would send them rushing to a doctor. (Incidentally, people seem to be more reluctant to consult a doctor about the two ends of their bodies, the feet and the mind, than they are about any of the parts in between!)

Although certain foot conditions require the attention of a doctor, most of them can be prevented or helped by things you can do yourself.

First of all, wear *correctly fitted shoes.* If your foot is normal, choose a flexible shank shoe with round toes and a straight inner border. It should be long and wide and deep enough not to cramp the toes or restrict the circulation. The cut of the vamp, and the trimmings and straps of women's shoes often interfere with the circulation. Shoes should be small enough to fit snugly around the heel and provide some support. Medium heels are best, and rubber ones provide good "cushions" for walking on hard surfaces. Wearing spike heels puts your weight on the big toe instead of on the heels where it belongs. However, alternating between high and low heels won't, of itself, cause any damage, and it is certainly better than wearing high heels all the time. In the summer your feet need better ventilation, so your shoes should be roomier and made of lighter, more porous material. Have two pairs of shoes in regular use and wear them alternately, keeping the other pair on shoe trees so they will hold their shape while the perspiration they have absorbed dries out of them.

FOOT TROUBLES. If you think your feet are *not* normal, *don't* buy any kind of "remedial" shoes or get arch supporters without consulting a doctor. You may be "correcting" the wrong thing; or your troubles may be due to something entirely apart from the shoes you're wearing. Your socks or stockings may not fit properly, thus bending or cramping the toes or causing calluses and blisters. Your feet may be swelling because your garters restrict the circulation. You may be putting too much of a burden on them because you are overweight (p. 44).

You may have to stand or walk too much on hard surfaces. Walking around a little helps to relieve the strain of standing; and getting your feet up on a couch or footstool for even a few minutes' rest at a time often does wonders. You may not be standing or walking properly. When you stand, your feet should be parallel with each other, not toeing out. When you walk, your footprints should make tracks that would almost touch a straight line drawn between them, with the heels just a trifle further away from the line than the toes. This is not walking pigeon-toed, but it certainly isn't toeing out, which is fortunately no longer fashionable.

Your foot troubles can be due to *flat feet* or *fallen arches.* Both these conditions should be diagnosed by a doctor (*not* a shoe salesman) who can help you to cure them. Flat feet can be inherited or caused by overweight or wearing improper shoes in childhood. If you think you have flat feet or fallen arches, the following exercises may help; they won't hurt you if your diagnosis is wrong, provided you do them in moderation.

With your shoes off, sit in a chair and pretend there is sand on the floor, and that you are heaping it into a pile between your feet by drawing them together in a scooping motion.

Put some marbles on the rug in front of you; pick one up with your toes and throw it forward.

Repeat these exercises, but stop if your feet become tired.

*Figure 6–16. Fallen Arch. The angle (indicated by dotted lines) is wider, the "bridge" is lower, and the footprint is solid.*

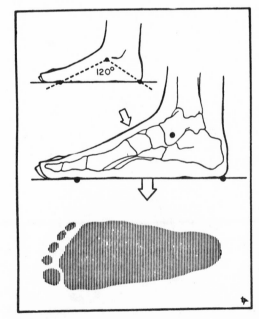

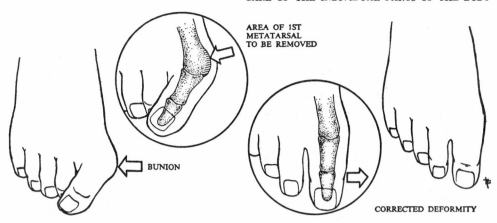

*Figure 6–17. A Bunion, Before and After Surgical Correction.*

*Corns* and *calluses* can cause a great deal of suffering. The best way to avoid them is by wearing shoes that fit. Corns are of two varieties: *hard corns,* usually found on the outside of the little toe, and *soft corns* between the toes. They are hardened or thickened skin which, unlike a callus, have a central point or core.

I have seen so many people get into trouble by using corn remedies or cutting their own corns that I wish everyone would have them removed by a podiatrist (a person who specializes in care of the feet). However, common sense tells me some of you are going to go right on attending to your own corns, so I'll give you directions for the best way to do it—with the following provision: anyone who is not in good health, who suffers from poor circulation, and, above all, *anyone who is a diabetic should never treat his own corns.* In addition, never treat corns or warts on the *soles* of your feet, as they usually require expert care.

For hard corns, soak the toes in warm water for about fifteen minutes, apply a drop or two of 10 percent *salicylic acid in collodion.* Cover the corn with a plain cornpad of the right size, and leave it on for three or four days. Then soak the toe again; the corn will probably lift out easily. If it doesn't, see a podiatrist. For soft corns, pare down the horny rim *very* carefully with a razor blade or scissors (which has been thoroughly washed and scalded, or left for a few minutes in alcohol), taking great care not to cut too far. If you should nick the skin, apply

iodine and *leave the corn alone.* After you have pared the corn, cover it with a plain pad or piece of adhesive plaster, to protect it from pressure, and keep it as dry as possible. It will probably get better; if it doesn't, see a podiatrist. *Calluses* can be removed by paring them off carefully.

A *bunion* is a deformity of the big toe, almost always caused by wearing shoes which force it to turn toward the other toes. It is frequently associated with flat or weak feet. In mild cases, the pain can be relieved by heat, and the condition will correct itself after properly fitting shoes have been worn for some time. In more severe cases, a physician should be consulted, since a surgical operation may be necessary to correct the condition.

*Ingrown toenails* can be prevented by wearing good shoes and by keeping the nails short, with the sides a little longer than the middle. Badly ingrown toenails should *always* be treated by a doctor or podiatrist, since a serious infection may result. If you have a slightly ingrown toenail, insert a tiny bit of cotton that has been soaked in castor oil under the ingrown edge of the nail; protect the nail from pressure by a pad of clean gauze.

*Athlete's foot (dermatophytosis)* is another condition which frequently requires a doctor's attention. It is caused by a fungus which is a tiny form of plant life. This organism grows on the dead cells that make up the calluses and "old skin" of the feet, and thrives on warmth and dampness.

It causes itching or burning spots, and often blisters, usually between the toes. In addition to the discomfort it causes, it provides sites for more serious infections. If you insist on treating it yourself, the following method is safe:

Dry your feet thoroughly and keep them as dry as possible. Wear socks that will absorb moisture, without being so rough as to irritate the skin, and shoes that fit well without being "airtight." After drying your feet, apply a mild alcoholic solution—rubbing alcohol or toilet water. Dry again. Put some plain unscented talcum powder on your feet and in your shoes. Keep your toenails short. Gently remove all scaly, soggy, or horny material from between your toes and from the soles of your feet. Put pledgets of lamb's wool or absorbent cotton between the toes if they are too close together. And use Desenex ointment over the infected, itching areas morning and night.

If the condition is severe, it may well be, as recent research by Drs. James J. Leyden and Albert M. Kligman at the University of Pennsylvania Hospital indicates, that it has been complicated by bacteria. In such cases, they have found, applying a special aluminum chloride solution wice a day with a cotton-tipped applicator brings relief of itching and malodor within forty-eight to seventy-two hours and marked abatement of all symptoms within a week. It would be well to see your doctor, who may suggest use of aluminum chloride, which a druggist can prepare when requested to make up "a solution of 30 percent aluminum chloride ($AlCl_3 \cdot 6\ H_2O$)."

It would be well, too, to see your physician if the condition is severe because you may not have athlete's foot at all, but some other skin condition that resembles it; or you may have an allergy or be sensitive to something with which your feet come in contact.

Other things that you can do to help care for your feet include: Keep them clean. Bathe them at least once daily, drying them carefully, and dust them with a plain talcum powder. It often helps to put them in hot water for a minute or two, then into cold water for just an instant, after which they should be rubbed briskly as they are being dried. Tired feet are often relieved by massage; use a kneading, rotary motion of the hands, with some plain cold cream, olive oil, or cocoa butter if they are dry or irritated. The following foot powders help check unpleasant perspiration and also reduce the danger of epidermophytosis. Use *Desenex powder* or a preparation made as follows:

Thymol, 0.5 grams
Salicylic acid, 2.0 grams
Talcum sufficient to make 100 grams

Apply either powder morning and night. If excessive perspiration persists, see a doctor.

## SKIN

The skin is the largest organ of the body. I shouldn't wonder if it seems strange to you to think of it in this way, because it did to me when I was a medical student.

### Function and Structure

The skin has many functions, the first and most obvious of which is to serve an as envelope, a *protection* against germs and cold and against the drying out of the body's vital fluids. The skin is resilient and tough enough to protect the soft underlying tissues from bruises and other mechanical injuries. In addition, it helps to *regulate* the body's temperature by the evaporation of perspiration and by contracting or relaxing the superficial blood vessels; it acts as an *organ of sense* because of the many nerve endings it contains; it can *absorb* certain substances; and it plays a part in the process of *elimination*. It's fortunate indeed that the skin is able to "grow back" and renew itself quite well when a portion of it is destroyed.

The *skin* is made up of two layers, the outer (called the *epidermis* or *cuticle*) and the inner (called the *dermis*, the *corium*, or the *true skin*). The amount of pigment in the lower portion of the epidermis determines whether the skin will be black or yellow, brunette or blond. *Hairs* are epidermal growths, and *nails* are a modification of the epidermal cells. The *sebaceous glands*, which open into the *follicles* from which the hairs emerge, produce lubricating and protecting oils.

The *sweat glands* lie coiled about in the dermis with ducts leading to the surface.

The skin reflects a great deal about the state of the body, as you have undoubtedly noticed in some sick people; and also the state of the mind, as you can plainly see when someone is blushing from embarrassment, or pale with fear.

## Care of the Skin

Normal skin requires chiefly to be kept clean with soap and water. Always use a *clean* washcloth or complexion brush. Don't massage the soap into your skin. Always rinse thoroughly. Normal skin tends to become dry with middle age, so that a plain cold cream or oily lotion is helpful. In the winter, use less soap than you do in warm weather, and always dry your skin thoroughly. Germicidal soaps and antiseptics are not necessary for either men or women. They can be irritating, and healthy skin isn't bothered by the germs that land on it. Of course, you should take care of cuts and abrasions.

The most important thing to do for your skin is to observe the suggestions in the chapter on general care of the body (p. 13). Avoid infections and irritating substances while you are at work (p. 142) and in the preparations you use on your skin (p. 498 on allergy).

## Shaving (for Men)

Almost every man I know is absolutely certain that his method of shaving is the best ever devised. I think that is true of mine, too! I give it here for those who are starting to shave, or who are troubled by frequent cuts or infections.

Because infections can be carried from the hands onto the face, I always start by cleaning my nails and washing my hands carefully. Then I wash my face briskly with warm, soapy water, and dry it gently with a clean cloth. Now I start applying the shaving cream. Having a really tough beard, which frequently must be shaved twice a day, I use very warm water, work in the brushless type of cream carefully, and then let it stay on, warm and wet, for 2 to 3 minutes. Now I shave, always using a fresh blade in a good-quality safety razor. I find it rare to cut myself since I adopted

*Figure 6–18. Structure of the Skin. The numbers indicate the sensory nerve endings: (1) warmth; (2) pain; (3) cold; (4) touch; (5) deep pressure.*

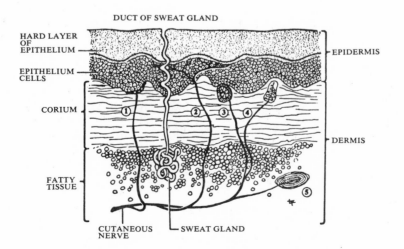

the following routine: to sit in a comfortable chair, using a good shaving mirror. I try to keep my mind, at least partly, on the shaving, rather than on the day's work ahead of me. It is helpful to stretch the skin in front of the path of a safety-razor blade, the way a professional barber does with his straight-edge blade.

After the shave is completed, I wash my face completely with warm water, and follow with generous amounts of after-shave lotion (ask your druggist to give you pure 70 percent alcohol if you don't react well to the perfumed solutions). Then I powder, especially over any areas that look chafed.

*For cuts:* The ordinary small cut will stop bleeding if you merely dab on *cold* water with pieces of clean tissue paper. Then stick on a piece of dry tissue paper. Usually by the time the shave is finished, you can remove the tissue gently with cold water, and the bleeding has been effectively stanched. If necessary, use a styptic.

*For infections:* I haven't had one in so many years after following the above routines that all I can say is that "prevention is worth more than cure." However, if you do have an infection on the face, shave around the area. (Skin infections are discussed on page 125). When infection is present, discontinue using a shaving brush if that is your method. Use a new blade each time, and shave the noninfected portions of the face first. If the infection covers a fairly large area, your doctor may want you to continue shaving daily, even over the infection, so that the medicine he prescribes can penetrate better into the infected hair follicles.

*Electric razors:* Men who use electric razors insist that anyone who gives them a fair try will be converted. For men with heavy beards whose work requires them to be free from "5 o'clock shadow" for late business calls or meetings, having a spare electric razor at work can be a godsend.

## Excess Hair in Women

Excess hair can be unattractive, and I don't blame anyone for wanting to get rid of it. But why not try bleaching first, using ordinary peroxide to which a drop of ammonia has been added? (Avoid bleaches containing sodium perborate.) If you must remove excess hair, the simplest way to do it is by shaving. If you use an electric razor (and there are some made especially for women), your skin won't become tough. Despite what you may have heard, shaving does *not* encourage the growth of hair or make it coarse. It's better and far easier than rubbing hair off with an abrasive such as pumice, and far less painful than pulling out hairs with tweezers. If there aren't too many excess hairs, you can cut them off very short with a pair of cuticle scissors.

Be very careful about the use of a *chemical depilatory* on the face; the waxes are safer, though painful. If you do use a chemical depilatory on your body, be very careful not to get it into your eyes. *Always try it on a small spot of skin to see whether it is irritating.* Don't use one more often than once every two weeks, and discontinue immediately if the skin becomes inflamed or itches.

None of these depilatories will remove hair permanently. The only permanent method is electrolysis, involving the insertion of a tiny needle into the hair follicle. An electric current is passed through the needle, and the root is destroyed. This difficult and tedious method is useful only for removing hair from small areas. Some women have had hair successfully and permanently removed in this way from their upper lip or from their cheek. Keep away from quacks or people who advertise miraculous methods for removing hair. Your doctor will help you find an expert who can do this work with safety to you, so that you won't find you have substituted ugly scars and pits for your excess hair.

## Wrinkles

Wrinkles must be the greatest skin problem of all, judging from the number of questions I have heard about it. Dermatologists place some blame for wrinkles on sunshine. This certainly doesn't mean that you should hide in the house! It does mean that you should exercise some care in the amount of direct or reflected sunlight you expose yourself to.

A close second in causing wrinkles is another of life's necessities, soap and water. The average housewife unthinkingly rinses her hands before she touches anything, and perhaps afterward. Without realizing it, she may rinse her hands dozens of times a day. I don't suggest that you give up cleanliness, but it is a good idea to do some of your housework wearing rubber gloves, or to rub on a good hand lotion from time to time. Bath oils have become popular because women have seen how nice their skin looks after anointing it with oil. Besides, a soaking bath is a good way to relax.

Massaging your skin won't prevent wrinkles. It won't do anything except, possibly, make you feel good. "Skin foods" won't do any good; your skin doesn't need these products because it, like any other organ, is fed by your body. Wearing "wrinkle eradicators" or "masks" to bed every night won't do any good either. In fact, once wrinkles or lines have made their appearance, the only way to get rid of them is by plastic surgery. This is expensive, lasts only a few years, and should be done *only* by a surgeon experienced in this field (a plastic surgeon). I consider it worthwhile in only rare instances, as in the case of an actress whose youthful appearance may be important in her profession. As far as the average woman is concerned—why not just avoid frowning and smile instead, so that when wrinkles or lines do appear they will add to, rather than detract from, your appearance?

If an obese person loses weight too quickly (more than three or four pounds a week), the skin can become loose. Weight loss should be undertaken at a moderate pace. If this careful loss is combined with exercise and possibly with massage, the skin will not become loose and wrinkled.

"Wrinkle removers" and "rejuvenating creams" *can be dangerous if they contain hormones;* most of them are useless. Exaggerated claims are made for many lotions, tissue creams, muscle oils, astringents, skin conditioners, and so on. If you find yourself sorely tempted to use one, consult your local Better Business Bureau or write to the American Medical Association, 535 North Dearborn Street, Chicago 10, Illinois.

## Cosmetics

Since I'm afraid I've been rather discouraging about "beauty aids," I'm glad to be able to tell you that most *cosmetics* on the market today will not hurt your skin and may improve your appearance. Lipstick, powder, and rouge are usually harmless unless you happen to be allergic or sensitive to them (often, to the perfume they contain). Some lipsticks dry the lips, but experimenting will help most women to find a suitable one. Pancake make-up and powder bases may clog the pores, and it is important to wash them off or remove them with cleansing cream every night.

There is usually no important difference, aside from the appearance, odor, and packaging, between expensive and inexpensive cosmetics.

## Common Skin Troubles

You've noticed that all skins are not alike. The amount of pigment varies, and so does the number of lubricating and sweat glands.

PIGMENTATION, SPOTS, AND FRECKLES. The less pigment the skin contains, the lighter its color will be; those rare people who have no pigment at all are called *albinos*. If your skin produces little pigment, you should guard against sunburn (p. 155). Some people have skin that will *freckle* on exposure to sun. If you are a freckler and have to spend a good deal of time in the sun, expose your skin as little as possible. A sunscreen lotion containing PABA (*p*-aminobenzoic acid) is helpful. White areas (vitiligo) that appear on the skin are usually due to a loss of pigment in certain areas. If they are conspicuous the best thing to do about them is to cover them, or avoid getting tanned, which makes them more conspicuous.

*Do not use a "freckle remover."* Anything that is strong enough to be effective may cause a severe inflammation unless it is used under a doctor's supervision. Usually, the best thing to do about freckles is to cover them with face powder or, if necessary, *Covermark*, or a similar preparation. Those people who have such disfiguring freckles that they are unhappy, should ask their doctors to refer them to a dermatologist or a skin clinic for a trial of more intensive treatments. The same is true of the "liver spots" (*chloasma*) which may occur in dark-skinned people. (These marks have nothing to do with the liver, and are simply increases in pigmentation.) Fortunately, many young people "outgrow" their freckles.

EXCESSIVE PERSPIRATION. This may be due to poor health; night sweats, for example, are characteristic of certain diseases. However, if you are in good health, but perspire excessively, especially under the arms, you can probably control it by a commercial antiperspirant deodorant. These preparations contain an aluminum salt, which is usually perfectly safe, unless you happen to be allergic or sensitive to this chemical. It is always wise to try any preparation cautiously for the first few times, using very little of it until you are sure it is all right for you, and stopping if repeated applications cause irritation. If you wipe off the excess after you apply commercial antiperspirants and deodorants, they usually will not harm the clothing, although they may discolor it. Chlorophyll preparations do not check perspiration, and while they are deodorants, they are no more effective than simply dusting your armpits with plain bicarbonate of soda (baking soda). It does no harm to check perspiration in the armpits, the hands, or the feet, as the rest of the body surface will do the work of eliminating it; but never apply an antiperspirant to the entire body. And don't take too seriously the "scare-propaganda" about "B.O."

The medical name for offensive body odor is *bromidrosis*. Truly offensive body odor is rare; it can usually be prevented by bathing and by using a deodorant or antiperspirant under the arms. No special soap is necessary. Men may prefer to wash under the arms regularly with soap, then follow with an application of rubbing alcohol which, when dried, can be covered with an absorbent powder such as the ordinary preparations for babies.

DRY SKIN. An insufficient production of fat by the sebaceous glands in the skin causes dry skin. This often occurs in middle and old age, encouraging wrinkling. If your skin is dry, don't wash it too often with soap and water; use a cleansing cream or oil or a soap substitute. Before going to bed, apply an emollient (lubricating) cream which usually contains lanolin or cholesterol, which is derived from lanolin, blended with vegetable fats and oils. Do not use plain lanolin. Olive oil or one of the commercial products such as

*Nivea* cream is satisfactory. Apply more frequently if necessary.

Dry skin is very apt to *chap* during cold weather or when the air is very dry. If your skin becomes chapped, treat it as I have just suggested that you treat dry skin. A commercial lotion or a hand cream is good for chapped hands.

CHAFING. This is caused by friction, usually from clothing or the rubbing together of body surfaces, such as the thighs, that are damp with perspiration. Keeping the parts dry, and using a good plain talcum powder, will usually clear up the irritation.

*Prickly heat* is often found in infants. It is due to retention of sweat. Treatment is directed at reducing sweating generally by as cool an environment as possible, light clothing, avoidance of tight garments. Bland powders may be helpful.

*Frostbite* is due to extreme cold, and usually attacks the nose, ears, fingers, or toes. The cold part should be warmed very gradually. *Don't* rub on snow or massage the frostbitten area, as this can damage the skin. If the frostbite is severe, see a physician, as gangrene can result unless treatment is started in time.

*Oily skin* can be more distressing than dry skin. To correct it, use plenty of soap and water, avoid creams and greasy lotions, and follow the rules I gave you for general care of the body. Go easy on heavy powder or pancake make-up, always washing it off thoroughly at night.

The main problem faced by many people with oily skin is *acne*, which I shall take up next.

## Acne

You probably call them pimples, blackheads, and whiteheads; we doctors call them *acne vulgaris*. This condition is so characteristic of youth that I can't help wondering who coined the slogan, "Keep that schoolgirl complexion." As boys and girls approach maturity, their glandular activity increases, including that of the sebaceous glands of the skin. In girls this may become pronounced at the time of their menstrual periods. Certain foods increase the activity of the sebaceous glands, among the worst offenders being chocolate, nuts, sharp cheeses, and fat or greasy food. If the pore opening is small or clogged by dirt or heavy cosmetics, the fatty material made by the sebaceous gland accumulates, and a "bump" appears under the skin—or perhaps a *whitehead* or a *blackhead* (a *comedone*). Blackheads are not due to dirt, but to the discoloring effect of air on the fatty material in the clogged pore. If this substance becomes infected, as it often does, a pimple results. The temptation to squeeze the unsightly pimple should be resisted. A hard push, and the membrane around the pimple is broken, so that the infection spreads to the surrounding tissue; it also spreads on the surface unless it is carefully washed off. The result —more pimples, and scar tissue or pits.

This story is all too familiar, especially to young people. All too familiar, too, is the suggestion that "you'll grow out of it, so grin and bear it." That is not good enough for the sensitive person whose appearance is disfigured by acne, or who is accumulating physical—and mental!—scars that will last a lifetime.

Fortunately, we doctors can offer a great deal better advice than that. First of all, try to discover and eliminate any food that encourages acne. For example, you yourself may know that chocolate is responsible. *Don't* arbitrarily cut out all desserts and fats, as they are an important part of the food you eat. Just go easy on rich foods, greasy foods, and chocolate—and search for the other ones which you should avoid entirely because they irritate *your* skin.

Keep the skin, particularly on the areas where acne is most apt to appear, such as the face, chest, and back, very clean. Plain soap and fairly hot water are best. Scrub with a *clean* washcloth, but not so hard you hurt the skin. Follow by a cold rinse. Change towels at least daily. Avoid all creams and greasy lotions. Do not plug the pores with heavy make-up or use "pore-closing" beauty aids. If you have pimples, *don't* squeeze them; I know this will take all your will power. Apply a compress wetted with hot water; this will encourage drainage and healing. Hide the offending spot with *Acnomel cake*, which will also help to heal the pimple. *Acnomel cream* is stronger, and

I think it should be used only under a doctor's direction. To get rid of blackheads, soak in warm sudsy water to loosen them, and press gently with a comedone extractor which can be purchased at most drugstores; don't use your fingers. If the blackhead comes out easily, touch the spot with rubbing alcohol (70 percent). If it doesn't come out, leave it alone for a while.

This is the best way to handle ordinary, mild cases of acne. Severe cases require treatment that only a doctor can provide. For severe cases, tetracycline antibiotics taken internally are often helpful. Alternatively, when carefully applied to the skin according to individualized medical direction, vitamin A acid and benzoyl peroxide may be dramatically effective. With expert care, the outlook for greatly diminishing or even completely controlling acne is excellent now. With such care, too, there is far less likelihood of permanent scarring.

Even if acne has scarred your face, medical science can help. "Planing" with a rotary, high-speed brush may be the answer. It consists in removing the outer layer of pitted skin, leaving the portion that contains the glands and hair follicles. New skin, rosy at first and then fading to a normal color, grows in from the bottom up.

Remember that "planing" is a *surgical operation*, although not a major one. It *must* be performed by a competent doctor, with the same aftercare that follows any operation. *Never* go to a "beauty specialist" for this kind of treatment. In fact, never go to anyone except a doctor, preferably a skin specialist (a *dermatologist*), for acne.

ROSEACEA (*Acne Roseacea*). Despite its name, this condition is quite different from acne. It is popularly known as "whiskey nose," a very unfair name because many people have it who never had a drink in their lives. It is due to a flushing of the blood vessels of the nose and cheeks, and drinking alcohol encourages this nervous reflex. After a time the blood vessels become pronounced, and the size of the nose may increase. Even the worst cases can usually be cured by a doctor. In its mild or early stages, the condition can be controlled by frequent application of cold water,

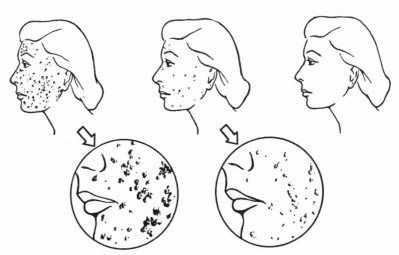

*Figure 6–19. Acne.* Left: *Severe case.* Center: *Severe case after having healed without treatment, leaving scars.* Right: *Properly treated case; no noticeable scars remain after healing.*

witch hazel, or ice, which contract the blood vessels. Pat or rub on gently—do not massage. And, of course, avoid alcohol, and also hot or spicy foods. More severe cases may respond to other measures, including antibiotics and topical preparations.

## Allergies and Sensitivity

In the past, many people used to suffer from rashes and other troublesome skin complaints that refused to yield to treatment; today we know that some of these are due to an allergy (see page 498). People have been familiar for generations with one form of allergy, namely *hives*. These are superficial areas filled with a watery substance, which appear and disappear on the skin, often itching quite badly. They may come out after a certain food has been eaten. *Nettle rash, drug rash,* and *urticaria* are other names for similar conditions. However, a great many medicines can cause drug rashes without hives.

*Itching* caused by allergic reactions can be relieved by applications of calamine lotion or by putting 1 cupful of bicarbonate of soda (baking soda) in the bath water. Of course, the best thing to do is to avoid the substance that causes the reaction. Sometimes this is easy. Many of us have been able to discover, by ourselves, that we get hives or "break out" after eating strawberries, taking a certain medicine, putting away winter clothes in moth balls, using a perfumed soap, wearing certain materials, and so on. It isn't hard to discover whether you, like most of us, are affected by poison ivy. However, in a great many cases physicians with special training in these fields (*dermatologists* and *allergists*) have to work like detectives to discover whether the condition is due to an allergy, and if so, which substance is responsible.

Recent studies have shown that among the leading causes of skin allergies are nickel sulfate (often used in making inexpensive watches, earrings, rings, and bracelets); potassium dichromate (commonly found in tanned leather); household antiseptics containing thimerosal (Merthiolate); *p*-phenylenediamine, an ingredient in many hair dyes.

Having skin that is sensitive to certain substances differs from being allergic to them. Here is an example: if your hands become sore after repeated use of a strong cleansing agent which doesn't irritate them when you use a weak solution, you are sensitive rather than allergic to it. The allergic person reacts to very small amounts of the materials that give him allergic reactions. Some skin is sensitive to many things, including the rays of the sun that cause sunburn. Tracking down a sensitivity can be difficult, too.

*Eczema* is a common and troublesome but *not* contagious skin disease which is at times of an allergic nature.

## Emotional Factors

It can be even more difficult to discover whether emotional factors are responsible for a skin condition, although here, too, some cases are fairly obvious. Perhaps you have known someone who gets a rash on the neck when embarrassed or angry.

There are indications that emotional factors may play a part in psoriasis. Neither this nor eczema can be cured as miraculously as claimed by any patented or advertised remedy, so don't waste any time or money before you see a doctor who, with skill and patience, can usually get good results.

## Infections of the Skin

Because of its exposed position, the skin can be infected by microorganisms, including *bacteria*, such as those causing *boils* or *impetigo; viruses* which cause *fever blisters;* parasites which are responsible for *scabies; fungi* which cause such diseases as *athlete's foot;* and the germ of syphilis, called the *spirochete*, which causes *syphilitic lesions.*

*Boils and carbuncles* are caused by pus-forming bacteria. These germs are often present on the skin, but are unable to do any damage unless its resistance has been lowered by such things as irritating friction, cuts, poor health, bad nutrition, or diabetes. A carbuncle is more serious than a boil because it is larger, goes deeper, and is accompanied by a general feeling of illness.

Boils and carbuncles respond readily to treatment by a physician who may incise and open them if necessary, and/or use penicillin—in addition to discovering and eliminating their cause. *Anyone suffering from a carbuncle should see a doctor;* so should anyone who has a number of boils or suffers from them repeatedly. They can be serious. Germs from the boil or carbuncle can get into the blood, with grave, or even fatal, consequences. This is particularly true of a boil or carbuncle on the nose or upper lip, because germs in these areas have easy access to the brain.

If you have a small boil which is *not* on the nose or upper lip, it is usually safe for you to try the following:

Wash the boil and the surrounding area with soap and warm water, several times a day, lightly dabbing on 70 percent alcohol afterward. Cover, not too tightly, with an antiseptic gauze pad to prevent irritation.

In addition, you should apply hot compresses—as warm as you can stand—every hour for 10 minutes at a time. Make these compresses by soaking an antiseptic gauze pad in hot water containing as much salt as will dissolve in it. This helps relieve pain and encourages the boil to drain. Cover with a fresh, dry pad.

If the boil does not get better within a few days, see a doctor. *Do not* open a boil yourself or let an "amateur surgeon" friend do it.

*Impetigo* is also caused by bacteria and is quite contagious, especially in infants. It is characterized by yellowish crusts, often on the face, that look as though they had been applied to the skin. A doctor can easily cure impetigo before other infections set in.

*Folliculitis* is similar to impetigo except that the infection occurs in the hair follicles or the pore openings of the skin. *Barber's itch* is a special case of folliculitis which affects the beard and makes shaving a problem for men afflicted with this frequently very stubborn infection. The medical name for barber's itch is *sycosis vulgaris.* It may take some time to cure even a mild case of folliculitis. You may need one visit to the doctor for instruction in removing the infected hairs.

*Fever blisters (herpes simplex)* are caused by a virus. They usually occur with a fever or cold, and appear around the mouth and nose; or they can follow exposure to sun and wind. Usually they clear up within a week or so. A drying lotion such as 1:500 aluminum acetate in cold water is comforting when applied with bits of cotton. Spirit of camphor is a helpful application in mild cases. Cold cream may help to bring relief during the onset. Troublesome, recurrent fever blisters should be seen by a doctor who may be able to remove the cause, or he may try to immunize you against them.

*Shingles (herpes zoster)* is also caused by a virus which infects part of a nerve, causing an eruption which appears on the skin. People used to say that a patient would die if the shingles completely circled the body, that is, if they "met." This is *absolutely untrue.* There are some potentially dangerous complications from shingles in the eyes and nerves. These should be treated immediately by a doctor.

*Athlete's foot* has been described on page 117.

*The itch* (*scabies*) is extremely contagious, but fortunately yields quickly to treatment. Hands, genitals, and folds in the skin are favorite areas for the tiny itch mite to burrow into the skin. However, almost any part of the body may be affected. It is not easy to tell whether or not one has scabies, and a doctor should always be consulted. The remedies used for scabies can aggravate other skin troubles sometimes confused with it. A doctor or health officer will tell you how to kill the parasites in bed linen and clothes.

Other parasites include *lice* and "*crabs*" (*pubic lice*), both of which can be quickly eliminated by powders or sprays containing certain chemicals— but again, this should be done under a doctor's supervision, as these materials are powerful. *Kwell ointment* is extremely effective in getting rid of pubic lice, usually with one application.

## Growths

*Corns* are caused by pressure, and may occasionally appear in places other than the feet (see page 117 for treatment of corns).

*Birthmarks* include *pigmented moles* and the *vascular birthmarks* such as "strawberry marks." Never attempt to remove either kind yourself. If they are disfiguring, they can be covered by a cosmetic preparation such as *Covermark* or, in many cases, removed by a surgical operation. Your doctor may feel it is best to remove moles located on the palms, soles, or genitals. Any mole that starts to grow or bleed should be seen by a physician.

*Keloids* are growths that do *not* become malignant. They appear in scars, and should not be cut out as they usually reappear in the new scar tissue. A doctor can remove them with radium or "dry ice." Deposits of fat in the skin cause harmless yellow tumors (*xanthoma*) which can be removed by a physician if they are unsightly.

*Keratoses* are soft brown spots that appear in middle age; in the aged, they may be hard, in which case it is usually wise to have them examined by your doctor. They may need to be re-

moved, as they may turn into cancers.

*Warts* are caused by a virus. Don't attempt to remove them yourself, for the only satisfactory methods of getting rid of them are not safe unless they are employed by a physician.

*Cancer* of the skin may be less serious than in any other part of the body because it can be diagnosed and removed early, provided no time is wasted on dangerous home "treatment." Always make certain that any new or changing growth or lesion—a lump, ulcer, or wart—is harmless by consulting a physician, rather than by "waiting to see." (See Cancer, page 429.)

## Other Skin Diseases

*Syphilis* may be the cause of any sore which appears on the genital regions, between three days to three months after sexual intercourse with an infected person. It may manifest itself again about six weeks later in the form of a rash resembling *measles,* accompanied by symptoms somewhat like those of a cold. Although it is not true, as some people believe, that a great many skin diseases are caused by syphilis, there is no time to waste before starting treatment if a sore should be a *venereal skin lesion* or a rash should be caused by this disease. *Be sure to consult a doctor immediately because he can cure this disease immediately*—or set your mind at ease by taking a test that will prove you do not have it. Syphilis does *not* cause pimples and itching. (See page 447 for complete description of syphilis.)

*Erysipelas* (St. Anthony's fire) is a streptococcal infection of the skin which produces a dull red to scarlet rash, chills, very high fever, severe headaches, and nausea and vomiting. It must be treated by a doctor, who can cure it with penicillin or other medication.

*Glanders, anthrax,* and *tularemia* are serious ailments contracted from animals suffering from these diseases. Skin lesions can be important symptoms.

*Rashes* can be caused by a number of contagious diseases such as smallpox, meningitis, measles, and many of the common diseases of childhood. Although I discuss these elsewhere, I want to impress on you the fact that *any rash or abnormal skin condition accompanied by a fever or a general feeling of illness is a danger signal.* If there is no fever, the rash may be due to an allergy or a toxic reaction to some chemical (see page 499 and page 145).

*Lupus erythematosus, pemphigus,* and *scleroderma* are potentially dangerous skin diseases. Lupus erythematosus is characterized by a red eruption of the nose and cheek, which takes the shape of a butterfly. It may follow exposure to sun. This disease frequently remains in its mild form especially if the patient follows the physician's recommendations. Pemphigus usually begins as a *number* of blisters often starting around the nose and mouth and gradually involving the rest of the body. Scleroderma, a hardening of the skin, is usually preceded by changes in the circulation of the skin, especially in the hands and feet, which become cold and bluish. Although these diseases are rare, I mention them in order to remind you that the skin is an important organ of the body, which can be affected by more than minor ailments!

### Never Neglect a Skin Disease

It is important to remember that, in addition to the serious diseases mentioned above, a skin condition can indicate the presence of a deep-seated disease of the lungs, liver, heart, and many other organs of the body, including the *endocrine glands.* It can also indicate general poor health or a *vitamin deficiency.* There are literally hundreds of skin ailments. You can't possibly learn them all. Some of them are difficult to identify. For this reason, and because their significance varies tremendously, it is necessary to consult a doctor. You can see how important it is to discover, for example, whether a rash is due to prickly heat or to a contagious disease.

*Always consult a doctor if anything unusual happens to your skin.*

## FINGERNAILS

These horny growths of skin cells also reflect your general health; the "white spots" that sometimes appear do not, as some people believe, indicate sickness. If your nails are *very* dry and brittle you may need medical attention. Your nails need

little care. In fact, most infections such as *abscesses, whitlows, paronychias,* or *"runarounds"* are usually caused by too much manicuring of the cuticle. Push it back gently. Do not use a sharp instrument for this or for cleaning your nails. Dryness encourages hangnails, and plain oil or a hand cream will help to correct this tendency. A hangnail will heal over in a few days if protected by a small bandage. Any nail polish you fancy is safe to use provided it does not cause irritation owing to an allergy or sensitivity. Always try out a new one on a single nail at bedtime, and make certain it is safe to use on your other fingers in the morning.

## HAIR AND SCALP

Like fingernails, hair is an epidermal growth. It, too, reflects the general condition of your body. For example, an underactive thyroid gland can cause dry, coarse hair.

### Care of the Hair

Keep your hair clean. Wash it no less than every ten days, more often if it tends to be oily. A pure plain toilet soap is the best, melted in a little water if you find it easier to use in liquid form. Good shampoos usually contain nothing more than soap or detergent, along with some perfume to which you may happen to be allergic. Poor shampoos contain borax or an alkali that is usually irritating to the scalp. Washing removes the natural oil in your hair, along with the dirt, and *no* shampoo I have heard of actually lives up to its claim that it restores these oils while washing your hair. For oily hair a tincture of green soap is satisfactory. For dry hair, a castile shampoo is good. Don't forget to wash your comb and brush at least as often as you do your hair.

Rinse your hair carefully after washing. If you have "hard" water, the soap you use is apt to leave a deposit on your hair. Perhaps you will want to use a soapless detergent if you have only very hard water and soap doesn't rinse off properly. Do not rub your hair too hard while drying it. Sunlight or a hair-dryer that blows air on the hair is good. So is brushing it gently as it dries. A little massage is helpful. Don't be drastic

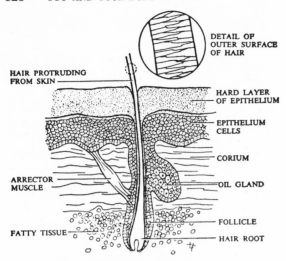

DETAIL OF OUTER SURFACE OF HAIR

HAIR PROTRUDING FROM SKIN

HARD LAYER OF EPITHELIUM

EPITHELIUM CELLS

CORIUM

ARRECTOR MUSCLE

OIL GLAND

FATTY TISSUE

FOLLICLE

HAIR ROOT

*Figure 6–20. Hair and Follicle.*

about it, though; just press the scalp with your fingers and move it about a little to stimulate the fatty tissue under the scalp. Do this once a day. The one hundred daily strokes with a hairbrush which our grandparents used to swear by is excellent for the hair, making it look sleek and glossy and stimulating the sebaceous glands that supply the natural oil.

If your hair is dry, rub in a little pure olive oil or other oil after shampooing, or more often if necessary. Lanolin has been very much overrated; it won't work magic for your hair. Brilliantines and similar pomades are usually made of mineral oil and keep the hair in place, but that is all they do. Sometimes these pomades are so heavy they clog the gland openings, and they may contain irritating substances. It is best to avoid them. If your hair is oily after shampooing, a little alcohol, *quickly rubbed off* (don't leave it on to evaporate) will correct this condition. Do not wet your hair repeatedly to keep it in place; your hairbrush will do this better without drying your hair.

Your hair does *not* need singeing, which you may have been told "seals up the ends of your hair, keeping in the oil, coloring and other vital fluids." It does not do this. Sunlight, while good for your hair in moderation, will not make it grow. Nor will cutting it off or shaving it increase its rate of growth. Keeping it clean and brushed is the best thing you can do for it.

## Dandruff

*Dandruff* is very common and troublesome. In this condition, the outer layer of the scalp peels off in little white scales. Usually these flakes eventually become larger, greasy, and yellowish if the dandruff persists. They may block the openings of the sebaceous glands so that the hair becomes dry. More often, dandruff is associated with an increase of the activity of these grease glands, so that the hair becomes oily. This latter condition is called *oily seborrhea*. The scalp condition may be associated with greasy patches of skin on the face, neck, and body.

You may best clear up mild dandruff by keeping your hair and scalp scrupulously clean by shampooing and rinsing every few days. Your comb and brush should be clean. A moderate amount of exposure to sunlight is helpful.

Almost every type of dandruff, including the severe cases accompanied by itching, scaling, crusts, or inflammation (seborrheic dermatitis), may improve or clear with use of special shampoos containing an ingredient such as sulfur, salicylic acid, or selenium sulfide. Full-strength selenium sulfide shampoo requires a prescription; half strength is available in commercial preparations. The prescription strength may be needed for especially severe cases.

## Gray Hair

The *color* of hair is due to pigment. *Gray hair* is caused by the fact that, for some reason not completely understood, air spaces form in the hair shaft. This usually takes place in middle age, although it can occur prematurely; it does not, however, happen overnight, as the old stories would have us believe, although illness has been known to cause rapid onset of grayness. As yet there is no indication that vitamins or anything else will prevent graying, or will darken hair that has turned gray.

## Bleaching Hair

Hair can be bleached by ordinary hydrogen peroxide to which a drop of ammonia has been added. Sodium perborate bleaches can be harmful, and all bleaching tends to alter the texture of the hair. Personally, I am not enthusiastic about bleaching, because the new hairs, and the new portions of hair around the roots, grow in with their original color.

## Hair Dyes

Hair can also be dyed or tinted. I know of *no completely safe hair dye* that will give your hair a *permanent, natural color*. If you wish to have your hair dyed, be sure to have a small lock tested first to find out whether the dye will irritate your scalp or cause a general illness. Some people have been made seriously ill by hair dye. Always repeat the test process each time you have your hair redyed because you can *develop* a sensitivity. Henna is safe but produces only reddish tones, and it may make the hair brittle. The "rinses" and "tints" such as you can buy in a reliable store are satisfactory. The U.S. Food and Drug Administration certifies many of them as harmless. Although they do not wash off if your hair gets wet, shampooing will remove them—but isn't that an advantage in case you change your mind or decide you like your hair after it has turned completely gray? Remember, too, that in many cases, white hair makes a person look younger rather than older.

*Never* dye your *eyelashes* or *eyebrows* because the skin about them, and your eyes themselves, are extremely sensitive. There have been cases of blindness resulting from attempts to dye eyelashes. A temporary darkener like mascara is relatively safe, but even that may produce irritation.

## Permanent Waves

Whether your hair is curly or straight depends on its structure, so of course you can't change it *permanently*, since it will grow back in its original form. However, hair is pliable, and it can be stretched and made curly (or frizzy) by a hot iron or hair curlers. Too much heat dries it out, or scorches it, and makes it frizzy. Hair that is kinky or too curly can be stretched and straightened.

How safe are permanents? The process depends upon the action of chemicals which make the hair more pliable, so that it takes the shape of the curler, and a "neutralizing" chemical that makes it hold its new shape. These chemicals probably do a *little* harm, at least to the hair, but this isn't important, as hair grows fairly regularly under ordinary circumstances. Far more important is the fact that many people become allergic or sensitive to these chemicals. *Always* have a "test curl" made first, to be certain you will not suffer a reaction which may be severe. Great care should be taken to keep the waving lotions from the eyes and any cuts or sores and to remove them promptly if they do touch any sensitive areas. Too strong a solution of the chemical can injure the hair, so it is important to make certain your beauty parlor operator knows her business. Don't have permanents more often than essential. Bleached and dyed hair is particularly sensitive. Almost all permanent-wave lotions are basically alike, but the skill with which they are applied varies with the individual operator.

*Home permanents* contain much the same ingredients as those used in beauty parlors. However, there is a greater danger, since you or the friend who gives you the permanent usually neglects to make a test curl; and you are more apt to be careless about keeping the lotion from your eyes and face—and from the children. All these lotions are dangerous, so be sure not to grow careless even if you have had no trouble with them in the past. Read the directions carefully. The American Medical Association, while recognizing these dangers, feels that home permanent kits are safe for normal use.

Nonneutralizing home-permanent kits depend for their neutralizing action on the oxidation that normally occurs when the waving lotion is exposed to air as it dries. So far there is no indication that this can cause any more damage to the hair than would occur if a neutralizer were used, but it may not produce so long-lasting a wave.

## Baldness

The time and money women waste on useless "hormone" creams and other beauty aids can probably be matched by that which men spend on "cures" for baldness. I am sorry to have to tell you that there is *no* cure for ordinary baldness. The miraculous ones you read or hear about have nothing to do with this type of baldness. For example, in *alopecia areata*, the hair suddenly falls out (often in patches); this disease is not fully understood, but appears to be connected with tension or other emotional factors. In many cases the hair will grow back again after the illness has subsided, and if the sufferer has been using a "hair restorer" he will sign testimonials crediting it with his new growth of hair.

Hair normally grows in "spells," a period of growth alternating with a rest period. On the head, its rate is usually about three quarters of an inch a month, although this varies in different people. If not cut, it grows to the length of about 25 inches, on an average. Hairs fall out—again the rate is different in different people—and new ones grow from the same follicles.

Baldness can be caused by general ill-health, infections of the scalp, nervous tension, and *temporarily* by a disease such as typhoid fever. Last, but by no means least, it can be due to the combination of sex, age, and inheritance which results in what doctors call *"male pattern alopecia,"* which simply means the ordinary baldness of men.

Frankly, we do not fully understand the factors that go into this condition. We know that the tendency to become bald runs in certain families, and that certain racial groups are more susceptible to it than others. We know that it is often associated with aging, perhaps because the layer of fat between the scalp and the skull tends to disappear, in men, with advancing years. We know that the male sex hormone has something to do with it, as it has with the growth of body hair. In this connection, I want to warn you *never* to take or use any preparation that has hormones in it, or is supposed to stop the action of a hormone. If the preparation so advertised actually has such an effect, it can be extremely dangerous to your endocrine glands.

If baldness is particularly distressing to you because of your business or profession—or for personal reasons—I strongly advise you not to waste money on hair "restorers" but to spend it on a toupee which, if carefully made to match your hair and skilfully fitted, cannot be distinguished from your own hair. Alternatively, hair transplantation is often successful now but expensive.

## Other Scalp and Hair Conditions

The scalp and hair can be affected by many of the conditions which afflict other parts of the skin. Protect your head from irritating chemicals whenever it is necessary. Never remove wens or growths of any kind. These require the attention of a doctor.

Children frequently pick up *head lice* (pediculosis capitis), the eggs of which are called *nits*. There are many time-honored methods of getting rid of them, including the laborious use of the fine-tooth comb. However, the new medicines are so effective that it is well worth your while to get a doctor to prescribe one and also give you directions for using it safely. Great care should be taken to avoid reinfection, by keeping the comb and brush absolutely clean by boiling or dipping in alcohol. This is also true of *ringworm*, a fungus infection of the scalp, to which children are quite susceptible. A doctor can cure this condition without much difficulty *after* he has determined exactly which fungus is causing it.

Remember that scalp infections can become serious, causing swollen glands and even blood poisoning. They can usually be avoided by taking the proper care of your scalp and hair, but if infection does occur be sure to see a doctor.

# 7
# KEEPING THE GERMS AWAY

If you had to choose between them, whom would you pick as a roommate, a leper or a person with tuberculosis? Ten to one you'd choose the person with TB. Yet, tuberculosis is *by far* more readily acquired than leprosy.

Until about a hundred years ago, tuberculosis (which was then called consumption) was not known to be contagious—doctors said it was due to an inherited "weakness of the constitution"—while they believed leprosy could be contracted simply by touching a leper's garment. At that time it was also believed that malaria came from breathing night air with its dangerous vapors or miasmas, that an epidemic of diphtheria would follow if locusts were prevalent, and that dysentery was due to becoming overheated.

Today we know the cause of germ diseases, how they are transmitted and how a great many of them can be prevented, avoided, or cured. There are more than a hundred contagious diseases to which you may be exposed during your lifetime. It would be far too big a task for you to learn the details of the cause, transmission, prevention, and cure of each of them. Even doctors don't know the exact manner in which *every* germ is transmitted.

However, there are only a *few* ways in which germ diseases can be contracted. By learning about them, you will be able to protect yourself and your family. Unfortunately, you won't be 100 percent successful. The chances are that everyone will contract at least one disease during his lifetime, if only a cold. That is why I describe a number of the common diseases, their symptoms and treatment, in other chapters. But even though

reading this chapter won't guarantee you complete protection, it will enable you to avoid many communicable diseases.

## GERM DISEASES

Communicable diseases are caused by germs—unlike, for example, the diseases I discuss in Chapter 5, which are caused by disorders of the endocrine glands. The words *communicable, contagious,* and *infectious* are used more or less interchangeably, although doctors do distinguish among them. We usually refer to the entire group as *communicable diseases*. The ones that children speak of as "catching diseases" we say are *contagious,* which means that they are transmitted by contact with a sick person, either directly or indirectly (for example, through the air into which he has sneezed or coughed). By *infectious* we mean diseases like lockjaw (tetanus) which aren't "caught" from a sick person, although they, too, are caused by infecting germs. However, since many diseases are both contagious and infectious, there is not much distinction made between the two terms.

### What Are Germs?

Medically speaking, a germ is a microorganism (too small to be seen by the unaided eye), especially one likely to cause disease. Although we naturally concentrate on the fact that they cause diseases, germs also perform many useful functions. Without them, there would be no wine, beer, cheese, or bread; and nothing would decay in the soil—with consequences it is difficult even to imagine!

*Micro* means small; germs are also known as *microbes*. Germs vary in many ways, and some of them are, comparatively speaking, very much larger than others; but they are all tiny. It was because of their size that scientists formerly ignored them. Even after doctors were able to see germs under their microscopes, they dismissed them as too little to amount to anything. It was not until 1865 that the French chemist Louis Pasteur discovered their importance. He proved that, although one germ by itself doesn't amount to much, these tiny organisms multiply rapidly under certain conditions and produce definite effects upon the "soil" in which they are growing—"soil" which may be a bottle of wine, or the body of a human being.

It seems difficult to realize that only a hundred years ago doctors didn't even suspect that germs have anything to do with wound infections or diseases. Now we know a tremendous amount about them: their various types and habits, the way they enter the body, how the body fights them, and how it can be helped in this battle.

## BACTERIA, VIRUSES, RICKETTSIAE, PROTOZOA, PARASITES, AND FUNGI

There are six types of microorganisms that cause communicable diseases. Knowing something about them will make it easier for you to stay healthy (see Figure 7-1).

### Bacteria

Bacteria are very tiny forms of life visible only under a microscope. To give you a rough idea of their size, imagine all the eight million people in the city of New York reduced to the size of bacteria. They would fit very comfortably into a drop of water!

Among themselves, the sizes, shapes, and habits of bacteria differ from one to another. Some swim about, others remain still. Some bacteria are little individualists, preferring to go it alone. The streptococci form chains like strings of beads, while others such as the ones found in boils live in clusters, like bunches of grapes.

Luckily, most bacteria, which are all around us, are more beneficial than harmful to mankind. Bacteria are very important in destroying dead matter. You might say that they are our most efficient department for garbage disposal. Bacteria help the growth of certain plants on which all other plants and animals depend. In fact, life without bacteria would not be possible, yet how pleasant it would be without the bacteria that cause tuberculosis (p. 441), pneumonia (p. 443), syphilis (p. 447), and diphtheria (p. 297), to name just a few!

### Viruses

These organisms are much smaller than bacteria, so tiny they cannot even be seen through an ordinary microscope but require a special apparatus, the electron microscope. Another reason they are harder to study is that, unlike bacteria, they are extremely fussy about where they grow, normally refusing to have anything to do with laboratory "food." It is only quite recently, and with the greatest of difficulty, that scientists have succeeded in working out ways of getting them to grow anywhere except in an animal body. Fussy as they are, they are extremely potent; very small numbers can start a disease. Some are very hardy. They cause a great many diseases, including polio (p. 464), yellow fever (p. 138), influenza (p. 476), infectious hepatitis (p. 444), rabies (p. 138), smallpox (p. 134), and such children's diseases as chicken pox, measles and mumps (Chapter 20). The common cold (p. 495), which affects just about everyone, is also caused by a virus.

### Rickettsiae

Smaller than bacteria but larger than viruses, rickettsiae are rod-shaped to round microorganisms found in the tissue cells of lice, fleas, ticks, and mites, and transmitted to man by their bites. They are responsible for such diseases as Rocky Mountain spotted fever (p. 138), typhus (p. 138), and Q fever (p. 593).

### Protozoa

These are microscopic creatures which may be fifty times larger than bacteria, but still cannot be seen without a microscope. Important diseases caused by these organisms are *malaria* and *amebic dysentery* (see pages 488 and 489).

## Parasitic Worms

Some of these parasites can be readily seen by the unaided eye, while others are so small they cannot be identified exactly without a microscope. The smallest are the size of a pinhead, while a tapeworm can grow to a length of thirty feet.

Many of these parasites, including the *flukes* (one of the two types of *flatworms*), are more prevalent in other countries, especially the tropics, than they are in the United States. The other type of flatworm, the *tapeworm,* is found in this country and is taken into the body by eating beef, pork, and fish containing this parasite. Inside the intestine, the tapeworm attaches itself to the intestinal wall and proceeds to grow. Some *roundworms* are also common in this country, especially in the South. They include the *pinworm,* the *intestinal roundworm,* and the *hookworm* (p. 300). Another roundworm which is found in pork causes *trichinosis* (p. 137), a disease in which the parasites eventually get into the patient's muscles.

## Fungi

These growths are related to mushrooms, only they are very much smaller. The green or white mold which forms on stale bread is a tiny fungus. A fungus causes athlete's foot (p. 117). Other types of fungi are responsible for various skin diseases. There are many fungus diseases, most of which are fortunately rare in this country.

## HOW THE BODY FIGHTS GERMS

"With all these unsuspected sources of disease around, it's a wonder that people manage to stay alive at all!" you may be saying.

In the past a tremendous number of people used to die annually from germ diseases. Less than a hundred years ago every fifth child died before reaching its first birthday, and almost as many more before reaching the age of two, the majority of them from dysentery and "childhood diseases." Epidemics of diphtheria were known to kill every child under twelve in an entire town, while plagues of smallpox, yellow fever, and other diseases would decimate the population. Until doctors learned about germs, there wasn't much they could do to help people prevent these diseases.

Fortunately, however, the body is not helpless against germs. It has filters, such as the tiny hairs in the nose, to keep them out, and secretions, such as the tears, to kill them or wash them away. If they do get in, the leukocytes (white blood cells) attack and devour them. The number of leukocytes in the blood increases rapidly when they are needed to fight infections. The fever usually caused by these diseases can help the body to destroy some germs which are unable to grow at a temperature much above normal (98.6° F.).

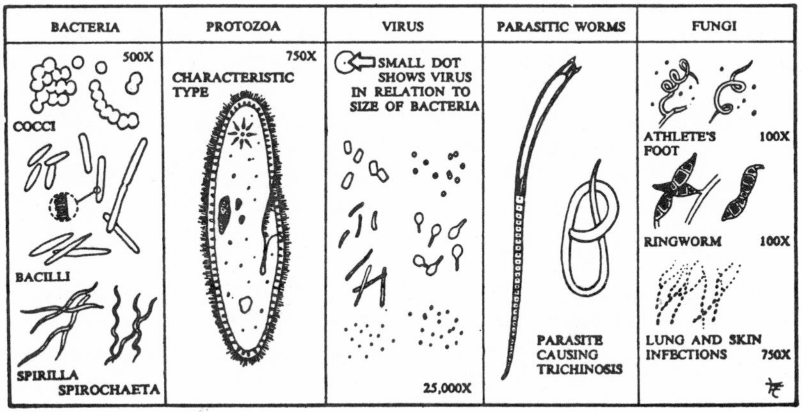

*Figure 7–1. Basic Types of Microorganisms. × means magnification; 500 × means the organism has been magnified 500 times its natural size.*

| BACTERIA | PROTOZOA | VIRUS | PARASITIC WORMS | FUNGI |
|---|---|---|---|---|

The body has still other resources. It manufactures substances which, in a sense, counteract the germs and render their poisons (toxins) harmless. These substances are called antibodies or antitoxins. After the body has won its battle against certain diseases, these substances remain in the blood and prevent the germs of that disease from getting a foothold again. This is what happens when you have measles, chickenpox, or any of the other diseases that people don't get more than once. We say that such people have become immune to the disease; this is called an *acquired immunity*. Many of us are immune to one or more forms of polio (infantile paralysis) because we have had an attack that was so mild we didn't even know we had it, usually mistaking it for the flu. Some types of immunity can be passed from a mother to her children. People who are immune to a disease without ever having had it are referred to as having a *natural immunity*. Many immunities are *partial* or *temporary;* that is, they don't *completely* protect an individual *during his entire lifetime.*

## How Doctors Help in This Fight

Doctors know how to make use of the fact that a mild attack of certain diseases prevents the illness from recurring. For example, vaccination has all but eliminated the terrible plague, smallpox. The doctor makes a tiny scratch on the person he is vaccinating, and applies some weak germs of a harmless disease called cowpox; the blood promptly creates antibodies which protect it against cowpox *and* smallpox for a number of years (see Figure 7-2). Introducing material that has been rendered harmless to the body but will cause it to create a resistance to certain germs is the principle involved in inoculations against many diseases.

The immunity acquired in this way is called an *active immunity;* the individual himself has made the substances that will protect him from the disease. When we speak of *passive immunity* we mean the immunity developed when an individual receives an injection of "antidotes" which have been created in the body of another person or an animal. Passive immunity usually doesn't last very long. *Booster shots* are given to revive an immunity, e.g., tetanus immunization. We might say that they cause the body to recollect the method by which it produced an immunity when the original injection was given.

Everyone *can* and *should* be immunized against the following dangerous diseases: *smallpox, diphtheria, polio* (infantile paralysis), *tetanus,* sometimes *typhoid fever,* and (in the case of children) *whooping cough, measles,* and *rubella* (German measles). The inoculations are easily obtainable and cause practically no discomfort. Your family doctor or pediatrician can give you these injections. They are also available free, or at very little cost, so lack of money must not keep anyone from being immunized. Any hospital, public health department, court, or health officer can give you information on this matter.

It is particularly important to protect children against these diseases, which are extremely dangerous to them. Diphtheria used to be one of the main causes of death in children, and whooping cough has a high mortality in infants, so don't put off having your child immunized because he is so little!

Measles now is recognized as a serious disease, one that children should be protected against by inoculation. It can lead to other and even more serious illnesses, like pneumonia. Multiple sclerosis and other diseases of the nervous system may be late-developing complications of measles.

I strongly advise adults who have not had the above inoculations to do so as soon as it is convenient. While being inoculated against tetanus and typhoid fever is not *essential* under all circumstances, why not have it done to be on the safe side? (See page 161-62). Other diseases against which adults as well as children should be immunized under special circumstances are: yellow fever (see page 138), tularemia (see page 137) and tick fever (Rocky Mountain spotted fever, page 138). Because of the effectiveness of the "wonder drugs" in curing this spotted fever, some doctors consider immunization unnecessary, but I think it is worthwhile if you live in or visit a place where it is prevalent.

Rubella occurring during pregnancy can be a threat to the unborn child. Vaccination of children against the disease can help prevent its spread to a pregnant woman. Nonpregnant women who are

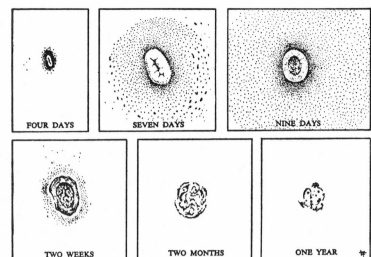

Figure 7–2. *Reactions from Smallpox Vaccination. Approximately life-size. The shaded areas indicate inflammation.*

not immune to rubella, as demonstrated by a blood test, should be vaccinated before becoming pregnant.

At the moment, there are no inoculations that offer *complete* protection against the common cold, some strains of influenza, and some forms of pneumonia. Flu shots in the fall of the year do give some measure of protection against the coming winter.

A very recent advance is the development of a vaccine to immunize against pneumococci, the bacteria that are a major cause of pneumonia, responsible for half a million cases annually in the United States alone, and a cause, too, of about a million cases of middle ear infections, mostly in children, as well as of meningitis, a dangerous inflammation of membranes enclosing the brain.

## Other Protections

Immunization will protect you from developing certain diseases even *after the germs have gained a foothold in your body*. For example, *rabies* and *tetanus germs* can be conquered by injections given between the time they start to grow and the time they cause symptoms of illness. But remember— the time is short, so never delay in getting treatment if you have any reason to suspect these germs have entered your body.

Injections will help the body to win its battle against certain diseases *even after the illness is under way*. For example, in *diphtheria* the anti-toxin can be injected to neutralize the toxic effect of the germs (p. 297).

A few types of germs can be destroyed by chemical substances which will kill them without injuring the other tissues of the body. Among these chemicals are quinine which attacks malaria germs, a compound of arsenic which strikes at the germ causing syphilis, and the sulfa drugs which destroy several kinds of germs. The "wonder drugs," or *antibiotics*, such as penicillin, act in a slightly different manner: they make it impossible for certain very dangerous germs to grow; the germs rapidly weaken and are overcome by the resistance of the body to microbes.

I explain which, if any, of these methods is effective in my description of the various diseases. At this point, I just want to emphasize the fact that they may save your life or that of someone in your family. It has been my sad experience, as a doctor, to see people die needlessly because they "didn't want to bother" with an injection or medicine, or because they "didn't like the idea" of having themselves or their children "stuck by a needle."

Although you can be immunized against many diseases, and saved from the disastrous effects of others by injections and drugs, the best protection of all is to keep germs from getting into your body. In order to do this, you should learn the ways in which they can enter.

# HOW GERMS GET INTO YOUR BODY

Your body has an excellent coat of armor in the skin, which keeps out germs. But cuts or other breaks in it, and openings such as the nose and mouth, provide opportunities for them to enter.

## Nose, Throat, and Lungs

Many bacteria and viruses are spread and taken into the body through the nose and throat. Most germs thrive in moisture, and spitting, coughing, and sneezing keep them circulating. Motion pictures show that a sneeze is composed of tiny droplets, and that when you sneeze, you may expel a spray of liquid to a distance of several feet (see Figure 7-3). Such diseases as the common cold, pneumonia, tuberculosis, whooping cough, scarlet fever, diphtheria, influenza, and meningitis are spread this way. These illnesses are circulated by diseased people, by people who are "coming down" with a disease, or by carriers of the germs who harbor them without being sick.

It is not etiquette alone that demands that you cover your nose and mouth when you cough or sneeze. The germs that are lodged in your nose and throat relish this free ride and the opportunity to spread and multiply. You should never spit in public or put into your mouth pencils or anything that other people handle. As much as you can, avoid crowds during the "sniffle" season or during an epidemic.

More people than you would guess have tuberculosis, which is one of the most serious diseases you can get by inhaling germs. *Any cough that lasts more than six weeks calls for a chest x-ray.* In fact, everybody should have periodic chest films to exclude tuberculosis—as advised in the section on the periodic medical checkups (p. 378). *Tuberculosis does not always reveal itself with outward signs. A healthy-looking, robust person may have it.* (See page 441.)

Sore throats, colds, and coughs should be treated with rest and plenty of fluids until they are cured. Prompt treatment of colds is necessary for the prevention of more serious diseases which are caused by viruses. Colds offer many bacteria, especially streptococci and pneumococci, a chance to get a foothold and infect your body with more dangerous diseases. See pages 496–97 on the treatment of colds.

It is best to rest until you are well and the fever is gone. Too many people with a contagious disease get out of bed too soon; they are so bored and so eager to get out and going that they immediately infect those trusting friends and relatives who no longer avoid them.

Nursing mothers with colds should ask the doctor about wearing a nose-and-mouth mask when handling the baby. And no kissing while sick with strep sore throats, pneumonia, etc.! No love is strong enough to withstand virulent infections.

## Infection from Food and Water

*Typhoid,* now fortunately an uncommon disease, is typical of the infections that can enter through the mouth. Other diseases of this group include *amoebic dysentery* and *dysentery* caused by bacteria.

Typhoid germs are found in food, milk, and water that have been contaminated by feces. Flies that have fed on body eliminations may also carry the typhoid germs to food and drinks. Every precaution should be taken to keep food, especially warm food, from being exposed to flies. Plastic covers for dishes are plentiful and cheap.

Habits of cleanliness should be encouraged by all members of the family. Washing your hands after going to the toilet and before eating should be a habit as automatic as breathing. This stress on cleanliness has a good purpose, since contamination can be spread by a person who is not himself ill, as in the case of the typhoid carrier. The famous story of Typhoid Mary is an example of this. Mary, a carrier of the disease, was a cook who went from job to job spreading infection to more than 100 victims.

While we may occasionally be at the mercy of such a person, we can accomplish a great deal by our own precautions. All the *milk* that comes to

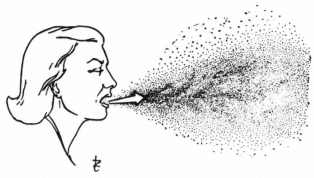

*Figure 7–3. How Germs Are Spread by a Sneeze.*

your table should be pasteurized. *Pasteurization* is the process of heating milk for 30 minutes at 142° F., or at 160° F. for one minute. You can do your own home "pasteurization" whenever in doubt about the milk by boiling it for three minutes. Another method of home sterilization is scalding the milk for half an hour in a double boiler. The milk should be 150° F. by a cooking thermometer for a half hour. At this temperature the milk simmers—there are small bubbles around the edge of the span.

*Certified milk* is *not* safe because the certification of the health of cattle is not foolproof; also, certified milk is handled before it is bottled. Of course, all milk is handled at the time cows are milked. But pasteurized milk goes directly after the heat process into sterilized bottles without being touched by human hands. Never drink raw milk, because the cow or the people who work with the milk may transmit disease. Smart farmers always drink pasteurized milk. Unpasteurized milk may carry not only typhoid, which is now rare, but also tuberculosis, streptococcal infection, brucellosis, and other diseases.

In most cities the *water* that comes from the faucet is safe to drink. But if you live in the country or are going there on vacation, be careful about the drinking water. Water drawn from wells or taken from lakes, ponds, or rivers may contain dangerous germs, no matter how clear it looks. To be on the safe side, boil the water for ten minutes before drinking it.

Amoebic dysentery, as well as dysentery caused by bacteria, is spread very much like typhoid.

Dysentery is a disease more common than typhoid, because these germs can live for longer periods outside the body. Typhoid and cholera germs have a very short life-span when they are not within the body. Cholera does not exist in the United States, and, thanks to modern sanitation methods, typhoid has been greatly reduced. In India, where people both bathe and eliminate their feces in the Ganges River, cholera has been very common.

Meats can carry disease. Some uncooked pork may contain the living parasite causing trichinosis. For complete protection, *pork should always be cooked thoroughly.* Any pinkness means that it is underdone. For roast pork, an hour to the pound at 350° is safe. Brucellosis (undulant fever) may be acquired from pork, beef, milk that has not been pasteurized, and also cheese and ice cream made from unpasteurized milk. *Raw fish and raw beef may contain tapeworms.* Although the U.S. Department of Agriculture inspects meats, you cannot always be certain they are still pure by the time they reach your dinner table. Thorough cooking of all meats and fish is the best preventive. In the tropics and in the Orient, due to poorer sanitation and health measures, many parasitic diseases are very prevalent.

Diseased rabbits cause *tularemia,* a serious disease which may be contracted even without the eating—just in the skinning and preparing—of the rabbit. It would be better if hunters confined themselves to the sport and abstained from eating their quarry.

*Canned food* that has been improperly prepared is dangerous. Bacteria can grow inside and cause food poisoning. Botulism is the name for a severe form of food poisoning which often results in a fatal paralysis (see page 331). The food and canning industries are extremely careful to avoid food contamination; botulism usually is the result of improper canning in the home. If you like to can food, boil it for at least three hours or steam-cook it under correct pressure. Boil again for fifteen minutes before eating.

Dangers may be lurking in *bakery goods,* especially those with custard fillings, such as eclairs, on which bacteria thrive. It is most important to buy your pastry from a clean, reliable bakery, and to put it in the refrigerator when you get it home. Make sure that the pastry has not been standing around in the bakery or in your home for a long time.

*Frozen food* is popular because, properly prepared, it can keep the original fresh taste. The home freezer is runner-up in popularity to the refrigerator. It can be a pleasure and a means of economy, but it can also be a source of danger if the food is not correctly frozen. Most meats, poultry, and fish can be quick-frozen and kept safely for long periods of time. Vegetables, bread, and cake are also popular freezer items. But many foods, such as concentrated fruit juices, should be used as soon as they are thawed and should not be refrozen.

The U.S. Department of Agriculture has some down-to-earth pamphlets about frozen foods and freezing equipment. They are all free. Some of the titles are:

*Freezing Combination Main Dishes*
*Home Care of Purchased Frozen Foods*
*Home Freezers—Their Selection and Use*
*Home Freezing of Fruits and Vegetables*
*Home Freezing of Poultry*

## VENEREAL DISEASES

Venereal diseases are spread mainly by sexual intercourse. The two main venereal diseases are syphilis and gonorrhea. In Chapters 33 and 34, I discuss in detail the treatment and cure of venereal diseases.

## INSECT BITES

Bites of insects are a source of infection because insects carry germs either in the mouth or in their excrement. An insect bite makes a tiny break in the skin, like the puncture of a hypodermic needle.

Rocky Mountain spotted fever is transmitted by the bite of ticks. Endemic typhus fever in Mexico and southern United States is transmitted by lice, ticks, and mites living on rats. Malaria and yellow fever are carried by certain mosquitoes. If you visit areas where malaria exists, protect yourself against mosquitoes. Use a salve with an odor that repels them (p. 160 ), and arrange mosquito netting over your bed at night, especially if your screens are inadequate. There is no immunization against malaria, but your physician can prescribe prophylactic measures before you go to a malaria area.

## ANIMAL BITES

Any animal bite which breaks the skin should be thoroughly washed with soap and water and cleansed or cauterized by a doctor (see First Aid, page 326).

*Rabies* (hydrophobia), a virus disease that affects the brain and nervous system, comes from the bite of mad dogs and other domestic and wild animals who harbor the virus in their saliva. If possible, the biting dog should be caught and studied by the health department. If the dog is infected, the person bitten must receive treatment to prevent rabies, a virtually 100 percent fatal disease. *If the bite is on the head, neck, or face, get the treatment started immediately because the virus can reach the brain very rapidly.* The virus travels along the nerves of the body to the brain, so that the farther away the bite the longer the trip to the brain. In bites on the foot, it has taken as long as a year for rabies to develop! Unless the dog is caught and found to be free from rabies, treatment *must* be given.

All warm-blooded pets—dogs, cats, monkeys—can now be vaccinated against rabies by a veterinarian. No pet owner should neglect this precautionary measure.

If a dog has to be shot because of viciousness due to his disease, he should be shot in the body so that the undamaged brain can be studied in a health department or police department laboratory.

Any dog that is acting queerly should be examined by a veterinarian.

## WOUNDS AND SCRATCHES

All cuts, wounds, and scratches are potential entrances for infections. They should be washed with soap and water and treated as explained in my chapter on first aid (p. 326).

One of the most serious dangers from wounds and deep scratches is *tetanus* (lockjaw). The tetanus germ is commonly found in the soil and wherever there are horses, cows, and manure. It is also found in the dust of city streets. A deep puncture by a nail is serious. Many people think it is the rust of a nail that causes the trouble. That is not true. The danger lies in the germs which may be on the nail.

The best preventive against tetanus is immunization by toxoid. Tetanus toxoid gives immunity for several years. A series of three toxoid injections, followed by a fourth about a year later, with boosters at four-year intervals provides the best possible protection. It is very wise to be protected by having been immunized with toxoid so you are prepared for any emergency. All doctors recommend it. Every man in the armed forces has received toxoid to protect him against lockjaw.

For the person who has not been immunized with toxoid, deep wounds or scratches require tetanus antitoxin (TAT) as an emergency measure to prevent tetanus. TAT is available in the emergency room of every well-equipped hospital, infirmary, or first aid station. This provides adequate protection against tetanus, but unfortunately some people suffer unpleasant reactions to TAT. For this reason, doctors will always test the patient for possible sensitivity to the horse serum with which TAT is made. Toxoid does not produce an unpleasant or dangerous reaction, which is an additional reason why you should have this important safety measure in advance of any possible accident.

## TAKE REASONABLE PRECAUTIONS

I hope that after reading this chapter you will take sensible precautions against possible infections. Make it a habit not to drink out of glasses or use towels that others have used, to stay away from "sneezers" as much as possible, and to keep yourself and your house clean.

But don't go overboard! We've all met or heard about people who are fanatics on the subject of germs. They are constantly scrubbing, boiling, or sterilizing their food, their homes, and themselves. They spray their noses and throats and the air about them with antiseptics, never touch a doorknob or sit on an unprotected toilet seat, shun others as though everyone had the plague, and generally wage a constant battle against contamination.

This is neither necessary nor effective. It is unnecessary because the odds are with us where germs are concerned. Most of them are harmless, and the dangerous ones seldom live very long under ordinary conditions. They soon die without the proper "food," sufficient moisture, the right temperature, and similar requirements. Most of them can't stand air and sunlight. Soap and water kill or remove them. Extreme methods of precautions are, as a rule, useless as well as unnecessary. Germicides, sprays, and disinfectants either (a) don't reach the germs they are intended for, or provide protection for only the few minutes they are actually in use, or (b) are too weak to kill germs or so strong they injure the skin and other tissues.

How about a household disinfectant? Personally, I feel that there is a danger of using such disinfectants as a *substitute* for cleanliness rather than as an aid to cleanliness. Sprinkling a little around makes everything smell so antiseptic that it is a temptation to go easy on the soap and water and elbow grease!

*Fumigation* after certain illness used to be required by law, and is still on the statute books in some states. However, scientific tests have shown that it is unnecessary and ineffective—except when it comes to destroying mice and vermin, which can be handled better in other ways. It was often substituted for the far more valuable thorough cleaning job. Soap and water, fresh air, and sunshine are the best aids in killing germs.

If you take reasonable precautions to keep germs away, you will find there is room enough in the world for you to get along very well in spite of them.

(See also Chapter 38, page 543, The Calculated Risk in Health.)

# 8
# YOUR JOB AND YOUR HEALTH

All of us who work for a living realize how important our health is to our job. To suffer from repeated illnesses or to feel continually below par is a great handicap in this competitive world. The healthy individual who can be depended upon, and whose capacity and skills are always at a high level, is in line for advancement, with better pay and greater security.

It is equally obvious that your job is vitally important to your health and that of your family. A good home, providing a proper health environment, depends to a great extent upon your income—either by itself or combined with those of other family members who are working. Up to a certain income level, wages tend to determine the amount and quality of nutritious food that can be purchased—to say nothing of clothes, recreation, medical and dental costs, and the many other things included in the total health picture.

In addition, one's work bears a close relationship to mental health. If the job is interesting and rewarding, we are apt to be happy and contented. This state of well-being is manifested in restful sleep, relaxed nerves, and a good appetite. This happiness is reflected upon all members of the family, whose emotional health then prospers, too.

We all know that accidents can result not only from inadequate safety measures on the job, but also from being jittery and tense. Doctors have learned that in certain illnesses, such as stomach ulcers and high blood pressure, nervous tension may play a part. (I discuss *psychosomatic illnesses* —that is, conditions brought about in this manner —on page 181.)

I am sure I need go no further to make the point that your job and your health are closely bound up with one another. That is why I am so anxious to have everyone take stock of his or her job, both with regard to the specific hazards associated with it and also with regard to its general health aspects.

## HAVE YOU A GOOD JOB?

First of all, a good job should bring in enough money to supply you and your family with the adequate diet described in Chapter 2. There should be funds enough to provide adequate housing of the type described in Chapter 22, with sufficient left over for clothes, recreation, health insurance, and other essentials.

If your job doesn't enable you to provide these essentials, can you get a raise? Are there courses you can take or other things you can do that will lead to your promotion? If not, can you find a job with better possibilities? Your supervisor, foreman, or shop steward might be able to give you helpful hints, and so might your doctor and clergyman.

Some cities have job counselors or offer opportunities for you to discover how to fit yourself for a better position. *Vocational guidance* has made great progress in studying the "square peg in the round hole" problem. I suggest that you write the United States Employment Service, Bureau of Employment Security, U.S. Department of Labor, Washington, D.C. 20210, asking for the nearest local office where you can obtain counseling, testing, and job placement services. Veterans are entitled to similar services from the Veterans Administration.

If your job provides sufficient income but leaves you unhappy and frustrated, vocational guidance agencies may help you solve your problem. A frank talk with your doctor, who may send you to a psychiatrist or psychologist, will help you to discover whether you should try to adjust yourself to your position or to find another one. Ideally, your job should be interesting and should provide opportunities for advancement.

Your work should be as safe as modern techniques can make it. A good job should not endanger your health. If you are frequently ill or have had accidents at work, it may be that you don't observe proper precautions, or it may also be the result of poor conditions in your place of employment. After reading this chapter you should be able to decide which it is. If it is the latter, bring the fact to the attention of your employers, either directly or through your foreman or union. If this fails to produce any improvement, the matter should be reported to the proper authorities, such as the department of labor of your state, or to your local or state department of health.

Of course, there are cases in which neither you nor the job is to blame. You may not be suited physically or temperamentally to the work you are doing. That is, even though you are healthy, you may not be strong enough for a certain job, you may not have a sufficiently good sense of balance, and so on. Your doctor can help you to decide this question.

# HOW TO STAY WELL
# ON YOUR JOB

All too frequently, *preventable* accidents or illnesses occur and result in the loss of health or earning capacity for varying periods of time. Different jobs have special health problems, and I shall take them up after I have discussed some rules to be generally observed.

## GENERAL RULES

*Come to work rested and relaxed.* Fatigue is a source of accidents; late hours are a danger to your health. Plan your late dances, card parties, and other entertainment on the night before your day off from work. The same applies to drinking. Never drink so much that you have a hangover at work the next day. And, of course, drinking alcoholic beverages on the job is particularly dangerous. If you cannot control your drinking, be sure to read and follow the advice on page 472.

Regular periods of rest are decidedly important. One or two days off each week are essential. So is your annual vacation. Being rested helps to decrease accidents and illness—in addition to making it possible for you to create a good impression on the job by being at your best physically and mentally. Be sure not to ruin these days off by doing things to overtire you or injure your health. (I consider vacations so important that I have devoted the next chapter to them.)

Don't be afraid of being considered a "sissy" if you *make a point of finding out and following all the safety rules on your particular job.* Be sure to discuss precautions not only with your employer and shop steward, but with the older workers when you go on a new job. Don't be ashamed to ask questions, especially about the particular hazards you face.

If a fellow worker is a danger to you or to others, take up the matter with your shop steward or anyone in authority. *There is no place in any job for the practical joker—particularly in dangerous industrial or farming work.* Every year workers are brought to hospitals, dying or seriously injured, because practical "jokers" pushed a compressed-air jet against them. I have seen people who have been crippled as a result of "playful gags" such as the "hot-foot." The worker who insists on practical jokes or who doesn't know how to handle dangerous equipment is the cause of many accidents and deaths.

Find out where the *first aid station* is located. Every place employing a large number of people will have a first aid room. Many of the big factories have a full-time nursing staff and sometimes a medical staff. Smaller ones have a first aid station and safety personnel who know how to use it. A squad of workers can and should be organized and trained to treat shock, minor burns, and cases requiring artificial respiration. Such easily arranged precautions can save lives. (Specific first aid measures are given in Chapter 23.)

*Electricity.* Exposed wires, crossed circuits, and carelessness can cause shocks or burns anywhere there is electricity. If you know of any wiring that is defective, be sure to call it to the attention of someone who can correct it. I discuss what to do for accidents caused by electricity on page 335, but I want to stress one fact in particular: *don't give up* if someone has apparently been electrocuted; artificial respiration plus cardiac massage continued over a period of hours have been known to save people who appeared to be dead.

*Sure footing* is essential, so be particularly careful if the floors or stairs are wetted by chemicals or liquids. If there is a danger of slipping, be sure you have a handhold. Take up the matter if no handholds are provided.

*Good lighting* is also essential. Poor lighting can cause accidents, eye fatigue, dizziness, and headaches. Any job, from that of a miner to an office worker, can be made unpleasant and even dangerous if the lighting is poor; this is especially true where the work involves handling machinery. If your eyes feel strained after a day's work, if they are inflamed or puffy, you may need glasses or a change of glasses. However, this may be due to the fact that you don't get enough light. See your doctor. If he says the lighting is to blame, and the company for which you work doesn't seem inclined to do anything about it, ask him to write them suggesting they inspect and improve the lighting of your work space. Sometimes simply keeping windows and light bulbs clean will be sufficient. Walls of light pastel shades help make a room light, and flat paint cuts down on the glare.

*Rest rooms* or lavatories will be inspected regularly by the department of health. If yours are not sanitary, or not adequately equipped with soap, etc., find out whether the health inspection has been performed. Workers should be given adequate opportunities to use these facilities.

*Dusts, fumes, and mists* are predictable hazards in many jobs. The dangers they present can be held to a minimum by a combination of ventilation and other measures taken by management, and by individual protective devices, such as I discuss later in this chapter.

## Learn the Particular Hazards of Your Job

Every job has its special health problems. Even sedentary occupations such as those of clerks and office workers are not entirely safe. Housework, too, is dangerous. Women who work at home should carefully read Chapter 22 in which I discuss danger spots in the home and tell how to avoid accidents which cripple and kill many people every year. They should also read Chapter 23 on first aid, and page 524 on the ailments associated with housework.

In addition, salespeople, librarians, teachers, and others who come in contact with large numbers of people during the course of a day's work or in going to and from work, should protect themselves against the increased danger of exposure to respiratory diseases such as colds (p. 496) and pneumonia (p. 443).

## SPECIAL PROBLEMS OF FARMERS AND RURAL WORKERS

It is not true that working on a farm is any healthier than in the city. Statistics show that the illness and disability rates are equally high in both places; in some rural areas, especially where doctors are scarce and hospitals poorly equipped, the residents may have even more health problems than the city dwellers do.

If you live in a rural area, be sure to learn the facts about the following diseases which may be found in some country communities:

Undulant fever (brucellosis) (see page 486)
Tularemia (rabbit fever) (see page 137
Typhoid fever (see page 136)
Tuberculosis of bones and joints (see page 462)

Dysentery (see page 488)
Malaria (in South) (see page 488)
Hookworm (in South) (see page 300)

Living in the country doesn't protect you against tuberculosis. Actually, the farmer needs to take every precaution listed in this book. And some extra ones, too.

For example, the milk obtained in cities is almost invariably pasteurized. This helps to prevent tuberculosis of the glands and bones and other diseases, such as undulant fever and septic sore throat, that are spread by milk. Unless the farmer goes to the extra trouble of pasteurizing the milk from his own cow, he and his family are constantly in danger from these diseases. A friend of mine who is both a doctor and a dairy farmer sells his milk to a dairy company which has a pasteurizing plant. He then buys milk from them and has it delivered at his farm, so that his family will be sure to have only pasteurized milk. Many wise farmers do likewise.

Home pasteurization of milk is described on page 137. This process is absolutely essential for all farmers who use their own milk.

## Accidents on Farms

Rural Americans have a high accident toll. The lessened danger from traffic is counterbalanced by the frequency of accidents from farm machinery and other hazards.

Because the accident rate on farms is high, and medical care often far away, the farmer should have a good knowledge of first aid. All farm vehicles should carry first aid kits, including instruction booklets. Even small wounds should be treated immediately, because of the danger of infection. Animal bites not only should be washed with soap and water, then treated, but should be reported to a doctor. The animal should be examined for rabies (see page 341).

*Tetanus* (lockjaw) germs thrive in the intestines of horses and other grass-eating animals and are therefore found around barns and in soil fertilized by manure. This terrible disease, which can result from any deep wound such as one caused by stepping on a nail, is a constant threat to people living in the country. It can be pre-

vented by inoculations. Everyone, particularly children, living in rural areas should be protected in advance against tetanus by inoculations. Never neglect a deep wound, however trivial it may seem; an immediate injection of protective serum may make the difference between life and death. Be sure to read the section on tetanus (p. 139).

Strenuous work in the open sun can lead to *heat stroke* or to *heat exhaustion*. Learn how to prevent these illnesses, how to distinguish between them, and how to apply emergency treatment if either of them occurs. (See page 335.)

The dry, leathery, heavily wrinkled skin often developed by outdoor workers is characteristic of many farmers. In itself, it is not a health hazard, but in general, farmers should be aware of any tendency to burn easily in the sun.

New chemicals are always being introduced to farmers, to kill weeds, enrich the soil, eradicate insects, get rid of rodents, and clean animal areas. Many of them are a real help to the farmer and make him more productive, but they must be used exactly as directed by the manufacturer. Your county agricultural agent or health department representative can advise and help you when you have questions about these chemicals. Be especially careful about touching or breathing them. Finally, if you have to dispose of some unused substances, bury them in their containers. Don't burn them, because they may give off harmful fumes. Don't pour them into the ground, because they might contaminate the water supply.

## Rural Medical Facilities

Medical care, hospital facilities, and, especially, the advice of medical and surgical specialists are difficult to obtain in some farming communities. Make every effort to get the best medical care, even if it means taking a trip of several hundred miles to the nearest medical center or medical school. Your local doctor, however good he may be, should not be expected to handle every type of medical and surgical problem. Your local physician will advise consultation with a specialist if he feels that it is necessary. He will also arrange for you to be admitted to the nearest medical center. If you go to such a medical center be sure your local doctor receives a complete report of the findings.

# HAZARDS ON THE INDUSTRIAL JOB

Some jobs are more hazardous than others, for example, those involving mixing chemicals, using a blowtorch, drilling, baking, handling meat, construction, mining, lumbering, and working with radioactive materials. Usually several sources of danger are involved, some of which are peculiar to the particular job while others are common to various forms of work. For example, welders have to be on guard against four major threats to health and life: (1) Electrical shocks and burns, (2) burns from gas flames or splashes of hot metal, (3) damage to eyes and skin from the rays of the powerful arc lights, and (4) bad air caused by chemical fumes during the welding process. Yet, during World War II, women and new workers were successfully trained to work safely at welding. It was simply a matter of making certain that all the proper precautions were taken. I am stressing this one occupation to impress on you the fact that it can be done. Not every job involves as many risks as welding does, so there is little excuse for many of the industrial accidents and injuries that do occur.

Your employer should supply you with the instructions and the equipment necessary to reduce or eliminate the risks you face. Your union may have further information to give you. The main thing for you to do is to acquaint yourself with the dangers you may be up against; and never become lax—it may result in serious harm.

## Nine Main Occupational Hazards

1. DUST. This can be a serious problem. Dust may come from the grinding, crushing, cutting, or drilling of metals, stone or coal. Industrial dusts are divided into the organic and the inorganic.

*Organic dusts* come from substances whose source is plant or animal life, such as coal, leather, flour, sugar, feathers, and cotton. Many organic dusts are not disabling or even harmful because the particles are too large to get into the finer and more delicate body tissues, or are not made of poisonous compounds. Organic dusts may produce allergies, skin irritations, or asthma. Miners of both soft and hard coal may develop a disabling shortness of breath because of the effects of coal dust on their lungs.

*Inorganic dusts* are in the main made from metals and minerals. One of the most dangerous, silica, may cause *silicosis*, with fibrous nodules throughout the lung tissue. It may also encourage development of tuberculosis. Asbestos dust also causes an inflammation of the lung, called *asbestosis*, and may increase susceptibility to lung cancer. Workers such as diamond cutters, rock drillers, asbestos-products workers, foundry and furnace workers, abrasive-soap makers, and packers are among those who may be exposed to silica and asbestos dust.

Textile workers exposed to cotton dust run some risk of *byssinosis*, a respiratory disease which may later lead to chronic bronchitis and emphysema. In some industries where beryllium is used, its dust poses a hazard of disorders of lungs, skin, liver, and other organs.

Workers exposed to these dangerous dusts will most likely be protected by the use of exhaust systems or suction devices which catch the dust at its place of origin, or by covering the dust with oil or water to keep it from rising, and by good ventilation and the use of helmets and respiratory masks. However well-protected they may seem to be, workers should have regular, periodic chest x-rays to detect early the presence of silica or asbestos in their lungs. They should be constantly alert for colds that don't seem to get better, prolonged coughs, or other symptoms of tuberculosis (see page 441).

2. SKIN DISEASES. Among the most widespread industrial illnesses are skin diseases. Chemicals, dirt, oil, germs—almost anything can irritate the skin. The chief skin troublemakers are *petroleum* products, such as machine oil, naphtha, or various cutting-oil compounds; *solvents,* which include degreasers like kerosene, gasoline, and trichlorethylene; *alkalies,* like lime, caustic soda, and strong yellow soap; and *plants,* including poison ivy, sumac, and poison oak. Florists are subject

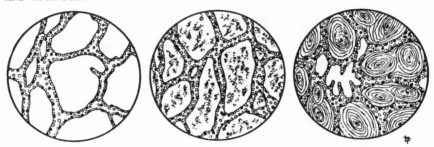

*Figure 8–1. Foreign Elements in the Lungs.* LEFT: *Microscopic section of a normal lung.* CENTER: *Similar section showing the presence of ordinary dust particles.* RIGHT: *Similar sections showing changes due to the presence of silica dust.*

to skin irritations from this group of plants. Furriers may be affected by paraphenylendiamine, and workers who use chromium in electroplating may develop chrome ulcers.

The list of skin afflictions is a long one. But there are several important precautions you can take to avoid having trouble with your skin.

Soap and water should be used generously right after finishing any dirty or oily job, and also before eating lunch and before leaving for the day. Special soaps may be needed to get rid of substances that cling stubbornly to or penetrate the skin. Don't rub away oils that get on your face and hands. They only seep into the skin and clog the pores, causing pimples and irritations. First wash off the oil with soap and water, and then dry with a clean towel. Special ointments can be used to cover the skin before contact with any offending agent.

Gloves, sleeves, and aprons offering protection against skin diseases should be worn. Pull your sleeves over the cuff of each glove to make sure no skin is exposed. Make sure your protective clothing is kept clean and changed often.

Dust, fumes, or gases harmful to the skin should be drawn off by suction hoods and the forced circulation of air.

Don't use advertised ointments for any skin disease you may develop. Visit your doctor and let him prescribe, because your skin ailment may require a very special prescription.

If you have taken these precautions and still suffer from certain chemicals or oils on the job, you may have developed an allergy to them. See your doctor, who may have to recommend another job if your skin is especially sensitive to the ingredients with which you are working (and if you can't be helped by precautions or desensitization; see page 498 on allergic diseases).

3. POISONS. These are a greater potential hazard to the health of workers in industries today than ever before, because of new inventions and the use of new chemicals and synthetic materials. *Lead poisoning* and the damage from inhaling *carbon monoxide fumes* are still common dangers. Although there are too many poisons for me to list them all, workers can familiarize themselves with the materials they are using and find out whether they contain poisonous ingredients.

The following general precautions should be taken. If necessary and feasible, masks, gloves, and respiratory devices should be worn for protection. Good ventilation is the best protection against carbon monoxide (CO) and other toxic gases. If the work produces a lot of fumes, wear an air-line respirator and a safety line. Be on the watch for headache, vomiting, dizziness, and a flushed face. Do not eat in rooms where poisonous substances are handled. Cleanliness is very important. Use plenty of soap and water, especially before eating and before leaving the plant. Be sure to have regular medical examinations, preferably on the job by the factory doctor.

The more common industrial poisons and some of the jobs in which they may be involved follow.

*Lead poisoning* can occur among bricklayers, color makers, dye makers, electroplaters, painters and paint makers, petroleum refiners, automobile workers, storage-battery workers, varnish makers, sheet-metal workers, lithographers, insecticide makers, explosives workers, rubber workers, and zinc miners. The more soluble forms of lead which may form particles in drinking cups are the more dangerous. Slow lead poisoning can result from small daily inhalations of lead dust over a period of time. The poison affects the stomach, the brain, and the nervous system. There may be paralysis of the muscles most frequently used, such as those of a painter's right hand. The precautions already mentioned, such as regular medical examinations, the proper clothing, and good ventilation, are of utmost importance.

*Carbon monoxide poisoning* presents a hazard to blast-furnace workers, firemen, cooks, petroleum-refinery workers, plumbers, welders, miners, compressed-air workers, and others. It can come on without warning. Abdominal pains, headaches, nausea, and dizziness are early symptoms. In very severe cases, death may result. Good ventilation is extremely important to prevent the fumes from accumulating. Carbon monoxide mixes with the hemoglobin of the blood, preventing the blood from circulating oxygen. For first aid, fresh air and, if needed, an oxygen tank and artificial respiration are effective in combating this poison.

*Benzol* and *carbon tetrachloride* are used, for example, by lacquer makers, leather workers, dry cleaners, soap makers, electroplaters, dye makers, paint and paint-remover makers. Benzol (or benzene) is a colorless liquid with a penetrating odor, used in making rubber goods, linoleum, celluloid, shellac, plastics, and artificial leather. The liquid evaporates fast, but gives off a very poisonous vapor. It is possible to get benzol poisoning by breathing concentrated fumes for just a few minutes, although gradual poisoning is more common. For protection, the worker should wear an air-line respirator and a safety belt. All machinery containing benzol should be closed and inspected regularly for leaks. There should be plenty of ventilation in the room, and, of course, you should get your regular medical examinations. Unusual bleeding, especially a sudden nosebleed, calls for immediate medical attention. People who have tuberculosis, heart disease, anemia, or a tendency to bleed easily should not work in plants where benzol is used.

In addition to symptoms of nausea, headaches, and irritations of the nose and throat, carbon tetrachloride presents a serious threat to health in that it injures the liver and kidneys. Be sure to take all the precautions described above for benzol.

4. INFECTIONS. Workers who handle cattle may get *undulant fever* (brucellosis). Those who work

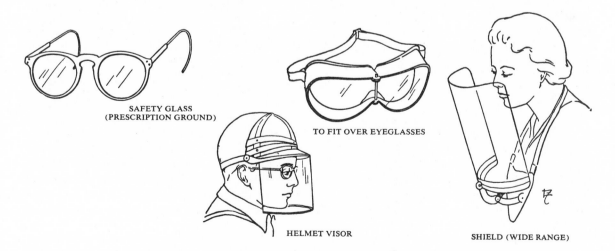

SAFETY GLASS
(PRESCRIPTION GROUND)

TO FIT OVER EYEGLASSES

HELMET VISOR

SHIELD (WIDE RANGE)

*Figure 8–2. Types of Protection for Workers Who Wear Glasses.*

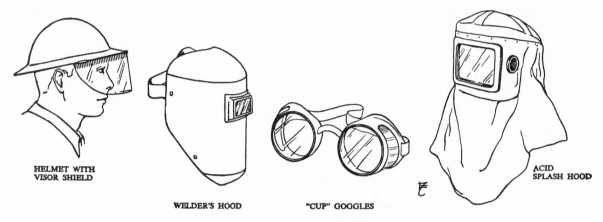

HELMET WITH VISOR SHIELD

WELDER'S HOOD

"CUP" GOGGLES

ACID SPLASH HOOD

*Figure 8–3. Types of Face Protectors.*

with hides may get *anthrax.* Slaughterhouse workers, as well as farmers, have to guard against *tetanus.* Dog-pound workers must beware of *rabies.* Barbers and beauticians have to guard against *ringworm (fungus* infections).

These are only a few of the many possible industrial infections. Frequent washing of the parts of the body exposed, and the wearing of gloves, are valuable protection against infections. Be careful about cuts. They should be washed immediately with soapy water and then treated with mild tincture of iodine or other safe antiseptics. As a general precaution, if your job involves handling living or dead animals get your doctor's advice on the best precautions to use against the specific infections you face.

5. RADIATION HAZARDS. The use of materials and devices that give off harmful radiation has increased greatly. Fortunately, more effective controls also have been devised, so that workers in industry can be protected.

One of these radiations, x-rays, has been used for many years, for a view of the inside of the body and, more recently, for cancer therapy. These same rays, if absorbed in too heavy a dosage, can *cause* cancer. In industry and in scientific laboratories, many other rays must be controlled, for they too can harm a human being, sometimes fatally. A person can receive a large amount of radiation, as from atomic fallout, without knowing it for years. The effects on his genes, which control heredity, may not affect him at all,

but may seriously damage his descendants.

X-rays, radium, and other radioactive substances give off different types of radiation, all of which require different kinds of protection. Here are some of the ways you can be protected if your job requires you to work with or near radioactive substances:

*Film badge.* The badge measures the amount of radiation you are exposed to. It is developed regularly, and the type and energy of the radiant source can be determined.

*Dosimeter.* Of the many kinds of dosimeters, the most common is the pocket-type device that is about the size and shape of a fountain pen. It can be held up to the light at any time and the person reading it can determine whether he has received a sudden or heavy dose of radiation, or if he is getting close to his maximum allowable exposure.

*Glove box.* The use of this enclosure, with its own air supply, exhaust system, and lighting, means that some industrial operations on radioactive materials can be performed directly, instead of with remote-control devices.

*Bioassay.* The amount of radioactivity absorbed by the body can be checked by analysis of the breath and urine.

*Instrumentation.* Proper instruments can record the amount of radioactivity in the environment, where human senses cannot detect it at all. Special instruments are available to detect and measure different types of radiation.

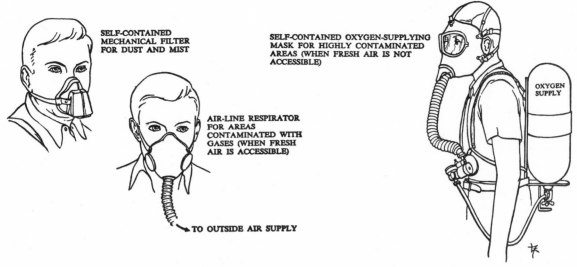

SELF-CONTAINED
MECHANICAL FILTER
FOR DUST AND MIST

SELF-CONTAINED OXYGEN-SUPPLYING
MASK FOR HIGHLY CONTAMINATED
AREAS (WHEN FRESH AIR IS NOT
ACCESSIBLE)

AIR-LINE RESPIRATOR
FOR AREAS
CONTAMINATED WITH
GASES (WHEN FRESH
AIR IS ACCESSIBLE)

TO OUTSIDE AIR SUPPLY

OXYGEN
SUPPLY

*Figure 8–4. Types of Protectors for Respiration.*

*Decontamination.* In spite of all precautions, accidents happen. If radioactive liquids or powders are spilled, or if an exhaust system breaks down, properly trained safety personnel can deal with the problem quickly. Their job includes getting rid of the contaminant immediately, getting affected workers, their clothing, and equipment clean, and testing workers for physical reactions.

Radiation can do great damage by (1) causing cancer or leukemia (malignancy of the bone marrow); (2) producing harmful effects on the skin, including "burns," loss of hair and fingernails, and darkening of the skin; (3) affecting the organs which produce the blood, thus causing anemia and insufficient white blood cells. Certain substances which make clotting possible can be affected, resulting in hemorrhages—bleeding from the gums, blood in the stools, and hemorrhages under the skin; and (4) producing sterility in either sex, owing to the action on the organs that produce the sperm or egg cells.

These effects usually do not occur until some time after exposure. In some cases, such as the development of cancer, they may not show up for years. Therefore, very great precautions must be taken, since you won't be warned of the danger by any immediate symptom such as pain. Skin burns, damage to the blood, and sterility were all

observed in victims of the atomic explosions at Nagasaki and Hiroshima.

6. DAMPNESS. Tankmen, vatmen, coal miners, and washers are among those who have to work exposed to the constant risk of dampness. This may cause coughs, colds, rheumatic diseases, and changes in the skin. Such workers should be as completely protected as possible by waterproof clothing, rubber boots, and gloves. Efforts should be made to control dampness by drain channels through which excess water is carried away.

7. ABNORMAL AIR PRESSURES. Divers and men who build tunnels have to work under unusually heavy air pressures. They can be subject to decompression sickness (the "bends"), resulting from too-rapid decrease in atmospheric pressure, as when a diver is brought too rapidly to the surface. The term "bends" is derived from the bodily contortions its victims undergo when atmospheric pressure is abruptly changed from a high to a relatively lower pressure. Partial paralysis may occur in severe cases. Only rarely is the condition fatal. Bends is treated by placing the victim in a decompression chamber, where the pressure is at the level to which he was originally exposed, and the pressure in the chamber is then reduced to normal at a safe rate.

Rising to a high altitude, which means entering a lower air pressure, can be just as harmful. Ascent as well as descent should be gradual. Pilots who rise too fast or take sudden dives may become dizzy, and the violent change in pressure may even burst their eardrums. Commercial planes are usually pressurized to prevent the effects of high altitudes.

8. ABNORMAL TEMPERATURES. Blacksmiths, welders, steelworkers, furnace men, and others may be exposed to very high temperatures. Such exposure may result in heat stroke, heat exhaustion, and cramps. Very low temperatures may cause frostbite, gangrene, or death. Insulation or air conditioning and protective clothing can help guard against these extremes in temperature. Additional salt, which may be taken in the form of coated salt tablets, is necessary to make up for that lost in perspiration. Relief periods—providing an opportunity to get back to normal temperatures—are extremely important. Workers should be on the alert for symptoms and should ask for relief the moment they appear. They should also report any colds or other disturbances to the company doctor or to their own physician.

9. NOISE AND VIBRATION. Technical advances in industry have been accompanied by new machines that are excessively noisy and produce a lot of vibration. Too much noise can damage your hearing. It can also cause pain. A related danger is that you may not hear orders or warning signals. Vibrations can have the same effect on a person as motion sickness. The heart, lungs, abdominal organs, or the brain may be damaged by excessive vibration. You may suffer injuries from being overexposed to excessive vibration, but not know it immediately. Many studies have been made to determine the tolerable limits of noise and vibration, not only to protect the workers against their serious effects, but to make the industrial operation as efficient and productive as possible.

I believe that everyone concerned in the major problem of industrial diseases—management, workers, doctors, and government and trade-union labor officials—should consider carefully these comments taken from the excellent book *Medicine,* edited by Hugh G. Garland, M.D.:

It has already been stated that there is no field of medicine which offers greater scope for prevention than the industrial medical field. . . . The late Sir Thomas Legge . . . after much practical experience in the field of prevention enumerated the following now famous axioms:

(1) Unless and until the employer has done everything—and everything means a good deal—the workman can do next to nothing to protect himself, although he is naturally willing enough to do his share.

(2) If you can bring an influence to bear external to the workman (i.e., one over which he can exercise no control), you will be successful; and if you cannot or do not, you will never be wholly successful.

(3) Practically all industrial lead poisoning is due to the inhalation of dust and fumes; and if you stop their inhalation you will stop the poisoning.

(4) All workmen should be told something of the danger of the material with which they come into contact, and not be left to find it out for themselves—sometimes at the cost of their lives.

Even though these axioms were based on the lead industry, they have wide applicability.

You may want more information about your job, occupational diseases, and health and safety standards. If so, you can write to the nearest regional office of the Occupational Safety and Health Administration (OSHA). The addresses are as follows:

9470 Federal Bldg.
450 Golden Gate Avenue
P.O. Box 35107
San Francisco, Calif. 36107

Room 15010, Federal Bldg.
1961 Stout Street
Denver, Colo. 80202

Suite 587, 1375 Peachtree Street NE
Atlanta, Ga. 30309

Room 3263, 230 South Dearborn
Chicago, Ill. 60604

18 Oliver Street
Boston, Mass. 02110

Room 3000, 911 Walnut Street
Kansas City, Mo. 64106

Room 3445, 1515 Broadway
New York, N.Y. 10036

Suite 15220, Gateway Bldg.
3535 Market Street
Philadelphia, Pa. 19104

Room 602
555 Griffin Square Bldg.
Dallas, Texas 75202

Room 6048
Federal Office Bldg.
909 First Avenue
Seattle, Wash. 98174

# 9
# YOUR VACATION

You probably look forward all year to your precious vacation—one, two, or perhaps more, wonderful weeks away from the office, the factory, or the routine of housework. You picture yourself lying on the beach, fishing in silvery brooks, climbing mountains, or driving through the countryside and stopping as the fancy takes you. Nothing to do but enjoy yourself and renew your strength, so that you will come home tanned and refreshed and eager for work!

Unfortunately the real picture is frequently very different. Vacations do not take place in a fairyland. The sun can burn as well as tan; the rolling billows hide an undertow capable of drowning the careless swimmer; poison ivy and stinging insects live in the green woods. As a doctor, I have seen too many vacationers who came home with a severe sunburn or in a state of physical exhaustion—or even with dysentery or typhoid fever. The saying, "I have to rest up from my vacation," is more truth than jest.

## WHY GO ON VACATIONS?

If the preceding has happened to you or to some member of your family, you may decide to swear off vacations for life. This year, you announce with determination, you're going to stay home and relax. You'll sleep late and go to ball games and the beaches and on picnics. In this way, you'll save money as well as disappointments.

It is true that you can have a good time and a good rest without leaving home, although even that requires some medical information and common sense. But you can usually have a better and

more profitable time by going away: a complete change of scenery and of people usually improves morale and makes for happier living. Don't be discouraged by the length of this chapter, or by the number of warnings I issue. Do remember that I cover a wide variety of vacations, both in this country and abroad; also, I include special information for those who take vacations to avoid illness, such as hay fever or asthma, and for those people who must take special precautions because of potentially serious chronic ailments. Only a few of the instructions will apply to you. If you follow them you will discover that vacations can be rewarding.

I have already mentioned the usefulness of regular vacations in your health program (p. 15).

## BEFORE YOU GO ON YOUR VACATION

I suggest that you see your doctor *before* you go on your vacation—so that you won't have to see him after it is over. I recommend that you have your annual checkup at this time so he can tell you how much and what kind of exercise you should undertake. If he says you are not in condition to climb mountains or play tennis, you can select a place where you won't be tempted to participate in such activities. You will have more fun lying on the beach or sitting in a boat pulling in the fish.

Deciding where to go for your vacation is important. Your doctor will advise you to avoid certain places at certain seasons if you have a tendency to hay fever. (Hay fever sufferers should read page 498.) Your doctor will find out whether a certain camp is close enough to good medical care to be safe for your small children. He will warn you that certain altitudes will force you to cut down on your activity until you become acclimated. Table 9-1 lists altitudes of popular vacation sites in mountain areas. This is particularly important for anyone who is suffering from impairment of the heart or lungs (see pages 416 and 439). If the place you are considering is not

---

## TABLE 9–1

### ALTITUDES OF VACATION AREAS

| EAST AND SOUTH | ALTITUDE IN FEET |
|---|---|
| Atlantic Coast | under 1,000 |
| Gulf Coast | under 1,000 |
| Green Mountains, Vermont highest point, Mt. Mansfield | 4,393 |
| White Mountains, New Hampshire highest point, Mt. Washington | 6,288 |
| Lake Winnipesaukee, New Hampshire | 504 |
| Cadillac Mountain, Maine | 1,530 |
| Moosehead Lake, Maine | 1,023 |
| Rangeley Lakes, Maine | 1,511 |
| Lake George, New York | 325 |
| Lake Placid, New York | 1,864 |
| Finger Lakes, New York | about 1,000 |
| Catskill Mountains | under 2,000 |
| Pocono Mountains, Pennsylvania | under 3,000 |
| Allegheny Mountains, West Virginia: | |
| valleys | 2,000 |
| peaks | 3,000–4,000 |
| White Sulphur Springs, West Virginia | 1,917 |
| Great Smoky Mountains, North Carolina and Tennessee peaks | over 5,000 |
| Florida resorts | under 350 |
| Blue Ridge Parkway, Virginia | 2,000–6,000 |
| Skyline Drive, Virginia: highest point | 3,680 |

| MIDWEST | |
|---|---|
| Ohio, Illinois, Indiana, Iowa, Michigan, Minnesota, Missouri, Wisconsin | 2,000 or under |

| WEST | |
|---|---|
| Pacific Coastline | under 1,000 |
| Phoenix, Arizona | 1,200 |
| Tucson, Arizona | 2,400 |

| Yosemite National Park, California: | |
|---|---|
| floor of valley | 4,000 |
| peaks | 9,000 |
| San Gabriel Mountains, California | 5,000–6,000 |
| Sequoia National Park, California: | |
| highest peaks | 14,000 |
| Death Valley National Monument | 0–5,000 |
| Colorado, altitude of state | 3,350 and over |
| Aspen, Colorado | 7,930 |
| Boulder, Colorado | 5,350 |
| Colorado Springs, Colorado | 5,980 |
| Glacier National Park, Montana: peaks over | 6,000 |
| Scotts Bluff National Monument, Nebraska | 4,649 |
| Nevada mountain ranges | 7,000–10,000 |
| Reno, Nevada | 4,490 |
| Las Vegas, Nevada | 2,030 |
| Sante Fe, New Mexico | 6,950 |
| Albuquerque, New Mexico | 4,945 |
| Carlsbad, New Mexico | 3,110 |
| Taos, New Mexico | 6,983 |
| Crater Lake National Park, Oregon | 6,000 |
| Bryce National Park, Utah | 5,000 |
| Zion National Monument, Utah: | |
| highest peak | 11,000 |
| Salt Lake City, Utah | 4,390 |
| Mt. Rainier National Park, Washington: | |
| general elevation | 4,000–6,500 |
| Mt. Rainier | 14,408 |
| Olympic National Park, Washington: | |
| peaks | 5,000–7,954 |
| Grand Teton National Park, Wyoming | 5,000–9,000 |
| Yellowstone National Park, Wyoming: | |
| general elevation | 7,000–8,500 |
| highest peak | 11,000 |
| Laramie, Wyoming | 7,159 |

| CANADA | |
|---|---|
| Lake Louise and Banff National Park | peaks over 9,000 |
| Quebec | 192 |
| Montreal | 48 |
| Toronto | 296 |
| Laurentian Mountains | less than 2,000 |

| MEXICO | |
|---|---|
| Mexico City | 7,800 |
| Acapulco | Seaport town |
| Taxco | 5,600 |
| Cuernavaca | 4,500 |

included, write to the Chamber of Commerce in the city or town nearest to it, and they will provide the information you request.

Although a vacation can't cure chronic diseases, some people are benefited by going to a "health resort" or spa. While the curative power of many famous mineral springs and baths has been greatly overrated in the past, the time spent in relaxing in an environment devoted to health, and under the care of a competent physician, can do a lot of good. Be sure to consult your doctor before you decide to take a vacation "cure."

Tell your doctor not only where you plan to go, but how you plan to get there, whether by train, plane, ship, or car. None of these modes of travel is in itself harmful, but each of them causes "seasickness" in some individuals. Your doctor has medicines to help *prevent* most cases of motion sickness (see page 511).

Your doctor probably hasn't the time to talk over every detail of your coming vacation with you. Undoubtedly you have already acquired some of the medical information you need: before going away on a "rough it" vacation, it will be well worth your while to reread Chapter 23 on first aid. If convenient, take this book, as well as the first aid kit described in Chapter 24, with you.

If you find it inconvenient to take along such a complete kit, the following represents a minimum for emergencies:

Aspirin, for headache, fever, muscle aches and pains
Antiseptic, such as hydrogen peroxide, tincture of iodine, or benzalkonium chloride
Skin lotion, to protect you against sunburn and windburn
Antinauseant, for motion sickness
Antacid, for mild stomach upset
Sedative, for emotional upset, overstimulation, or nervous upset
Broad-spectrum antibiotic, effective against a wide range of bacteria, in case of serious illness; to be selected by your doctor and used precisely as he instructs you
A container of small bandages
Sterilized gauze squares
Roll of adhesive tape, one-half inch wide
Pectin-kaolin compound (such as Kaopectate) for diarrhea

Pepto-Bismol, a preparation found in recent medical studies to be useful for the "tourist trots"

## RULES FOR VACATIONISTS

Wherever you go or whatever you plan to do, be sure to observe the following rules. Some of them seem so obvious you may wonder why I include them, but let me assure you they are broken regularly by even the most intelligent men and women. One very successful executive I know has never managed to get through a vacation on his sailboat without suffering from a severe case of sunburn! Somehow, people get the idea that they change themselves as completely as they do their appearances when they get out of their city clothes and into their sports outfits.

### Don't Overexercise

Don't plunge immediately into a full program of activity, especially if you do sedentary work the rest of the year. Going from a sea-level city to a high altitude and promptly indulging in a few highballs and a set or two of tennis can almost be guaranteed to bring about an immediate collapse. Take it easy the first day. Play ball or go swimming for only an hour or so and work up to a full activity *gradually*. In this way you will avoid muscular cramps and "charley horse" and the exhaustion that may spoil your entire vacation.

If you are over thirty you may have to be even more careful. Heart attacks can occur, especially in men who are overweight. Too much of even a "mild" sport can be dangerous. Stop as soon as you begin to feel tired. A good rule to observe is this: if you pant or get completely out of breath, cut down on what you're doing or eliminate it entirely.

### Don't Overeat

You will be tempted to do so when you sit down to a hotel dining table lavishly laden with food. It is true that you are paying for it and that you are ravenous because you've been exercising; but you're apt to pay for overeating. The extra food puts more strain on your heart, which will be pumping pretty hard as you dash around the tennis court later on. Never stuff yourself until your stomach feels distended. Avoid rich foods during vacations that may give you indigestion at home; don't count on bicarbonate, etc., to make up for your excesses.

Diarrhea often follows an overly rich diet, or one that includes foods strange to you. Contaminated water also can cause the "tourist trots." If you are plagued by this unpleasant problem, change to the softest, blandest foods available, such as boiled or poached eggs, custard, or rice with milk and sugar. After each movement, drink something hot (preferably soup, tea, or milk) to compensate for fluid loss.

A recent study indicates that Peptol-Bismol, an old patent medicine, is valuable for traveler's diarrhea, with one ounce every half hour for four hours leading to significant reductions in diarrhea, nausea, and cramps within twenty-four hours.

## SUNBURN AND SUNTAN

Almost everyone wants to come home from vacation "as brown as a berry." To accomplish this, many people would rather lie and broil in the hot sun than recline beside a shady brook; and they feel cheated if the days are crisp or cloudy. They tend to confuse a good time and a good tan.

Sunshine is healthful for most people; it makes them feel and look better. However, it is almost certainly harmful to people suffering from certain diseases. These include tuberculosis of the lungs (p. 441) which often becomes worse after injudicious exposure to the sun, nephritis (p. 422), and certain skin diseases such as lupus erythematosus. However, psoriasis and some other diseases are helped by sunlight (p. 506).

No matter how anxious you are to get a good tan, don't try to do it the first day. You are very apt to get a burn that reddens and blisters your skin or even puts you in the hospital. You can prevent painful and ugly sunburn if you are careful about a few things. They include:

1. *Learn when and where the sun has the greatest burning power.* Watch out for the noonday sun! When the sun is high overhead its rays are short, direct, and burning. Remember, when you are on Daylight Saving Time during the summer, 1:00 P.M. on your watch is really noon, the time of most severe sunburn. Late afternoon is a safer time to start your sunbathing. As the sun goes down, its rays are long and burn more slowly. Even when the sky is overcast, the sun can burn cruelly, so be careful on hazy days as well as on bright ones. Remember, too, that some of the worst cases of sunburn I've seen have been on people who went to the beach or to snowcovered mountains. This is because, *in addition to the direct sunlight,* there is a *reflected glare* from the sand and water, or the snow and ice.

2. *Know your own type of skin and how easily it burns.* Skins differ in their sensitivity to sunlight. Children burn more quickly than adults. Babies under two years and delicate children of any age need close watching when they start their sunbaths. Allow them only five or ten minutes at the start, Increase their time in the direct sun at the rate of about five minutes each day. People with fair skins are quicker to burn than are brunettes. Some people never develop a tan, and burn every time they stay out in the sun; others merely freckle.

For most people, *fifteen minutes is long enough* for the first sunbath. Each day after that, the exposure time can be lengthened by fifteen minutes. Time your sunbaths. Start with short ones and gradually make them longer so that you will get a good protective tan without burning. If you know that you burn quickly, start exposing yourself to the sun after four o'clock in the afternoon. The face, the skin in front of the elbows, and the legs are more sensitive to burning than are other parts of the body; they need extra protection.

3. *Use a suntan preparation.* Suntan preparations help to guard your skin against burning, but even the best ones give only partial protection, so don't fail to watch the clock just because you're using one of them. There are many such preparations, sold under trade names, and all are intended to promote a tan and discourage a burn. Some people prefer an oil; others like a cream or lotion. Before starting on your vacation, buy a good sun-

tan preparation. Some contain an ingredient, PABA (*p*-aminobenzoic acid), which acts as a sunscreen.

## Other Suggestions for Sunbathers

Drink plenty of water when you are suntanning. You will need it to make up for the fluid you lose, even though you may not realize that you are perspiring on a dry, sunny day. Take salt tablets or salty crackers, or tomato juice with salt in it.

Getting overheated in the hot sun is dangerous for anyone. It may put a strain on the internal organs, particularly the heart and blood vessels. An elderly person or one with heart trouble or any disease should always ask his doctor about sunbathing.

The fact that you are enjoying yourself is no protection against *heat stroke* or *heat prostration* (see page 335).

You may be called upon sometime to help a person who has been burned by the sun. Sunburn can make people very sick, with chills, fever, and even delirium. Be sure to call a doctor if the burn is severe. Extensive and large blisters always need the attention of a doctor; there is danger of infection. In mild cases where the skin turns red, use a dusting powder containing equal parts of zinc oxide, boric acid, and talcum. For moderately bad burns where the skin is red and slightly swollen, apply wet dressings of gauze dipped in a solution of aluminum acetate, 1 part in 500 parts of water. Another soothing dressing is made by soaking gauze in cold white mineral oil. After the swelling goes down, replace the dressings with a soothing cream containing: cold cream, 88 parts; methyl salicylate, 10 parts; and benzocaine, 2 parts. Any druggist will make these preparations for you. In very severe, extensive sunburn, your doctor may prescribe corticosteroid tablets.

The sun can help to make your vacation enjoyable, or it can spoil it for you. Don't let chance decide this important question.

## WATER WISDOM

Swimming is one of the most healthful sports. It exercises the body without overheating it. It develops strong, smooth muscles and good lung capacity. It can be enjoyed by healthy people from childhood to old age; and, properly supervised, it is even recommended for people recovering from certain diseases such as polio (infantile paralysis). However, don't decide for yourself that swimming is "good for what ails you." *Be sure to get your doctor's advice* if you have been ill recently or are suffering from a chronic ailment.

The health and enjoyment you will gain from swimming far outweigh its dangers, provided you acquire some "water wisdom." Many people have taught themselves to swim, but a few hours of instruction will be worthwhile. Drowning ranks among leading fatal accidents, so don't confuse the joys of the moment when you plunge into the water with your ability to swim.

## Is the Water Clean?

First of all, find out whether or not the water you plan to swim in could be polluted. A silvery brook or clear blue lake may be contaminated by germs that can give you typhoid fever or dysentery; a swimming pool may be too crowded or its water changed too seldom to protect you against a number of diseases. The local health department will know about the condition of pools and bathing beaches in its territory. Feel free to *check with them*. This is particularly important if there is an epidemic of some disease.

## Swimming Time

Don't go into the water immediately after meals or when overheated or tired from other exercise. Always come out *before* you get tired or chilly. A swim should leave you relaxed and comfortable. If it doesn't, you have stayed in the water too long. Take a shorter swim next time. Remaining in the water when you feel chilly lowers your resistance to infections such as colds, pneumonia, polio, or sinus or ear infections. Getting overtired is dangerous, too. It puts a strain on your heart and blood vessels.

## Double Safety

On a long swim have someone row along beside you, or go with another good swimmer. Be sure that you both know lifesaving methods. The most expert swimmer may drag you down if he gets a cramp. Rescue training will teach you how to avoid his clutches while you tow him to shore. Unless you both know lifesaving methods, better swim parallel to shore or stay within rescue distance.

No matter how well you swim, stay very close to shore if you are swimming in an isolated spot. The races you won in high school will not protect you against cramps!

Don't attempt a long swim on the *first few days of the season.* Your swimming muscles have lost their strength through the winter. Give them time to get strong again before tackling rapid currents, a heavy sea, or a long-distance swim.

Someone else may not be as sensible as you, so familiarize yourself with the first aid instructions for applying artificial respiration given on page 331.

## Feet First

Before diving in a new place, test the water for depth and hidden logs or rocks. Lakes and rivers change in depth according to rainfall. In salt water, there are high and low tides to consider. *Find out for yourself* whether your dive should be a shallow one. Don't risk a broken neck.

If you have trouble with your sinuses or ears, give up diving and underwater swimming. Water in the nose washes away protective secretions that help prevent infection. In addition, infections can wash into the sinuses through the nose or reach the middle ear through the eustachian passage from the throat (see Figure 6-14, page 113).

## POISON IVY

One or more varieties of poison ivy appear in many parts of the United States. These plants are responsible for about 350,000 cases of skin poisoning every year. It is well worth your while to learn how to avoid joining these sufferers!

Poison ivy grows in the form of climbing vines, shrubs which trail on the ground, and erect shrubbery growing without any support. It clings to stone and brick houses, and climbs trees and poles. It flourishes abundantly along fences, paths, and roadways, and is often partially hidden by other foliage. The leaves vary in length from one to four inches. They are green and glossy in summer; in the spring and fall they are red or russet. The fruit is white and waxy, resembling mistletoe. Although poison ivy assumes many forms and displays seasonal changes in leaf coloring, it has one constant characteristic which makes it easy to recognize. *The leaves always grow in clusters of three,* one at the end of the stalk, the other two opposite one another. The old jingle, "Leaflets three, let it be," has helped children and adults to recognize poison ivy at a glance, and to avoid it "like poison." (See Figure 9-1.)

### Poisoning

The irritating substance in poison ivy is the oily sap in the leaves, flowers, fruit, stem, bark, and roots. The plant is poisonous even after long drying, but is particularly irritating in the spring and early summer when it is full of sap.

Most cases of ivy poisoning are due to direct contact with the plant, at any time, even in the winter. Some are caused by handling clothing, garden implements, and pets which have been contaminated by the oily sap. People differ in their sensitivity to poison ivy. Some people are so sensitive that exposure to smoke from a brush fire containing poison ivy can result in a severe inflammation of the skin. Too many people suffer from ivy poisoning because they haven't learned to recognize poison ivy; they walk through it, brush against it, and even gather its attractive foliage. They usually transfer part of the irritant on their hands to their faces and other parts of their bodies. I have seen some really serious cases of poisoning in the mouth because children—and, occasionally, adults—have eaten the leaves or berries of this poisonous plant.

If you realize that you have accidentally handled poison ivy or brushed against it, wash your skin as soon as possible. Yellow laundry soap is best for this purpose. Lather several times, and rinse in running water after each sudsing. This should remove or make less irritating any oil which hasn't already penetrated the skin.

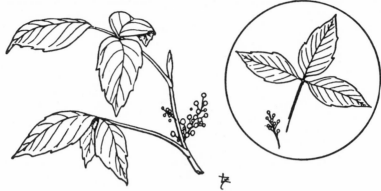

*Figure 9-1. Poison Ivy. Common east of the Rocky Mountains. Three leaflets; grayish berries in season.*

## Symptoms

The first symptom is a burning and itching sensation. This is followed by a rash and swelling and probably small or large blisters. The length of time elapsing between contact with poison ivy and the first symptom varies from a few hours to seven days.

## Severe Cases

If there are large blisters, severe inflammation, or fever, or if the inflammation is on the face or genitals, a doctor's help is needed. He will know how to relieve discomfort and guard against secondary infections until the attack subsides, as it eventually does.

Stubborn cases which do not respond to proper treatment may be due to repeated contact with contaminated clothing. Any suspected garments should be dry cleaned or washed with plenty of soap.

## Treatment of Mild Cases

When there are only a few small blisters on the hands, arms, or legs, the following treatment may bring relief: Apply compresses of very hot, plain water for brief intervals. Or apply calamine lotion or a compress soaked in a dilute Burow's solution (1 pint to 15 pints of cool water). Your druggist will supply you with Burow's solution.

If these methods don't help, consult a doctor.

## Precautions

Most people will be safe if they learn to recognize the "leaflets three," and let them be. Campers, field men, and others whose activities take them through underbrush and into the deep woods require the further protection of clothing which really covers the body. This means trousers, long sleeves, and gloves. It should be remembered that garments worn for such work as digging up poison ivy become contaminated with the irritating oils. They are not safe to handle or to wear again until they have been laundered or dry cleaned.

Several methods of inoculating against poison ivy have been developed, but they are of varying effectiveness. Consult your doctor at least three months before you expect to be exposed again. He will test your skin to determine the extent of your sensitivity. Your doctor may decide to try to desensitize you with an oral preparation. Series of injections are sometimes tried, but they may be painful and not necessarily successful.

## Eradication of Poison Ivy

Poison ivy should be eradicated wherever and whenever possible. Growing and spreading through school grounds and parks, it is responsible for much needless suffering and expense. Communities and civic groups should insist that poisonous plants be removed, especially from grounds where children play. Find out whether, and where, your vacation resort has eliminated poison ivy.

## OTHER POISONOUS PLANTS, BERRIES, ETC.

The method of preventing ivy poisoning, and the treatments for it, are effective for oak-leaf poison ivy, western poison oak, and poison sumac. These are the most common of the sixty varieties of plants in the United States that can irritate the skin.

There are a number of poisonous berries, and over eighty kinds of poisonous mushrooms. Every year people die or become seriously ill because they have decided that one of these "looks good enough to eat." Children are frequently tempted by poisonous holly berries or the berries that grow on privet (the shrubs often used for hedges). Adults are apt to place their faith in some incorrect notion, such as the old superstition that you can tell mushrooms from toadstools by cooking a silver coin with them, which is supposed to tarnish if the variety is poisonous. Pay no attention to these old wives' tales; they cause a number of deaths every year. Although it is possible to learn to identify poisonous mushrooms and berries, it isn't easy. It is much wiser to play safe. Train your children not to eat things they find in the woods or fields, and set them a good example by not doing it yourself.

What to do in case of mushroom or berry poisoning is described on page 331.

Be sure to check with local authorities before you decide to bring home a mess of clams or oysters for dinner. The beds they grow in may be contaminated by typhoid and other germs! Not only that, but mussels, clams, and certain other shellfish are dangerous during some seasons of the year. They become poisonous as a result of feeding on microscopic organisms that appear in the ocean during the warm months, particularly in the Pacific.

## INSECTS

Insects run poison ivy and sunburn a close second in ruining vacations. Pest control programs have helped to reduce their number and ferocity, difficult as this may be to believe when a mosquito is ruining your night's rest.

Spraying with insecticides will help get rid of most insects. The "space sprays," such as aerosol bombs, kill insects in flight and are useful in rooms that are screened to prevent more pests from entering. If you want to prevent insects from entering, use a residual-type spray that covers surfaces with a coating which remains effective for

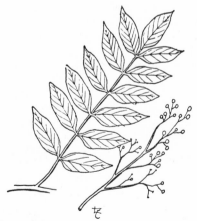

*Figure 9-2. Poison Sumac. Seven to thirteen leaves; pale waxy berries in season.*

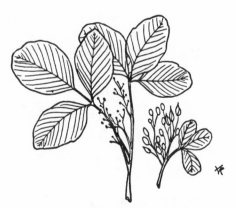

*Figure 9-3. Poison Oak. Found mainly on the Pacific Coast. Three leaflets; white berries in season.*

up to a month outdoors, two months indoors. To do this, apply the spray to screens, porches, shrubbery, etc. The same type of spray is also useful for getting rid of cockroaches and bedbugs, but be sure to air the bed and mattress thoroughly after spraying.

*All insecticides contain material poisonous to human beings, especially children.* Be careful how you use them. Read the directions on the label. Don't spray foods, dishes, or anything infants or children may touch or put in their mouths. Wash your hands and face after applying insecticides. *Many insecticides are inflammable;* unless the label definitely states that this is not the case, don't use them around open fires.

## Insect Repellents

The United States Department of Agriculture has spent years studying the best way to keep insects from biting human beings. They have produced formulas containing combinations of chemicals, applications of which will repel insects for about two hours. The following materials have been found to be safe and generally effective. They can be used separately, although combinations of them provide more protection against a larger variety of insects:

> dimethyl phthalate
> dimethyl carbate
> Indalone
> 2-ethyl-1, 3 hexanediol
>   (Rutgers 612)

Most druggists can supply you with dimethyl phthalate. They may also be able to provide you with the following combination, or formula, which is marketed by several firms; it is sometimes referred to as "6-22": dimethyl phthalate, 60%; Indalone, 20%; dimethyl carbate, 20%.

Always try these materials or formulas on a *small area* of your arm or leg before using them liberally, to see whether you happen to be sensitive to them. As a rule, they will not cause any irritation. However, they are poisonous if taken internally and harmful if they get into the eyes. Be careful with them. They will also damage plastics and some synthetic materials, especially rayon—but not nylon. Fortunately they do not hurt cotton or wool, so they can usually be rubbed on socks as well as on ankles, for double protection. Some people object to the oily consistency of these insect repellents, but most people find that a small price to pay for protection against black flies, gnats, mosquitoes, and other pests.

## Insect and Tick Bites

Scratching bites irritates them, sometimes causing infections. Bee and hornet stings can be dangerous, if a person is especially sensitive to the venom. Try to keep children away from holes in trees and other places where bees and hornets may gather. Chigger bites can be annoying on a vacation trip. The best protection against insect bites is proper clothing, but if you are a little careless, as we all are at times, a paste of baking soda and cold water will soothe the bite. See page 341 for more detailed information on bites of bees, wasps, ants, and other insects.

*Ticks* fasten their heads into the skin of their victim and suck his blood. Ticks should be extracted whole. If they are carelessly pulled off, all or part of the mouth may be left in the skin. To

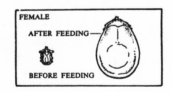

*Figure 9-4. The Common Wood Tick (Shown Greatly Enlarged).*

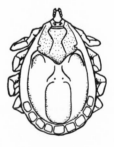

FEMALE
(BACK VIEW)

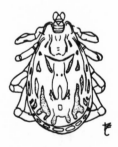

MALE
(BACK VIEW)

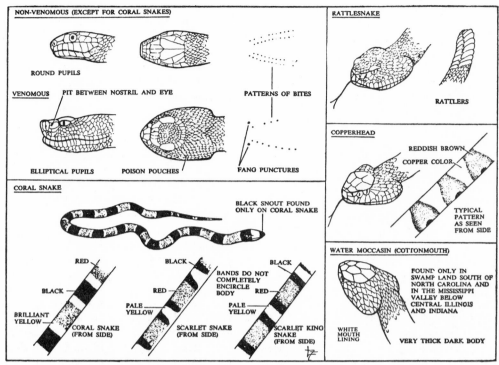

*Figure 9–5. The Four Major Types of Poisonous Snakes in the U.S.A.*

loosen the tick's grasp, you can apply petroleum jelly, baby oil, gasoline, or turpentine to the area and leave it for half an hour. Once the tick has relinquished its hold, it should be carefully removed with tweezers and destroyed, but not with bare hands. The site should be washed with soap and water, and an antiseptic applied to help prevent infection.

The only really dangerous *spider* in this country is the black widow. It, and *scorpions* and *centipedes*, are discussed on page 341.

## SNAKES

There are poisonous snakes in many parts of the United States (see Figure 9-5). However, in many vacation resorts a snake is as rare as it would be on the streets of a large city. If you are going to a snake-infested part of the country, be sure to read carefully page 336, and *take along the snakebite kit which your doctor will help you*

*to obtain.* In case of snakebite, keep the affected area cold if at all possible. An icepack will numb the pain and slow down the process of damage to the tissues.

## INOCULATIONS

If you were in the armed forces you probably feel as though you have been inoculated against every existing (and a few nonexistent) diseases. Nevertheless, you should discuss the matter with your doctor, because time passes and you may need a booster shot.

### Tetanus (Lockjaw)

I advise my patients to be immunized against lockjaw, especially if they are going to be in areas in which there is a special risk of being infected by the tetanus bacillus. As this tiny germ thrives in the intestines of grass-eating animals, particularly horses, it is found in and about stables and in garden soil treated with animal manure. It usually enters the body through a deep wound such as is made by stepping on a nail, which frequently happens to children who go barefoot. Any punctured or torn wound, especially one soiled by dirt or having bits of clothing or other contaminated material forced into it (which often happens in Fourth of July accidents with firecrackers) is dangerous.

Tetanus is easy to prevent, but *one half of the people who develop it die from the disease.* The longer treatment is delayed, the less chance of recovery. Read carefully the section on tetanus (p. 139) and remember: *any deep wound requires the immediate attention of a doctor.*

## VACATIONS IN FOREIGN COUNTRIES

If you are going abroad, be sure to tell your doctor where you are going. He may advise smallpox vaccinations: you will run into difficulty if you try to reenter the United States from certain countries without an International Certificate of Vaccination saying you have recently been protected against smallpox. Typhoid "shots" are essential for some countries; and your doctor will tell you how to protect yourself against amebic and bacterial dysentery, which are prevalent in many parts of the world.

## ANTIBIOTIC FIRST AID

Travel to isolated places can now be made safer as far as such diseases as pneumonia, acute appendicitis, blood poisoning, meningitis, and many other illnesses are concerned. The "wonder drugs" have made "first aid" possible for these dangerous diseases.

*I do not believe in the careless, indiscriminate use of these antibiotics.* Like other medicines, they have specific functions and hazards. First aid is

*emergency* therapy, and should be followed as soon as possible by supervised medical care. No one who treats an injured person for a fracture on a hiking trip would do more than apply splints and other first aid measures. This in itself is often lifesaving, minimizing damage during the trip to the doctor by preventing blood vessels from tearing. Similarly, if you were traveling in an isolated part of Mexico or in some of our own forests, and your traveling companion experienced a cough, chill, fever of 104 degrees, rusty expectoration, and pain in the chest, it wouldn't take you long to suspect that pneumonia had set in. A two-day carry of such a person over rough trails might cause his death. But, given the right amount of antibiotics, his illness could be brought under control, and he could be safely transported to the nearest doctor or hospital. There the treatment would be supervised by a physician until the disease was completely cured.

If you are going to an isolated spot, *ask your doctor* for instructions in antibiotic first aid. These should include (1) a prescription for one of the antibiotics having a wide range of activity, (2) exact directions for when it should be used (definitely not for mild colds and fevers), and (3) an agreement that when you return you will make a complete report to your doctor regarding when and why you used the antibiotic; let him decide what to do with any unused medicine.

## WHEN YOUR VACATION ENDS

People often start for home feeling happy and relaxed, only to arrive tense and exhausted after a long bumper-to-bumper drive through Sunday traffic. You can undo much of the good your vacation has done you by trying to prolong it till the last minute. Allow time enough to take it easy the way home. Get there in time to unpack, read your mail, and make those phone calls you simply have to attend to before you can go to bed. In that way, you will get the full benefit of what ought to be the happiest and healthiest weeks of your life.

# 10
# CLIMATE AND ILLNESS

If you or other members of your family have a long-lasting illness, you have undoubtedly at some time considered moving to a better climate. Before you decide to make a major change for the sake of a more healthful climate, my advice is: think not twice but three times! Then stop and reconsider. The chances are very high that you are making a mistake, and once the change has been made—and jobs given up and connections severed—the road back may be impossible.

It is true that certain climates are better than others, especially where individual tastes are concerned. People who hate the cold wonder why anyone lives in Maine except from sheer necessity, while those who suffer from the heat feel the same way about the inhabitants of most of the southern states. There is no doubt that many people feel better in a high, dry climate than they do by the damp seaside. Also, some diseases are benefited by certain climates.

"Then why," you ask, "do you warn us against moving?"

The answer is: man is a complicated being. He is never just a "case" of tuberculosis, asthma, rheumatism, heart disease, and so on, but rather an individual who happens to suffer from an ailment. A number of factors, therefore, should be taken into consideration before uprooting one's self or one's family. Changing location for the climatic treatment of health is far too often done hastily or recklessly, without proper consideration.

At one time, doctors were much more ready to recommend a change in climate for health's sake than they are now. There are so many more controls over the climate in our own homes and places of work, and so much more understanding of the new problems that a move to another part of the country can create, that we doctors now are extremely cautious about recommending relocation. In the next few pages, I describe some of the serious kinds of questions you should ask yourself (and your doctor) before you think of uprooting yourself from your home, family, and friends.

## SOME PROBLEMS INVOLVED IN MOVING

Take the case of one of my own friends: Mr. A, a lawyer, is troubled with serious sinusitis. There are days when headaches make life close to unbearable, but he manages to carry on a remunerative practice despite the difficulties. It is true he has developed a violent distaste for the frequent and sometimes painful visits to his nose-and-throat specialist, his family doctor, and his allergist. They all help him, but nobody can provide consistent or complete relief.

One day Mr. A meets a business acquaintance from the Southwest. This booster for his own good climate tells him that sinusitis doesn't exist there, and urges him to move out "where we're all healthy." Mr. A. is in a particularly bad period of his sinusitis. In desperation—and hope—he closes his office and moves to southern Arizona.

There is profound and immediate improvement in his sinusitis. He is overjoyed.

But he soon discovers that he has merely traded

one headache for another! The legal profession in some southwestern cities is already oversaturated by the native sons plus the lawyers afflicted with tuberculosis, arthritis, sinusitis, hay fever, and other complaints who have migrated year after year from other parts of the country.

Mr. A. has a difficult time. His attempts to earn a living in business and as a salesman don't work out. He suddenly realizes how much his profession means to him. The hot summers bother him.

The experiment has been a failure. He returns to his home, two thousand miles away, and starts to rebuild his practice.

The decision to move had appeared so sound to Mr. A that it would have seemed juvenile to consult anyone about it. Yet if he had discussed it with his trio of doctors, they would probably have given him some sober advice. I say "probably" because climatology is rarely taught in our medical schools, and many physicians are not well informed on this complicated and important subject.

Assuming Mr. A's doctors had thought seriously about climate and health, they would have said to him, "Look, we know you suffer excessively from your sinus headaches. There is a good chance that you may actually have fewer symptoms in the Southwest. The headaches and the annoying drip in the back of your throat may trouble you less, and you may feel better generally.

"But," they might have continued, "how will your nerves hold up if you can't make a living at your tried and beloved profession? There is no point in exchanging your sinusitis for a stomach ulcer which might result from your tension and worries! Besides, you know you have a tendency toward coronary artery trouble. How is your heart going to react to the relentlessly hot summers in the desert country?"

A compromise could have been arranged. Mr. A had reached the point where he was so desperate about his illness that he was willing to consider drastic measures. This would give his doctors the opportunity to get him to accept a program that could safeguard his profession while preventing or overcoming the worst attacks of his illness.

For example, a long winter vacation could be arranged in the Southwest or some other region where his sinusitis would improve temporarily. During the summer months he could spend his weekends away from the humid city in a high, dry atmosphere. At home and in the office, the nearest thing to Arizona climate could be provided—a filtered, air-conditioned atmosphere with temperature and humidity controls he could adjust to his own comfort. Expensive? Of course. But far cheaper than the plan Mr. A actually followed.

## ILLNESSES IN WHICH CLIMATE IS HELPFUL

You are probably asking, "But aren't there illnesses that demand a change of climate, where any amount of sacrifice is justified?"

There are some, but they are very few, and fortunately they are becoming even less numerous because of air conditioning and because of newer treatments.

Many people have uprooted themselves because of tuberculosis. Yet, contrary to popular legend, tuberculosis does not require a change of climate.

The problem is less clear-cut in cases of asthma. This disease may originate in various ways. In a fairly large number of patients there is a psychosomatic factor. (See Asthma, page 454.) This means that attacks are precipitated by emotional factors. A dry, warm climate may benefit the disease if there is no serious emotional disturbance involved. But an injudicious change to a strange area, the loss of a job the patient values, and loneliness for family and friends may be so disturbing that they throw the balance the other way.

The same reasoning applies to the patient with arthritis. The severest joint troubles are clearly physical, but an emotional element can enter into the disease picture. If the change of climate benefits the emotional as well as the physical part, the patient may improve greatly. But if only one and not the other is helped, then the move may prove to be a serious error.

Some chronic infections of the lung, such as *bronchiectasis,* and severe forms of bronchitis may benefit from a mild climate.

## HOW TO DECIDE ABOUT CHANGE OF CLIMATE

How does one steer a safe course in such a complex field? Painful symptoms and, especially the threat of irreversible damage from potentially crippling diseases like arthritis and asthma demand the most careful thought and decisions. I think it is possible to reach the correct decision by evaluating a few facts about climatology and by following some simple rules.

1. Go slowly. The diseases benefited by moving to a mild climate are mainly chronic, slow-changing ones. Your decision need not be hurried. It can be made after months of deliberation.

2. Review the entire situation with a panel of medical experts. Your family doctor will welcome an appointment with a specialist to go over the details of your illness. The cost may appear to be high, but it is always small compared to the expense of changing your whole way of life.

New treatments are constantly being developed. The specialist may suggest a trial period with a new treatment that may promise as much relief as a change of climate. The specialist may even suggest discussions with a psychiatrist to ease any nervous tensions that may be exacerbating your problem.

Perhaps the specialist will take the view that a change of climate offers the only hope for relief. In that case you have the assurance that the drastic change in your life is really necessary. Your family doctor will welcome the specialist's aid in making the decision about the climate that will be best for your particular condition.

I recall a friend who moved his family from the East because of his wife's asthma. Someone had told them, "Los Angeles is the place for you." Friends there rented them a house and they moved out.

Several months later my friend's doctor received a distressing, almost frantic letter saying that the patient was very much worse than when she had left home. The situation seemed desperate. The husband had located a job and cut himself off completely from his work in the East.

The doctor communicated with physicians in Los Angeles. They knew the answer, which is obvious to old residents of Los Angeles County: there are actually several distinct climates there. The patient had settled on the coastal strip and was exposed to weather as damp as that which she had left. When she moved twenty miles inland, closer to the desert and behind mountain ranges which protected her from the ocean, she found the warm, dry semidesert air that greatly benefited her particular type of asthma.

When a child has asthma, a careful review of the medical situation is necessary, sometimes requiring the combined judgment of a pediatrician, an allergist, a nose-and-throat specialist, and perhaps a child psychologist. Even if you live on a farm or in a small community, it will be worth the time and money to travel to the nearest medical center for a consultation with specialists.

If the specialists and your own doctor agree that the change of climate is essential, then take their advice—but act in gradual steps! I urge you to remember that we doctors may merely be expressing an opinion when we say, "I think this is a wise step. I hope it will prove beneficial." No one can guarantee absolute success.

## TRIAL PERIOD

It is best to qualify your optimism and *give yourself a trial period.* If you are the sick person, take a relative or friend along and try the suggested location for a few months in the winter *and* the summer. You may find that you feel wonderful all year. On the other hand, the beneficial effects of a dry climate in winter may be completely nullified by the blistering heat of summer. Only actual experience can answer this.

A sick child can be placed in a special school in the selected climate for a year, if the family can afford the expense involved. If the asthma, rheumatic fever, or other illness shows marked improvement, the other members of the family can take time to make the move.

## SHOULD ELDERLY PEOPLE MOVE TO MILDER CLIMATES?

Elderly, retired people often wonder whether changing to a mild climate will be desirable for their health. I recommend the same careful program for them that I have outlined for sick people. Consultation with their doctors and a trial period are equally important for them, for a change of climate is splendid for some and very bad for others. To many of us, intellectual and emotional climate is more important than physical climate. Old people often become lonely and miserable when they move away from their home towns, and happiness is essential for their well-being. They should act carefully and experimentally before changing their homes in the hope of prolonging their lives (see my chapter The Later Years, page 530).

# PART TWO

## You and Your Mind

# 11
# THE HEALTHY MIND

During the generation since World War II, we Americans have grown up in our attitude toward mental illness. That war started the maturing process by showing us dramatically that of the men drafted, more than a million were unfit for military service because of personality problems or more serious types of emotional disturbance. The rate of such rejections was higher than for heart trouble or tuberculosis. The war also showed us how frightening or shattering experiences could hurt the mind, even though the body was still healthy.

Americans started to look at mental illness more honestly, just as they were able to think about and talk about other serious health problems more openly. There is still much misunderstanding about mental health and mental illness, but just one proof of public interest is the great number of books and magazine articles on every aspect of this topic.

We know from the oldest records of human history that people have always suffered from mental illness. For centuries, they were "punished" or, at best, neglected. Only during the past two hundred years have understanding and humane treatment come about. By now, we can see real progress in many ways. Drug therapy has made it possible to help many more mentally ill persons. Scientists and physicians are developing other new techniques for care and treatment. Communities are accepting more responsibility for preventive programs as well as for care, treatment, and rehabilitation of the mentally ill. From my own associations among doctors, I can vouch for the fact that increased interest and experience with patients' emotional problems has resulted in earlier recognition and more effective treatment. I call this chapter "The Healthy Mind" because I know of the great interest in emotional as well as physical problems. Americans are asking their family doctors many questions about mental health and illness. They want to know such things as what constitutes a normal person, how emotional problems arise, how they can be prevented, and what can be done to relieve them. They want to safeguard mental health for themselves and their families. They know how their home environment affects them and their children. They also know how important it is to recognize the early signs of emotional illness and to ask for a doctor's help.

Such questions are not indications that the people who ask them are morbid or abnormal. On the contrary, interest and frankness are steps in the right direction. Facing their emotional lives and problems honestly and seriously is a normal way for most people to enrich and deepen their understanding of their own personalities and those of others. This makes for better relationships with friends, family, and children.

But, despite these healthy trends, many misconceptions persist. How many of them do *you* subscribe to? Take out your pencil and jot down "True" or "False" to each of the following statements:

1. Only a very few types of mental illness can be inherited.  _____
2. Masturbation does not cause insanity. _____
3. A certain amount of daydreaming is perfectly normal.  _____

169

4. Unusual impulses in regard to hatred, murder, or sex—including homosexual ideas—occur *occasionally* in normal people.   _____

5. Homosexuality is not "degeneracy."   _____

6. A person who is mentally ill should be regarded in the same way as a patient who is suffering from a physical disease.   _____

7. Marriage rarely improves emotional illness.   _____

8. Mental problems are not cured by sexual experience.   _____

9. There are better outlets than anger or temper tantrums for "nervousness," anxiety, or conflicts.   _____

10. Normal young children have considerable curiosity about sex.   _____

11. Even the "ideal child" is occasionally disobedient.   _____

12. Emotional illness may start early in childhood.   _____

13. Chronic drunkenness is a deep-seated psychological illness.   _____

14. Emotional difficulties, rather than inherited criminal tendencies, account for much criminal behavior.   _____

15. Modern psychiatrists deal with many emotional problems that have nothing to do with insanity.   _____

*If you wrote "True" to all of these statements, your attitude is healthy and modern. If you took a long time to decide on most of them, or if you answered eight or more "False," your attitudes toward mental hygiene need to be changed. Should you be discouraged? Not in the least! The quiz was made up from statements which a specialist in psychiatry prepared for doctors because he had found that even physicians held many erroneous ideas. Now you can be doubly proud if you answered most of them right!*

And even if you were wrong on all of them, it should merely encourage you to read this chapter and learn the right answers. (After all, you did not spend eight years getting an M.D. degree, and many doctors, after those eight years, still did not know all the right answers!) It isn't easy for us to discard worn-out ideas any more than

it is to get rid of those worn-out clothes that clutter up a closet or attic!

This section of the book, on emotional problems, will enable you to replace threadbare ideas and attitudes with ones that will serve you well in solving problems you may have to face in yourself or members of your family. It will tell you about many kinds of mental disorders, how they arise and how some of them can be ameliorated or even cured. It will give you some understanding of *mental hygiene,* which is as important as knowledge of general body hygiene (which it can influence tremendously). When mental health is understood, and the principles of mental hygiene are applied by parents and teachers, as well as by doctors specializing in this field, current thinking suggests that a great many cases of mental disturbances will be *prevented* or cured at an early stage.

*A word of caution.* The information in this section of the book is not intended to make you an "amateur psychiatrist"—one of those justly unpopular characters who know all the answers, "diagnose" people from across the room or on the basis of one piece of information, "psychoanalyze" their friends, and so on. No good psychiatrist would attempt what the parlor amateurs do so blithely. Human behavior is complex. When I give an example, it is only an *example;* and many of my explanations are given only to show you some possibilities. So don't say, "Why, he's talking about Mary" or "That means me," and get upset as a result. It certainly isn't my purpose to alarm you. On the contrary, I feel that this is perhaps the most encouraging section of the book, for tremendous progress is being made in understanding, preventing, and curing mental problems.

When I speak about the outworn ideas to which many people cling, I don't mean that you should discard everything you've ever thought or observed. That might prove to be a case of "throwing out the baby along with the bath water." If your answers to the questionnaire were wrong, it may only be because of misplaced emphasis or a misinterpretation of certain terms. Doctors, like people in all specialized fields from baseball to electrical engineering, use some words in a way that differs somewhat from the way they are generally used. I shall define some of them as I go along, but if a meaning isn't clear to you, a glance at the Dictionary of Medical Terms (p. 551) will help.

First of all, I should explain that in discussions of this kind, doctors give the word "mind" a slightly different meaning from the one that is generally given to it. We don't use it as though it were simply the organ of intelligence, but give it some of the qualities one thinks of as associated with the words *emotions, personality, nerves,* and *soul.* These meanings are all embodied in the term *psyche* (as in words such as psychiatry, psychology, and psychoanalysis).

Then, too, there are many definitions for the word "normal." Unless you and I use the same one, we probably won't arrive at the same answer to any question about "the normal person."

## WHAT IS NORMAL?

A dictionary defines this as "in accordance with an established law or principle; conforming to a type or standard," and gives as synonyms: "regular, natural, standard, model, common, ordinary, typical, unusual."

According to the law, anyone who is able to distinguish between right and wrong is sane; and normal behavior is regarded as responsible behavior. For centuries it was believed that insanity was due to demons. Even today there is a tendency to define as normal that which is in accordance with "what God intended," so that anything varying from the Gospel is unnatural and abnormal. Some people believe that normal behavior is practically the same thing as abnormal behavior except that it "doesn't go too far." Others define normality as being like the majority (despite the fact that history has shown that in a decadent society such as Nazi Germany the majority can be brutally sadistic). Similarly, people often feel that to be normal is to be happy, without taking into consideration the fact that some obviously insane people are "happy." "Maturity" is another word used as a synonym for being normal, although adolescents can certainly be normal without being mature. However, all of these definitions play some part in describing the word as psychiatrists use it.

We doctors think of a normal person as one who adjusts himself to his surroundings—the world he lives in and the people in it—and also to his own potentialities for living, making realistic efforts to change the world about him, if necessary. By abnormal behavior we mean that which results from an inappropriate or ineffective manner of getting along in one's surroundings. For example, a person who was afraid of being run over by an automobile might refuse to go outdoors, or he might spend his life in bed; this would appear to solve the problems of his fears, but obviously it would not be a satisfactory solution at all. When we examine abnormal behavior carefully, we see that it consists of a technique or set of techniques for adjusting to situations—techniques which are inadequate but are retained because they are in some way satisfying or, at least, more rewarding than anything else the individual has tried.

Because doctors who deal with mental problems use the word normal in this manner, some people believe we tend to dismiss ethical and religious values. They even feel that psychiatrists advocate immorality. It is true that some extremists among the early psychiatrists used to overemphasize "getting rid of inhibitions," but psychiatry has long since discarded any such tendency, as you will see when I talk about "inhibitions" a little later. It is not true that we "dismiss" good and evil or "explain away morality" in our effort to understand everything. (Of course, there is some truth to the saying that "to understand is to forgive.") While we doctors recognize moral responsibility (each in our own fashion), we feel that our contributions, as scientists, are in the area of *understanding* and *explaining* rather than moralizing. I feel strongly that these contributions can and do help people to lead far better and more moral lives.

## WHAT IS A NORMAL PERSON?

Although I have explained what we mean by normal, I have not yet begun to answer the first question people usually ask: *What is a normal person like?*

## Personality Structure of the Normal Person

1. REALISTIC ATTITUDES TOWARD LIFE. The normal, emotionally mature adult faces facts whether they are pleasant or unpleasant. For example, he likes to drive his car, but realizes that there are definite dangers attached to driving. Because he is mature, he takes special care to check the brakes, tires, lights, and all the essential parts of his automobile at reasonable intervals. The immature person may say, "Accidents never happen to me," and refuse to take any precautions. Or he may be the other type of immature individual who checks his brakes every day and still loses sleep at night worrying about the fact that "accidents always happen to me."

2. INDEPENDENCE. The mature person forms reasoned opinions and then acts on them. He is not reckless or headstrong, and seeks a reasonable amount of advice. Once he has the facts, he is capable of making a decision. He is willing to face the consequences of his decisions.

On the other hand, the immature person often has difficulty making up his own mind. He wants his relatives or friends or business associates to tell him how to proceed. When he is forced to make decisions alone, he may become upset, nervous, "rattled," or even vicious. Many immature people don't want to accept the responsibility of the decisions they have reached, but blame others if something goes wrong, and demand inordinate praise if the decision leads to success.

3. ABILITY TO LOVE OTHERS. The mature adult gets pleasure out of giving love to children, mate, close relatives, and friends. Such a person is selective in his love relationships and doesn't need a huge circle of people to be intimate with. On the opposite side, the immature person finds it difficult to love others and wants always to be loved, to be fussed over, and to be the center of attention. If you observe young children, you will notice that they want to be loved and to be the center of all affection. Seldom does a little child show sustained love for others. This is part of normal development in children, but when such traits appear in adults, they interfere with healthy personal relationships. The adult person expects to give more love to a child than the child returns.

4. REASONABLE DEPENDENCE ON OTHERS. A mature person can give a great deal of affection and love, but he also enjoys receiving these things. A good love relation between grownups must be based on the capacity of both partners not only to give love and sexual pleasure, but also to experience pleasure in receiving them. In this way two people build a shared emotional life. The ability to share, to give, and to receive love and friendship indicates that a person is flexible and adaptable.

The flexible, truly strong person will seek a reasonable amount of advice when important decisions must be made. He will accept just criticism about mistakes or faults.

5. MODERATE REACTIONS OF ANGER AND HATRED. The normal person gets angry, of course, but he restrains his anger to reasonable limits and doesn't indulge in temper tantrums. At work, or in other situations which he may not be able to control, he may have to curb his temper in the face of petty annoyances because of the "long-term values." The normal person can get stirred to fierce anger when the occasion demands, as enemies of humanity have learned to their own cost. Such anger is a sign of normality. This type of anger reaction is very different from that of the person who goes into a temper tantrum because a store can't provide a desired item.

6. ABILITY TO MAKE LONG-RANGE CHOICES. The mature person can forego an immediate gratification for the sake of more lasting values. For example, a mature young couple may decide to put off marriage for a few years in order to complete their education and get started in life. Immature individuals rush into marriage without thought of the greater happiness that a delay might bring.

A mature student working hard before examinations will refuse invitations and will indulge in pleasures when the work is finished. He foregoes the immediate pleasures for the deferred gratification of making a good showing in his studies.

Later, when it is appropriate, he will probably take a vacation and go to dances and entertainments. That would be good judgment and would indicate a flexible, healthy personality.

7. A RELAXED CONSCIENCE. The normal person accepts responsibility, does his job well, but insists on and enjoys his leisure hours and vacations. He and his conscience are at home with each other. The poorly adjusted person always feels driven to accomplish things, rarely enjoys his work, and is frequently the unfortunate type who is always worrying during Sundays and vacations about how things "could have been done better." The mature person enjoys his leisure in restful ways so that he returns to work with refreshed strength and interest. He may do many things during his leisure, but he looks upon them as hobbies, not as more work.

8. GOOD ADJUSTMENT AT WORK. A normal person usually likes his work and does good work. He does not change jobs often. When he does, it is on the basis of a realistic appraisal of the job and of the chances of finding something else. He will give up a job when there are health and accident hazards which are not being corrected, or if the rate of pay is substandard. But the normal individual will not change jobs simply because the foreman has a nasty disposition or a fellow worker is difficult to get along with. He doesn't go from job to job, or from city to city, seeking some other type of employment merely because the "other fellow's grass looks greener."

9. LOVE AND TOLERANCE FOR CHILDREN. The mature adult likes children and takes time to understand their special needs. He can almost always take a few minutes off, no matter how busy he is, to build blocks with a three-year-old or to answer the many questions of an older child. (There is more on adult attitudes toward children in Chapter 19.)

10. GOOD SEXUAL ADJUSTMENT. The normal adult makes a good sexual adjustment. He or she is not prudish and enjoys the sexual act with a loved one. Such a person doesn't need additional stimulation from love affairs or prostitutes. The normal adult achieves a pleasantly satisfying orgasm during the sexual act and can relax completely afterward.

Sexual adjustment has broader implications as well. It means accepting oneself as a male or female without conflict about this accident of birth. It includes understanding the special problems of the other sex, and accepting with tolerance and sympathy some of the emotional difficulties these create—in oneself and in others. I am referring to the still-existing "inferior status" of women and to the "bread-winner" role of men, and the tensions these cause in our excessively competitive business world. Incidentally, this tolerance toward, and appreciation of, those who are different from oneself should extend not only to the opposite sex, but to people of different racial, national, and cultural backgrounds.

11. CAPACITY FOR CONTINUED EMOTIONAL GROWTH. The ability to learn and grow emotionally is characteristic of the normal individual. This makes it possible to "age gracefully," for understanding increases even though the aging person has reached or passed his prime in other ways.

A friend of mine, reading this description of the normal person, turned to me with a rueful smile, "Anyone who satisfied these qualifications would be quite somebody! *I'm* not like that, and I don't know anyone who is."

Can you think of anyone you know who possesses all of these qualities? Probably not. And that is as it should be; these are goals to seek throughout life. No one is *perfectly* normal, because perfection is seldom reached by human beings.

Perhaps you will see a greater resemblance between yourself and this idealized normal person when I round out the picture. I don't want to give the impression that to be normal you must be a complete conformist, untouched by fears and conflicts.

## The Normal Person Is Human

There is a limit to what even the normal, healthy person can "take." The well-adjusted person is not absolutely secure from all danger of "cracking up," at least temporarily. During wartime it was fairly clearly established that there was a limit to the number of bombing missions on which even the best-adjusted pilots could go without suffering from what is called combat fatigue. However, the normal men recovered quickly after being relieved of the unbearable tension. Certain forms of stress are difficult for almost anyone to endure—for example, the kind to which mechanics on an airplane base were subjected when they had to give all of their attention, time after time, to saving the planes on the ground from bombs, without being able to fight back or protect themselves. Some forms of pressure can easily be endured by one normal person and not by another. A colleague of mine recently went to a psychiatrist because he was facing a situation he knew would be terribly difficult for even a doctor—the fatal illness of his only child. He wanted help so that *he* could give the best help of which he was capable to his wife and others of their family.

Pressures are sometimes dramatically extreme, but everyday life also can be frustrating, to the point of explosion. The businessman under pressure to make a profit, the student obliged to achieve good grades, the assembly-line worker forced to meet a quota—people in many situations must find acceptable outlets for life's daily pressures.

*All normal people aren't alike.* The reason why some situations are harder on certain individuals than on others lies in the fact that human beings aren't like a simple chemical combination. Obviously, all well-adjusted people are not equally intelligent, physically endowed, and talented. "It takes all kinds to make a world," as the saying goes. In fact, you have undoubtedly noticed that there are different personality types. Different psychiatrists have described them in various ways. Dr. Carl Jung divided people into *introverts,* who are absorbed in what goes on inside their own minds, and *extroverts,* who are more concerned with the things happening outside than they are with their own experiences. Another psychiatrist, Dr. Karen Horney, speaks of three basic character types—those who "move toward people," those who "move against people," and those who "move away

from people." These might become, respectively, a successful salesman, a competitive athlete, and a philosopher. Under unfortunate circumstances the same types might produce, respectively, a playboy, a gunman, and a recluse.

*Normal people are influenced by unconscious motivations.* People suspected that there was an "unconscious" part of the mind before Dr. Sigmund Freud, the great Viennese psychiatrist, made his contributions to understanding its influence and the way it worked in actual cases of emotional illness. People noticed, for example, that they sometimes forgot things that they didn't want to remember—even though they *thought* they wanted to remember them. They knew that one could fall in love in spite of a conscious intention not to. In short, they knew that "something" went on under the surface of their awareness.

Even the well-adjusted person doesn't (for example) fall in love in a completely conscious manner, although he isn't ruled by his unconscious to such an extent that he falls in love with someone he knows to be completely unworthy of affection.

A well-adjusted person may be "afraid" of a snake even though he knows it is harmless. He may go through periods of emotional distress—as, for example, during puberty when he is faced with the problem of tearing himself away from the dependence of childhood and of solving his sexual needs. He, too, is distressed by tensions, sometimes seeking foolish ways (such as smoking) to relieve them. He even has periods of depression, for example, when he has lost a dear one, or his health is below par; women may regularly experience a brief "premenstrual depression."

Healthy, well-adjusted men and women are subject to human tensions, but they are able to find ways to relieve them without excessive anxiety. I am sure you have already found some of these ways yourself, but here are my suggestions:

*Talk over your worries,* with a sympathetic friend, relative, doctor, or anyone else whose judgment you respect.

*Get away for a while,* even if only for a walk.

*Work off your anger,* preferably in some physical activity.

*Take one thing at a time,* especially if you feel overwhelmed by the pressures of too much to do.

*Give in sometimes,* even if you are certain that you are right. But face the fact that you might be wrong.

*Help others.* Preoccupation with your own troubles can become a vicious circle.

*Be slow with criticism.* Awareness of your own shortcomings and of others' is no excuse for harsh criticism.

*Cooperate.* We live in a competitive society, but many situations call for a cooperative effort. If you compete all the time, you might be too weary and worn to enjoy success when you achieve it.

## "ALL BUT THEE AND ME"

"Everyone seems to be more or less peculiar!" you may say at this point. Perhaps that reminds you of the remark the old Quaker made to his wife: "All the world is queer save thee and me, and sometimes I think thee's a little queer."

Until fairly recently even the medical profession tended to ignore the people who are "a little queer," dividing minds into two groups, the normal and the abnormal. Like the law, medicine used to be concerned only with the sane and the insane. During the last seventy-five years, however, it has become plain that those divisions are scientifically inaccurate and meaningless. Now doctors have come to see that divisions should be made between those who are a little upset (the "maladjusted," "peculiar," "neurotic," "troubled") and those whose mental condition is such that they cannot function in society.

We do not consider this former group as standing midway between the first (the "sane," "normal," "well-adjusted") and the third (the "insane," "psychotic"). It is closer to the first than it is to the third. Perhaps the difference between the people in Group 1 (normal) and Group 2 (psychoneurotic) can be described as a difference in degree—*in quantity*—while the difference between Group 2 and Group 3 (psychotic) is a difference in kind—in *quality*. We can compare those in the first group to people who possess good physical health; those in the second to people whose illnesses, however severe, involve only a part or a few parts of the body, so that they can usually manage to be up and about; and those in the third group to people with an incapacitating illness affecting the entire body.

All types of human minds can't actually be divided into three groups. I'm dealing with them in that way because it is the most nearly scientifically accurate of any convenient division.

Now, having described the healthy mind, I will take up the partially sick mind and the sick mind in the two following chapters.

# 12

# THE PARTIALLY SICK MIND

A person whose mind is "partially sick" may be extremely intelligent, successful in his or her career, and able to function responsibly in society. The signs of the illness may not be apparent, or may reveal themselves in such a way that one would not suspect their mental origin—for example, in fancied or *real* physical symptoms. In other cases the illness takes such forms that people call it "lack of will power," "degeneracy," "laziness," "cowardice," and so on—never realizing, for example, how great may be the demands on the "will power" and "courage" of the victim of fears and phobias.

During their studies of the more severe forms of these illnesses, psychiatrists have learned a great deal not only about their cause and cure, but also about *all* human behavior. In this way, great advances have been made in *psychology* (the science which deals with the nature and functioning of the mind) as well as in *psychiatry*.

## WHAT IS PSYCHIATRY?

"Psychiatry is the bunk!" a businessman I know informed me at lunch one day. It seems he had mislaid his watch, a gift from his wife, and she had accused him of not loving her. She had just read a psychiatry book, she said, and it explained that people lost things because they wanted to; therefore the loss of the watch she had given him meant that he wanted to get rid of *her!*

Or take an elderly woman who talked to me about a forty-year-old daughter with no social life —she always got sick headaches that prevented her from going out. "My daughter wants to con-

sult a psychiatrist but naturally I won't hear of it," the old lady said vehemently. "There's never been any insanity in *our* family. Besides, he'll give her a lot of ideas about sex."

"Psychiatry is not a science," I overheard a young laboratory worker announce. "And so I don't want to have anything to do with it."

You probably know better than these people did. You realize that the wife of the man who mislaid his watch had interpreted the psychiatry book too literally (if it was a good one, it undoubtedly merely *suggested* some of the unconscious motives people may have for losing things). You know that the elderly lady was foolish to talk about insanity or worry about the psychiatrist giving her daughter "ideas about sex." You may understand, as the laboratory worker didn't, that psychiatry *is* a science. It is the science of prevention and treatment of disorders of the mind—even though, as in all fields of medicine, every question has not yet been answered. You know that it is possible to accomplish many wonderful things in medicine even before all the questions have been answered; after all, vaccination saved countless people from smallpox long before doctors were able to give a scientific explanation of immunity.

However, psychiatry is a young branch of medicine. Whenever a new field is opened, "fools rush in where angels fear to tread"; so it is only natural that psychiatry at first attracted its quota of individuals with more enthusiasm than common sense —as well as the inevitable quacks and fakes. Since there are also people who avoid anything new, it is not surprising that there are those who look down on psychiatry as the "Johnny-come-lately" of the medical profession. I feel that I can best straighten

176

out some misconceptions about psychiatry by giving you a brief account of its background.

## A THUMBNAIL SKETCH OF PSYCHIATRY*

For centuries, mental disorders were problems for the devil-doctors, magicians, or priests. This was logical, for all illness was supposed to be of supernatural origin. The *supernatural theory of mental diseases* persisted long after it was suspected that physical ailments were not caused by forces from the other world. (The word *lunatic*, for example, comes from the Latin word for the moon, which was supposed to cause madness.) Yet even in early days there were indications of some insight into psychology, such as the interpretations of dreams, the treatment of the insane by music, the rituals of mourning for the dead, the confessing of sins, and so on.

As long as people believed that mental disorders were the work of evil demons who inhabited human bodies, the mentally ill were treated with extreme cruelty. Although the supernatural theory has been discarded, some traces of the old attitude still persist.

By the sixteenth century, some connection between the human brain and human behavior began to be suspected. But it was not until the French Revolution in 1789 that a French doctor, Philippe Pinel, advanced the revolutionary theory that the *insane should be treated as patients* and not as loathsome or amusing monsters. This idea formed the foundation for modern psychiatry, although it did not of itself explain very much.

Soon after this, two other French doctors made great discoveries. Dr. Paul Broca showed that an injury to a portion of the brain (the speech center) caused a man to utter unintelligible sounds, so that he *seemed* to be insane, although he was not. The other doctor, Jean Marie Charcot, showed that he could hypnotize certain patients who would then produce the actual physical symptoms he suggested, such as a swelling of the legs. These dis-

* From here to page 179 I give a brief history of psychiatry and sketches of the leading psychiatrists.

Turn to page 179 if you are familiar with this historical background.

coveries opened the door to an understanding of the relationship between the body and the mind.

Because doctors were learning how to use the microscope, the emphasis during the later years of the nineteenth and the early ones of the twentieth century was placed on studying the *physical* origin of mental disorders, particularly those in the nerves. Rapid advances were made in *neurology* (the study of the nervous system). The theory that all mental diseases had an *organic-structural* origin became popular. A great deal was learned about hereditary defects, head injuries, and bacterial infections. Now it is generally agreed that only a small portion of all mental illnesses can be accounted for in this manner.

In the early years of the twentieth century a German doctor named Kraepelin advanced the *disease-entity* theory, according to which mental diseases differed from one another as much as, for example, measles differs from appendicitis. Although this theory was not very important, Kraepelin did some excellent work in classifying mental diseases.

The *conditioned-reflex* theory was presented by a Russian, Dr. Ivan Pavlov. He discovered that dogs could get so accustomed to associating the ringing of a bell with being fed that saliva would eventually flow from their mouths when the bell was rung, even though no food was present. For a time doctors were inclined to believe that most "peculiar" human behavior could be explained by the theory that it was due to conditioned reflexes —the "conditioning" having taken place so long ago that it was forgotten. Modern psychiatrists are not in agreement about how much this can explain the reactions they observe in the mentally ill.

Toward the end of the nineteenth century, Dr. Sigmund Freud of Vienna discovered that when he hypnotized an hysterical patient, she talked of things about which she obviously had no conscious knowledge. He worked out techniques for getting at this "unconscious material" without resorting to hypnosis. One of his methods consisted of getting the patient to say anything that came into her mind (*free association*). By means of his new techniques, he worked out what was actually the first explanation of the deep roots and motivation of human behavior. He took into account both unconscious and conscious motivation.

His contributions were invaluable. Even though all of his interpretations may not be universally accepted today, it is true that most modern psychiatry is based on the same general theory to which Freud subscribed—that is, the *functional* theory. This places emphasis upon the patient as a whole—his past life in addition to his present symptoms—the *person* and not just the disease.

## Some Specific Contributions by Noted Psychiatrists

*Dr. Sigmund Freud* emphasized the importance of disturbances of the sexual life in causing neuroses. He developed a comprehensive theory of personality as well as a method of treatment. His *libido theory* included such concepts as that of *infantile sexuality;* also the *Oedipus complex,* which means the attraction of the child to its parent of the opposite sex and the rejection of the parent of the same sex; and the *castration complex,* which is the fear of the genitals being severed or injured as punishment for the emotions involved in the Oedipus complex.

*Dr. Alfred Adler* considered sex a less important factor; he regarded man's main problem as the struggle for power in order to overcome feelings of inferiority. The idea of *repressed aggressiveness* and the *inferiority complex* were among his contributions.

*Dr. Carl Gustav Jung* felt that there was a higher nature in man which conflicted with his instinctive animal side. He felt that this higher nature was part of a tribal or racial *"collective unconscious"* —that is, "the unconscious of the human race."

*Dr. Otto Rank* believed that the baby's painful experiences while being born were a source of neuroses. His major contribution was the development of new and useful techniques of therapy.

*Dr. Sandor Ferenczi* also contributed new techniques. He emphasized the constructive value of the patient's relationship with the psychoanalyst; the therapist, by accepting the patient wholeheartedly, gave him what children want from their parents.

*Dr. Wilhelm Reich* contributed, in his early work, to the understanding of the individual by his analysis of character structure—the *personality pattern.* (The value of his later work is highly questionable.)

*Dr. Karen Horney* stressed the role that culture and environment play in causing neuroses, giving attention to the present situation—the problems immediately facing the patient.

*Dr. Erich Fromm* felt that the significant problems are those of man's relationship to the world which, in its present state, prevents him from being free.

*Dr. Harry Stack Sullivan* also discarded the instinct theories. He stressed the relationships between people, particularly those between an individual and his mother, father, and others who are significant when he is young. This is the *interpersonal theory.*

*Dr. Adolf Meyer,* the Swiss-born "father of American psychiatry," had the greatest influence on psychiatry in this country. His psychobiology, also called "common sense psychiatry," stressed the practical approach to the combined mental and physical life of the patient, and emphasized the cure more than the search into the cause. In general, Meyer's methods form the basis for much of modern work with psychotic patients while Freud's form that for dealing with the problems of neurotic people.

By studying the individual as a whole, psychiatrists learned that people have basic needs—involving security, affection, independence, and sexual activity—which vary according to the stage of their development. They found, for example, that a baby is not "a little vegetable" who will thrive as long as he is kept warm and well fed. On the contrary, a baby may become listless and apathetic —and even die through lowered resistance to infection merely because he has received *no* affection. They found that a baby can be upset, even though he is given adequate care, if his mother is always tense or "in a state of nerves."

It was clear that a child has to check (repress) certain impulses because of their consequences; for example, he must learn to check his desire to touch the pretty flame because it will burn his fingers. Certain *inhibitions* are necessary. But if the child's *basic emotional needs* are frustrated, unfortunate repressions and inhibitions result, causing unconscious conflicts. Forbidden impulses are forgotten or excluded from awareness but continue to exert an influence from the unconscious part of the mind. In other words, the child arrives at a solution to his problem that doesn't actually solve it, although it makes things seem bearable. (We do this as adults, when we repress our grief at the loss of someone dear to us, in the hope of avoiding unhappiness.)

Take a four-year-old boy whose normal interest in sex is expressed by comparing his own organ with that of a little girl. Let us assume he is discovered by horrified parents who tell him he's wicked, punish him, and frighten him with threats that the doctor will cut off his penis. From then on, the little boy may indeed "behave properly" by repressing his sexual instincts. Unconsciously, however, they still exist. These unconscious desires conflict with his desire for love and approval, and he feels anxious, afraid, and guilty without knowing why. I don't want to give the impression that the unconscious represents the "bad" side of one's nature which struggles with the good; unconscious drives can be healthy ones.

## THE IMPORTANCE OF CHILDHOOD

I could describe countless problems that arise at an early age. They would all be intended to stress the point that a *great many mental illnesses are initiated in this period*—or, at least, that the soil is prepared for them. Psychiatrists emphasize that the child's emotional life—his sense of security, his feeling of being loved, and so on—is far more important to his development than are the factors we call hereditary, that is, the qualities he inherits.

*It is for this reason that I have devoted an entire chapter to our children's emotions* (see page 275). Every parent or prospective parent should read this. I hope others will, too, because childhood helps to explain adult life.

The development of a normal emotional life is a continuous problem. Childhood experiences are extremely important, but life is never static and everything that happens leaves its imprint. Adolescence is an important period in emotional as well as physical development. That is why *I have devoted a chapter to the problems of adolescence* (see page 308).

Marriage is another great step forward in the development of emotional life. While it is a valuable experience for most people, some are unable to benefit from it or even accept it. I hope every young adult will study the chapter on emotional attitudes toward marriage (see page 207).

To return to the subject of this chapter, the *maladjusted person:* as I said in the last chapter, the borderline between the badly adjusted and the well-adjusted individual is not so clear that we can always determine in which group an individual belongs. However, a boundary does exist.

## DIFFERENCES BETWEEN THE NORMAL AND THE MALADJUSTED INDIVIDUAL

Everyone has fears, worries, tensions, and emotional discomfort. However, those of the neurotic person have special characteristics.

1. They are usually exaggerated, continual, or of long duration, or they are not realistic.

Here are some examples. Any normal person may be afraid of catching a disease, being struck by lightning, or run over by a car; the neurotic person may be terrified or panic-stricken. The normal person gets over his fear of being hit by an auto when he reaches the other side of the street; the neurotic person starts immediately to anticipate the next time. The normal person may worry about failure in business or in love when he has evidence that things are not going well; the neurotic person does so when things are going beautifully—for example, interpreting the most casual glance of his loved one at another person as a sign of infidelity.

2. These fears, worries, and tensions prevent the neurotic individual from reacting to his best interests. They interfere with his ability to work and to get along with people.

For example: the fear a normal person experiences on going into battle makes him alert and cautious (i.e., a good soldier); the neurotic person may become panicky and be unable to protect himself. A well-adjusted mother knows her older children face certain risks, but she doesn't refuse to let them out of her sight on that account. A neurotic mother may keep her children with her even though she knows it hinders them from developing a healthy degree of independence. A well-adjusted person may dislike unfair criticism of his work, but he'll put up with a certain amount of it if the job is excellent in other respects; a neurotic individual may quit work because he is spoken to in only a moderately critical tone.

3. Neurotic people experience feelings of fear, anxiety, and depression without knowing why. This sometimes makes them fear they are becoming insane. Right here I want to state emphatically that *it doesn't mean anything of the kind.* Quite the contrary, there appears to be some truth to the saying, "The best way to keep from going crazy is to be neurotic!" Of course, it isn't the *best* way, any more than the best way to avoid breaking your arm is to keep it in a sling.

In each of these illustrations that I have selected, the explanation of the neurosis lies in the unconscious mind of the neurotic individual. Let me suggest a few interpretations to show how this could happen.

## THE TYRANNY OF THE UNCONSCIOUS

Some understanding of the unconscious is necessary for the comprehension of the reasons people think, feel, act, and talk as they do. The concept of the unconscious was developed to explain how events, feelings, and ideas of the earliest years seem to disappear into forgetfulness, but in fact are submerged and are able to influence us throughout life.

Think of the unconscious mind as a storage place for past thoughts and experiences. This part of the mind releases the past to the present slowly and reluctantly, because our human tendency is to forget what was unpleasant, fearful, or undesirable in any other way. Because of feelings of guilt or inferiority, the unhappy, neurotic person behaves in ways that may puzzle him as much as his friends. He can no more peer into his unconscious mind than you can gaze into a mirror to see how you look with your eyes closed. The unconscious of the healthy person is not (or is very seldom) in serious conflict with his conscious desires; but the conscious of the neurotic person is always being forced to surrender to his unconscious. The neurotic person becomes the slave of his unconscious.

Now, it is quite possible for slaves to be contented—if they are submissive, or can get around their masters, or if their masters are consistent and not too demanding. But this isn't the same thing as being free to make one's own decisions without any limitations except those imposed by society for the protection of others.

## SOME CHARACTERISTICS OF NEUROTIC INDIVIDUALS

As a group, these people are able to recognize reality. They may see it through dark or distorting glasses, but they do see it. They do not have hallucinations, as do some of the psychotic people I discuss in the next chapter. Only *part* of their personality is disturbed. They are all able to function, more or less, in society. Almost all of these people have a certain amount of insight; they know, although they won't always admit it, that there is something wrong with them. Neurotic individuals show a great range of behavior. It is a rare person who does not at some time display some trace of neurotic symptoms or behavior. At the other end of the spectrum, some people are so overwhelmed by neurotic ways of behaving that they need intensive treatment, in a psychiatrist's office or possibly in a hospital.

Although these characteristics apply in general to people whose minds are partially ill, there are many varieties of disorders from which they may be suffering. Among the most important are the following:

### Character Disturbances

Classed as *neurotic personalities,* people with these disturbances are not neurotic in the full sense of the word, since they are not suffering from any of the neuroses described on pages 181-82. They have no actual mental illness; yet they are not in perfect health. I sometimes compare them to people who are about fifty pounds overweight and, while there's nothing specifically wrong with them, are too fat to enjoy perfect health or to be statistically speaking, "good risks."

These people have *character problems*—not merely the ordinary problems of life but those stemming from or exaggerated by traits in their characters, such as shyness, timidity, irritability, depression. You know such individuals. Probably you have heard some of the following things said about them:

"Mary would have heaps of boy friends if she could only realize how good-looking she is."

"You get the feeling Jack doesn't quite trust anybody; he always seems so wary."

"Tom's great fun when things are going his way, but he's a very bad loser."

"We really ought to ask Joan because she's so sweet, but she kind of puts a wet blanket on things by being always in the dumps."

"I bet Dick'll be the last one to get a raise even though he's the smartest one in the office."

"It's a shame Dotty flies off the handle the way she does; she feels awful about it afterwards."

"Anne's so jittery she makes me nervous."

The world has always realized that these people are "their own worst enemies." But not until recently, with the development of psychiatry, have we begun to understand why, and (as I'll explain on page 183) how they can be helped to lead fuller, more useful, and happier lives.

## Neuroses (Psychoneuroses)

1. ANXIETY NEUROSIS. In this condition a person experiences episodes of anxiety which vary from mild uneasiness to panic. Sometimes they manifest themselves by physical signs such as sweating, dizziness, diarrhea, difficulty in breathing, a pain in the heart. The individual may feel extremely tense and irritable; he may awaken in the night in a state of terror. The characteristic feeling is one of "anxious expectation," the way one normally feels when something dreadful is about to happen, except that there is no idea as to what the dreadful thing might be.

This state is often associated with a fear of losing love, as, for example, when there is conflict in the unconscious mind between a desire to hurt the loved one (perhaps to get even for having been hurt) and a desire to win that person's love.

Sometimes the anxiety is "shunted off" by associating it with the situation in which it was experienced. That is, if the anxiety first occurred in an

elevator, the individual may "blame" the elevator, which he then fears and avoids in the hope of avoiding the anxiety.

Some psychiatrists feel that there is no such thing as a *pure* anxiety neurosis.

2. PHOBIAS. These are divided into *common phobias*, or exaggerated fears of things most people are afraid of, such as death; and *specific phobias*, or fears of things that aren't in themselves frightening, such as open fields or elevators. Phobias are usually rooted in anxiety, in the fear that, having been "bad," something is bound to "get you." The phobic person projects anxiety onto some external situation which he or she then feels has to be avoided.

Included in the almost endless list of phobias we find: *acrophobia*, the fear of high places, *agoraphobia*, open spaces; *aichmophobia*, sharp and pointed objects; *anthropophobia*, of people; *astrophobia*, storms; *batophobia*, falling objects; *claustrophobia*, enclosed spaces; *climacophobia*, falling downstairs; *dromophobia*, crossing the street; *hypnophobia*, fear of sleep; *kleptophobia*, of stealing; *mechanophobia*, of machinery; *monophobia*, of being alone; *mysophobia*, of dirt and contamination; *necrophobia*, of the dead; *nyctophobia*, of the dark; *pantophobia*, of everything; *potamophobia*, of running water; *phagophobia*, of swallowing; *syphilophobia*, of syphilis; *topophobia*, of situations (stage fright); *xylophobia*, of the forest; *zoophobia*, of animals.

3. HYPOCHONDRIA. In this neurosis, the mind's illness is expressed through a preoccupation with body functions or organs. The patient is afraid of, or believes he suffers from, physical disease. He notices body sensations, such as normal fatigue, that do not concern or bother other people. There is no physical cause for this condition. However, telling him he's all right physically won't cure the hypochondriacal attitude.

4. CONVERSION HYSTERIA. This differs from hypochondria in that the mind's illness is expressed in a physical symptom or symptoms, which, although not *real* in one sense of the word, are certainly real to the patient. Hysterical paralysis is one example. A soldier undergoing a severe conflict between his desire to be brave and his desire not to be killed,

finds his legs suddenly paralyzed. He is not "faking"—he actually feels nothing when pins are stuck into his legs. However, there is absolutely nothing wrong with his nerves—usually the loss of sensation is not even anatomically possible, a section of one nerve being "dead" while other sections beyond the "dead" point remain sensitive. When the conflict is resolved, either by circumstances or within the soldier himself, his paralysis vanishes.

5. OBSESSIVE-COMPULSIVE NEUROSIS. This causes people to perform actions without knowing why or without wanting to perform them. The impulse stems from an idea or set of ideas that have no relationship in the individual's conscious mind. For example: a person always has to put on a certain undergarment inside out. This is similar to the way some of us feel about having to "knock on wood." It is a sort of ritual, an appeal to magic powers. However, the normal person who knocks on wood does so as a kind of joke because he has been told it is lucky; but it is no joke to the victim of such a neurosis. He performs his rituals because he is extremely insecure. As a child, he may have turned to his own "magic" in a desperate attempt to cope with problems too great for him to handle.

6. NEURASTHENIA. Literally, this word means nerve weakness. It was once believed that the nerves in the brain could actually get tired, and "brain fatigue" would result. Now we know that, like hypochondria and conversion hysteria, this is a product of the patient's psyche. It is real to him, even though it is medically and scientifically "impossible." The patient honestly feels and *is* too weak or tired to get out of bed, or even to think coherently. He can sleep for periods that would be impossible for a well person, or simply lie for hours doing nothing. Yet he is not physically ill. Resting doesn't cure him, but solving his problems does.

7. DISSOCIATIVE NEUROSIS. Sometimes, parts of the memory and personality become separated from one another. Anxiety may cause a person to forget for a time who he is and what he is doing. When he regains his self-awareness, he has forgotten what took place during his forgetful period. An extreme example of this neurosis is *amnesia*. A less severe condition is *somnambulism,* or sleepwalking.

## Psychosomatic Illnesses

In recent years we have heard a great deal about psychosomatic illnesses (*soma* means body). These are different from conditions such as those I described under 3, 4, and 6, which vanish completely when the psyche recovers. Psychosomatic illnesses result from the interaction of the mind and the body. They usually affect only those parts of the body under the control of the involuntary nervous system, such as the digestive tract, the endocrine glands, the heart, the lungs, the urinary bladder, and the skin.

I can best illustrate this by describing an ulcer of the stomach. Observations were made by two physicians (S. Wolf and H. Wolff) who were able to watch the digestive processes of a patient who, because of a previous accident, had to be fed through an opening made directly into his stomach. They could actually see that inflammation occurred when the patient became angry or upset.

When food is present in the stomach, digestive juices are put out to "work on" (digest) it. However, certain emotional reactions can also stimulate the flow of these juices. If there is no food in the stomach, the acid juices may irritate the stomach itself, sometimes eventually causing an ulcer (open sore). Now, it is important to remember that this ulcer exists as an organic disease of the stomach. Unless it is treated by medicine and diet, it may cause a hemorrhage or it may perforate. However, unless the emotional tension is relieved, the patient won't be giving his ulcer its best chance to heal; and, of course, he'll have to continue his diet and medicine in order to minimize the risk of getting another ulcer. Thus, *psychosomatic diseases require treatment of both the body and the mind.*

In addition to ulcer of the stomach and of the duodenum, the following are regarded as diseases in which emotional factors may play an important part:

migraine headache
mucous colitis
ulcerative colitis
asthma
high blood pressure

THE PARTIALLY SICK MIND — 183

arthritis and rheumatism
skin disturbances

Undoubtedly others will be added to this list. As yet the evidence is not as clear-cut in any of these diseases as it is in the case of certain ulcers. We do not know, for example, to how great a degree a patient's asthma is due to his having inherited an allergic constitution and how much to his having emotional problems. However, we do know that asthmatic patients generally improve far more rapidly when their emotional difficulties are relieved at the same time that they are being desensitized to the pollens or other allergens which set off their attacks of asthma.

Less dramatic, but at least as important in its effects on the body as the preceding diseases, is everyday stress. When you have to make a physical or emotional effort beyond what is usual for you, in response to some difficult situation, you are under stress. This can be a source of worry, anxiety, and fear. Stress can be so serious that a mere tendency to illness may develop into an active health problem, or new illnesses may result. Trying to live on too low an income is one of the most stressful situations I can think of. An inadequate education, lack of spare time, lack of privacy, severe pressure on the job—all are stress situations that can affect the body.

In our complex society, it is not possible to remove all causes of stress. It is not desirable either, because some degree of stress is often necessary if we are to accomplish specific goals or protect ourselves from danger. The body has many ways of adapting itself to difficult situations, such as increasing the output of the adrenal glands, changing the blood sugar level, or adjusting the digestive tract. But when a part of the body is *overwhelmed by stress* and cannot react as it should, or overreacts, then the resulting ailment is psychosomatic.

## THE PEOPLE DESCRIBED IN THIS CHAPTER CAN BE HELPED

Probably I am saying this just in time to keep you from being completely discouraged by what you've been reading! It is depressing to hear about all these unhappy, frustrated people. But fortu-nately, there is a bright side. *All* the people I have been talking about *can be either cured or helped.*

## THERAPY (TREATMENT)

Although the word therapy means *treatment*, I like to remember that its original meaning includes the idea of *service*.

There are many kinds of treatment for mental ailments. The most effective for the people I have been discussing in this chapter is *psychotherapy*. It means treatment by psychological methods. The term covers everything from the simplest "spilling out" of troubles to a spiritual adviser or wise friend, to the long, involved process of psychoanalysis.

Almost every doctor practices some form of psychotherapy, sometimes without knowing it. In dealing with a patient who has an exaggerated fear that he is ill, the doctor's examination, explanation, reassurance, and firmness are forms of psychotherapy. Or, when he helps a tense and nervous person to find a hobby—that is psychotherapy, too.

## FORMS OF PSYCHOTHERAPY

### Guidance and Counseling

There are times when *simply putting one's problems into words* helps to clarify them and make them seem less alarming. It may reveal what the *real* trouble is. Though this may be painful, it usually is encouraging to know where one stands.

*Confessing* one's weaknesses, failures, and sins is valuable, provided the person to whom they are confessed understands their importance (however trivial they may actually be). He must also be able to make the person who is confessing feel that he is not condemned, but that he is still worthwhile, despite his faults and frailties. Doing something constructive to make up for his past is far better than brooding about it.

*Receiving information* is sometimes most useful in equipping an individual to solve his own problems—especially if they were due, wholly or in part, to ignorance or misinformation.

These are some of the techniques utilized in various forms of counseling—which include marriage counseling (see page 218), child guidance (see page 285), and vocational guidance (see page 141). These methods can be successfully employed by doctors in general practice and also by clergymen, social workers, and others who do not have medical degrees but have been trained in this work. They know the types of problems that can benefit from counseling, and when more expert help is required. At one time there was a fairly sharp division between the *directive* and *nondirective* approach to this type of therapy. In both forms, the individual was encouraged to talk about his problems, but in the *directive* he was told what he should do, and in the *nondirective* he was never given any advice. The present tendency is to combine the two methods, being careful not to give too much advice, since this does not help the individual to become independent, yet at the same time realizing that he is apt to become confused if he gets no advice at all.

## Behavioral Therapy

In this technique, a specific symptom such as a phobia is selected as the target for change, and the patient is led, or conditioned, through a series of steps, to change his or her behavior.

The steps may include progressive relaxation, using breathing exercises, and picturing in the mind pleasant scenes to introduce a state of calm.

Systematic desensitization may be employed and is somewhat like allergic desensitization, in which small, gradually increasing doses of an allergen such as a pollen or other allergy-producing material are used to increase tolerance. Thus, in systematic desensitization, a person fearful of flying, for example, may be led through a whole hierarchy of situations in his mind—imagining going to an airport, inspecting a plane, going into the cockpit, being aboard while the plane taxis on the ground, and then while the plane flies. Later, as he accepts these imaginary situations without difficulty, he may be led through a series of real-life steps until he progresses to the point of being able to fly without fear.

## Hypnotherapy

Hypnosis induces a state of altered consciousness which permits intense concentration on ideas and suggestions. While in this state the patient can be given active suggestions by the therapist to break undesirable habits such as smoking or to change some forms of neurotic behavior. Some therapists use hypnotherapy in conjunction with other forms of therapy as well.

## Adjunctive Therapies

These forms of help play the same kind of role in psychotherapy as nursing care does in medical care. The most common of these is *occupational therapy*. This term is apt to make us picture insane people weaving baskets. Actually, it means far more than providing methods of relieving tension. People whose emotional problems are associated with the fact that they do not feel useful (perhaps because of old age, ill health, or lack of opportunity) are often tremendously benefited by doing something that makes them realize they are creative, successful, and independent—on even a small scale. *Sports, diversions,* and *hobbies* make many people happier and more relaxed simply because they are enjoyable. They, too, bring with them the benefits of increased confidence in one's capacities, including the capacity to have meaningful social relationships.

## Medicines

Medicines such as tranquilizing agents and sedatives may be given in some instances to relieve tension. Stimulants are occasionally prescribed. Medications should be taken *only* on a physician's recommendation. As a general rule, they are given in connection with other treatment, but a doctor may find them sufficient under certain circumstances: for example, he may prescribe a tranquilizer or sedative to relieve the tension in a person awaiting news of a dear one who is critically ill.

Medicines such as sodium amytal are sometimes used to put a patient into a state that enables him to realize, and tell, what is troubling him. It has been used successfully on soldiers who "cracked up." This was often found to be due to guilt feelings connected with the death of a comrade or comrades; the incident that caused these feelings had been "forgotten" (being too deeply disturbing) but was recalled during the sleepy state. Once brought into the open, these feelings could be coped with. I discuss treatment of severe mental illness by medicines in the next chapter, The Sick Mind.

## Forms of Psychoanalytical Therapy

Freud was the originator of psychoanalysis. There are very few psychoanalysts who practice it today exactly as Freud did. On the other hand, there is no psychoanalysis that does not derive from him. Nevertheless, we usually speak of *Freudian* and *non-Freudian* psychoanalysis. An important difference lies in the fact that Freudian psychoanalysis usually consists of as many as five hourly sessions a week over a period of several years, whereas in the non-Freudian forms, shorter, less frequent, and less protracted sessions are considered sufficient. In the latter form, more emphasis is placed on the immediate situation of the patient and his relationships with others.

PSYCHOANALYSIS. This process consists of (1) uncovering the unconscious forces influencing the patient, which he cannot, simply by will, bring into his consciousness. The patient does this by "free associating" (saying anything that comes into his head), by telling about his dreams, and so on. The psychoanalyst makes this as easy as possible, by having the patient recline on a couch where he is scarcely aware of the doctor's presence, and by prompting him with an occasional question, such as, "What does that make you think of?"

In the course of these sessions, *transference* takes place. That is, the patient tends to react toward the psychoanalyst in ways that he reacted, or still reacts, to important figures in his life, usually his parents. Because the psychoanalyst is a neutral sort of figure, the patient can see his own patterns of reaction. For example, a patient might be able to rationalize his fear of his neighbors, John Jones and Bob Brown, by saying "Jones is after my job and Brown is after my wife." In psychoanalytic sessions, unable to find a "reason" for his similar fear of the psychoanalyst, he may then discover that it springs from his unconscious mind. He might later learn it was actually a concealed fear of his father, stemming from childhood days.

(2) Once the unconscious material has been brought out, the patient begins to feel relieved. Insight makes him stronger, his unconscious less powerful. He can then begin reacting in a new way.

Anyone who has been psychoanalyzed will probably say at this point, "It sounds quick and easy when you tell about it—but believe me, it isn't. Reacting in a new way is a long drawn-out process. At first everything went fast; I felt as relieved as I would if a boil had been lanced. But the rest of it took a long time."

That is quite true. The person who undertakes psychoanalysis has usually spent many years reacting in the old way, and habits are not easily changed even when one understands how they came about and wants very much to change them. When you've been on your knees for years, it isn't easy to learn to walk on your feet!

PSYCHOANALYTICALLY ORIENTED PSYCHOTHERAPY ("Brief Therapy," "Analytic Interviews"). While employing some of the techniques of psychoanalysis, these forms of therapy are much shorter. They also concentrate on everyday problems of reality rather than on the patient's unconscious. It is felt that this therapy does not encourage the patient to become dependent on his analyst (or his sessions with him) but to do the work on his own. Brief therapy may be used where psychoanalysis would not be helpful or feasible.

GROUP THERAPY. Usually four to ten patients are treated during the same therapy period. Some psychiatrists combine it with individual sessions, others use it alone. It is considered valuable because the patients react to each other as well as to the doctor, and because their self-confidence is increased by being with people whose problems are like their own. For example, obese people who overeat for psychological reasons (see page 49) often respond well to group therapy. Some of its principles are used successfully in *Alcoholics Anonymous*.

Group therapy has become a successful technique in many kinds of institutions, such as rehabilitation centers for adolescent boys, veterans' hospitals, and prisons. There are many approaches and theories, but all forms of group therapy rest on the principle that we humans are social beings who are influenced deeply by the groups we belong to. In group therapy, the healing influences that have always been recognized in an intuitive way are brought to the aid of troubled people through the skill of psychiatrists and psychologists.

FAMILY THERAPY. Like an individual, a family has its problems, its values, principles, and goals. Perhaps only one member of the family appears to be in trouble, but the relationship within the family may have to be examined. Because the psychologically maladjusted person may be the product of an unhealthy family situation, many psychiatrists and other therapists have turned to family therapy as a method of help. In such therapy, the entire family may work out its conflicts and difficulties through discussions, much as an individual does in the more conventional type of therapy. Family treatment has attracted the interest not only of psychiatrists but of social agencies and of the federal government, which supports research projects in this area.

PLAY THERAPY. This is a form of psychotherapy adapted to children. Anyone who has tried to help an emotionally disturbed child knows how hard it is to get him to talk about his problems. Play therapy provides a solution. The child reveals himself, far better than he could by talking, when he plays with toys and acts out his fantasies. The therapist helps him "get things out of his system," accepting him warmly as he is, and guiding him toward the solution of his problems. Since these are related to the way he is treated at home, play therapy is usually combined with some form of therapy (often group therapy) for the parents.

Some of these forms of treatment take longer than others, and require a greater degree of professional training. I shall not attempt to say which forms will be of most benefit to various types of people who need help. I think you'll see why if I draw a parellel from the field of surgery.

Lancing a boil is a simple surgical process as compared with correcting a congenital dislocation of the hip. Your family doctor would probably feel quite competent to handle the first, but not the second. Yet the person with the boil may be suffering acutely, while the person with the congenital dislocation may get along quite well. In other words, the distress caused by a condition does

not always indicate how long and complicated a method is necessary to relieve it, or whether it should be undertaken only by a specialist.

I have known soldiers who had very severe emotional disturbances but who recovered after only a few sessions, such as those I described, under narcosynthesis. I also know some parents who were very much concerned because their daughter seemed to be "on the verge of a nervous breakdown" when they visited her at college. (Incidentally, "nervous breakdown" is not a term doctors use, as it has no precise meaning; some people consider it a polite way of saying "insane," while to others it describes any emotional illness that comes on suddenly.) As I learned later, this girl had fallen very much in love and wanted to get married, a desire that was in conflict with her wish to complete her education—which she knew meant a great deal to her parents. Her hesitation precipitated a quarrel with her sweetheart who said things that hurt her badly. Angry at him, she unconsciously blamed him for the predicament she was in, yet she loved him intensely. She began to experience anxiety feelings. Fortunately, she discussed her problem with a very fine clergyman at college. As she was basically a well-adjusted person, she quickly recovered from this temporary *situational neurotic condition,* and was able to face the real problems confronting her and her young man.

Both the girl and the soldiers I described were in acute distress, yet found relief quickly. In the case of the girl, no doctor was required.

The next case can, I think, be compared with that of a person with a congenital dislocation of the hip.

George Gray was an extremely intelligent man in his forties, the owner of a successful business established by his father. An early marriage had terminated in divorce. I had met him several times at the home of some mutual friends where, on one occasion, we had talked about psychoanalysis.

Some years later he told me that, following this discussion, he consulted a psychiatrist who recommended that he be psychoanalyzed. Like others who had known Gray slightly, I had no idea that there was anything wrong with him. Yet he had been suffering from a well-concealed "emotional dislocation." To put it briefly, he was extremely lonely but unable to establish any close relationships with other people, especially of the kind that might lead to marriage, although he considered marriage desirable. His fears and suspicions of people had reached the point, he said, where he would refuse invitations he wanted to accept, walked or took taxis because he dreaded being close to people in the subway, and found it increasingly difficult to have dealings with his business associates.

"My psychoanalysis has taken five years, but it's worth it!" he told me enthusiastically. "I can't tell you how different, how much better, my life has been since I no longer feel the way I used to —as though I was living on enemy territory and had to be constantly on guard."

I mention these cases to show you that the form of therapy required depends on many things: on the individual and how deep-rooted his problems are, and also on the goal that is desired. In some cases a cure will be rapid, since eliminating a few symptoms is the aim, as, for example, in the case of a person who is well-adjusted except for a recent tendency to insomnia. In other cases a basic change in attitudes is essential. Only a qualified person can evaluate the situation correctly.

## DON'T BE RELUCTANT TO SEEK HELP

When people fail to ask for help, or refuse to accept it, I have found that it is usually for one of the following reasons:

1. *Some people lack information, or are misinformed about mental illness,* particularly the milder forms. I've often heard them say such things as: "I think it's right to go to a doctor if you're crazy, but I'm not, and I should be able to help myself. I got into this state and I ought to get out of it by using my brains and my will power."

I appreciate these feelings. It is admirable to want to solve one's own personal problems. However, it is even more admirable to admit honestly that one isn't always capable of doing it alone. Please remember that the psychiatrist doesn't solve your problems *for* you; he can only help *you* to solve them. I won't argue with you about whether you "should" have taken some other course along the road of emotional development, rather than the one which "got you into this state." But I do want to remind you of the fact that you probably began to get off the course when you were very young. The thing to remember is that you have lost your way, and the psychiatrist has a map to help you find it again. Don't feel it is your duty to spend years trying to find it by yourself when your talents and ability should be spent in making a good life for yourself and others, particularly your children.

2. *Some people are afraid of help.* Why? Well, imagine a young savage who breaks his ankle while he is alone in the jungle. His life is in danger, his suffering is intense. But he makes a crude cast for it; he can get around; and eventually it ceases to hurt very much. Many years later he learns that his ankle can be repaired. By now he doesn't want to part with the cast; he has grown accustomed to it, even proud of it because it makes him different. Having it removed will be a lot of trouble and will probably hurt. Besides, there is no guarantee that his ankle will be absolutely perfect.

There is no reason to be frightened if you think you resemble any of the people I've described in this section more than you resemble the well-adjusted individual in Chapter 11. On the contrary, if you do need help, you can get it, and be better off than you imagined possible. Getting rid of your "cast" will be no hardship when you've reached the point where you don't need it any more!

3. *Some people don't know they need help.* I want to caution you against trying to convince anyone that he or she needs help. This is difficult at best; and there is a real danger that you might be talking to someone with a serious mental illness such as those I describe in the next chapter (in which I discuss what you should do in such cases —see page 200). Talk the matter over with a responsible person who has had some training or experience in this field, such as your doctor or clergyman.

If someone comes to you because he or she is disturbed or has an emotional problem, don't try to solve it on the basis of the information I've given you. The best thing you can do is to tell your friend in a tactful, natural manner that trained help is available, with some suggestions (which I give in the next section) about how to find it. If someone you know well and believe to be maladjusted tries to get you to assure him that he is "perfectly all right," be reassuring on the question of sanity. But be honest. Explain that you aren't any more qualified to decide about questions of mental health than you are about physical health. Recommend his talking to his own doctor or to a psychiatrist, making it clear that you do this in just the way that you'd suggest his having a chest x-ray taken to detect possible early signs of tuberculosis. In trying to help such a person—or in any dealings with a neurotic individual—remember that he feels insecure, unwanted, and inferior, regardless of the front he may assume. Accepting him warmly as a human being with potentialities as well as problems is genuinely reassuring (as it is to a well-adjusted person, too).

The *psychopathic personality* is usually convinced that not he, but everyone else, is out of step. (I describe this group of people in the next chapter; it actually belongs in a special category, rather than with the partially sick mind or the sick mind.) These individuals seldom accept help and, being legally sane, cannot be compelled to have treatment. Unfortunately they can do a great deal of damage to their children and others who have to live with them. I think anyone, however well adjusted, who has to live with such a person should see a psychiatrist for guidance in minimizing the difficulties of the relationship and to keep the home situation as satisfactory as possible.

4. *Some people consider psychiatric help too expensive and too much trouble.* They would be reconciled to spending time and money to cure themselves of tuberculosis or to have a surgical operation, such as the removal of a tumor—especially one that might become cancerous. Surely it is worthwhile to invest the same amount of time and money to overcome a long-standing, crippling emotional illness! I can't emphasize too much the fact that such an illness—even when the individual suffering from it feels he can "take it"—can have a serious effect on others, especially the children of such a person. Also, it is unwise to put off seeing a doctor to save money, because delays usually increase the amount of treatment that will be required.

However, it is true that some people just don't have the money for psychiatric treatment. I'll discuss that in the following section.

## HOW TO FIND PSYCHIATRIC HELP

Consult your doctor. Make mental health a part of your health program of regular checkups as I have suggested (see page 379). Don't hesitate to talk about yourself—your real self—to your doctor. He will be as interested in your emotional problems and symptoms as he is in the fact that you had scarlet fever and pneumonia as a child.

Often your family doctor himself can help you. Pent-up emotions are sometimes released in only a few interviews, especially if they are due to unusual stresses and strains of recent development. Many general practitioners are qualified to provide some of the forms of psychotherapy I have described. Medical schools teach psychiatry as a major part of the doctor's training.

However, do remember that physicians are human, and we are not all emotionally constituted to be able to help with all the kinds of problems our patients face—even if we had the time. Try to size up your doctor. It is important for you to find someone with whom you will be personally in sympathy. Give your doctor a chance, but if you find you aren't going to "click," you have a perfect right to find someone else. Few doctors will be unduly sensitive about this. The best psychiatrists realize that it is not possible to establish a good relationship with every patient. Knowing how important this is in the success of the treatment, they sometimes even suggest that a patient change to someone else if they don't happen to be personally compatible.

Usually your own doctor can find a good psychiatrist for you in the same way that he does a good specialist in any other field. Sometimes, he may suggest that you see a therapist who does not have the degree of M.D. but who usually has a Ph.D. in psychology, and is a member of the American Psychological Association.

Your doctor or the psychiatrist may recommend a psychiatric social worker, a clergyman trained in counseling, or a marriage counselor, if he feels they are competent to help you; or he may suggest one to supplement his treatment.

NEVER accept treatment for an emotional difficulty from an advertising "psychologist" or "psychoanalyst."

Your county medical society will supply you with the names of specialists in psychiatry and psychoanalysis who have been awarded diplomas by the National Boards which examine and certify specialists in the various fields of medicine.

Clinics at the large hospitals and medical schools, and mental hygiene clinics operated by various social agencies, can often give you therapy you might otherwise not be able to afford.

In specific instances, the following organizations may be helpful:

American Association of Marriage and Family Counselors, 41 Central Park West, New York, N.Y. 10023
Alcoholics Anonymous—listed in your local telephone directory
The National Save-A-Life League, 815 2nd Avenue, New York, N.Y. 10017 (This organization offers help to people who consider suicide a way out of their difficulties.)

## Psychotherapy in Rural and Small Communities

I realize that your difficulties will be very much greater if you live in a rural community or small city rather than in a large one. You may be lucky enough to have a family doctor who is interested in emotional problems and capable of handling many of them. You may be close enough to a medical center or large city to drive over once a week, or once in two weeks, for treatment by a specialist or at one of the hospitals or clinics there. With modern transportation it is usually possible to get to a medical center if you have enough determination to do so. This is not easy, of course, for someone who is working or tied down with young children. In such cases you have to use all sorts of ingenuity in sizing up the possibilities for treatment in your own community. Talk the situation over with your doctor, your county health officer, or your clergyman. All of them should be interested in emotional problems and emotional illness if they are doing their jobs properly. If they cannot help you, write your State Mental Health Association explaining your problem; they may be able to provide help for you in some way, perhaps by recommending a book on mental health that deals with the type of situation you face. If it is impos-

sible for you to seek any help outside your community, it may do some good to talk to one of your friends who is a *trustworthy, sympathetic, and well-adjusted person*. This is much less satisfactory than talking to someone who has had training, but it is often better than keeping all the tensions bottled up within yourself until they reach the explosive point.

## NEW HORIZONS

I hope this chapter has broadened your understanding of "the troubled people," and how psychiatry can help them to achieve peace of mind and break the chain that makes people visit upon their children the mistakes (*not* sins) of their own parents. I hope, too, that you have caught a glimpse of the possibilities the future holds for us, individually and collectively, when our energies are no longer dissipated in the squirrel cage of maladjustment. Then we can go ahead as normal, mature people, to solve the real, and fascinatingly complex, problems of living in the modern world.

## A SPECIAL WORD ABOUT DEPRESSION

Almost all of us, quite normally, have our minor ups and downs of mood. There are days when we feel particularly good; other days when we feel less so. There are times, too, when quite naturally we may feel particularly unhappy or depressed—for example, when a loved one dies or we experience another loss or a separation from a familiar person or place.

Ordinary everyday "blues" are usually brief and self-curing. And, with a loss, too, we normally "work through" our grief and mourning and before long are back to our usual selves and activities. But for many people, depression is a more serious problem. It may be unremitting or recurring. The National Institute of Mental Health has estimated that each year upward of four million Americans suffer depressions severe enough to keep them from performing regular activities or to compel them to seek medical help. And millions of others are believed to have only somewhat less severe depressions that make them unhappy and interfere with their lives.

Depression can be either undisguised and fairly obvious or "masked" and not immediately obvious at all.

For these reasons and also because it is so common, I am treating it here under a separate heading.

In its undisguised form, depression has these characteristics: a chronic change of mood, an extended lowering of the spirits, a loss of enjoyment of things and activities that have usually made life enjoyable. A dull, tired, empty, sad, even numb feeling pervades.

There are behavioral symptoms, too: irritability, excessive concern with small annoyances or minor problems, impaired memory and ability to concentrate, loss of sexual desire, difficulty in getting going in the morning, excessive feelings of guilt.

And there are physical symptoms: appetite and weight loss, disturbed sleep, fatigue, headache, dizziness, indigestion, sometimes heart palpitations, chest constriction, pain in the area of the heart.

But depression can also be less obvious. Some psychiatrists say that the "exhausted housewife," the "bored adolescent," and the "occupational underachiever" may be suffering from depression. They also consider that depression may be disguised, in some cases, in sexual promiscuity, overeating, excessive drinking, or possibly even some phobias.

Moreover, quite often the physical complaints —the headaches, fatigue, chest discomfort, other pains and disturbances—may be so much in the forefront that they are the prime concern, submerging the "blue" feelings. They may mask the depression not only from others but from the victim himself, and even on occasion from a physician whom he may consult for the physical troubles.

Disguised or undisguised, depression may be linked to an external event such as a loss of loved one, job, promotion, money. But quite often it may be "endogenous"—meaning that it comes from within, without apparent external cause. Suddenly, a person may decide that he or she is a failure in life, when that is not really true. Unaccountably, self-esteem and self-confidence vanish, and depression blooms. It is possible that endogenous depression may have a biochemical cause.

Mild, self-limited depressions can often be managed without professional help. Giving yourself a special treat, keeping busy, trying a change of scene or pace, helping others, tackling difficult or satisfying work, or physical activity may help.

But extended severe depression warrants medical attention. Simple measures you may use on your own are not likely to work. In some cases, there is danger of suicide.

Today, depression can almost invariably be overcome, no matter how severe. Drug treatment is often effective, although it may take three or more weeks to work. Psychotherapy is not considered the most effective treatment, although it may be needed and useful for some patients to help them alter life patterns that may precipitate depression. For the suicidally depressed, electroconvulsive (shock) treatment may be used for quick results.

MANIC DEPRESSION. Depressive illness such as I have just discussed—all in one direction, down— is known as *unipolar*. But *manic*, or *bipolar*, depression affects an estimated four million Americans who experience episodes of severe depression alternating with other episodes of great elation (manic behavior). Some in the manic phase are given to flamboyant speech and actions; they have feelings of being incapable of doing anything wrong.

Treatment for manic depression has been discouraging in the past. In their depressed state, patients have responded to antidepressant drugs, the same kind used for unipolar depression. For the manic phase, treatment has relied on electroshock or heavy doses of potent tranquilizing agents. Neither has been entirely satisfactory. The heavily sedative tranquilizers have kept manics in a kind of chemical straitjacket until their high episode has passed. Electroshock has produced only temporary benefits. Most bipolar victims have had repeated recurrences.

More recently, however, improved results have been obtained in many cases with a drug, lithium. It is used to prevent or reduce manic episodes and is helpful also in preventing the depressive periods of manic depression.

Lithium should be used expertly, with care. It may produce side effects such as nausea, vomiting, and diarrhea, which often disappear as the body adjusts to the drug or as the dosage is reduced. Sometimes, there may be more serious undesirable effects: confusion, tremor, impaired speech or vision and, if these are not heeded, still more serious consequences such as seizures and coma. Usually, however, when blood levels of the drug are checked regularly, and the dosage adjusted so the levels are satisfactory, the patient will not have serious reactions.

If you suspect that you or a member of your family has a depressive illness, consult your physician. He may have the experience to be able to treat the problem successfully. Otherwise, he can recommend an experienced psychiatrist in your area, or you can contact the American Psychiatric Association, 1700 Eighteenth Street, NW, Washington, D.C. 20009.

# 13
# THE SICK MIND

You may hesitate to read this chapter because anything having to do with "insane" people makes you feel uncomfortable. If you feel that way, don't let it worry you, because it is a perfectly normal reaction. And don't worry, either, if you find a certain fascination in reading about these things; that, too, is normal. Almost everyone reacts in one of these ways when first coming in contact with psychotic people—in books or in real life. Just remember that here, as in so many instances, the light of honest information will dispel the mysterious shadows.

## PSYCHOPATHIC PERSONALITIES

I shall deal with the group of people included in this general category in this chapter, although they do not actually belong here, but in a chapter of their own.

Those persons who fail to develop a conscience, who know the difference between right and wrong but don't care, and who have little or no sense of what is socially acceptable, we call *psychopaths* or *sociopaths*. They are generally antisocial, aggressive, and impulsive. They feel little guilt about their actions, or none at all. Free of worry or concern for the present or the future, the psychopath may lie, cheat, steal, swindle. He may physically harm others or even commit murder.

These people have a good sense of reality, yet they may have abnormal ideas and behavior patterns. For example, persons with psychopathic personalities may bring one lawsuit after another

because they feel, without justification, that they have been wronged; yet they do not suffer from true *paranoia*, which I describe on page 197. They may lavish all their love and affection on a pet animal, indifferent to the needs of friends and relatives. Occasionally they can be quite charming. Often, if they do something wrong, they are "sorry," and feel that ought to end the matter even though what they did caused a great deal of damage. This is not due to insincerity but to the fact that their own emotions are extremely shallow. They don't seem to learn from experience, probably because experiences do not affect them very much. Certain kinds of criminals belong in this group.

Psychopaths may be quite intelligent. So far as we know, their particular form of sickness is not caused by organic damage. However, they have not grown emotionally. In every other way they appear mature, but so far as their emotions are concerned, they are about at the level of a two-year-old. They may perform criminal acts and are remorseful if they are caught, but not because of what they did. There is no easy way to predict when the psychopath may break the law, nor is it true that only psychopaths are capable of sexual criminality. (I discuss other types of sexual criminality on page 196.)

In neurotic individuals, the unconscious conflicts carried over from childhood may show themselves in specific symbolic symptoms, like compulsory hand-washing. But psychopathic persons are affected throughout their personality, so that everyone else appears wrong. The psychopath or sociopath may really believe that anyone who tries to live honestly, maintaining good relationships with other people, is stupid.

## PERSONALITY DISORDERS

Disorders of personality are difficult to define. A person who drinks too much, for example, may have his problem under partial control and be considered a neurotic. He may be a psychopath, practically without a conscience. Or alcoholism itself may be his most serious problem, so serious that he can hardly function in society and may eventually have to be hospitalized. Because I feel that the following personality disorders are so serious that they affect a person's mind and personality completely, I have included them in this chapter. In a very real sense, such people are crippled, but they need not always be treated in hospitals. Their illnesses are often difficult to diagnose and to treat, but modern psychiatry has new techniques and new drugs that make the outlook for these unfortunates brighter than it was even a few years ago.

### Alcoholism and Drug Addiction

Alcoholics and drugs addicts are chronically sick people whose ailment shows itself in their behavior, which is generally disorderly and antisocial. Unlike many other maladjusted individuals, they have turned to something *outside* themselves to find the characteristic "inadequate but temporarily satisfying solution" to their problems. As in the case of other maladjusted people, this does not solve their difficulties. But, in addition, they face the problems that result from excessive drinking or from taking drugs. In advanced cases, their physical condition is very poor; in fact, deterioration often sets in. In many cases, hospitalization is necessary if a cure is to be effected.

Much of the progress in treating alcoholism and drug addiction has been made possible by the recognition that these are diseases, not crimes (although crimes are often committed by addicts). They have physical as well as psychological aspects, and there is growing belief that chemical abnormalities within the body may play a significant role. Also, alcoholism and drug addiction are recognized as social problems. More research and more treatment facilities are being made available on the local, state, and national levels.

### Sexual Deviations

I want to make it clear that we doctors do not include among the deviations all forms of sexual activity that vary from the usual. Broadly speaking, we consider a man or woman normal if he or she derives greatest pleasure from insertion of the male genital organ into that of the female. But this does not mean that experimentation to obtain satisfaction by other means is abnormal. For example, there is certainly nothing abnormal for a man who reaches climax rapidly, before his wife does, to make it possible for her to achieve climax by manual manipulation. There is nothing abnormal about any caress, in the foreplay before coitus, that both partners find pleasurable.

The oral zone—mouth, lips, and tongue—is, to a greater or lesser degree, a sexual one. Some couples find the genital kiss important for fullest sexual satisfaction. This does not constitute abnormality.

More and more psychiatrists, though not all, now consider sexual deviations to be reflections of mental illness only if they cause unhappiness for those who practice them or interfere with their ability to function normally. Homosexuality (see later) is increasingly being viewed in this way.

Certain deviant behavior, it is generally accepted, results from emotional difficulties which must, if possible, be corrected—while at the same time the actions of the deviates may need to be controlled to prevent them from harming themselves or others.

Right here I want to remind you that mature people often carry about with them certain "holdovers" from their childhood. You may, therefore, find in yourself traces of some of the sexual deviations I shall describe. Don't decide, for that reason, that you are perverted!

Let me give you an example. A Peeping Tom who gets his greatest sexual pleasure from watching a woman undressed or undressing or watching a couple engaged in sexual actions is undoubtedly maladjusted. (A woman, too, may be a "Peeping Tomasina!") Perhaps, in his childhood, Tom had a shocking experience connected with his parent's sexual relations, or perhaps he had been so strongly convinced of the wickedness of sexual intercourse that he could not permit himself to be involved actively in such a thing, but had to get his pleasure as an "innocent bystander." This does not mean, however, that you or I are perverted if we have not entirely outgrown our childish fascination in the forbidden. Most men, no matter how mature, find the glimpse of an accidentally revealed shapely limb more exciting than the extensive areas of the feminine form which are frankly displayed by a bevy of girl athletes!

Deriving the highest, or only, sexual satisfaction from watching or peeping (voyeurism) is one form of sexual deviation. Following are some of the others:

FETISHISM. This is a deviation in which some material associated with the body, such as a shoe or underwear, becomes the necessary condition for sexual arousal. A part stands for the totality in order to overcome the influence of an old, often hidden wound.

HOMOSEXUALITY. Sexual attraction toward persons of the same sex is found in both men and women. Some individuals may have sexual relationships with members of both sexes and are known as bisexuals.

I should like to emphasize here that during a child's emotional development, his sexual energies are directed at various times toward those of his own sex and toward those of the opposite sex. As he matures, these energies focus on the opposite sex, but traces of the earlier attitudes usually remain. As a result, occasional homosexual feelings or dreams may occur. Homosexual experiences also may occur in a normal person who is put in an unusual situation, such as continued isolation from members of the opposite sex. He usually returns eventually to normal relationships. These isolated experiences should not be confused with homosexuality as a continued, preferred sexual outlet.

Homosexuality is complex. Many theories have been suggested to explain it. Children normally identify with the parent of the same sex; a little girl wants to be like and rival her mother; a boy, his father. If, for some reason, identification is with the parent of the opposite sex, a child may be oriented toward homosexuality.

Homosexuality may also develop another way. Usually, for a time shortly before and during early adolescence, children prefer members of their own sex. Boys enjoy being together, have male heroes, look down upon girls; girls "detest" boys, have crushes on girls, and love some "best friend" intensely. With the advent of sexual maturity, sexual drives are directed—not always without some conflict—toward members of the opposite sex.

During this difficult period, unfortunate experiences may have a devastating effect on some young people who have emotional problems. Whether the experiences are obvious or subtle, they may set up a barrier on the road to normal sexual development so that homosexuality may become, in effect, a detour on that highway, and some people never find their way back to the main road.

Homosexuals are often depicted as inevitably lonely, unhappy people. Not by any means are all of them so. And certainly they are not to be regarded as wicked or depraved. Some homosexuals are unhappy about their condition and would prefer to be heterosexual. Achieving this is not easy. Psychiatric help can be valuable for homosexuals who wish to seek it.

"Amateur psychiatrists" have done a great deal of harm by speaking glibly about "latent homosexuality," "bisexuality," and so on. I hope I can prevent them from causing you needless worry by stating emphatically: (1) A homosexual experience (or experiences), especially in adolescence, does not mean that an individual *is* homosexual; and neither does a homosexual dream or fantasy. (2) There is a certain amount of basic homosexuality in the normal individual, as well as some holdovers from the period during which one preferred the company of one's own sex. (A high-school girl expressed this when she said to her mother, who was a friend of my wife's, "I'd ever so much rather be with girls except for the fact that men are so attractive.") (3) Homosexuality is a complicated problem and in itself is only *one* factor of the maladjusted individual's personality.

EXHIBITIONISM is the act of revealing one's body, usually the genital organ. This is, in its essence, similar to "peeping." A certain amount of "showing off" is normal. This is not to be confused with the exhibitionism of the maladjusted individual. Such a person may be attempting to reassure himself against fears of sexual inferiority; or the maladjusted one may be expressing defiance toward a supposedly hostile world by shocking people in this manner.

NARCISSISM OR SELF-LOVE. This is quite different from *self-respect* and from the satisfaction which normal men and, more particularly, women derive from looking well. The term comes from the name of a Greek youth who, according to the myth, saw his own reflection in a pond and was so enamored of it that he fell in and was drowned while attempting to embrace himself. Most children go through a period of being attracted to their own images in a mirror, stating frankly, "You're pretty" or "I love you." People who do not outgrow this stage are often basically so insecure that they feel no one else will ever love them. This exclusive preoccupation is frequently accompanied by a preference for masturbation to sexual intercourse. Such people are incapable of loving anyone else. They may marry for money to spend on the beloved person—namely, himself or herself.

NYMPHOMANIA AND SATYRISM. These conditions, the excessive desire for intercourse in a woman and a man, are rare. Although the terms are often applied to people who are promiscuous or highly sexed, they should be reserved for *compulsive* sexuality, which cannot be satisfied. Like compulsive eating, it often springs from insecurity and may be indulged in to ward off anxiety. Unable to find the hoped-for release in sexual intercourse, such people must desperately try, try again. A nymphomaniac is often unable to experience an orgasm, remaining unsatisfied no matter how often she has intercourse; or she may be attempting to satisfy something that cannot be satisfied by coitus. She may be unconsciously homosexual and will not find what she is looking for in any man; or she may be trying to compensate for feelings of inferiority; or she may (unconsciously) feel that intercourse is wicked and she must not enjoy it fully. The male equivalent of the nymphomaniac may be similarly maladjusted; he may be an unconscious homosexual, or have intense conflicts due to feelings of guilt, fear, or inferiority.

BESTIALITY (the act of having intercourse with animals). The Kinsey reports indicate that about 17 percent of all males raised on farms have had some sexual experience with animals. The practice is fairly common among shepherds and others who are isolated from women. However, *preference* for sex relations with animals is due to an emotional maladjustment usually springing from feelings of inferiority. Even the woman who showers her affections on a pet animal is apt to be afraid to bestow it on a fellow human being. She may tell herself people are unworthy of her love, but she is actually afraid they will not appreciate her because she is unworthy.

SADISM AND MASOCHISM (deriving pleasure from giving or receiving pain). Sadists may inflict pain on animals or upon people, usually their sexual partners. They wish to dominate, to prove their strength or virility by being aggressive or, for example, by being like their dominating fathers who used to punish them. Sadism need not be expressed in the form of a sexual deviation. Teasing is one of its mild forms, although this may be far from mild, as those of us who have known practical jokers can testify. Children are often sadistic in their drive to assert themselves—although I believe some actions which are called sadistic in children are due to curiosity and lack of understanding; a child who pulls the wings from flies *may* have no idea he is being cruel, since he may be acting from the same impulses that make him examine an inanimate object.

Masochists derive pleasure and satisfaction from being treated cruelly, from being hurt physically or emotionally, or from hurting themselves. This usually has its roots in the (often unconscious) desire to be punished for some "sin." Masochism has been called neurotic submissiveness, and sadism, neurotic aggressiveness; but since they spring from similar maladjustments, they may both exist in the same person. Masochism appears in a nonphysical form, as a character attitude, far more frequently than it does as a sexual deviation.

SEXUAL CRIMINALITY. The unscientific term *sex maniac* covers people who, like Jack the Ripper, commit violent sex crimes, such as rape and murder. They are suffering from emotional illnesses or defects, however well concealed these may have been before the crime was committed. Many of us have peculiar sex impulses, usually of a transient nature, which we do not actually consider carrying out, any more than we would put into action any number of notions that pop into our minds—from jumping off the top of a high building to tripping up a pompous fat man. In some sex criminals, the mechanisms that control healthy people are defective or break down. In others, deep-rooted feelings of guilt, inferiority, or insecurity may cause their sexual instincts to be shunted off in abnormal directions, some of which are socially dangerous.

## PSYCHOSES

People suffering from psychoses are called psychotics, or psychotic persons. They are, to a greater or lesser extent, out of touch with reality some, if not all, of the time.

A psychotic individual may live in his own private world, not seeing or hearing anything that goes on around him. He may not even feel it if he is suddenly slapped, or if he does feel it, it may bring a happy smile to his face. He may go into a *catatonic* state, standing absolutely motionless for hours in a position no normal person could maintain for more than a few minutes; on recovering from this state he may be able to report on things that happened, to which he had appeared completely oblivious. He may suffer from *hallucinations,* that is, see and hear things that have no existence outside of his mind, or *delusions* which are unreal beliefs. A person, for example, may be strongly convinced that he is the King of England.

This distortion of reality is one of the main differences between neurotic and psychotic people. Something may *seem* real to the neurotic, but it *is* real to the psychotic. This is what I mean: George Gray, whom I told you about on page 186, said he used to feel as though he were living on enemy territory; however, he knew exactly where he was living, using those words to describe his uneasiness and fear of people. A psychotic person saying the same thing would be convinced that he *was* actually surrounded by enemies who wanted to kill him, force him to do certain things, "gain control of his thoughts," and so on. The "evidence" which the psychotic person presents is quite different from that by which someone who is neurotic reaches his conclusions. If, for example, the latter believes he is unattractive to women, he may support his theory by the evidence that a girl refused to accept his invitation, ignoring the fact that he invited her so late she might well have had a previous engagement. A psychotic person, however, "proves" that people are trying to get into his thoughts by pointing to a television aerial on the roof or citing the way someone looked at him in the subway. The entire *quality* of reality is distorted to the psychotic person.

Like neuroses, psychoses may have their roots in the individual's early life. Perhaps we can say that the psychotic person's inadequate or inappropriate methods of dealing with his difficulties are *complete,* while those of a neurotic person are *partial.* Or we might say that the latter takes unwise courses in struggling with his problems, whereas the former is overwhelmed by them. If we compare the neurotic person to an imaginary man who goes through life with a cast on his ankle because he once broke it, we can say that the psychotic person puts his entire body in a cast because he can't endure the pain in his ankle.

The psychotic person lacks insight. His disorders are so intense or inclusive that any compromise with normal social requirements is impossible. In other words, he fails *totally* to adapt.

Because of his distortion of reality and the fact that his entire psyche (rather than just a portion of it) is ill, such a person may need to be protected from himself and society, and society protected from him. Otherwise he may fail to guard himself from the ordinary hazards of life or may deliberately mutilate or kill himself or some other person. It requires the judgment of a trained psychiatrist, often after a period of observation, to determine whether or not a psychotic person is likely to constitute a danger.

## Types of Psychoses

The psychoses may be classified in different ways, but they are usually divided into *functional* and *organic* (with brain damage). The functional psychoses are considered under the headings of (1) *schizophrenia*, (2) *paranoia*, and (3) *manic-depressive psychoses*, including *involutional melancholia*.

SCHIZOPHRENIA. This disease was formerly called *dementia praecox* (early loss of mind), because it usually appears between the ages of fifteen and thirty. It is the type of psychosis most frequently seen. Schizophrenia means split mind, and, indeed, the individual suffering from it does not appear to be a "whole person." The type of child most apt to develop this disease is usually shy, dreamy, bored, and lacking in physical and mental "pep." Unable to cope with the world he tends to withdraw from it, and the added difficulties of adolescence may drive him into a world of his own creating. (But *a certain amount of daydreaming is perfectly normal*, especially in adolescence, so don't decide your teen-age daughter is going to be a schizophrenic because she's so immersed in a romantic dream that she doesn't hear you call her to dinner!)

As a rule, schizophrenia manifests itself slowly, although sometimes it makes its appearance abruptly in an acute attack of confusion. The patient becomes more and more withdrawn, his emotions fade or become distorted. The "split" personality of the schizophrenic seems quite apparent when with a happy smile he says things like, "I'm going to be shot by a firing squad within the hour," or cries over something that a normal person would consider good news. He may have difficulty in comprehending even the simplest abstraction such as "a stitch in time saves nine"; it is as though he were incapable of making the slightest mental effort.

Schizophrenia is divided by psychiatrists into four types, the *simple*, the *hebephrenic*, the *catatonic*, and the *paranoid* types. Although certain types of schizophrenia respond more readily to treatment than do others, early diagnosis and treatment are extremely important. Of course, this is desirable in all cases of neurotic and psychotic illness, but it is particularly true with schizophrenia, as the chances of recovery appear to be closely related to the duration of the condition.

PARANOIA. This psychosis is also called *monomania*, *delusional insanity*, and *persecutory insanity*. The patient suffering from it may sound and act fairly normal, although he is very ill. That is, his memory may be adequate, his confusion not apparent, and his reasoning logical, although his premises are false and his judgment impaired. It usually occurs between the ages of thirty and fifty, particularly among people who have always been self-centered, jealous, and suspicious. A person suffering from it becomes more and more deluded, seeing hidden meanings to support his conviction that he is being plotted against—by such means as x-ray or hypnotism. This type of psychotic person feels quite justified in "defending himself" by lawsuits or antisocial acts including murder. Some of these people are commonly referred to as *maniacs:* for example, a man may be spoken of as a *pyromaniac* if he sets fire to a building, as a paranoid person might do in order to "destroy the evil people in it."

A paranoid person is quite different from a neurotic individual who believes "everyone's against me" or "everything happens to me," for the latter merely places undue emphasis on certain things that happen, whereas the former distorts them completely.

MANIC-DEPRESSIVE PSYCHOSES. I have discussed manic-depressive illness earlier (p. 190 ).

The "cyclic personality type" of individual is not to be confused with a true manic-depressive. Normal people have their ups and downs, which may be of a fairly rhythmical nature. Their moods may alternate during the course of a day, so that they feel wonderful (or terrible) in the morning, and quite the opposite at night. Some women feel depressed before each monthly period; many people get "blue" in bad, wintry weather, while each spring day makes them bubble over with high spirits. These moods are quite different from the periods of wild elation and the ones of profound unhappiness which the person with a manic-depressive psychosis goes through.

Other personality types also show traits that are

somewhat similar to the symptoms of the major types of psychosis. The *schizoid* personality keeps to himself as much as he can, and is nervous or uncomfortable in company. He daydreams extensively and may find more pleasure in his fantasies than in the real world. The *paranoid* personality is suspicious of other people, although he is not convinced that others are actually plotting to harm him. It is extremely difficult to decide at what point these personality traits begin to pass over to genuine psychosis.

*Involutional melancholia* is a state of depression which may occur in the later periods of life, during the change of life (menopause) in women and its emotional counterpart in men. It is always accompanied by the danger of suicide.

## THERAPY (TREATMENT)

Many of these illnesses are not hopeless although their severity may make them appear to be. New methods have been devised and are constantly being discovered to restore mental health to people who used to be regarded as incurably insane.

The various forms of *psychotherapy* I described in the last chapter are used on psychotic patients if and when their condition is such as to make it feasible. You can see for yourself how ineffective it would be to employ methods based on verbal communication when patients are out of contact with reality, completely absorbed in their own fantasies and hallucinations.

*Adjunctive therapies* are very useful in the treatment of psychotic people. In addition to occupational therapy, they have been helped by *music therapy* and by *hydrotherapy* (wet packs, immersion in warm water for several hours at a time, etc.). *Psychodrama*, like play therapy, provides a means of communication for patients who are not up to the more articulate forms of expression, as well as a way to "get things out of their systems."

*Shock therapy* may be employed when a psychotic patient remains out of contact with the real world. This method has proven effective, sometimes bringing about spectacular improvements, although frequently it must be followed by psychotherapy to be permanently effective. *Electrical shock* and *insulin coma* are the most frequently employed forms of shock therapy. The patient is rendered unconscious by a carefully controlled electric shock or a dose of insulin, usually repeated several times a week. Several theories have been advanced to explain how these treatments restore the patient to reality: that the shock breaks through the barrier the patient has erected to keep out the real world; that whatever portion of his mind remains healthy responds to the threat of annihilation represented by the shock and "takes over" in the emergency; that there are physical reasons, such as the fact that the supply of adrenaline is suddenly increased by the shock. However, shock therapy was not developed as a result of theories, but rather because of observations made by doctors who had seen its astonishing effects when it occurred by accident—as, for example, in the case of a psychotic patient who happened to have diabetes and had an accidental overdosage of insulin resulting in shock or coma (see page 78).

Shock therapy has been successful in patients suffering from depression, particularly involutional melancholia, and in schizophrenia. Extreme care is taken to prevent any injury to the patient from the shock, so that the incidence of accidents is extremely small.

In some cases the patient is given a light shock —*subcoma insulin*, for example—or is put to sleep for a comparatively long period by means of electricity or drugs.

MEDICINAL THERAPY. Treating mental patients with medicines has opened a new era in psychiatry. This form of therapy not only has benefited the patients but has drastically changed the kind of care in mental hospitals and has steadily lowered the number of long-term patients. The savings are enormous, both for the individual patient and for the local, state, and federal governments that build and maintain mental hospitals.

Tranquilizers can make belligerent, overactive patients manageable and responsive to other forms of therapy. In the opinion of many psychiatrists, the potent tranquilizers used for psychoses—as distinguished from milder ones employed for anxiety and tension—are misnamed and are, rather, not so much tranquilizers as antipsychotic agents.

Depressed patients may be treated with antidepressant drugs. Many such agents are now available, and usually it is possible to find one that is most likely to help an individual patient.

## SOME PHYSICAL CAUSES OF PSYCHOSES

The psychoses I have been discussing are the result of *functional* disorders. That is, they have (as far as science can discover) no basis in the physical, organic structure of the mind, although body chemistry may be significant in some illnesses, like schizophrenia. However, similar conditions can arise from physical causes. These include:

*Infectious diseases* involving the brain itself, such as encephalitis and tubercular or syphilitic lesions. Most diseases such as acute meningitis and mastoiditis are controlled by the "wonder drugs" before they can reach and injure the brain. *Paresis,* which causes a form of paranoia, used to be prevalent in the past, before syphilis (which causes it) could be prevented and cured. Paresis itself can be cured today.

*Certain diseases involving the nervous system.* *Huntington's chorea,* which usually occurs first at thirty to forty-five years of age, can cause mental deterioration. It should *not* be confused with the form of *chorea* known as *St. Vitus Dance* from which children may suffer (see page 292).

*Deficiencies.* For example, *pellagra,* which is due to a vitamin deficiency, can eventually affect the brain. This disease responds quickly to treatment, mainly consisting of Vitamin $B_2$.

*Poisons.* Some substances, such as lead, affect the brain. The poisons, called *toxins,* formed by the bacteria causing some diseases can bring about delirium, which very much resembles a temporary psychosis, in patients who have very high fevers.

*Tumors* involving the brain or affecting the central nervous system can cause psychoses.

*Interference with the brain's blood supply,* which may result from a cerebral hemorrhage or hardening of the arteries, can interfere with the brain's normal functioning (see page 427 on arteriosclerosis).

*Epilepsy.* In a very small percentage of all cases of epilepsy, some mental deterioration will result. (See page 465 for a discussion of this "stepchild of all diseases.")

*Wounds and blows.* Obviously, the brain can be injured by gunshot wounds and damaged in various ways by blows.

*Senility.* There are psychoses which are associated with aging of the brain.

## MENTAL DEFECTIVES

The majority of mental illnesses from which people suffer do not stem from a lack of intelligence. However, there are conditions in which the intellect is involved. We use the term mental defective to describe people whose intelligence is below normal. Lowest in the scale are the *idiots.* Their brains are, from birth or shortly thereafter, so defective or so badly damaged that they do not progress beyond the level of intelligence of a child of three. Next come the *imbeciles* with a mentality of, roughly, from three to seven; and then the *feebleminded* (also called *retarded* and *morons*) who go all the way up the scale from the mental age of seven to the "low normal."

Idiocy and imbecility exhibit themselves early in the child's development. (I describe the normal development of babies on page 273.) Feeblemindedness may not become apparent immediately. Sometimes it is not easy to recognize the higher grades of feeblemindedness. Methods of determining the intelligence (such as the *intelligence test,* which establishes the *intelligence quotient*—the IQ) are excellent. But they deal with human beings and not with material things that can be weighed and measured exactly. No matter how carefully allowances are made for emotional factors, they cannot always be completely separated from the intellect. There have been cases in which a child's IQ has "changed"; it was low due to apathy, which resulted from an emotional state and disappeared with treatment. There have also been children whose general physical condition was below par and caused them to do badly on intelligence tests. Once in a while we even see a child who has survived in spite of practically complete neglect, and whose apparent mental deficiency is due to a lack of any education whatsoever, using the word "education" in its broadest sense.

Some types of mental deficiency are due to a constitutional defect, producing what used to be called "monsters" or "nature's mistakes." Such abnormalities are fortunately rare, and when they occur in the brain and nerves the deformed infant often does not survive very long. We do not know the reason for some of these defects. A few of them are hereditary.

This certainly does *not* mean you shouldn't have children because you have heard that "there's feeblemindedness in the family" or "insanity runs in the family." In the first place, "poor Great-Aunt Martha" (or Cousin Horace) may not have been feebleminded at all but, for example, suffering from the effects of an infectious disease contracted in infancy. In the second place, if insanity actually did "run" in the family, it may very well have been due to the fact that a mentally ill parent was allowed to remain in the home, creating an atmosphere which encouraged the children to develop unhealthy attitudes.

I do not mean to say that mental defects and illness cannot be inherited, but I can't overemphasize the fact that *only a very small fraction of all mental cases are primarily due to inheritance.* If you have any cause to worry about your family or that of your spouse, talk it over with your doctor. Provided you can give him accurate information, he can probably assure you that you are in no danger of having a defective or mentally ill child. Or he may wish to have you consult one of the centers specializing in the study of heredity.

Incidentally, marrying a cousin does *not* mean that your children will probably be defective; it simply means that there is an increased chance of their inheriting family characteristics, from blue eyes to the fortunately very rare hereditary mental diseases.

Some defects causing mental deficiency can be corrected before any permanent damage is done if the infant is treated early enough: for example, *cretinism* (see page 81).

Mental deficiency can be caused by certain things that affect the infant while he is still in his mother's womb: for example, if she is subjected to excessive radiation or if she has syphilis (but not gonorrhea) or, sometimes, if she has German measles during the early months of her pregnancy. It is not caused by things we used to hear about—like being frightened by a mouse or thwarted in her desire to eat lobster.

Mental deficiency can result from birth injury—that is, damage to the baby's brain while he is being born. *Cerebral palsy,* caused in this way, used to be considered a form of mental deficiency. Now, however, it has been discovered that the injury is usually not in the portion of the brain and nerves involving the intellect, but rather in the parts involved in muscle control. Because these children were unable to control their muscles—including those having to do with speech—they were formerly treated as though they were imbeciles; this, of course, had a disastrous effect on their development.

## HOSPITALIZATION

Many of the cases I have discussed in this chapter should be treated in hospitals. The mistaken notion that "it would be cruel to send a psychotic patient to an institution when he would not hurt a fly," or "it's my duty to look after him," has caused needless tragedies and suffering. A psychotic person *may suddenly become* capable of hurting himself or others; and the entire family, especially its younger members, may suffer severe emotional disturbances as a result of his presence. Perhaps equally important is the fact that the patient may have a very much better chance of improving or getting well in a hospital or sanatorium equipped to treat and to care for him than he has in any home.

Don't try to handle the problem of hospitalization yourself. Get medical advice as to whether it is really necessary. If the condition comes on suddenly, and the patient becomes violent or homicidal or suicidal, you may have to restrain him, if possible with the help of others, until the doctor or the police arrive. In less acute cases, a doctor, *not* a member of the family, should take over. There are several reasons for this. In the first place, an untrained person is not capable of telling whether or not anyone is psychotic, and a mistake in either direction can be serious. Nor can an untrained person handle anyone who is seriously ill mentally. A psychotic person may kill himself or someone else even though he seems to be quite docile.

If you notice that a dear friend or member of your family is undergoing a marked change in personality (if he loses interest in his friends, recreation, or work, seems to be "off in a dream," incoherent, depressed, or overly suspicious), talk it over with your doctor or at a hospital clinic. Do not discuss the matter with the person himself unless he asks your advice. Then say it would be wise for him to have a complete *medical* checkup by his regular physician or one you suggest (see page 368 on how to choose a doctor).

The second reason for you to avoid taking the matter into your own hands concerns your relationship to the patient. If you should trick him into going to some mental institution, it will interfere with the help you could otherwise give him during his stay there and even after his cure. The period following a patient's release from a mental institution is a difficult one, and he will require your sympathetic understanding. People may be reluctant to accept him as cured, and many employers refuse to employ someone who has been institutionalized. They feel his sickness may recur. It is true that it may—but on the other hand, *any* employee may become physically or mentally ill, or have an automobile accident. Great efforts are being made to educate the public regarding mental illness. Detailed suggestions for helping a discharged patient are given by his doctor or the social service department of the institution, and by government and private organizations, such as your state or community mental health association. Through them you can also get useful books and pamphlets, some free and some at a nominal cost. But by far the greatest help you can give lies in establishing a good relationship. The basis of such a relationship must be *your complete understanding and acceptance of the fact that there is no stigma attached to mental illness.*

Finally, there are laws which make it very difficult for an individual who attempts to handle a psychotic patient on his own. The average person usually has no idea of what is involved in the *legal aspects of commitment.* These vary in different states. Often they seem unnecessarily complicated, even "unfair," but we must remember that it is hard to work out a simple method covering all the requirements for safeguarding the individual and protecting society. Relatives of the mentally ill naturally want to avoid publicity, and in most states it is possible to keep this to a minimum if the facts are known to the family doctor or the committing physicians.

Patients are usually committed for a period of observation (around a week) after which time they are reexamined. Under certain circumstances, alcoholic persons can be committed in this way. As they are usually released quite soon, it is especially important to have the help of an understanding doctor so that the alcoholic person won't feel some member of his family is trying to punish him, but will be receptive to the idea that he is ill and can be cured.

It is not easy to see someone dear to you enter a mental institution, even when your doctor says it is necessary. Try to remember that he or she has a good chance of coming out again, cured or improved.

## Types of Hospitals

Mental hospitals, like other hospitals, vary as to *type* and *quality.* In recent years, many new types have been developed, and the quality has, with few exceptions, been rising. Some hospitals provide up-to-date treatment while others limit themselves to caring for the patient's basic requirements (*custodial care*). In some cases, the latter is all that can be done. When selecting a mental institution, you should find out which type it is, in addition to making certain that it meets the requirements I have given on page 390 when I tell you how to select a hospital. A private "custodial" sanatorium may be ever so much "nicer" and less depressing in appearance than a state institution, but in many instances the treatment which the latter offers is most important. Remember, too, that mental illnesses may sometimes require comparatively long periods of hospitalization, in spite of the advances being made through psychopharmacology (treatment by drugs). I have known families that failed to take this into consideration, making great sacrifices to pay for a few weeks in a private institution when the same amount of money should have been stretched over a longer period in a state hospital.

Just as drug therapy has helped bring about a decline in the total number of persons in mental hospitals and the length of their stay, so have other new methods of treatment, like group therapy and family therapy (which I discuss in the preceding chapter), led to the development of smaller and more flexible hospitals.

Not so many years ago, the mentally ill person faced the extreme of full-time care in a large hospital or little or no care at home. Now, many communities have organized *halfway houses*. Just as the name implies, these are centers where the patient may be helped along the road from serious illness to recovery. He may sleep there and go to his job during the day. Or he may go to the halfway house at regular intervals for the attention and help he still needs as he continues to recover. There are no barred doors or windows in these centers, and the rules are much more relaxed than in the large, public hospitals.

These new facilities, whether they are part of a community mental health center or an independent establishment, are increasingly important for the care of mentally ill persons. Not only do they provide the continuing, but less intense, care that a patient needs, according to his progress, but they can provide mental health services on a clinic or outpatient basis, establish programs for preventing mental illness, and promote community programs for mental health. They fit in with the goals of medicine—prevention and individual care.

## Severe Cases

Some of the cases I have discussed in this chapter do not respond to treatment, and the emphasis is placed on making the patient as safe and comfortable as possible. Families of such patients face difficult decisions which I think many of us, including some physicians, tend to dismiss glibly.

As yet, there is little that medical science can do to repair a defective brain or brain degeneration. There are times, therefore, when we doctors must honestly tell parents that a child cannot be

normal, and that the only wise thing to do is to place him in an institution. Unfortunately, however, this is sometimes said in a tone that implies "and forget you ever had him." Quite understandably, many parents react to this by saying, "No, never," closing their minds and consequently ruining their lives and those of their other children.

Doctors should always help these parents to explore the situation thoroughly and arrive at the best solution. It is not always easy for a parent to realize that the mentally defective baby will not remain physically a child. His intelligence will not progress beyond the level of the three- or five- or seven-year-old, but his physical development will continue—with all the problems this entails not only for the family but for the defective child himself. Even the most loving of parents cannot always spare such a child the unhappiness which often adds emotional disturbances to his mental deficiency. In many cases, placing him in an institution is the only way to be fair to him, as well as to his family and to society.

However, some types of defective children *can* be brought up in the home. Occasionally there are circumstances which make it possible to do this —not without sacrifice, of course, but without serious injury to the family. These defective children include a small percentage of idiots and an increasingly larger percentage of the higher grades of mental defectives. Skilled and patient teachers in schools for the mentally retarded are able to teach some of these children enough to enable them to live safely in the world and even to attain a degree of social usefulness. Before any decision is made, the entire situation must be carefully evaluated, including the child's condition, the home situation, the availability of help in education, and so on.

The parents of a *psychotic* child face an even more complicated situation. In the first place, it is often difficult, sometimes impossible, to determine whether or not, or to what degree, a psychotic child is also mentally deficient. In the second place, there are as yet very few day "schools" where such children can be helped or, at the least their parents relieved of the difficulty of caring for them all day long.

I think it is advisable for all parents who face

the problem of placing their children in institutions to have some form of psychiatric help in making their decision. No matter how much information is obtained and how wisely the decision is arrived at, the emotions are bound to be involved. If feelings of uncertainty and guilt are brought into the open before the decision is made, it can be "lived with" far more successfully than if these feelings are repressed.

What I have been saying about defective children naturally applies in many instances to older incurables. It is particularly difficult to "put away" a beloved parent even when one realizes that his or her presence in the home is injuring the children in the family. One mother I know felt so unhappy after visiting her father (who had lucid periods during which he used to beg her to take him home) that she upset her children almost as much as his presence would have upset them. Talking to an understanding psychiatric social worker enabled her to find an outlet for the sorrow she thought she could conceal from her children.

The fear that their dear ones will not be handled with consideration or receive the best treatment in an institution is particularly hard for families to bear. It is true that some state mental institutions are overcrowded and understaffed, as you may have read in articles exposing the conditions in mental hospitals. Fortunately some of the conditions described by these investigators are being remedied. Fortunately, too, many state institutions do excellent work even when they lack the money that would make them far pleasanter places for the patients—and for the doctors and other personnel.

The type of institution your community provides depends largely on the attitude of your community. If its citizens understand the importance of mental health, if they are sufficiently interested to find out the qualifications of candidates for elected and appointed positions, if they support progressive legislation in this field—including the granting of adequate funds—their institutions will be able to provide the best that medical science can offer.

Your understanding of mental illness will enable you to find the best ways of preventing it in your own family circle or helping to cure it if it should occur. It will also enable you to do your share, as a citizen, in bringing the benefits of mental health to the entire community.

# PART THREE

## You and Your Home

# 14
# EMOTIONAL ATTITUDES TOWARD MARRIAGE

---

What do most people seek when they marry? The answer, which is *happiness,* may seem obvious, yet there was a time when a consideration of happiness had no part in marriage plans.

In the past, most marriages were based on custom and tradition. Every step, from finding a mate to the wedding ceremony, was controlled by the families of the young couple. Even today, this is the accepted procedure in many parts of the world.

Havelock Ellis, the eminent authority on love and marriage, put it this way, "One may doubt if the happiness today demanded in marriage— whether or not often found—had any existence in ancient days. . . . If marriage often appears less happy today it is because we are less willing to submit to unhappiness or to the make-believe of convention."

Nowadays, in America, people usually marry because they have fallen in love. The choice of a spouse is up to the individual.

While young people no longer depend completely (if at all!) upon parental advice, many of them want guidance. There is an increasing demand all over the country for scientific knowledge of sex and the psychology of successful marriage. This is a good sign, and it should be encouraged and satisfied by schools, churches, social agencies, and particularly parents.

While there is no such thing as a blueprint for a happy marriage, it is wise, before taking the step, to be aware of the conditions that best lead to such happiness. Scientific studies have been made, examining thousands of marriages, to discover the reasons for their success or failure.

Experts in the field of marriage list the ensuing factors as most important in choosing a mate. Because falling in love is an emotional process, it is ridiculous to expect anyone to go around with this list in hand and check off each item! However, it is a good and sobering idea to consider these factors before actually marrying. Young people need all the reliable information about sex and marriage that is available, because in spite of the fact that contemporary American society appears liberal about sex, there is still much ignorance and misinformation about sexual activity and reproduction. Unfortunately, there is also a lot of hypocrisy, fear, conflict, and guilt. A healthy attitude toward sex does not mean there are no rules. It means that you learn to understand the significance of sex in everyday life, in its true perspective.

EMOTIONAL ADJUSTMENT. It is obvious that people who are normal in the sense that I use the term in Chapter 11 have the best chance for happiness in life, which naturally includes happiness in marriage. Be sure to read Chapter 11 for an overall picture of the normal person.

Within the broad framework of that description, which types make the best husband or wife? The following list gives certain characteristics which should be considered before marriage. Authorities suggest that at least two of the good characteristics should be present.

| GOOD | BAD |
|------|-----|
| Optimistic personality | Pessimistic personality |
| Cooperativeness | Dominating personality |
| Consideration and sympathy | Inconsiderate and unsympathetic |
| Some degree of emotional dependence | Too self-sufficient emotionally; too much "narcissism" or self-love |
| | Dependent personality: too strong an attachment to parents |

CULTURAL BACKGROUND. The best chances of success lie in finding a mate of the same race, philosophical outlook or religion, and economic and social class. Most people feel more at home with others who have had a similar childhood and have similar customs, manners, and tastes. While marriages between people of different groups can be successful, they usually face additional problems due to social disapproval or to the number of adjustments which must be made, and which often create tensions and irritations. For example, a rural Southern boy and a city-bred Northern girl may find it extremely difficult to find a way of living that suits them both.

EDUCATIONAL LEVEL. School provides experiences in learning and in being with others; these are extremely helpful in making marital adjustments. It is desirable for both partners to have, roughly, the same amount of formal education—or the informal equivalent.

ECONOMIC AND JOB STATUS. More important than the size of a man's income is the fact that he has a steady job which does not require him to move about, leaving his wife and family for prolonged intervals of time. The more educational preparation he has put into his job, the better candidate he is for marriage. Most important is the fact that he has put aside savings before marrying.

NUMBER OF FRIENDS. Generally speaking, men and women who have had many friends of each sex before marriage are apt to be types that will make satisfactory mates.

MEMBERSHIP IN ORGANIZATIONS. It is considered a good sign if an individual is a member of a social, labor, or any other kind of club or organization. It indicates the fact that he is accepted by, and accepts, a large group of people.

## COURTSHIP

No matter how much your pulse beats at the sight of your beloved, don't rush into marriage. Give yourself and your future mate a chance to know each other. It will save a lot of trouble later on. Don't marry anyone with the idea in the back of your mind of reforming him or her. Remember, you are marrying an adult whose tastes and habits are pretty well fixed. If Mary takes John for what he is, and not for what he may become, it will save her a lot of disillusionment. So use the valuable time before marriage to discuss, and try to reach a basic understanding on, all important matters. Questions such as the following should be faced before marriage: Shall the wife work? For how long? Can you live on the husband's earnings? Who will manage the family income? How many children? How should they best be brought up?

The following questionnaire will serve as a helpful guide:

Answer *yes* or *no*.

°1. Do you like to spend most of your leisure time together?

°2. Do you agree on whether or not to have children? Agree on their upbringing?

3. Do you both enjoy the same friends?

4. Do you have similar tastes in books, movies, art, and the kind of home you want?

5. (For the prospective husband) Do you like to putter around the house, build and fix things, do gardening? (For the prospective wife) Do you like to cook, sew?

°6. Do you both have the same basic philosophy of life? Same religion or agree on attitudes toward religion?

°7. Do you like, or share his (her) attitude toward, his (her) parents? Is there agreement on ways to deal with them?

Some comments are necessary on the above questionnaire. Answering "yes" to all the questions would indicate a situation which we are not likely to find often. A carbon copy of yourself is neither expected nor desired. Disagreement on minor matters makes for stimulating conversation. Danger exists only if there are basic antagonisms. Certain questions are more important than others. There should be a positive "yes" on the questions which are starred. In regard to question 6, it is found that religious disagreements play a small part in disturbing a marriage. These differences tend to be worked out satisfactorily during the courtship. After marriage, the problem is usually centered on the religious upbringing of the child. Question 7 involves the in-laws, who have been the cause of many marital upsets. The courtship period is the ideal time to get to know them and make every attempt to like and be liked.

The courtship period usually goes through several stages:

*Dating.* This is the time when you play the field, meeting the opposite sex at dances, school, clubs, the Y's, and church gatherings. Dating, however, should be constructive. The normal person dates the opposite sex with the ultimate goal of marriage in mind. When something "clicks" between two people, then all other dating falls off.

*Keeping company.* While no serious commitments are made, dates are concentrated on one person.

*Going steady.* The attachment has become stronger.

*Private understanding.* An avowal of love has been exchanged. Each has, if possible, been introduced to the other's family.

*Engagement.* This is the final test before marriage. It is the time for practical talk, freely and honestly exchanged, for a decision on compatibility, for examination of personality defects. For the average couple, one year has been suggested as the minimum time for engagement. Of course, this is not an ironclad rule, since some people need more time than others to get acquainted or have had more time to get acquainted before becoming engaged. But a whirlwind courtship should be avoided. Most of them lead to divorce.

# LOVE VERSUS INFATUATION

Many people ask "Shall I marry for love?" or, "I am very fond of someone who would, I feel, make a good husband (or wife). But I am not in love. Shall I marry anyway?"

On the other hand, a strong sexual desire for another is often mistaken for love. Psychologists and marriage counselors call this "infatuation" if it is not accompanied by other feelings such as sympathy and tenderness. In adolescents this is called "puppy love" and is usually outgrown in time.

An adequate definition of love has troubled poets and philosophers from time immemorial. However, for the practical purposes of successful marriage ask yourself these questions:

1. Do you feel a sense of oneness, each with the other? That is, do you consider the other person a part of yourself?
2. Do you feel you can trust the other person? Does he or she give you a sense of security?
3. Are you concerned about his or her welfare and well-being? Do you try in all ways to make the other person happy?
4. Have you found that being apart from the person for a period of time, you still feel the same emotional attachment?
5. Do you find that the longer you know each other, the desire to stay together grows stronger and that you do not grow bored as time goes by?

If you have answered "yes" to these questions, you may safely say you are in love. If you look over these questions again, you will also notice that they describe true companionship. A physical attraction is not enough to guarantee a happy marriage. Sex is of basic importance in the relationship, but as one authority puts it, it is the sturdy *foundation* upon which the house must be built.

# MARRIAGE

What is the best age to marry? Generally speaking, it would be the age when one has reached physical and mental maturity. Naturally, this will vary with each person, but experts put it between the ages of twenty-two and thirty. This has been found to be the average age in most successful marriages, with the husband from four to seven years older than the wife. Here again, exceptions are found. In many a happy marriage the wife is from one to five years older. The point is that the couple should be emotionally stable and mentally mature enough to withstand the stresses and strains of marriage. Since there is a somewhat subtle change in the quality of the relationship after the days of courtship, the adjustments that may be required after marriage involve a deeper and more intelligent attitude.

Many people must postpone marriage for economic reasons. However, we can assume that, in most instances, a bachelor of over thirty-five has remained single from choice. This may indicate character traits which are not compatible with those of a good husband and father. (In many instances these can be changed, though not without trained assistance.) The "bachelor girl" or spinster may also be a bad marital risk, although we must realize that women often adopt this pose because they are unable to find husbands. I should like to caution people against rushing into marrying a "confirmed bachelor" of either sex!

I should also like to urge people to take into consideration the marital history of a prospective partner. Don't dismiss the fact that he or she has been divorced with "It wasn't his (or her) fault," but be certain you have a good reason for believing that history will not repeat itself. Men and women who have been married and divorced several times are not good marital risks.

Determination to make the marriage a success is one of the most important weapons against divorce. As one authority says, "Tolerance, understanding and good humor are more valuable assets in marriage than a starry-eyed idealization of the other partner."

Neither party should expect the other to give in on all points, to make all the sacrifices. It should be a mutual undertaking. Sacrifices will have to be made at one time or another, but they should be made without resentment, with the larger view in mind: the happiness of both.

One doctor wisely said of the happy marriage, "Surely this is success in life. It would be better to fail in all else and succeed at home than to succeed in all else and fail at home."

Love between a man and a woman can be the most beautiful and thrilling human experience.

If we were to define married love in its simplest terms, we would say it has three parts: (1) a sexual attraction, (2) a deep feeling of companionship, and (3) a desire for parenthood. The first two are essential, the third very valuable for emotional fulfillment and complete enduring happiness.

Most of us have experienced the joys (and, of course, the difficulties) of companionship. We have been close to our parents, our brothers and sisters, our friends. We have probably even felt some parental emotions for the baby in our own or another family. These experiences are vitally important in preparing us to make good homes of our own.

We have also had the opportunity to discover some of the things that go into making a good marriage. "I won't nag at my husband when I get married." "I think a man is entitled to good cooking and a nice house if he works hard all day." "I won't expect my wife to bring up the kids all by herself." "Husbands should want to be with their wives and not keep going out with the other fellows." Remarks such as these, which children frequently make in discussing marriage, show that they have been able to see for themselves some of the things that are necessary for a good married life. But the regular day-to-day life and the intimacy of a relationship between two people of the opposite sex has been a closed book. This is the new factor in marriage—the one for which people have unfortunately been least prepared by their other relationships and observations. As though that weren't enough, difficulties have been added in the form of ignorance and misconceptions, all of which flourish under the taboos of society.

How unfortunate it is that the act of sexual intercourse with its natural beautiful consequence, the birth of a baby, should be clouded by fear and darkened by shame! The poet Goethe said, "Whatever you cannot understand, you cannot possess." Possession, each of the other, is the essence of both sexual intercourse and marriage.

Education, training, and experience are necessary if the sexual relationship is truly to be the perfect physical expression of love.

# IS SEX EDUCATION NECESSARY?

Some of you may consider me out-of-date for feeling that sex education is necessary in this enlightened day and age. According to most parents, today's young people know as much as—if not more than—they should about sex. And I'm sure that many young people will smile in a superior manner at the very idea of being educated in such matters by any old fogey who writes books!

However, from the questions that are still asked us, we doctors know that a great deal of ignorance and misinformation remain, at least in certain areas of this subject. Both young and older couples frequently ask us whether their sexual relations are "all right." They would like to have the boundaries of normal sex relationships defined, and they are concerned with problems of frigidity and impotence.

Of course, a great deal of progress has been made. Wives of the Victorian era almost never consulted physicians when they were unhappy in their sexual relations. Most doctors of that day would have been deeply shocked if a woman asked them whether there was anything to be done because she failed to achieve an orgasm during sexual intercourse. Today, few physicians are so old-fashioned as not to want their patients to enjoy a full and happy marital relationship.

However, there are some people who feel that too much emphasis on sex education is a mistake. Take the case of a young married woman who said to my wife, "I'm sorry Bill and I ever read that book about sex in marriage! It just made him feel guilty because he can't live up to what it says a man should do to satisfy his wife; and *I* feel guilty because I'm upsetting him! I'd rather be ignorant than become self-conscious trying to follow a lot of blueprints!"

It is true that some books dealing with sex education have been written in a manner that tends to destroy the spontaneity of this delicate relationship. Because matters concerning sex techniques and skills were taboo for so long, some writers tend to go too far in the other direction, exaggerating their importance and minimizing the importance of the physical attraction existing between two people who love one another.

Yet attraction and intuition are not enough to enable people to solve the problems which may give rise to, or result from, an unsatisfactory sexual relationship.

Many a man has seen nothing wrong in using his wife for his own erotic gratification, without considering her needs, perhaps because of unawareness of their existence. Many wives have been brought up to think of sex in marriage as something they owe their husbands, a duty that they tolerate. Because their emotional life should have an outlet, they have become frustrated and perhaps turned to their children, whom they throttle with neurotic attention. Is it any wonder that the husband of such a wife strays into the arms of a responsive mistress?

These are extreme, though unfortunately not rare, situations. Many marital problems are due to less obvious sexual causes; these, too, can only be solved by a better understanding of sex.

## The Purposes of Sex

You notice I use the plural rather than the singular. Biologically speaking, reproduction is the purpose of sexual intercourse—the means by which life is created. There has been some tendency in recent years to pass over this aspect of the sexual act, perhaps because of the fact that it was, at one time, regarded as the only purpose of sexual intercourse. While a great deal has been written about men and women who want to have children because they think they should, or to prove they can, or for any one of a number of neurotic reasons, most people who feel that life is worth living want to pass on the precious gift of life, to create a new life with the beloved partner.

But sexual intercourse is also an expression of love in the most intimate manner. Giving and receiving the greatest pleasure (and experiencing the release which accompanies it) is a natural and healthy desire. A man and a woman are bound to one another most securely when they share this deepest of all attachments.

## Satisfactory Sexual Relations

Since sexual intercourse can lead to great happiness or great misery, it is important that it be understood by both husband and wife. In discussing this subject, I shall not attempt to deal with the moral aspects of some questions that arise, for in my opinion this would be going outside the province of the physician.

*Should a couple have sexual intercourse before marriage in order to find out whether they are compatible?* Whether or not to have premarital sex relations is a matter for each couple to decide. However, it seems naïve to me to believe that one can successfully "test" so subtle and delicate a matter. A satisfactory sexual adjustment is seldom achieved immediately, far more often developed gradually.

*Does the size of the respective organs of man and woman play an important part in the success of their relationship?* Again, no—at least, far less often than is generally imagined. A great many men have worried unduly because they feared they were too small, as have women because they thought they were too large to give pleasure or so small as to make intercourse painful. Except in very rare cases, the relative size of the sex organs is not a major problem, because of the possibility of employing techniques that will minimize any difficulties.

*Does having practiced masturbation affect the ability to have successful sexual relations?* The harmful effects of this practice are due to the fears and guilts associated with it. Physically, no damage is done by it. Almost everyone has practiced some form of masturbation; 92 percent of all men interviewed by Dr. Kinsey recalled having practiced masturbation at some time; 88 per cent of all (unmarried) men practiced it between the ages of 16 and 20, and some 50 per cent at the age of 50. The practice among females is scarcely less general.

*Does youthful "petting" interfere with satisfactory sex relations later on?* Most normal young people engage in some sort of lovemaking that does not terminate in intercourse. It is the usual way for them to discover, or demonstrate, their physical attraction for each other. Prolonged or habitual petting, which requires the exercise of

great self-restraint, may have a temporary bad effect. For example, a girl who is accustomed to being on guard against letting herself "go too far," may find it difficult, when she is first married, to relax and enjoy the sexual act.

*Is sexual experience with others in the past helpful (or harmful) to the establishment of successful sex relations with one's spouse?* It is certainly not necessary. Experience in the art of lovemaking should, ideally, be obtained with one's chosen mate. It is often distressing, especially to a man, if his loved one has been intimate with someone else. However, since our civilization often makes it impossible for people to marry and establish a home until long after they have reached maturity, premarital sex experiences do occur. I think it is important to realize that loving someone as he or she *is* requires an understanding of the fact that even past relationships have contributed to creating the person one loves. On the other hand, promiscuity —and also the coldness that comes from repressing sexual desire—are indications of a neurotic attitude toward sex. They may be only a phase of the difficult emotional period of adolescence, but they may be so permanent and deep-seated as to require the help of a trained person, as I explain on page 183.

*Does having a homosexual experience mean a person cannot have normal sex relations?* According to the Kinsey report, a great many men and an appreciable number of women have had some sort of homosexual experience which did not interfere with normal sexual relations later on. However, I feel that everyone who is concerned about such an experience should discuss it frankly with a doctor or a competent counselor, since homosexuality is a complicated problem (see pages 194 and 315).

*Is the wedding night a crucial one in the establishment of satisfactory sexual relations?* It can be. The bride may be tense and overwrought, especially if the wedding was a large one. She requires the utmost consideration from the groom, who is usually nervous himself. There have been cases in which the shock of wedding night experiences has created a lasting injury as far as a girl's attitude toward sex is concerned. However, I am inclined to believe that this danger is less great than it was in the past, when many brides had no idea of the nature of sexual intercourse. A groom sometimes finds it difficult to avoid causing his bride some physical pain, but his tenderness for her at this time is apt to be sufficient to compensate for it.

Some of the difficulties of the wedding night can be avoided if the bride has had a preliminary medical examination. In some but by no means all virgins, the hymen, the membrane at the opening of the vagina (see Fig. 14-1), does not rupture easily. This makes intercourse extremely painful or even impossible. In such cases it can be removed by a physician, a procedure so minor as hardly to be called an operation. The hymen can also be stretched, according to the doctor's directions, prior to the marriage.

Before the wedding night the marriage partners should discuss birth control with each other (see page 223 on contraception). Also, your doctor or marriage counselor will answer questions about contraceptive methods.

*If the husband is considerate and gentle, will the bride enjoy sexual intercourse?* Some young women derive no more pleasure from it than they would from any intimate caress. This may be due to the fact that sexual desire sometimes develops slowly in women. They may not reach sexual maturity until they have been married for quite a while. This awakening may be gradual or it may take place suddenly.

Generally speaking, women are less quickly and spontaneously aroused than are men. Both partners should realize this fact. A woman should not feel that her husband is "crude" or "oversexed" if he desires intercourse with her because he has seen her partially undressed or because she has given him an affectionate kiss. A man should not consider himself rejected or decide that his wife is cold if she fails to be aroused so readily.

Many women need a "warming-up" period before they feel a desire to have intercourse—in many cases, before they are physically ready for it. When a woman is sufficiently aroused, her vagina is well lubricated and naturally receptive to the insertion of the penis. Many women respond best to lovemaking that begins with verbal expressions of affection, kisses, and gentle caresses, and proceeds to stimulation of the breasts, the nipples, the clitoris (the small projection outside the vagina, which is composed of erectile tissue similar to that of the penis), and the vagina itself. Each husband

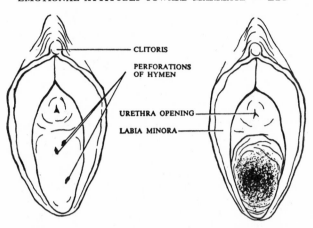

*Figure 14-1. The Hymen.* LEFT: *A characteristic hymen, with small perforations.* RIGHT: *Complete absence of hymen.*

should learn to know the degree to which his wife is excited by caresses of different parts of the body.

*Will a wife always achieve sexual satisfaction if her husband is sufficiently skillful?* Some women do not, even under the most favorable circumstances, experience an orgasm (the climax of the sexual act). Some experience an orgasm only after they have been married for some time. Some women experience this climax only occasionally, perhaps only at certain periods of the month, as their desire may be of a cyclical nature, reaching its peak before, during, or after the menstrual period. Although in men the orgasm is clearly defined, it may be vague or "diffuse" in a woman. Its degree of intensity varies. It may be centered in the clitoris, it may appear to involve the internal portion of the vagina, or a woman may experience both types of orgasm. While some psychiatrists believe that a "clitoral orgasm" indicates immaturity, there seems to be little scientific evidence for making a distinction between it and a "vaginal orgasm" in most women.

Often, failure to achieve an orgasm does not prevent a woman from having great pleasure in the sexual act; *it does not necessarily cause her to become tense and to feel frustrated*—this, too, varies in individual women. While it is extremely important for a man to help his wife experience the complete sexual satisfaction he enjoys, I know of instances in which couples have become disturbed and tense because of this failure—which often has the effect of postponing satisfaction or creating psychological barriers to it.

Men often reach the climax of their sexual excitement more rapidly than women do. This discrepancy in "timing" can usually be compensated for by making certain that the woman is highly stimulated *before* intercourse actually begins. While many couples find it particularly satisfying to reach this moment simultaneously, others see no objection to having the woman have her climax first. As a general rule, a woman's desire fades rather slowly after she has had an orgasm, whereas that of a man is apt to vanish immediately. It is not unusual, especially if a man is young or greatly excited, for him occasionally to have an orgasm immediately upon beginning the sexual act (this is called *premature ejaculation*). However, if it occurs habitually, he should consult a doctor. Failure to have an orgasm during coitus is rare in men (except when they are under the influence of alcohol) and should be discussed with a doctor or other trained adviser.

*What causes frigidity in women?* As I have indicated, failure to have an orgasm does not necessarily mean a woman is frigid. Doctors speak of true frigidity in women as the inability to derive pleasure from sexual relations. This may be caused by insufficient lubrication or lack of adequate stimulation. More likely, frigidity is the result of psychological factors. Failure to enjoy intercourse, or distaste, dislike, and actual abhorrence of it,

can be due to conscious or unconscious feelings of guilt, inferiority, or fears—such as the fear of pregnancy, of growing up, of surrendering to a man. In such cases help is usually required to discover and remove the underlying cause.

*What is impotence in men, and what causes it?* By impotence doctors mean the inability of a man to have an erection. (It does not mean *sterility*, which is the inability to have children: see page 232). Impotence can be, but rarely is, due to physical causes. Even when an adult male is castrated (has his testicles removed) he is usually not impotent. Impotence may be due to such psychological difficulties as hostility to women, guilt, and fears—for example, the fear of catching a venereal disease or of being sexually inferior. Some men are able to have intercourse only with women whom they do not respect and are impotent with a woman they admire or love. This is usually due to their often subconscious division of women into two groups: madonnas (good mothers), with whom sexual intercourse is forbidden, and harlots, with whom it is permissible. This stems from the idea that sex is wicked or from an overveneration of the mother. In most cases, psychiatric help is required to solve the problems causing impotence.

But many cases of impotence start from a commonplace cause. It is natural for every man to have an occasional episode of impotence, usually as the result of fatigue, preoccupation, or alcohol. Some men, especially those over forty,

*Figure 14-2. Exterior Female Genitals.*

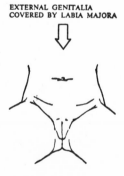

EXTERNAL GENITALIA
COVERED BY LABIA MAJORA

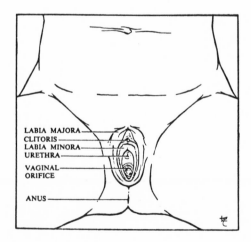

LABIA MAJORA
CLITORIS
LABIA MINORA
URETHRA

VAGINAL
ORIFICE

ANUS

worry unduly about such an episode and develop a "fear of failure" cycle. It is the fear, not the aging, that leads to their chronic impotence.

*How often should one have intercourse?* This is a question I can answer in only the most general terms. Statistics that have been compiled by Dr. Kinsey and others indicate that the average is about twice a week, more often in young or newly wedded couples, less often in older ones. But so many factors—such as opportunity, physical fatigue, compatibility, and temperament—enter into these figures that they mean little to any individual. The best "yardstick" I can suggest is: if both partners feel well, if coitus does not cause discomfort or fatigue, and is followed by physical and emotional relaxation, there is no need to worry about overdoing things. Repeated failure to be satisfied after experiencing an orgasm is an indication of some problem which should be discussed with a physician or trained counselor.

The desire to have intercourse usually declines in people as they reach middle age. Yet some women reach the height of sexual vigor quite late in life, even after they have passed the menopause; and some men retain virility into their old age.

Whether or not to have intercourse while the woman is menstruating is a matter for each couple to decide. It may cause the wife some discomfort, especially if she has "cramps" during her period, but it will do no physical damage to either the man or the woman. I discuss the question of intercourse during pregnancy on page 243.

Having intercourse does not "use up" one's potency, and abstaining from it does not increase virility. However, having sexual relations several times a day regularly may decrease the amount of sperm a man produces, thus lessening the chances of having a child. Too much sexual activity does not cause insanity. Too little does not cause it, either, although distressing emotional tension may result from frustration. Lack of interest in sex or excessive interest in it—both of which I mention on page 217—are indications of difficulties that require expert help. Occasionally these difficulties are of a physical nature, but the overwhelming majority of them spring from psychological problems.

In this connection, I want to warn you: *never*

take any medicine, pill, or injection in order to increase or decrease sexual desire, unless a competent physician has discovered a physical condition that requires it. "Potency pills" that contain hormones can be extremely dangerous (see page 83). *Aphrodisiacs* such as *cantharides* ("Spanish fly") are actually poisonous irritants. Alcohol does not increase desire, although it may appear to do so because it releases inhibitions. Occasionally, a tense or shy person finds it easier to relax after having a glass or two of wine or some other alcoholic beverage. But anyone who remains *dependent* on an artificial aid will probably find some form of psychotherapy (see page 183) a far wiser way of getting rid of repressions.

Too much alcohol eventually decreases sexual potency as it does health in general, so drinking too much is obviously an unwise way of attempting to modify sexual desire. Do not use drugs, injections, or remedies of any kind, and don't give them to your children—not even saltpeter (nitre) which used to be dealt out lavishly in boys' schools and other institutions.

A well-balanced diet, enough rest, and general care of the body, which I discuss in Chapters 1 and 2, are essential to your health, of which your sexual health is an important part. Incidentally, there are no special foods that can increase or decrease potency. When abstinence is necessary, keeping busy and avoiding erotic stimulation as much as possible may relieve sexual tensions.

*Is intercourse ever harmful or dangerous?* It is, of course, dangerous when either partner is suffering from a venereal disease (see pages 447 and 485). Intercourse, and all other forms of close contact, should be avoided in cases of contagious illness. Certain noncontagious diseases make intercourse inadvisable or even dangerous. This depends on their severity and the general health of the individual. It is impossible to give a yes or no answer except on the basis of a medical examination. Anyone who is not in good health should discuss this matter frankly with his or her physician, who will be able to decide whether or not coitus is permissible.

However, I want to make the point that it is often possible to relieve strain or prevent overexertion on the part of either the man or the woman, or both, by assuming certain positions during intercourse. I know of more than one couple that have refrained from having sexual relations because, for example, a fragile wife could not endure the weight of her robust husband, or a man found the exercise too much for his weakened heart. They thought it was not "nice" or "normal" to assume another position which would alleviate their difficulties.

The majority of people in our culture assume a certain position during coitus; but this, again, is only a matter of custom. There is no reason to believe that any position is the "right" one if another method is desirable because of health, relative size, or individual preference.

## Positions During Intercourse

There are two main possible positions in coitus. The first is the face-to-face posture; the second is that in which the man faces forward but the woman turns her back. Everything else is a variation of these basic positions. The purposes of the different positions are to increase sexual pleasure and to prevent hygienic dangers or injuries.

Also, a person who has a disabling illness such as certain forms of heart disease may want to use the positions that require the least amount of physical exertion, e.g., the side positions.

MAN ABOVE WOMAN. In our Western culture this combination is considered the normal or standard position. The woman lies on her back and spreads her thighs until there is room between her legs for the man's thighs. By bending her legs, she allows for deeper penetration. The man lies upon his partner's abdomen, supporting his knees and elbows as far as possible on the bed so that he will not be too heavy a burden. If the woman holds her thighs together after entry, it will be helpful in cases where the penis is too small or the vagina too large. It will also increase friction against the clitoris. By holding the thighs tightly together, the woman can prevent the penis from entering too deeply, if this is needed to prevent pain.

If the vagina is large or has been stretched, the following technique may be very helpful: The woman lifts her thighs high enough to encircle the man's neck with her legs or to rest her feet on his shoulders. Thus her body is almost at right angles,

with her shoulders flat and her torso lifted as vertically as possible.

WOMAN OVER MAN. The woman can assume a kneeling position over the man and let herself down gradually until the penis is inserted. The advantage of this position is that the woman has full control of the movements, quickening or slowing down as she pleases. It also enables her to adjust herself to the penis by bending forward so that full contact with the clitoris is made. Properly carried out, this position can lead to sexual delight. It is advantageous if the man is tired. Its disadvantages are: it requires a good deal of exertion on the part of the female while the male is passive; it is not recommended if her vaginal passage is unusually short; and it is also not recommended for the sick or convalescent male because it is apt to be more stimulating than the position described in the next paragraph.

LYING ON SIDE, FACE TO FACE. The man and woman lie on their sides, facing each other. The woman raises her upper thigh, resting it on the man's upper thigh. This is excellent for those who wish to perform coitus during pregnancy, as there is little pressure on the woman's abdomen. For couples who wish to relax, this side attitude will be appealing and restful.

REAR ENTRY. This method is also recommended especially for pregnant women or in any other case where deep penetration and weight on the abdomen are not safe. The woman is placed with her back to the man, usually in a kneeling stance. The man enters the vagina from behind. This position does not give the woman as much pleasure as some other ones, as the clitoris is not touched by the penis during the union. The man can correct this by fondling the clitoris (and also the breasts) with his hands.

## What Are Abnormal Sex Practices Between a Man and a Woman?

Broadly speaking, a couple is sexually normal if each derives the highest sexual pleasure and satisfaction from the insertion of the male genital organ into that of the female. This does not preclude experimenting in obtaining satisfaction by other means. For example, there is certainly nothing abnormal in the case of a man who has reached his climax rapidly and, if his wife has not reached hers, makes it possible for her to do so by manual manipulation. There is nothing abnormal about any caress, in the foreplay preceding coitus, that both partners find pleasurable.

In adults the oral zone (the mouth, lips, and tongue) is, to a greater or lesser extent, a sexual one. Some couples find the genital kiss important for the fullest realization of sexual satisfaction. Without attempting to draw an exact line defining the normal limits of this practice, psychiatrists tend to agree that maladjustment is indicated only when actions involving the mouth, rather than the genitals, are the main or only source of sexual pleasure and climax.

I describe true sexual perversions (deviations) on page 193. In discussing them, I make the point that mature people usually carry with them some holdovers from childhood. These can cause problems in marriage if they happen seriously to conflict with those of a partner—if, for example, the man derives great pleasure from seeing his wife's body, and the woman feels distaste for exposing it. Such difficulties can usually be resolved *provided* both partners approach matters concerning sex in an open-minded, intelligent way, and not with shocked or self-righteous indignation or guilty shame.

However, in some cases it may be impossible to reconcile the immaturity or maladjustment without trained assistance. Here are some examples. The medical words I use are defined on pages 194-195. Of course, I am not referring to people who have a *trace* of the following characteristics but to *extreme* cases.

NARCISSISM. These women (or, a little less often, men) can love only themselves. If their partners love them—well, they have that much in common, namely, devotion to the same person! But the partner usually wants (and quite rightly) more than that. A successful marriage, including successful sex relations, is usually impossible as long as the partner remains extremely narcissistic.

SADISM AND MASOCHISM. We've all seen marriages in which the husband or wife seems to enjoy being dominated, even badly treated, by his or her partner, while the partner enjoys treating his or her spouse badly. However, things seldom work out so neatly, and even if they do, they don't spell "happiness."

EXCESSIVE SEXUALITY (Nymphomania and Satyrism). I am not referring to instances in which one partner is more highly sexed than the other, since the consideration springing from love will find ways to bridge differences ordinarily. But *compulsive* sexuality, which cannot be satisfied, has deep roots which cannot be reached by love. Fortunately this condition is very rare.

PROMISCUITY. The truly promiscuous person has intercourse as readily with one individual as with another, attaching no wish for intimacy, in the real meaning of the word, to the sexual act. It is by no means the same thing as *infidelity*, although the two may overlap. The former is more serious, the latter more common and causes many unhappy marriages. I say "causes" although both infidelity and promiscuity are actually *signs* that there is something wrong, usually in the individuals but perhaps in the marriage. I wish every husband and wife who is faced with the problem of infidelity would *not* blame the "other man" or the "other woman," but would honestly face the question, "What is wrong with yourself, your husband (or your wife), or your marriage?"

REPRESSION. We call people sexually repressed when they have pushed their normal sex instinct so far under the surface of their consciousness that they feel indifference, distaste, or even abhorrence for sex. Of course, there are degrees of repression and, in mild cases, it may melt away in the warmth of love. But in extreme cases, happiness in marriage is impossible.

THE UNRESOLVED "OEDIPUS COMPLEX." A man who is seeking only his mother when he chooses a wife, or a woman who only wants her husband to take the place of her father, will not find what either is looking for. Sometimes a degree of marital happiness is possible for the "little girl" wife who needs to be fathered or the "overgrown boy" husband who needs mothering. But marriage will not bring true happiness, because such people cannot be good husbands or wives, and certainly not good parents.

## HOW TO GET HELP IN SOLVING MARITAL PROBLEMS

As I have indicated earlier in this chapter, some sex problems are due to ignorance or misinformation. These often clear up readily in the light of truth. Others, such as those I have mentioned in the above section and at other places in this chapter, are more complicated. If you need any information I have not given (and, of course, it would be impossible to answer in a single book every question that might be asked) or if you are worried about yourself, your spouse, or your marriage, be sure to talk things over with a trained person. I suggest you talk to your doctor first, if that is possible. If not, consult a marriage counselor who will probably be able to help you or will advise you to see a doctor or psychiatrist.

Marriage counselors are relatively new (see page 188). They concern themselves with every aspect—not only those related to sex—of marital and premarital problems. Marriage Council Institutes call upon the services of physicians, psychiatrists, sociologists, anthropologists, and clergymen. Every large city has a Family Service Association, supported by the Community Chest, which is interested in marriage counseling. If one is not available in your community, write the nearest large city for suggestions. Your doctor, clergyman, the YMCA, YWCA, or a local health officer can usually help you find a marriage counselor. The American Association of Marriage Counselors, Inc., 41 Central Park West, New York, N.Y. 10023, will provide the names of trained, accredited marriage counselors in or near your community.

Expert sex therapy is increasingly available and effective. Designed basically for couples whose sexual life is marred yet who still have a reasonably intact relationship, sex therapy makes use of psychotherapeutic, behavioral, and physiological methods. It seeks to demystify sex, encourage couples to see their sexual problems as something outside themselves that they can attack jointly. It includes various exercises for enhancing arousal and diminishing undesired behavior. Among the problems for which it is used are premature ejaculation, impotence, inability to achieve orgasm, and involuntary spasm of the vaginal muscles, making penetration difficult or impossible.

More and more sex therapy clinics are being established. Many are associated with hospitals. In the clinics, specially trained psychologists, psychiatrists, and other physicians provide effective, expert help. But not all sex counseling being offered today is expert. Your physician will usually be able to recommend a worthwhile clinic that may be nearby or not too difficult to get to.

If yours is a sex problem, don't be ashamed to ask for help. It isn't easy to solve all the problems involved in expressing one's sexual drive in such a way as to bring about lasting happiness in marriage. You may find that you have been worrying unduly and your difficulty can be solved with relative ease before it develops into anything serious. But even if it cannot be solved easily, it is worth solving. A satisfying sexual relationship is part of every truly happy marriage. It can be achieved by any physically and emotionally healthy man and wife who care for one another.

# 15
# HEALTH PREPARATIONS FOR MARRIAGE

---

Let us assume you have made your choice; you have found *the* person with whom you wish to spend your life. When two people marry, they promise to live together in sickness and in health. To help them start off in good health, to reassure them that their marriage will be built on a solid foundation, the young people owe it to themselves, and to their children to come, to see their doctor. Not only will he perform a physical examination, but he will try to answer the couple's questions, about themselves and about the family they are planning.

To ensure that a man and woman are not endangering one another, and possibly the next generation, many states require a blood test, such as the *Wassermann test,* before issuing a marriage license. This should be mandatory in order to detect syphilis which can be cured—and must be —before anyone has a right to marry. I wish the laws would also require an examination for the other common venereal disease, gonorrhea, which is also curable. In addition I believe that everyone should have an x-ray test made of the lungs to detect tuberculosis, before getting married. Tuberculosis is not, of course, a venereal disease, but it and syphilis are two major communicable illnesses; tuberculosis can be checked and usually cured by prompt medical attention.

Whether your state requires only the Wassermann test, or whether additional physical examinations are necessary, you and your partner should ask a physician to test your blood for compatibility. It is important to know whether the prospective mother and father have different Rh factors, because this difference could create a health problem for children. (The Rh factor and its importance in parenthood are explained on page 241.)

## THE BLOOD TEST FOR SYPHILIS

Thanks to the excellent educational campaigns of recent years, the public is at last beginning to adopt an enlightened attitude toward venereal disease. People accept blood tests for syphilis as a matter of routine. Today nobody, however saintly, would think of saying, "You needn't test my blood for syphilis," when giving a blood donation or being inducted into the armed forces.

It is extremely unusual to acquire syphilis except as a result of intercourse with an infected person. But it is *possible.* And this disease can have the most serious consequences, including disablement or death. Still worse, even unsuspected syphilis in a woman can cause her to give birth to children who are blind, crippled, or deformed. Therefore there is no excuse for refusing or neglecting to have a routine blood test to detect syphilis, which *is a curable disease.*

The power of medicine to cure syphilis is no reason to ignore this terrible disease or to minimize its importance. I suspect that the public tendency to take the curing power of penicillin and other medicines for granted is one reason that, all over the world, the incidence of syphilis began to rise sharply in the early 1960's. It is certainly not "as easy to cure as a cold." (This serious disease is discussed in detail on pages 447-49.)

## THE EXAMINATION FOR GONORRHEA

Unlike syphilis, gonorrhea cannot be discovered by a routine blood test. It starts as a local infection of the genital organs, and its detection requires inspection of these areas and perhaps a microscopic examination of their secretions. If untreated, it may spread and affect other parts of the body. Though not transmitted to unborn offspring, it may infect a baby's eyes during or after birth, and can be a cause of blindness. *Gonorrhea, too, is entirely curable.* (See page 485 for a discussion of gonorrhea.)

## THE X-RAY FOR TUBERCULOSIS

Tuberculosis may go undetected for a long period of time while insidiously injuring the body and being contracted by others, especially those who have close contact with a tubercular person. Children are especially vulnerable to this disease. There are numerous instances of adults who, not realizing they had tuberculosis, outlived the children they unknowingly infected. It is possible to harbor and spread tubercle bacilli without having any symptoms such as a cough, chest pain, loss of weight, or noticeable amount of sputum.

A chest x-ray often detects hidden tuberculosis. It reveals any suspicious areas which will make further tests necessary. Largely because of the public's growing enlightenment regarding the need to have chest x-rays made at regular intervals, countless cases of tuberculosis have been discovered in time to arrest this disease which was formerly so deadly.

I discuss tuberculosis fully on page 441. If you don't take the time to read about it now, *don't neglect* to have yourself checked for this and other diseases before you get married. It's the least you can do for yourself, your loved one, and your children.

## OTHER HEALTH PRECAUTIONS

In addition to the examinations for syphilis, gonorrhea, and tuberculosis, you should have a thorough medical checkup to determine whether you are suffering from any ailment that should be corrected before the wedding.

Getting married is like starting on a journey that should last the rest of your life. Isn't it sensible to have a thorough medical checkup before you embark? It will enable you to discover whether you're coming down with something that may spoil what should be the happiest time of your life, or whether you should change some of your plans for the sake of your health. Certain heart conditions, for example, make it foolhardy for a man to stay on some jobs, although he could safely do another kind of work. Some illnesses make it extremely dangerous for a woman to have a baby, although she could do so with safety after the disease has been brought under control. Isn't it wise to find out before you're married?

A checkup also provides an opportunity for the prospective bride to discover whether she happens to need a very minor "operation" in order to prevent difficulty and pain in having sexual intercourse (see page 213). She and the prospective groom should ask any questions and discuss any sex problems with the doctor at this time. He, rather than a friend or relative, is best able to provide accurate information.

It is a good idea, especially if you and your fiancé are related, to give your physician all the information you possess concerning the physical and mental ailments from which members of your family have suffered. He will probably be able to set your mind at rest regarding the chances of having children who might inherit a physical or mental defect.

Your doctor may feel you should consult an expert in this field. Many questions naturally cannot be answered simply by correspondence with an expert. However, a visit is well worth your while if you are worried about getting married because of fear that you may pass on some hereditary disease to your children. If there should be a real danger of their inheriting a serious condition, it is much wiser for you to know in advance, so that you can agree to adopt children or, if the risk is slight, accept it (as I suggest on page 543 in discussing calculated risk in health) in the same way you accept other risks in life, including the risk of being run over every time you cross the street.

You notice I said you should tell your physician about the mental as well as the physical illness in your family. I'm sure you realize that mental health is as important as physical. Why not discuss that, and ask your fiancé to do so, with your doctor?

You may tell me, "My goodness, I couldn't possibly ask John (or Mary) to bring me a note from the doctor saying 'This certifies that the bearer is not crazy!'"

You're quite right. Yet I do want to tell you that I have known many a married man and woman who have said after a "breakdown" has brought suffering to the family: "If only I'd known that something should have been done about Max's drinking or Maxine's spells of depression. I thought we'd be so happy together that everything would work out all right." How much wiser it would have been to get help while Max or Maxine was still young and their problems comparatively easy to solve, and before they had families and children who were bound to suffer!

Naturally no doctor can give anyone a slip of paper guaranteeing freedom from all problems of an emotional or "nervous" nature. But it is possible to discover and eliminate the seeds of many problems that may cause trouble in the future.

I urge every couple contemplating marriage to read and discuss Part Two of this book, or at least Chapter 11, which deals with the normal mind. I also hope all young couples will talk freely and frankly to a doctor, a psychologist, or a marriage counselor. Certain tests can be made to determine mental and emotional health.

The Army tests everyone to discover whether he or she is a good physical and mental risk before acceptance. Surely getting married is as important as joining the armed forces!

What better dowry can you bring to, or receive from, the person you marry than the guarantee of good *physical* and *mental health?*

## 16
# THE STRATEGY OF BECOMING GOOD PARENTS

Most married couples want and expect to have children. It is part of marriage. They may know exactly how many they would like to have, and at what intervals they want to have them. Frequently, they are not so sure, and ask me what I consider best, and how to arrange things to suit their wishes.

Let us assume you have asked my advice. If I know you are physically and emotionally ready for parenthood, here is what I would advise.

I would recommend that you first get completely adjusted to each other and to being married before you have your first child. I would probably suggest that you wait a few months or a year before embarking on the venture of bringing a child into the world. It might be longer. This would depend on you—how long you've known each other, how many rough edges there are to be rubbed off, and how old you are. That's not because a woman has to be young in order to have her first child in perfect safety, but because I'd like you both to be young enough to enjoy your *grandchildren*, too. How long to wait would also depend on the length of time required to get your home settled and to be financially prepared for the baby. At the same time, I would like you to remember that people generally tend to become less fertile as they grow older. If they wait too long, they may find it difficult to have children when they want them, or to have as many as they want.

I would not select any special season of the year for your baby to be born, provided you live in a moderate climate or have modern conveniences. If the climate is severe, it would be better to have mild weather during the baby's first few months in order to give him a good start and simplify things for his mother.

I say "him," but I would not care whether your first child was a girl or a boy. I disagree with people who feel it's best to have a girl first because "girls are easier to handle." My mature, adult couple is going to be able to bring up either a boy or a girl with equal ease!

When your first child is two or three years old, I would like you to have another baby. There is no magic interval at which to space your children. However, a child is usually in a comparatively "settled" stage of development at about three years of age (see page 276), and this is a good time to add a little brother or sister. How you space your children depends a good deal on your income. If you can afford help with the household, the mother (and, indirectly, the father) will be able to enjoy a second child comparatively early. In other words, I wouldn't want you to have a second child, any more than I would want you to have the first, before you were physically, emotionally, and economically ready for it. Being an only child for a while will not hurt your firstborn. Having parents who are tired and worried and harassed might.

How many children should you have? I think the answer to that question is: as many as you want and can afford—and again, I mean physically and emotionally, as well as financially. Large families are nice, but so are small ones, and if I *had* to choose, I would put quality before quantity. My only suggestion regarding the "ideal" number of children is this: keep an open mind about it, for your ideas may change. We, ourselves, change with each child we have, because it is a unique experience, and we change with experience. This is to be expected, and natural.

"Speaking of nature," you may say, "why not let nature decide how many children we should have, and at what intervals?"

Being a doctor, I appreciate nature's wonders. But I also devote a great deal of time and energy trying to control some of the things that nature does. Nature works in a large-scale, lavish manner, without concern for the individual. Nature made microbes, some of which are very useful: for example, we would have no cheese without them. But nature also made some microbes that kill people in the prime of life, and we doctors are constantly working to control these microbes. Similarly, nature has made man and woman, most wonderfully, to bear children, many children, so that some will survive the hazards nature puts in their way. Since we have eliminated a number of these hazards, many of us feel it is not necessary to have so many children.

In ancient days, unwanted babies were left on mountain tops or in the open fields to perish. Civilization has wisely put a stop to that. But civilization will have to go even further, and not permit unwanted children to be cast out, figuratively speaking, so that they perish emotionally and spiritually.

The major religions in this country have recognized the wisdom of controlling nature's lavish manner of providing children. Some form of birth control, they agree, may be desirable or even necessary. I would like to describe the various methods without, of course, attempting to make any decisions of an ethical or moral nature.

## METHODS OF BIRTH CONTROL

In addition to total abstinence, conception can be controlled by mechanical or chemical means and by the rhythm method, and it can be prevented by surgical sterilization of either the man or the woman.

THE ORAL CONTRACEPTIVE PILL. Since its introduction in 1960, the oral contraceptive pill, commonly called "the pill," has become the most commonly used form of birth control among American women. Studies have shown its effectiveness to be as high as 99.5 percent.

Various types of oral contraceptives are available. Most work on the same principle. They contain chemicals similar to natural female hormones that control ovulation, or egg release; and by preventing ovulation, they produce infertility as long as they are used on a regular schedule.

The most common type, marketed under many brand names, is the combination pill. Along with estrogen to prevent ovulation, it contains another female hormone, progestogen, to thicken the mucus at the mouth of the uterus and make the uterine lining incapable of sustaining a fertilized egg. This type is taken for 21 days; for another 7 days, no pills, or pills without hormones, are used; and the cycle begins again in the fifth week.

Another type, the sequential, is no longer available because of risk to health. It delivered estrogen alone for the greater part of the cycle and progestogen alone for the remainder. Its higher estrogen content made it less safe.

Also available is the mini-pill. It contains no estrogen, only minute amounts of a synthetic progestogen. It does not usually interfere with ovulation but seems to work by thickening the cervical mucus so it becomes a barrier to sperm. It must be used daily; omission of even a single pill could lead to pregnancy. Its efficacy rate of about 97 percent is not quite as good as the combination pill's but still high enough to be an alternative for women unable to tolerate estrogen. In some women, the mini-pill produces nuisance side effects such as nausea, weight gain, headaches, or irregular bleeding which often disappear after a time.

Oral contraceptives have their advantages, including convenience as well as high efficacy. But they have drawbacks, too, for some women. Despite the most careful testing of any new drug or other measure before its release for general use, it is virtually impossible to know what undesirable effects may arise with use over long periods by millions of people. And with such use of the pill—among eight to ten million American women and fifty million or more worldwide—reports have appeared in recent years suggesting possible relationships between pill use and increased risk of various disease states.

Only very recently, an important large-scale, long-term study has been made. It compares the health consequences and benefits of use of oral contraceptives and also of two other commonly used contraceptive methods, the IUD (intra-uterine device) and the diaphragm. I present the results of that study for your guidance. Undoubtedly, your physician will be aware of them and will be abreast, too, of any subsequent information as it may be reported in the medical literature.

I should like to emphasize here that for many women the advantages of the pill far outweigh any risks—and, indeed, for many, the risks may be very, very low. That may be true for you in particular. Your doctor, after examining you and considering your medical history, can determine whether it is advisable for you to use the pill or another method of contraception, and if the pill, which one. He undoubtedly will suggest, too, that if you use the pill, a medical examination at least once a year is advisable, and he will provide you with a list of symptoms that could possibly develop and let you know which of these indicate that you should stop use. It's important to pay close attention to his instructions.

INTRAUTERINE DEVICES (IUD's). Intrauterine devices have been gaining in acceptance. Several types are available. They are small metal or plastic devices which must be inserted into the uterus by a physician or other professional. Most have an appendage, or tail, to permit the wearer and the physician to check the IUD's position and make its removal easier.

IUD's are highly effective in preventing pregnancy but a little less so than the two-hormone pill, with a failure rate running in the range of 1 to 5 conceptions per 100 women a year.

Among possible hazards are pelvic infections and perforation of the uterus. Both problems rarely occur if the device is inserted properly and the woman has had a thorough medical examination beforehand.

Spontaneous expulsion of the IUD or excessive bleeding and cramping are more common consequences. Both these difficulties can often be alleviated by substituting an intrauterine device of a different size or shape.

THE DIAPHRAGM. Before the pill became available, the diaphragm was the number-one birth control method. When properly used, it can be about 97 percent reliable. It is finding increasing use again today.

The diaphragm is a flexible, dome-shaped rubber hemisphere that comes in different sizes and must be fitted by a physician. It covers the cervix and helps to prevent sperm from entering the uterus. But in itself a diaphragm is not enough. A contraceptive jelly or cream should be used with it. Only a small amount of jelly or cream is needed, but it must cover the entire inner and outer surfaces and the rim of the diaphragm. The jelly or cream acts to kill sperm.

If the diaphragm is fitted carefully by a physician and directions for its use are followed exactly, and if it is regularly inspected for possible holes or tears by holding it up to the light and stretching it gently, it should prove reliable, safe, and comfortable to wear. I have found that there is a risk of impregnation while a woman is first learning to use the diaphragm method. During this period, I recommend that the husband use the condom, perhaps for several weeks, until his wife feels completely sure about the diaphragm method.

A LONG-TERM STUDY OF PILL, IUD, AND DIAPHRAGM. The study, an ongoing one, was begun in 1968 by a medical team headed by Dr. Martin Vessey of Oxford University in England. It includes 17,032 white married women who were attending 17 clinics of the British Family Planning Association.

At the time they joined the study the women were between the ages of 25 and 39. Some 57 percent were using the pill at entry, 25 percent were using the diaphragm, and 19 percent were using the IUD. A detailed record of each woman's medical, obstetric, contraceptive, and other history was made, with special attention given to conditions known or suspected to be related to any method of contraception.

After seven years of the study, an interim report of the results to then was issued.

Of greatest concern to women using the pill and to their physicians is the possibility that the pill may be associated with development of cancer. The study has found no evidence of any cancer-causing effect, and the cancer rate among pill users appears to be somewhat lower than among the other two groups. The investigators note, however, that there may be a long delay between first exposure to any agent capable of causing cancer and the actual appearance of cancer, "so that the present lack of evidence, though reassuring, is not conclusive."

The study found an increased risk of stroke and of gallbladder disease associated with pill use. It also found that IUD users are more likely to develop iron-deficiency anemia and diseases of the reproductive tract, such as inflammation of the fallopian tubes (salpingitis) and pelvic inflammatory disease, than are users of the other two methods. It found no serious health hazards associated with diaphragm use.

The investigation also determined that pill users had considerably less benign breast disease than did women in either of the other contraceptive groups—and fewer menstrual disturbances as well. On the other hand, those on the pill had more migraine headaches, and irritation and ulceration of the cervix were diagnosed more often among them than among women using the other methods.

Women using the pill were less likely to develop some types of ovarian cysts than those using the other methods. Those who became pregnant while using an IUD were much more likely than the others to have a miscarriage or an ectopic pregnancy.

There were some other findings, but the evidence for them is still not sufficient to justify firm conclusions. The findings: that women using the diaphragm had markedly lower rates of abnormal cervical cell development, those on the pill had a lower rate of duodenal ulcers but had more hay fever and skin diseases.

Still another finding—on impairment of fertility for a time after discontinuation of oral contraceptives in order to become pregnant—needs further and more refined study.

What the present study indicates is that of 1,037 women not previously pregnant who stopped using the pill in order to become pregnant, about 16 percent had still not given birth 30 months after discontinuation of contraception. Of 681 women, also previously not pregnant, who stopped other methods, about 11 percent had not given birth at 30 months. Among women who had been pregnant before and who discontinued contraception to become pregnant again, return to fertility was also delayed, but by 30 months only

about 8 percent in all three groups had not yet succeeded in giving birth. Why the same oral contraceptive should appear to affect the fertility of the previously pregnant and previously nonpregnant differently is a puzzle that needs clarification.

The British investigators conclude that "the available evidence does not yet allow a final balance to be struck between the benefits and risks associated with the new methods of contraception that have become widely used during the last two decades." They note, however, that "there are no material risks associated with the use of the diaphragm apart from the risk of pregnancy and that there may be some unintended benefits."

THE PILL AND SMOKING. Another recent study has produced results which can be important to some women. It indicates that cigarette smoking combined with use of oral contraceptives can increase the chance of having a fatal heart attack.

The study was carried out by Dr. A. K. Jain, a research analyst at the Population Council, an international family planning research organization headquartered in New York City. In it, Dr. Jain analyzed death rates among women, especially among those aged 40 through 44.

The analysis revealed that the annual death rate for American and British women aged 40 through 44 who neither smoke nor use oral contraceptives is only 7.4 per 100,000. In contrast, for women who use the pill but do not smoke, the death rate is 10.7 per 100,000. For women who smoke but who do not use the pill, it is 15.9. And if women both smoke and use oral contraceptives, the death rate is 62 per 100,000—almost a ninefold increase over that for women who neither smoke nor use the pill.

Even for women in their thirties, Dr. Jain found that there is an increased heart attack fatality risk from smoking and using the pill. For women aged 35 through 39, the death rate for those both using the pill and smoking is 23 per 100,000, and for those aged 30 through 34 it is 16 per 100,000.

The new study presents women and their physicians some additional choices to make about the pill. Those who are smokers, especially if they are over 40, may want to use another method of contraception. But women who do not smoke may now feel less anxious about the pill.

Your physician will take into account the studies I have just mentioned and other studies as well which provide indications of which women may and may not do well on the pill. He may, for example, recommend that you not use the pill if you have high blood pressure, suffer from migraine, have had blood-clot troubles (thrombosis) or a stroke, certain kinds of cancer, or have a liver disorder or certain heart problems.

THE CONDOM. The condom, a thin flexible sheath, is worn by the man over the penis, in order to prevent sperm from entering the woman's vagina. There is little danger that it will break during intercourse because condoms have been greatly improved since the Federal Food and Drug Administration placed them under its control as medical materials. However, it is important to buy condoms at a good pharmacy and to select a recognized brand. To be absolutely certain, the condom should be tested before it is worn. The "cigarette test" can be made by inflating the condom like a balloon and then blowing cigarette smoke into it. If any trace of smoke is seen curling out, the condom should not be used, for sperm can pass through the most minute hole. The inflated condom can also be placed under water for testing. If there is a leak bubbles of air will arise.

The condom is highly recommended as a birth preventive, as well as a protection against disease. Some men dislike it because they feel it lessens the amount of sensation that can be experienced during intercourse. Most men find it satisfactory.

The condom should be in place before the male organ enters the vagina. It is risky to use the condom only just before the male orgasm because some sperm may leak out before ejaculation actually takes place. The condom should be applied in such a way that there is a loose space at the tip, in order to permit room for the ejaculated semen. Usually it is advisable to lubricate the condom with K-Y jelly, or some other bland lubricant, before intercourse is attempted, in order to facilitate entry.

Unless the condom is forbidden by religious precepts, I believe it should be used during intercourse with a virgin partner, who is not ready to employ the feminine techniques for birth control, if conception is to be prevented. Similarly, it should be used while the woman is learning how to use contraceptive techniques.

THE RHYTHM METHOD. This is a method of partial abstinence, based on the fact that women are unable to conceive during part of each month.

Approximately once a month, the human female *ovulates*. During ovulation, one egg cell is liberated from the ovary so that it may be fertilized by the sperm (see Figure 5-4, page 85). The egg cell leaves the ovary and travels down one of the fallopian tubes toward the womb. If a sperm unites with the egg, conception takes place. For about two weeks after ovulation, the lining of the womb is prepared, having built up the tissues with an enriched supply of blood, to nourish the future embryo. If conception does not take place, the

*Figure 16-1. Diaphragm.*

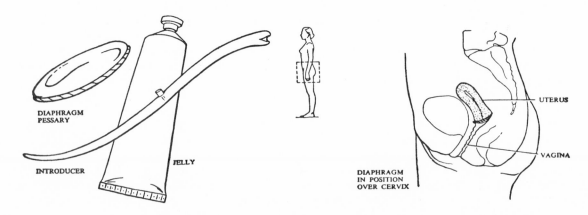

DIAPHRAGM PESSARY

INTRODUCER

JELLY

DIAPHRAGM IN POSITION OVER CERVIX

UTERUS

VAGINA

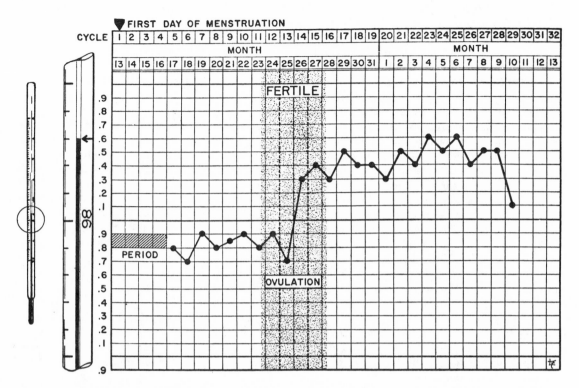

*Figure 16-2. The Rhythm Method. A sample chart, showing how to determine the period of fertility. Because the factors involved are apt to vary, this method is not reliable, and a doctor should be consulted before using it to avoid conception. The normal temperature range is shown on the thermometer.*

unused, built-up tissue breaks down into the bloody discharge known as menstruation. Menstruation occurs fourteen days after ovulation, on the average, although it varies in different women.

The "safe" period is, on the average, about twenty days long. It starts ten days before menstruation and lasts until approximately ten days after the onset of menstruation. Usually, pregnancy can result only when coitus is performed during the middle days of the menstrual cycle, the period four or five days before to four or five days after ovulation takes place.

As the "safe" period varies according to the menstrual cycle, each woman must determine it for herself. Some women are able to determine when ovulation occurs. At that time, midway between periods, they may experience an "intermenstrual" pain, a peculiar, sudden, spasmodic sensation opposite one of the ovaries, followed by a heavy feeling in the lower abdomen, which may last several hours. If they are alert to it, most women will observe an unusual mucous secretion at that time. These indications are helpful in determining the exact day of ovulation. Far more accurate, however, is the rise in temperature which occurs in women at this time, usually between 0.6 and 0.8 of a degree Fahrenheit. To determine the period of ovulation, you should keep a temperature chart for no less than three months. A five-minute temperature should be taken every morning after awakening, while you are still in bed.

The accompanying chart indicates the "safe" period for menstrual cycles of different lengths.

In even the most regular women, ovulation may be hastened or delayed if they are ill or emotionally upset. If this should happen, the calculations will be in error. Because of this possibility, the rhythm method cannot be considered as reliable a means of preventing conception as the condom or the pessary. Of course, it also has the disadvantage of limiting the days for having intercourse.

Its advantages lie in the fact that it does not depend on either the man or the woman alone. It is a partnership responsibility. Also, it is not dependent upon a mechanical or artificial device, but on regular periods of abstinence. This makes it morally and ethically acceptable, not only to Roman Catholics but to members of certain other religious denominations.

For absolute safety—when, for example, pregnancy would constitute a serious threat to health or life—I feel that all couples whose religious scruples permit *should use both the condom and the diaphragm-contraceptive-cream technique, and should not have intercourse on the days when conception might take place.*

OTHER METHODS OF BIRTH CONTROL. These consist of *douches, suppositories, jellies* and *creams,* and *coitus interruptus,* all of which are, to different degrees, unsatisfactory.

(*a*) *Douches.* Douches are used to wash out or kill the sperm before conception can take place. Since it is usually impossible to wash all the sperm from the vagina, the emphasis is placed on killing them by means of a chemical. In many instances, sperm have already entered the uterus before the woman has a chance to wash out the seminal fluid. By then it may be too late. Women may find it unpleasant to rise and douche after intercourse, when they want most to relax. As explained on page 214, sexual desire does not terminate abruptly in most women, and they want, and need, some relaxation and affection after coitus is completed.

I advise you not to use any of the advertised douches which contain chemicals such as creosol or hypochlorite. As I explain on page 106, I consider it best not to use anything except a little salt or vinegar in a douche except on a doctor's prescription. So-called feminine hygiene douches are not effective for contraception and are not necessary for cleanliness.

(*b*) *Suppositories.* These are small capsules that are made of cocoa butter or gelatin and con-

tain a chemical ingredient that destroys sperm. The suppository is inserted in the vagina a few minutes before intercourse and is melted by the body heat. The melted, greasy base coats the opening of the uterus and forms a blockade against the entrance of sperm, while the chemicals kill the sperm. Although the principle of the suppository is sound, it has not been found completely reliable in action. Sometimes it does not melt properly before ejaculation takes place or, when melted, does not completely cover the mouth of the womb.

(*c*) *Jellies and creams.* These work on the same principle as the suppositories, being inserted into the vagina with a special applicator. The cream or jelly is intended to block the opening into the uterus and at the same time to destroy the sperm. Since the jellies and creams are already in semi-fluid form, they have an advantage over the solid suppository in that they do not have to melt before the crucial moment. Still, they are not entirely reliable.

(*d*) *Coitus interruptus.* This consists of withdrawing the penis from the vagina just before the semen is ejaculated. It is one of the oldest methods of preventing conception and is mentioned in the Bible in the story of Onan who "spilled his seed upon the ground." It is still widely practiced.

I never recommend it because (1) even if it is successfully practiced, it is not an adequate safeguard against conception because sperm may leak out before the actual ejaculation takes place; (2) it is usually a cause of tension and strain, placing a heavy responsibility upon the husband, who finds it difficult to control his actions while he is highly excited. As a result, he may become irritable or emotionally disturbed, feeling guilty if he fails. The wife's concern lest he should fail to withdraw at the proper moment is a source of fear, tension, and emotional difficulties in her as well; and (3) at best, coitus interruptus does not permit the development of the full tenderness and love during the sexual act that comes when intercourse is completed while the sexual organs are united.

The birth control techniques, devices, and preparations described in this chapter are the most common, but others exist. Every family must decide for itself which, if any, to use. Young couples who have decided to limit and space their family should discuss the subject with their doctor or with a qualified person at a birth control clinic or family planning agency. Most large cities and many smaller ones have such services. Or you may write to the Planned Parenthood Federation of America, 810 Seventh Avenue, New York, N.Y. 10019, for information

## ABORTION

Except in circumstances making them essential to safety or health, abortions were illegal in the United States prior to 1973. Now, at any point within the first twelve weeks of pregnancy, a woman may, in consultation with her doctor, decide to end her pregnancy. During these twelve weeks—the first trimester of pregnancy—abortion is relatively safe and simple but thereafter becomes more complicated with risks increased.

Abortion has been performed by dilating the cervix and scraping out the contents of the uterus. More recently, a new technique is being used increasingly. It is called *vacuum aspiration* or *menstrual extraction*. The abortion is achieved by inserting a thin tube into the uterus and gently withdrawing the contents by use of a pump at the other end of the tube.

Some people feel that destroying a human life is never justified. Personally, I respect the religious, ethical, or moral convictions on which their opinions are based. However, as a doctor, I do not agree with them, and I am sure they will respect my viewpoint as I respect theirs. I feel that the life of a mother should not be sacrificed or endangered, with all that it means to her present and future children, for the sake of maintaining the life of an unborn infant, whose chances of survival are often very slim.

I fully realize the measure of responsibility this places upon the doctor. He must decide whether or not it is necessary to perform an abortion. In some cases this decision is not a difficult one—for example, in the case of a tubal, or ectopic, pregnancy. This is a rare condition in which the embryo develops outside the uterus, in the fallopian tube which leads into it (see illustration on page 126). Such embryos cannot survive; they die in one way or another, often by bursting through the tube in which they have been growing. At that point the danger to the mother's life is great. Therefore tubal pregnancy is considered a clear-cut indication for terminating a pregnancy by removing the embryo, instead of waiting for it to die and endanger the mother's life.

Most cases are not so clear-cut. The doctor's decision may be a difficult one. But most doctors are forced to make difficult decisions in other circumstances, too. We must do our best to decide wisely.

That is why it is so important for the woman to have a complete medical checkup *before* she becomes pregnant. In most cases, this will indicate whether or not she can safely have a baby, and there will be no difficult decision for her or the doctor to face after she has conceived.

As for use of abortion under other circumstances—to end unwanted pregnancies—certainly contraception is preferable.

## STERILIZATION

Although it was once regarded as an extreme and undesirable form of birth control, sterilization has become, especially since 1970, the fastest-growing contraceptive technique.

The number of married couples who have chosen it as a means of contraception has doubled in the last decade. As many as 23 percent of couples seeking birth control are now selecting sterilization. Among white couples, sterilization appears to be about equally divided between the sexes; among black couples, mostly women thus far have been undergoing the procedure.

For all practical purposes, a sterilization procedure, once performed, cannot be reversed. A man who has been sterilized may never again impregnate a woman, and a sterilized woman is unable to conceive.

Sterilization, therefore, is not something to be entered into lightly. It may, however, be the solution for women for whom pregnancy may be hazardous to health, couples who do not want to risk passing on a grave hereditary disease, and other couples whose families are complete.

Sterilization has no deleterious effect on sexual desire or ability to enjoy sex.

The sterilization operation for women is called *tubal ligation* and involves cutting and tying of the fallopian tubes to prevent the passage of eggs between the ovaries and the uterus. It has been most easily and safely performed in a hospital. More recently, in a newer technique, a doctor uses a laparoscope, a plastic tube equipped with lights and a lens, and works through a tiny opening either in the abdomen or vagina, avoiding a large abdominal incision. This operation may be done under local anesthesia without hospitalization.

The sterilization operation for men, a *vasectomy*, involves cutting and tying the ends of the vas deferens, a small tube through which sperm travel; there are two of these tubes, one on the left and one on the right. A vasectomy may be done in a doctor's office under a local anesthetic in about half an hour. Small incisions are made on both sides of the scrotum. A man is not instantly sterile after the operation but must wait several weeks until all sperm are eliminated from the seminal vesicles. He still continues to produce sperm but they are absorbed rather than joining the semen. Postoperative discomfort is seldom severe. Techniques for reconstructing the vas have been developed (for men who change their minds), but even if sperm reappear in the semen, fertility is not necessarily restored. Evidence suggests that, as a consequence of vasectomy, sperm may be altered by the body's immune system.

# BIRTH CONTROL METHODS OF THE FUTURE

A number of new types of contraceptives are under development.

Possibly the first of the new kinds to become available will be longer-acting hormone contraceptives for women. These would consist of synthetic versions of female sex hormones just as present oral contraceptives do. However, they would be given by injection every month, three months, or six months. Such contraceptives, in fact, are already being marketed in Europe and some developing countries. Some women may find them more acceptable than oral contraceptives that have to be taken daily. And some investigators believe the injectables would have fewer side effects than the orals, since it would take less of them to achieve comparable effects.

Also being tested are sex hormone contraceptives that exert their effects from six months to six years. A tiny capsule containing the hormones is implanted under the skin of the forearm. The capsule then releases the hormones at a constant rate, preventing ovulation.

Another method of birth control now under study is an antipregnancy vaccine. It would immunize women against human chorionic gonadotropin (HCG), a hormone that is produced by the egg when it is fertilized. The hormone signals the body to avoid menstruating and thus to maintain pregnancy. Otherwise, the fertilized egg would be washed out as the uterus is cleared by menstruation.

Ordinarily, a woman would not make antibodies against a hormone or other chemical that is natural to her body. But investigators recently have purified a chemical subunit of HCG, linked it to tetanus toxoid, and injected the chemical packet into animals and human volunteers to determine if it would provoke formation of antibodies not only to the toxin but also to HCG. It does. And thus far in early animal studies, the vaccine appears to be effective, safe, and reversible.

There have been efforts to find a contraceptive for men that would be the equivalent of contraceptives for women that switch off ovulation, in the case of men switching off sperm production. The problem until recently has been that libido has been destroyed at the same time. However, there are early indications that the problem may have been surmounted by use of a small amount of testosterone, the male sex hormone, along with the contraceptive. The quantity of testosterone is not enough to cause sperm production but enough to keep sex drive intact.

How soon any of these or other newer birth control measures will become available is unknown. The process of development, testing, refinement, establishing safety, and obtaining approval is a long and expensive one.

## DISEASES THAT MAY MAKE IT DANGEROUS TO BECOME PREGNANT

Heart disease
Kidney disease, especially Bright's disease and chronic pyelitis
High blood pressure
Diabetes
Tuberculosis
Venereal disease

Some of these illnesses can be cured completely. Others, if they are not too severe or can be controlled, will not necessarily endanger the life of the mother or baby. Even heart disease does not, in many instances, constitute too serious a problem if proper care is taken. But only a doctor can decide, after a careful examination, whether pregnancy will be harmful or dangerous in each individual case.

## OTHER MEDICAL CONDITIONS AND GENETIC COUNSELING

I feel it is most unfair to bring a child into the world if the mother is mentally ill. In most cases, it is scarcely less unfair to do so if the father is suffering from severe emotional illness.

I doubt very much, too, the wisdom of having children if they are apt to inherit a disease that may make their lives miserable. Many genetic diseases, which may be passed to children even though the parents themselves are not ill but only carriers, have caused early deaths in infants and suffering in many of those who survived.

Among genetic diseases are hemophilia, or bleeding disease; Down's syndrome, or mongolism, with its mental retardation; cystic fibrosis; sickle cell anemia; Tay-Sachs disease; thalassemia major or Cooley's disease; and PKU or phenylketonuria.

Increasingly effective treatment is now available for some of these and other genetic diseases, and there may well be more advances in the near future.

If one or both parents come from a family with a history of genetic disease, it is possible in some cases through relatively simple blood or other tests to determine whether either or both are carriers of the disease.

Help is available, too, in the form of genetic counseling for parents who have been afflicted or are carriers. Skilled genetic counselors—and your physician can direct you to one—can provide information about the risks of having offspring who may be afflicted and what the alternatives may be. I want to emphasize that counselors will not make decisions. Only parents can do so. But with the help of counseling, a decision can be an informed one.

Today, too, a technique called *amniocentesis* can be used during pregnancy to discover defects in an unborn child. Usually done during the fifteenth or sixteenth week of pregnancy, amniocentesis involves taking a small sample of the amniotic fluid surrounding the fetus through a hollow needle inserted through the mother's abdomen into the womb. The fluid contains castoff fetal cells that can be analyzed for signs of disorders. It can be performed on an outpatient basis by an experienced obstetrician.

Amniocentesis can determine the sex of the child, particularly helpful for such male disorders as hemophilia and Duchenne muscular dystrophy. It can reveal Down's syndrome. And it is now capable of detecting a rapidly lengthening list of genetic disorders, including Fabry's disease with its kidney failure and death in young adulthood; Lesch-Nyhan syndrome with its severe mental and physical retardation; Hunter's syndrome, which often produces death in the first decade; disorders of fat metabolism (the body's handling of fats in the diet), which frequently lead to death in early childhood; Tay-Sachs disease; maple syrup urine disease; and others. The safety of the test is high.

## ADOPTION

Many couples need not be childless because they are unable to have children of their own. Fortunately, adopting a baby is no longer a very risky

232 - YOU AND YOUR HOME

matter. Responsible agencies eliminate practically all the risk by obtaining information about the real parents and by examining and testing the child. They try to match the child and the adoptive parents, as far as is possible. Of course, there is a considerable risk if one obtains a baby through unofficial agencies, so stay away from the baby rackets!

## CAUSES OF CHILDLESSNESS

Probably you have noticed that, up to now, I have been talking about couples who feel it would be unsafe or unwise for them to bear children. You may even have said to yourself, "He sounds as though everyone who wanted a baby could have one—and the minute they decided on it, too!"

Of course I realize that this is not so. Many couples who want to be parents and are ideally suited for the role are, temporarily or permanently, unable to have children.

### Miscarriages

Some women become pregnant but are unable to carry a baby, and repeatedly experience miscarriage or spontaneous abortion.

There are a great many reasons why this happens, including nature's carelessness in not guaranteeing that all seeds are planted properly. Emotional stress, general ill health, malnutrition, and illnesses, including infections, and glandular disorders, can cause miscarriages. In some cases, it is comparatively easy to cure these conditions.

As I explain in discussing pregnancy (p. 241), some miscarriages can be avoided by refraining from sexual intercourse during the days on which the woman's menstrual periods would occur if she were not pregnant. Sometimes, a week's rest in bed at these periods, especially during the first months, may save the embryo. Rest during the week or so which corresponds to the time of a previous miscarriage is also important.

Other more difficult cases may yield to treatment and care. It is true that some women miscarry easily, and others do not. But don't be alarmed or discouraged by a miscarriage, especially if it is your first pregnancy. It has been estimated that about 16 percent of all married women in the United States under the age of thirty-five have had at least one spontaneous abortion. Undoubtedly the figure would be higher if we could determine how many "late" menstrual periods were actually early miscarriages.

### Low Fertility

To be *sterile* means to have no reproductive power, to be barren. I prefer to use the term fertile which can be qualified, that is, one can be relatively fertile, extremely fertile, and so on, rather than the word sterile which has such a final ring to it! Actually, many people who consider themselves sterile can reproduce, and often do so to their own surprise.

Doctors can usually determine a man's or a woman's fertility. A man may produce few or many fertilizing cells. These may have a long or a short life-span, and may be either very active or too inactive to make the necessary journey to the reproductive cell, or egg, of the woman. The woman's secretions may be injurious to the sperm, or her tubes may be narrow, or her uterus incapable of forming tissues needed for the egg after it has been fertilized. There are many, many factors that can interfere with fertility. Fortunately, the majority of them can be corrected today, although it often takes time and the skill of specialists to do so.

This is what I suggest, first of all, to childless couples wanting a baby. Since either one or both of you may not be very fertile, give yourselves the best possible chance of conceiving a child. This means that you should have intercourse at the time when it is most apt to result in conception. In other words, *study the rhythm method of birth control on page 226 and practice it in REVERSE.* Many couples have considered themselves to be sterile when they have never actually had intercourse at *exactly* the time conception could take place. The act of intercourse should be performed in such a way as to allow the semen to reach, and be retained in, the inner portion of the vagina. This will be facilitated if the woman elevates her legs and keeps them raised for a short time after the act is completed. No douches of any kind should be used. It is not necessary for the woman to have an orgasm in order to become pregnant.

Some men fail to produce a sufficiently large number of sperm cells to impregnate a woman if they have intercourse frequently. Therefore I urge infertile couples to refrain from coitus for a week before the day of ovulation. On that day, they should have intercourse in the morning and again at night.

Be sure to follow these suggestions before you start wondering whether either of you is sterile. If you still don't have a baby, *both* of you should consult a doctor or a *fertility clinic* which he, your nearest hospital, medical center, or medical school will help you locate.

It is possible that in some cases a period of rest and relaxation may improve fertility. In others, a minor surgical procedure may be called for. In still others, hormone medication may be of value. Sometimes, medication may solve the problem by promoting ovulation if the difficulty has been

there. Such medication does, however, often have a tendency to result in multiple births. In some cases of lowered fertility in men, the physician may have the husband collect sperm by masturbation and then inseminate it deep within the vagina; this is similar, in a way, to artificial insemination.

ARTIFICIAL INSEMINATION. When the husband cannot produce healthy sperm, the physician may obtain it from a carefully selected healthy donor and inseminate the wife with it. The identity of the donor is always concealed and, in turn, the donor never knows the identity of the recipient. The husband is indicated as the father on the child's birth certificate. Medically, artificial insemination is safe and often effective. But there may be emotional and other problems which deserve careful consideration before it is used.

## 17
# PREGNANCY AND CHILDBIRTH

When I was a medical student I used to wonder why any doctor would specialize in obstetrics. On one occasion I asked an elderly obstetrician about this, commenting on the fact that he had to be ready to go out at any hour of the day or night, and that there was no time that really belonged to him and his family.

This was his answer: "Obstetrics is the pleasantest as well as the most satisfying of all specialties. Did you ever stop to think that *our* patients aren't sick and miserable, but are going through a normal experience which, with some help from us, is the richest and most thrilling in their lives? *We* almost never have to see a patient die. In fact, when it's all over we usually have not only one patient who is living and well, but three—the mother, the baby, and the father!"

In those days, forty years or so ago, about 65 mothers died in every 10,000 births in the United States. Today, less than 2 deaths occur in 10,000 deliveries. The discomfort and pain of pregnancy and childbirth have also been tremendously reduced. So forget the horror stories of the past, and be glad you are having your baby now. As the old doctor said, it is the richest and most thrilling experience in a woman's life. And the father? Like the obstetrician, he can have the satisfaction of helping make it so.

234

## PREGNANCY BEGINS

Conception, the act of becoming pregnant, has all the ingredients of a most exciting drama, carried out on a microscopic scale.

In coitus, a healthy man puts forth about a teaspoonful of semen. This semen contains from *300 million* to *400 million* spermatozoa, or male germ cells, which are also called sperm. Any one of these can fertilize the egg cell of the woman, but *only* one. As the writer, Aldous Huxley, put it, "but one poor Noah may hope to survive."

The spermatozoa face their first hazard in the vagina, whose acid secretions kill millions of them. However, many escape, swimming up through the vagina by means of their whiplike tails. Those with sufficient energy proceed through the cervical canal into the womb, and on into the fallopian tubes. In one of these two tubes, an egg cell may be waiting, if the female has ovulated, a process I describe on page 84. There is only a short period, no more than two days or so, when this egg cell, or *ovum*, will be in the right place and in the right condition to be fertilized. Sperm can retain their potency for only about forty-eight hours within the woman's reproductive tract, except in some rare instances. But if all goes well, that is, if intercourse occurs at or near the time of ovulation and the sperm are of normal activity, the chances are that a male cell will reach the female cell. It penetrates the female cell, and in that moment a new life is created.

Once the head of the sperm has penetrated the egg, the tail, now unimportant, disappears. The vital material which is the father's contribution to the heredity of the offspring is in the forepart of the sperm. The moment a particular sperm has penetrated and fertilized a particular egg, all the characteristics which a child can inherit are determined. Whether your baby will be a blond or a brunet, whether its eyes will be blue or brown, is settled. Nothing you can do will change it. Whether your baby will be a boy or a girl is settled, too. Which it will be depends on the sperm: an egg cell can develop into either a boy or a girl. I hope all prospective fathers will take note of this fact if they are inclined to blame their wives for giving them a girl when they want a boy, or vice versa. Not that there is anything they can do about it, or that science, so far, is able to do either!

Whether or not you will have twins or triplets is also decided very soon after this important moment. They occur more frequently in certain families than they do in others. Your chance of having twins is, on the average, one in 88, of triplets one in 6,000, and of quadruplets, one in 500,000.

Soon after this magical moment of fertilization, the egg cell begins to divide. More cells appear. About five days to a week later, the tiny embryo travels to the wall of the uterus. There it digs out a little hole for itself. Soon a cover forms over it so that it is attached to the wall of the uterus in a protected, completely enclosed pocket. At this stage it begins to grow rapidly. By about the twenty-eighth day after fertilization the embryo is large enough to be seen without the aid of a microscope.

## HOW A WOMAN KNOWS WHEN SHE IS PREGNANT

At this stage, the embryo is still far too tiny for anyone to detect its presence. Nevertheless, the average woman is aware of its existence at this time, or suspects its existence. Some women know even earlier. Occasionally, a woman insists she knows almost immediately, before she has had any symptoms definite enough to describe. Perhaps she does. Most women, however, have to wait for the appearance of some of the following signs and symptoms:

Frequently their first clue to pregnancy comes when they observe that their breasts are enlarging, that the nipples are becoming larger or pigmented, that is, darker in color, and that tiny new blood vessels are forming on the breasts. There may be new sensations of tingling and fullness.

Another early symptom may be an overpowering drowsiness, which is not related to fatigue but is a simple, acute sleepiness. Some women awaken early in the morning. Others feel suddenly dizzy. There may be an increased desire to urinate, with a feeling of pressure in the bladder.

The best-known sign of pregnancy is a missed menstrual period. However, menstruation is sometimes delayed or absent for reasons other than pregnancy, and in rare instances women menstruate for several months after conception. The presence or absence of menstruation is therefore not absolutely reliable as an indication. In fact, all of the symptoms I have been describing can be due to other causes. They can and do arise from purely emotional factors such as the fear of, or the hope of, having a baby.

## HOW THE DOCTOR KNOWS WHEN A WOMAN IS PREGNANT

In making an early diagnosis of pregnancy, the doctor is guided, as he is in making most diagnoses, by the symptoms which the patient describes to him. If she experiences all the symptoms I have mentioned above, he can be fairly certain she is pregnant. His training will enable him to evaluate some of them better than she can. For example, an experienced doctor can tell a great deal by examining the breasts.

At about the tenth week, his examination will enable him to detect pregnancy with a fair degree of accuracy. By pressing the abdomen in the proper place he can feel the slight enlargement caused by the swollen uterus. The tissues at the entrance to the vagina have a bluish hue. If the fingers are inserted into the vagina, the cervix, or mouth of the womb, can be felt, and it is definitely softer than it was in the nonpregnant state.

However, you can be absolutely certain of pregnancy at the middle of the fourth or the beginning of the fifth month. At that time, an x-ray will reveal the baby's bones; its movements can be felt, and its heartbeat detected.

Even as early as the eighth week, a sonograph —a picture produced by sound waves—may reveal the presence of the baby.

Tests have been devised which make it possible to determine pregnancy, in most cases, within two weeks after the first missed menstrual period. If you have any reason for wanting to be certain immediately, it is very simple to have such a test made. All it requires is a small quantity of your urine or blood.

## THE COURSE OF PREGNANCY

This is what happens to the baby and to the mother after conception has taken place. Incidentally, doctors use the word *fetus* or *embryo* in talking about an unborn baby, usually saying *embryo* when it is in its early stages, and *fetus* later on. Some women seem not to like these words, especially *fetus,* but I hope you won't mind if I use them occasionally instead of the cumbersome "unborn baby."

| END OF MONTH | THE BABY | THE MOTHER |
|---|---|---|
| 1 | The embryo has passed the microscopic stage and is now visible, a tiny piece of tissue. | May be sleepy in the early evening. Frequently has to get up to urinate at night. Breasts may be larger, and the pigmented area increased. Nausea and vomiting may occur. |
| 2 | A little over one inch long. The face is formed, the limbs are partly formed. Has the definite appearance of an infant. | Nausea and vomiting may persist. Breasts continue to enlarge, increased blood supply, and bluish veins appear. |
| 3 | Three inches long and weighs one ounce. Limbs, fingers, toes, and ears are fully formed. Sex can be distinguished. Nails are beginning to appear. | Abdomen may show signs of enlargement. Tissue at entrance to vagina is bluish. Mother may experience dietary cravings, emotional upsets. |
| 4 | About eight inches long, weighs nearly half a pound. Movements can be felt by mother; heart sounds can usually be heard, bones detected by x-ray. Eyebrows and lashes are formed. Skin is pinker, covered with fine hair. | Nausea and vomiting and drowsiness are over. Begins to feel unusually well, very energetic, with a sense of well-being. |
| 5 | Twelve inches long, weighs one pound, has hair on head. | |
| 6 | Fourteen inches long, weighs nearly two pounds. Skin is wrinkled, and fetus looks like an old man. Will usually die if born at this stage. | Pink or silvery white lines, called *striae,* may appear on the abdomen and breasts. |
| 7 | Sixteen inches long, weighs about three pounds. More fat under the skin. In the male infant, the testicles are in the scrotum. | |

| END OF MONTH | THE BABY | THE MOTHER |
|---|---|---|
| 8 | Eighteen inches long, weighs about five pounds, has a good chance to survive if born now. | Breathing may become difficult. The baby is pushing the diaphragm up and causing shortness of breath. |
| 9 | Average length about twenty inches, weighs about seven pounds. | Increased desire to urinate may return, especially at night. The baby's kicking may cause pain. Much shifting and moving about. |
| At Birth | The head is as large around as the shoulders are across. The infant is less wrinkled than previously, almost smooth, and is covered with a cheese-like material. | (described on pages 250-51) |

This chart is intended to give you only the most general idea of the course of pregnancy. Naturally, you want to know a great deal more about it. I hope you will understand that the facts I shall give you are not intended to *replace* the information you will receive from your doctor, but only to provide the background for it. Your doctor's advice may differ in some details from mine. There usually are several equally good ways of handling situations during pregnancy. Remember, your doctor knows *you*. If you have confidence in him, you should follow his advice. If you don't, you should get another doctor!

## WHY YOU SHOULD HAVE A DOCTOR

Until recent years, women often had their babies with the help of only a female relative or midwife. Not too long ago, women who were expecting babies would choose the doctor they wanted to handle the confinement, and that was usually the last the doctor and the patient saw of one another until the baby arrived. Unless something definitely "went wrong," a woman would not expect to "bother" the doctor during her pregnancy.

One of the chief reasons things seldom "go wrong" today is that the doctor sees the patient frequently from the earliest stage of her pregnancy. *He knows her physical condition and can detect even the slightest indication of a complication.* This, together with his knowledge of how to handle such problems, accounts for the present increased safety and ease of pregnancy and childbirth. Even during a normal, uneventful, and uncomplicated pregnancy, a doctor's advice is invaluable to the mother. He supervises her diet, the amount and kind of activity she can engage in, and many other aspects of her day-to-day life. A doctor knows how to alleviate most of the discomforts that might otherwise plague a pregnant woman.

I feel that the best advice I can give you is this: as soon as you are fairly sure that you are pregnant, put yourself in the care of a well-trained obstetrician, and do what he, not your grandmother or a neighbor, says you should do. I suggest that you choose a specialist instead of a general practitioner, if this is at all possible, because you will feel much safer in his experienced hands if complications should arise.

If you have a doctor of your own, ask him to recommend an obstetrician. If not, and you live in a city, you can easily find a good obstetrical specialist by following the suggestions outlined in Chapter 26. If you feel you cannot afford a private doctor, find out about the clinics at the nearest hospital. The best and most highly paid obstetricians usually contribute some of their time to the clinic patients at a maternity hospital. Your choice will be more limited in rural areas, but by all means pick a doctor who has had a good basic training (see page 368) plus plenty of experience in delivering babies. Your general practitioner may be very skilled in obstetrics. Realizing the responsibilities they will have, general practitioners in rural areas often take postgraduate courses in obstetrics to prepare themselves.

## The Unmarried Mother

Every prospective mother has the right to good care for herself and the child she is bearing. This is just as true for the mother who is unfortunate enough to bear her child out of wedlock. Many tragedies could be avoided if these girls, who are often very young, realized that good care is available in most communities. The Salvation Army and other agencies run by various religious denominations provide, or help the girl to find, medical aid. They offer advice and guidance as well. So, too, do other organizations such as the Florence Crittenton Homes Association, Inc. There are about fifty branches of this organization in various parts of the country, with headquarters at 608 S. Dearborn Street, Chicago, Illinois 60605. Information can also be obtained by writing the Children's Bureau, U.S. Department of Health, Education, and Welfare, Washington, D.C. 20201.

## YOUR FIRST VISIT TO THE DOCTOR

Many women dread the first visit to the doctor, and leave the office wondering what they were worried about. It is true that this is a very important visit, but don't be disturbed because of that. You are going to see a good deal of your doctor, so it won't matter too much if you don't know the answer to some question he asks you, or make a mistake in answering another.

Your doctor will probably go into considerable detail in taking your medical history: what diseases or surgical operations you have had, diabetes, rheumatic fever, heart disease, kidney disease or tuberculosis. He will question you closely about previous pregnancies, whether you have had a miscarriage or premature birth, and whether your previous labors and deliveries were normal. Answer the doctor's questions as fully as you can, but don't be reluctant to admit that you don't know or can't remember. He will realize that you are flustered rather than scatterbrained! On the basis of the information you give him, he can tell you with a fair degree of accuracy when your baby will arrive (see page 240).

The doctor will then weigh and examine you completely. Perhaps this is the first time you have had an internal, pelvic examination. You may be embarrassed and tense. The doctor will understand this, and try to cause the minimum of distress and embarrassment. He will drape you in sheets as completely as he can, and will proceed in a straightforward, objective manner. If you are tense, you may find that breathing in and out hard, with your mouth open, tends to relax your muscles and make the examination less uncomfortable for you and easier for the doctor.

He will examine you from top to toe, listen to your heart, and determine your blood pressure. He will check your breasts carefully, and examine your abdomen. At about the tenth week he may be able to detect the baby's presence as he feels your abdomen. He is almost certain to be able to do so by the fourth to fifth month, at which time he can also probably hear the baby's heartbeat. It differs from the mother's in that it beats nearly twice as fast.

Your doctor will take great pains with the vaginal, or pelvic, examination. It is very important for him to know the size and shape and position of your uterus. The examination will also tell him whether there are any tumors in the uterus, or if there is any venereal or other disease. Any marked abnormality such as a tubal pregnancy (see page 246) will be revealed. He will probably also take your pelvic measurements. This helps him to decide whether the hard bony structure through which the baby must pass at birth is large enough to let the average child through. If it is too small, or otherwise abnormal, he will consider the possibility of a caesarean operation.

Several laboratory tests usually accompany the first interview. Your doctor is most anxious to discover any diseases that can be checked before they interfere with your health or that of the baby (see page 231). He will test your urine, mainly to discover whether it is free of sugar and albumin; sugar may be an indication of diabetes, and albumin is sometimes a sign of kidney damage. He will test your blood, routinely, for syphilis and for anemia. He will also type your blood to see which group you are in—A, B, AB, or O—since you might need a blood transfusion at some time during your pregnancy or at the time of delivery. Whether or not you are Rh negative (see page 241) will also be determined. He may want you to

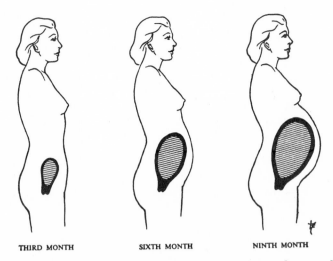

THIRD MONTH     SIXTH MONTH     NINTH MONTH

*Figure 17-1. Pregnancy. Three stages, showing changes in the position and size of the uterus.*

have a chest x-ray taken, if you have not had one in recent months.

As you can see, this first examination is a very important one. It will probably be followed by routine monthly visits during the first five or six months of pregnancy. After that, your doctor may want to see you every three weeks and, in the last two months, about every two weeks. He may possibly ask you to send in a sample of urine by mail between checkups, so that he can be certain there is no new development in the interim.

## Talk Things Over with Your Doctor

During these visits, your doctor will give you advice about your life as a pregnant woman. In these talks, he will undoubtedly dispel most of your fears and the ghosts of old superstitions that may have been haunting you. He will be able to do a far better job along these lines if you tell him what is on your mind. An obstetrician friend of mine once had a very intelligent patient who was having her first baby when she was thirty-six. It never occurred to him, until the subject came up at the eighth month, that she was convinced her labor would be long, difficult, and dangerous. If she had mentioned this earlier, he could have spared her a great deal of worry. Although it has been estimated that a woman who has her first baby at this age will be in labor about an hour

and a half longer than if she were in her twenties, labor is not "a terrible experience" in these days. Women of that age, and even older, can now have babies without difficulty or danger.

Don't be afraid your doctor will think your questions are silly. He would much rather answer them than have you worry needlessly. It will save time and trouble if you make a list of things you want to know, so that you can ask about them at the end of the interview if they have not been cleared up already.

## YOUR PREGNANCY

Although the majority of pregnancies run a very smooth course, most women expect to feel different, as well as look different, during the period of *gestation;* this is the technical name for the time the baby spends in the uterus.

One of the first things you will probably want to know is, exactly how long will that be? The period of gestation differs enormously from species to species. The human baby requires nine months, the opossum's baby eleven days, and the elephant's nearly two years! In humans, this period also varies, probably influenced by the length of the mother's menstrual cycle. Most doctors agree that a baby will almost never live if it is born before the 196th day after the last menstrual period, while a pregnancy lasting more than a few days after the 300th day is rare. The *average* pregnancy lasts 280 days.

This means that a fairly high percentage of women will have their babies a week or two before or after this date. It is sometimes difficult to determine the exact date when the baby was conceived. Your doctor will make a rapid calculation when you tell him the time of your last menstrual period, and come out with the date when you may expect your baby. Suppose you say that your last period was November 16. He advises you to make a date with your maternity hospital about August 23. This is how he does it: he adds seven days to the date of the last menstrual period, and then counts back three months.

This will give you a pretty good idea about when to buy the things you will need for the baby (see page 258) and to settle the question as to arrangements for your confinement, or lying-in, as it was once called, which I discuss on page 247.

## Care of Your Unborn Child

There is little you need to do specifically for your baby. Taking care of yourself is the best way to take care of him. Your thoughts, your activities, and the food you eat will not alter his mental or physical characteristics. If you enjoy museums and concerts, by all means go to them while you're pregnant, but don't drag yourself around in the hope of having an artistic or musical child! Similarly, a craving, fright, or emotional experience during your pregnancy is not going to mark him in any way. The little boy next door did *not* get his buck-teeth because his mother was frightened by a horse, and the mole on your cousin's back is *not* due to the fact that his mother had a craving for strawberries!

Don't worry, either, about hurting your baby if you should happen to bump your abdomen, and don't be afraid to sleep in certain positions because you think it will crush him. Your baby is well protected inside your womb.

Just as we doctors know that these old wives' tales are foolish, so do we know that, in some ways, the fetus in the womb *is* subject to outside influences. Doctors have noticed that if a woman is very tense during her pregnancy, full of irritations and complaints, her unborn child may be unusually active. And in more specific ways, the pregnant woman's diet and the general state of her health will have an important bearing on her baby's physical condition. Then, the pregnant woman must be on guard against some specific illnesses and conditions, like those that follow.

GERMAN MEASLES. Any serious disease or complication of pregnancy and childbirth is dangerous to your baby *and* to you. However, there is one disease, German measles, which is mild in its effects on the mother, but can seriously affect the unborn child, especially if the disease is contracted during the first three months of pregnancy. A certain number of babies whose mothers have had German measles may be born with an abnormality, such as cataracts, deaf-mutism, heart disease, or mental retardation. This disease may also cause a miscarriage.

*It is very important for pregnant women who have never had German measles to avoid anyone who has it. If you have been exposed to German measles, notify your doctor at once.* He may want to give you an injection of gamma globulin that can lessen your chances of getting it, although there is no complete certainty of prevention.

MEDICATION. I want to reemphasize here that during pregnancy especially, you should never take any medication except what your doctor prescribes for you and in the precise dosage. It has become evident that the fetus can be affected adversely by some drugs, including certain antibiotics, tranquilizers, barbiturates (sleeping pills), diuretics, vitamins in excess, and amphetamines.

VENEREAL DISEASES. These can have a tragic effect on the baby, even though it is possible for a woman to experience only minor symptoms at the time. *Syphilis* is particularly dangerous. Unless they are treated while the disease is in its earliest stages, nearly half of the women with syphilis deliver stillborn or infected babies. The babies that do survive are apt to be physically or mentally defective. There is no excuse today for bringing such a child into the world, since early syphilis can be cured by penicillin. (See page 447.)

*Gonorrhea* is less dangerous to the unborn child, but inflicts its damage when the baby is actually being born, while it is passing through the birth canal. If the germs responsible for gonorrhea get into the infant's eyes, they may cause blindness. The routine use of silver nitrate in the eyes of all newborn babies has prevented this disaster in most hospitals and home deliveries. However, there is no excuse for running the slightest risk that it may occur, since gonorrhea, too, can be readily cured. (See page 485.)

THE RH FACTOR°. There is a risk to some newborn babies if the mother happens to be "Rh negative" and the father "Rh positive." A certain substance is present in the blood of about 85 percent of all white people, and they are called Rh positive; the remaining 15 percent who lack it are called Rh negative (the percentage is different in other races). Problems will usually not result unless the mother is Rh negative and the father Rh positive. Even then, the first child will probably experience no difficulties. After that, a real danger exists in a small percentage of cases.

This is what happens. The baby of such parents has a very good chance of being Rh positive, like his father. If he is, the mother will react to the Rh substance in her baby's blood by producing "antibodies." With each new child, she will produce more of these antibodies. In addition, if she has ever had a transfusion of Rh-positive blood, she will produce antibodies which remain in her blood. If there is a high concentration of these antibodies in her blood, they will injure the blood cells of the baby. The doctor can determine if the concentration of these antibodies is rising to dangerous levels by repeated tests on the mother's blood. When the baby is born, he may suffer from a severe anemia.

The danger to the child is greatly minimized if the doctor has typed the mother's blood, and, if she is Rh negative, the father's as well. He will then know whether to be prepared to give the baby a special kind of transfusion that will, in most cases, save his life and fully restore him to health. In these transfusions, the baby's blood is almost completely replaced with Rh-negative blood.

Thanks to an important advance, it is now possible to immunize Rh-negative mothers (after their first pregnancy) against Rh-incompatibility reactions. Immediately after delivery, anti-Rh antibody is injected into the mother and combines with Rh-positive red blood cells or substances from the fetus that have entered the mother's circulation, rendering them inert, no longer capable of causing maternal antibody formation.

MISCARRIAGES. If a baby is lost during the first 16 weeks of pregnancy, doctors refer to this as an *abortion*. *Miscarriages* occur from the 16th to the 28th week. A baby born after the 28th week and before the full term of approximately 280 days is considered *premature* (premature babies are discussed on page 254).

It is hard to estimate how many abortions and miscarriages occur, because many of them are not reported. It may be as many as one in every five conceptions.

If you have never had a miscarriage, your doctor will probably tell you not to worry about it, although he may suggest that you refrain from having intercourse during the days when your first three menstrual periods would occur if you were not pregnant. He may also suggest that you take things fairly easy during those days.

If you have had a miscarriage, he will probably suggest that you take additional precautions on those dates, and especially at about the time your previous miscarriage occurred. Women who have had many miscarriages may present a variety of problems which can be solved only on an individual basis. In order to do this, an obstetrician may need the help of a specialist in another field, such as an *endocrinologist*.

Remember, most women do not miscarry easily or often. It is astonishing what the majority of women can endure without miscarrying! So don't worry about it. It is desirable for you to be familiar with this and other possible complications of pregnancy (which I discuss on page 245). But they are the exception, not the rule, and modern science can cope with them.

## YOUR HEALTH AND HYGIENE

Unlike your grandmother's, your life is not going to be very different now that you are preg-

---

° Rh is pronounced as two separate letters—*R* (arrh), *h* (aitch).

nant. Your appearance need not be unattractive, your activities will not be much restricted.

## What Can You Do During Pregnancy?

This varies a great deal with different individuals. Those who enjoy their work, or who must work because of financial reasons, can usually stay at their jobs, provided these are not too strenuous or physically exhausting—for example, office work or some other reasonably sedentary position. If your doctor does not object and your health is good, you may even be able to continue to work until the eighth month, provided, of course, that your boss has no objection! Many women feel that working keeps their minds off their "symptoms." Others, unfortunately, find it too tiring. I would advise against starting a new or strenuous job after you have become pregnant.

Whether or not you work, your activities need not change a great deal. Many doctors feel that it is safe to engage in sports such as golf, riding, tennis, and dancing, as long as you do not become overtired. Some doctors feel that it is wise to engage in only mild forms of exercise during the early stages of pregnancy, when the danger of a miscarriage is greatest. They almost invariably recommend walking, housework, and a normal social life for the healthy pregnant woman.

There is no reason why a pregnant woman cannot drive a car or take motor trips as long as her figure does not become too cumbersome. However, if you go on a long trip, stop the car at least every hour and a half, and get out and move around for a few minutes. And, of course, obey the cardinal rule—"Do not overtire yourself." This holds true for all forms of travel. If you have a tendency to seasickness, or if the weather is apt to be uncertain, don't take a trip by boat or airplane.

Always consult your doctor before undertaking anything new, or when you are in doubt.

Keep occupied. Try to get some fresh air and exercise every day; but don't overdo it. Get as much *sleep* as you need.

Instead of being a boring time, full of real or imaginary indispositions, pregnancy can be a time for a woman to develop new skills or to catch up on those she gave up after marriage. Sewing, painting, playing a musical instrument, experimenting with new recipes—these are all ideal during these nine months of waiting.

## Clothing

Fortunately, the modern woman can dress becomingly in clothes that conceal her condition during the early stages of her pregnancy and keep her from looking ungainly later on. Practically the only prohibition about clothing is that it should not be too tight or uncomfortable in any way. Round garters constrict the blood vessels of the leg, so wear a garter belt instead. There is a comfortable type of belt which is worn below the protruding abdomen. Wear comfortable, safe shoes. Remember that the extra weight you are carrying is highly localized and will shift your center of gravity considerably, so that high heels will not support you properly during the last months of pregnancy.

Whether or not you wear a maternity girdle and what care you give your breasts depend entirely on your doctor's judgment. Some doctors recommend a girdle after the fourth month, while others leave it up to the patient. A well-designed maternity girdle is not intended to disguise your figure. It may even make you look larger. Essentially, it is a sling to support the abdomen. A good girdle can do wonders in relieving back strain and fatigue. Most women are more comfortable if they wear a firm brassiere that supports but *does not flatten* the breasts. However, wearing a girdle or brassiere usually makes little or no difference in the way a woman feels or looks after she has had her baby. The recovery of a youthful, prepregnancy figure depends mainly on the tone and elasticity of her muscles, and on how much weight she has gained.

## Personal Hygiene

There are no prohibitions about washing or bathing the entire body, including the genitals. Tub baths are sometimes forbidden in the last months of pregnancy because of the danger of infection. Shower or sponge baths are always safe.

Douches are unnecessary (see page 107). *Never take a douche during pregnancy unless your doctor recommends it.*

Some doctors recommend rubbing lanolin or cocoa butter into the nipples in the last few months of pregnancy. This helps to soften them and prevent cracks from occurring during the nursing period. However, most obstetricians consider this unnecessary and merely advocate ordinary cleanliness.

## Alcohol and Tobacco

Most doctors permit their obstetrical patients to drink alcoholic beverages occasionally and in moderation. Until recently, they adopted the same attitude toward smoking, but with the new information available on the effects of smoking, some physicians now advise their ladies in waiting to stop altogether. I also suggest that now is the time to stop smoking. If you cannot, it is important that you at least smoke only moderately, for there is evidence that the fetal heart beats faster when the mother smokes, a smaller baby is likely to be born, and the prematurity rate is higher.

## Sexual Relations

Aside from the possible danger of miscarriage during certain days of the month (see page 241), sexual intercourse is safe during a normal pregnancy. Again, moderation is wise. During preg-

*Figure 17-2. How a Baby Develops. The umbilical cord has been omitted in these pictures, which show an unborn baby in a characteristic position, at various stages of development.*

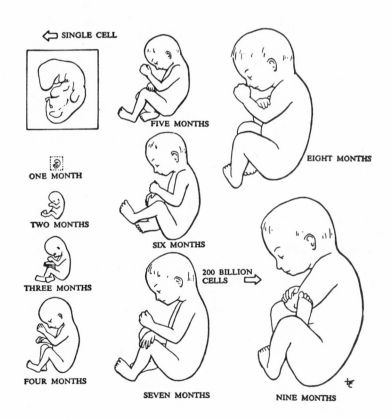

nancy, a woman's sexual desire is unpredictable. It may be heightened or decreased. Don't worry about it. Whether or not you have an orgasm will make no difference to your baby. You may find, especially during the later stages, that you prefer some position other than the one you usually assume.

## Emotional Reactions

You may find that you are on edge and emotional, especially during the early months of pregnancy. You may be unusually sensitive and irritable, so that you become upset and cry if your husband seems to speak crossly to you. The demands and fretfulness of your other children may seem almost too much to bear.

Try to take this in your stride. It isn't anybody's "fault." Our bodies and emotions are influenced by special chemicals called hormones. During pregnancy, the body has more of certain hormones than it had before, and less of others. This imbalance may cause exaggerated emotional reactions. Remind yourself that they are only temporary. After the first few months, if you are reasonably stable emotionally, you will recover your calm disposition. However, pregnancy may be a strain if a woman tends to be highly unstable, and severe nervous reactions may result. If you are at all concerned about this, consult your doctor, who will reassure or advise you.

## DIET AND WEIGHT

In the first few weeks of pregnancy there may be a slight loss of weight, especially if there is any "morning sickness." After this passes, the increase begins, and it usually becomes a problem to keep the weight down.

Being overweight puts a strain on everyone. This is especially true of the pregnant woman. You will be much more comfortable, too, if you are not carrying around excess fat in addition to your baby. Besides, it is much easier to avoid getting fat than it is to reduce. Many young women never recover their trim figures after pregnancy because it is so difficult to get rid of those extra pounds after the baby has arrived.

If you are of normal weight, twenty pounds is a good amount to gain during the course of your pregnancy. If you are underweight, the doctor may decide that this is a good time for you to pick up a few permanent extra pounds. But if you are already too heavy, he may actually put you on a reducing diet!

Many pregnant women overindulge themselves because they feel they have to "eat for two." Actually, you should continue to eat for one, enough but not too much. Watch both the quality and the amount of food that you eat. You should consume about two thousand calories a day. These should come mainly from meats and other proteins, green vegetables, and fruits. Starches, fats, and sugars —bread, rice, potatoes, spaghetti, butter, and desserts—should usually be restricted. Many nutrition experts believe that the pregnant woman needs one and a half times as much protein as the nonpregnant one. This is to supply the demands of fetal and maternal growth and tissue replacement. The value of fruits and vegetables lies in their mineral and vitamin content.

Your doctor may give you a prescription for capsules to supply extra iron and thus prevent anemia. He may urge you to drink a certain amount of milk a day because of its vital calcium content, suggesting skimmed milk if you need to watch your weight. This contains just as much calcium as whole milk. Many doctors prescribe vitamin capsules to guarantee that you consume ample amounts of the essential vitamins.

## Fluid

Drink plenty of fluid. This may be water, but anything liquid—milk, coffee, tea, fruit juices, and soups—counts too. Avoid fattening beverages like sodas and soft drinks. You need a large amount of fluid to flush the kidneys and bladder frequently. This greatly reduces the danger of infection in the urinary tract. You may have heard of women who retain an unusual amount of water and suddenly become large and puffy in appearance. This is not due to the fluid they have been drinking, but is a sign that something is wrong, and it requires the immediate attention of the obstetrician (see page 246). He may be able to control it simply by having you cut down on or eliminate *salt*. But it may be something serious.

## "Problems" of Diet

You may experience acute *cravings* for certain foods such as pickles, lobster, candy. Almost any food may be the guilty one. In recent years, this craving seems to be less common. Maybe our diets are more adequate today. However, don't be upset if you have an intense desire for something you may never have been interested in before. Provided it is edible, it will do no harm to eat it. Also, it won't hurt you or the baby if you *don't!* At any rate, the capricious taste will surely pass.

NAUSEA AND VOMITING. "Morning sickness," the nausea and vomiting which usually, but not always, appear in the morning, is very common in the early months of pregnancy, although more than a third of all pregnant women escape it completely. Sometimes it consists of little more than a mild intestinal uneasiness or indigestion. In severe cases, the pregnant woman vomits and feels miserable. It seldom lasts beyond the third month, although in rare cases it can persist, or be so extreme as to require hospitalization.

There are many ways to prevent or minimize morning sickness. If possible, try not to think about it, and it may pass. I say "if possible," because a middle-aged mother I know tells me she still dreams that someday she will find her obstetrician in the throes of seasickness and get her revenge by telling him brightly not to think about it! Here are some suggestions of a more concrete nature. Select the ones that you think will apply to you.

Have some dry crackers, a thermos of weak tea, or whatever appeals to you, on your bedside table ready for you to eat before you get up. Lie still afterwards for a while. Then get up and have breakfast. Or, if possible, have breakfast in bed!

Eat small meals frequently, six or even seven times a day, instead of three big ones.

Although you need fluids, they may not "stay down" on an empty stomach, so eat "dry" foods first, sipping fluids in small quantities.

Rest after eating. Lie down for twenty minutes or so after even a small meal. If nausea is worse in the evening than it is in the morning, try getting more rest. Some women need a great deal of sleep in the early months of pregnancy. Lying down whenever you feel squeamish often staves off nausea and vomiting.

Avoid sights and smells that seem nauseating to you. Even if you used to like cigarettes, they may disturb you now.

Greasy foods, butter, and fat are apt to cause distress. Plain baked potatoes often turn out to be least offensive. Wheat germ may help nausea, so try to include whole-wheat bread or cereal. Cucumbers, cabbage, cauliflower, spinach, and onions are frequent offenders.

"HEARTBURN" OR INDIGESTION. Heartburn has nothing to do with your heart. It is a burning sensation you feel behind your breastbone. Omitting gas-forming foods such as cucumbers and cabbage often helps. Try cutting down on desserts and rich foods, too. Heartburn can sometimes be prevented by taking a tablespoonful of cream half an hour before a meal. You may find relief by taking a level teaspoonful of milk of magnesia.

CONSTIPATION. Most women are no more prone to constipation during pregnancy than they were before. Usually it can be corrected by diet. Fruits, including the time-honored prunes, vegetables, and a coarse cereal like oatmeal are good. Cold fruit juice or a glass or two of cold water before breakfast is helpful. A mild laxative like milk of magnesia is not harmful, but don't get into the habit of taking laxatives, and *never* take any stronger laxative without consulting your doctor. *It isn't necessary for you to have a bowel movement every day.* Too many people worry about their bowel movements. Try to be relaxed and casual, as well as regular. (See Constipation, page 504.)

TEETH. Many women still believe the old saying "a tooth for every child." This is not true. Don't blame your baby if you find an unusual degree of tooth decay. It is probably due to the fact that you are indulging a fancy for sweets or that your diet is inadequate. Be sure to visit your dentist so that your teeth will be in good shape while you are pregnant.

## DISCOMFORTS AND COMPLICATIONS OF PREGNANCY

HEMORRHOIDS (PILES). These may appear or become exaggerated during pregnancy. Your doctor can help you. See page 509 for suggestions.

VARICOSE VEINS. As I suggest on page 511, avoid round garters or anything that restricts the circulation in your legs. Get off your feet as often as you can, and avoid standing still for any length of time. If these veins are marked or troublesome, your doctor will probably recommend an elastic bandage or elastic stockings.

BACKACHE. This condition may be due to many things, as I explain on page 458. If it is caused by unusual muscle strain because your heavy abdomen is pulling on unused muscles, it will be relieved by rest, a maternity corset, and sensible shoes.

SWELLING OF THE FEET AND ANKLES. If this does not disappear after you have taken extra rest and remained off your feet for a day or two, your doctor should be consulted. It can mean something that requires medical attention.

SHORTNESS OF BREATH. If this becomes so extreme, at any time during your pregnancy, that you cannot climb a short flight of stairs without discomfort, be sure to see your doctor. If a mild case interferes with your sleep during the later stages of your pregnancy, using several pillows so that you are half-sitting and half-lying will bring relief.

## DANGER SIGNALS

Like all the rest of us, you may develop some illness while you are pregnant. Because pregnancy is an added strain, and because you have your baby to consider, it is most important for you to be familiar with the *danger signals* I discuss in Chapter 28. There are a few conditions to which pregnant women are more than usually susceptible and some, such as miscarriage and complications of childbirth, which the rest of us are spared.

CYSTITIS AND PYELITIS. *Cystitis* is an infection of the bladder, in which bacteria, pus, and sometimes blood are found in the urine. The symptoms are a desire to urinate often, and pain and burn-

ing sensations on urination. It responds quickly to sulfa drugs and specific antibiotics and drinking large quantities of fluid. It should be treated immediately, as it may lead to pyelitis. *Pyelitis* can develop into a very serious condition if not treated, because it is an infection of the kidney (see page 424). Luckily, the sulfa drugs and penicillin or other antibiotics are very effective. The symptoms are *chills and fever*, back pain in the region of the kidneys, and sometimes pain on urination and too frequent urination.

ECTOPIC (TUBAL) PREGNANCY. In this condition, the fertilized ovum has burrowed into the fallopian tube instead of the womb. Since the tube is small, the egg is apt to burst through after it reaches a certain size. This is called a *ruptured* ectopic pregnancy. The tube may also abort the fetus by pushing it out. The symptoms are *vaginal bleeding* and severe pain on one side. Usually surgery is necessary to remove the damaged tube and stop the hemorrhage. With *prompt* recourse to surgery, mortality in this type of pregnancy is greatly reduced. Removing one tube does not prevent a woman from becoming pregnant again, although in a small percentage of cases she will have another ectopic pregnancy.

Since bleeding can indicate an ectopic pregnancy, a miscarriage, or premature labor, it is essential to report it immediately to your doctor. Delay in seeing your doctor for even the slightest amount of bleeding can endanger your life or that of your baby. He can often prevent a threatened miscarriage.

TOXEMIAS AND ECLAMPSIA. These conditions are fortunately very rare. Very little is known about their cause. *Eclampsia* is the more serious form, and can be very dangerous. There is no specific medicine to cure eclampsia, but careful medical attention along a number of lines has saved many women with this condition. Even more important, prompt attention to the symptoms of toxemia will usually prevent the patient from developing eclampsia. This treatment varies in individual cases, but usually depends to a large extent on the regulation of salt intake and on rest.

Because these conditions can be serious, it is important to notify your doctor immediately if you observe any of the following danger signals of toxemia, *even if you are feeling well:*

*Puffiness about the face and hands*
*Persistent vomiting*
*Severe, persistent head-ache*

*Disturbances in vision (blurring, dimness, spots before the eyes)*
*Very rapid gain in weight*

The doctor has other ways of detecting toxemias in advance, by taking your blood pressure and examining your urine. That is why you should have these tests made, and cooperate with him wholeheartedly, even if he gives you instructions that seem unduly cautious to you. These illnesses are usually associated with the last three months of pregnancy, and are more common in women who are pregnant for the first time. Serious trouble is prevented by good care.

PLACENTA PREVIA AND PREMATURE SEPARATION OF THE PLACENTA. These complications are also rare, and little is known about what causes them. Both occur in the last three months of pregnancy, and are accompanied by vaginal *bleeding*.

In *placenta previa,* the placenta or afterbirth is misplaced. Instead of being attached high up on the uterine wall, it is down near the cervix. If some of the placental tissue is torn by the expansion of the cervix, which is the mouth of the womb, pain and premature labor will result. The bleeding which results can be serious for the baby.

*Premature separation of the placenta* is caused by a hemorrhage just below its point of attachment. A blood clot forms and loosens the placenta from its mooring.

Maybe you have almost decided you don't want a baby, after reading all the complications that can occur. Don't be dismayed. These complications are the exception rather than the rule. For example, the danger from the Rh factor is about 1 in 600; from placenta previa and premature separation of the placenta, about 1 in 200. Now that you know about them, you will run even less risk. You will be prepared to cooperate with your doctor and avoid even the slightest danger by either preventing any complication or, in the very unlikely event that one does occur, taking care of it in time.

In both these conditions, immediate medical care is necessary, for they are apt to be fatal to the baby. Fortunately, the danger to the mother has been greatly reduced by the use of blood transfusions. With immediate care it is frequently possible to save the baby as well.

# PREPARATIONS FOR CHILDBIRTH

Long before your baby is due to arrive, you will undoubtedly have made arrangements for your confinement. The tentative date your doctor gave you at the first interview has been confirmed or corrected on the basis of later indications. You have talked over the actual childbirth with your doctor, settling the question of preventing or controlling pain.

## Home versus Hospital

Most of our grandmothers had their babies at home. Some of our mothers did too. But the trend to hospital births has continued, until today about 95 births out of every 100 take place in hospitals. Two generations ago, most home births went perfectly well, but we doctors are now used to working in hospitals where everything we need is ready, even in the most unlikely complication. Even if, for some special reason, you are thinking of having your baby at home, I still am sure that you will be more comfortable in a hospital and will get better care. However, if you and your doctor decide that a home delivery is all right, be sure to follow his instructions most carefully.

*If you are going to the hospital,* decide well ahead of time, in the first months of your pregnancy, if possible, how much you can afford to spend, and make your arrangements accordingly. If you can afford a private room, are you sure you want to spend the money on it, instead of on something else? A semiprivate room may suit you just as well. I hope you will read at least part of the next chapter before you make up your mind about expenses.

THE ROOMING-IN SYSTEM. You may have heard of the rooming-in system which some hospitals provide. Like many doctors, I think it is an excellent one.

Many of us believe that the act of birth is probably a shocking experience as far as the child is concerned. Having lived comfortably in his mother's womb for nine months, he is suddenly on his own, forced to adapt to a great many new stimuli in a strange world. He is exposed to light, air, drafts, hunger, pain, and many other new sensations. The rooming-in system makes this transition easier for him.

In the rooming-in system, the baby shares his mother's room, from a day or two after he is born until they leave the hospital together. The crib is arranged so that she can reach her baby without getting out of bed. She helps to care for him, changes and dresses him, feeds and comforts him, and in general learns to understand him. We can only guess, but with some degree of accuracy, that this makes the baby happier than he would be in the nursery. The mother, too, profits from this intimacy. The husband, also, comes to feel at home with the baby.

Of course, the system imposes certain hardships on the mother. She does not have the vacation she probably needs. But I feel the advantages usually outweigh the disadvantages.

The rooming-in system is still not available in all hospitals. Chiefly for their own convenience, most hospitals keep all the babies in one large nursery. Every three or four hours, the baby is brought to the mother for a feeding, by breast or by bottle. Some babies are hungry more often, and may cry for an hour or two. In the rooming-in system, the baby is fed on demand.

Even if your hospital does not provide the rooming-in system, don't worry. If the birth was normal, as almost all are, you will be in the hospital less than a week. Once you are home again, you (with your doctor's advice) can decide on your baby's routine for feeding and everything else.

## Pain During Childbirth

Whether or not a woman admits it, she can hardly fail to give some thought to the question of the pain connected with having a child. How bad will it be? From what some women have told her, it must be unimaginably terrible, beyond description, although they usually manage to describe it in great detail! Others say they didn't feel a thing. Still others say it was unpleasant but perfectly bearable. Where does the truth lie? *Don't* be reluctant to talk this over with your doctor. There is no doubt that fear and tension aggravate pain, especially labor pains, and that they are far less intense if the patient can relax.

NATURAL CHILDBIRTH. An English doctor named Grantly Dick Read worked out a method called natural childbirth or childbirth without fear. Women in primitive countries usually have their babies with little difficulty. They may stop working in the field to have a baby, and almost immediately return to their tasks. Why, he reasoned, shouldn't civilized women be just as well off?

In order to make this possible, he advocated helping the prospective mother, from the earliest stages of her pregnancy, *emotionally* and *physically*.

Emotional preparation consists in ridding the mother of all her fears. She learns exactly what happens during her pregnancy and at each stage of the delivery. She knows just what to do to keep the pain at a minimum.

Physical preparation consists in doing exercises to limber up the muscles she will use when she delivers her baby.

During the entire pregnancy, she has the help and support of her doctor and his staff. Someone is with her throughout the actual period of labor —her husband, the doctor, or a nurse, to massage her back, tell her what to do, and in general give her warm, friendly support and encouragement. Anesthetics are available if she wants them.

Doctors who use this and other similar methods report that nearly half their patients do not want an anesthetic during the labor period. Some require it at the final moment of delivery.

Women who have had their babies by this method are usually very enthusiastic. They find it deeply satisfying to be conscious throughout the delivery, and thrilling to know the exact moment they have given birth, and to see and touch the baby the instant he is born. Without doubt, it is an incomparably beautiful experience.

However, the use of this technique does require a great deal of time from the doctors and the nursing staff, who must be well-trained and convinced of its advantages.

If you have a choice, and decide to use this system, be sure you are making your own decision. Don't do it because you think you should. There are valid arguments against it. As one young mother put it, "I am not a primitive woman. I can't imagine myself doing a day's work in the fields under the best of circumstances—or my husband, either, for that matter!" It is true that most of us are not accustomed to hard physical work of any kind, and let me remind you that childbirth is work! That is why it is called *labor*.

I feel that Dr. Read and those who have advocated other, similar systems have taught, or reminded us of, some very important ways to make childbirth easier, and that the techniques are very helpful. That is one reason why I am going to tell you exactly what happens when a baby is born. Of course, you can skip that section if you'd rather not know! Before I do that, however, I will discuss other methods of reducing or preventing pain.

ANESTHESIA. If you are interested in anesthetics, or pain killers, turn to page 400, where I describe the major methods of preventing pain. Most doctors use some form of anesthetic, or analgesic, or both, during childbirth. An *analgesic* lessens the sense of pain: aspirin is a mild analgesic.

All these methods have their virtues and their faults. With skillful administration, the faults can usually be avoided. That is why an experienced doctor is needed during childbirth. Many doctors use analgesics during the first period of labor, to help the mother relax and sleep or doze between pains. Most doctors use an anesthetic during the period when the baby is actually coming into the world.

Your doctor will know what to do for you. Have confidence in him. But, by all means, talk things over with him before the delivery, so that your mind will be at ease. While you are in labor, let him know if your pain is so intense or unbearable —to you, not to some mythical "strong woman"— that you need relief. He will give you something to lessen it or to "put you out" completely.

## What to Take to the Hospital

Having made your arrangements with the hospital, you may as well get ready the things you will need. Pack the following:

A sanitary belt. The hospital will furnish the pads.
Toilet articles: tooth brush and paste, comb, brush, hand mirror, toilet water, cosmetics, and so on.
Some nightgowns. The hospital will furnish these, but after the first day or two, you'll want your own.
Bed jacket, bathrobe, bedroom slippers.
Some brassieres that you can wear while nursing. These fasten in front.
A few articles for your spare time: books, pen, writing paper, and stamps; a pad on which to make lists for your husband of all the things you didn't get around to doing before you left!

Of course, it is a good idea to do everything yourself if you can, so why not make a list ahead of time and attend to the items on it before you are ready to go?

How will you know when the time has come?

## LABOR BEGINS

Usually you will know you are in labor by one or more of the following signs:

1. "Show." This is the passage of blood-tinged mucus, usually only a small quantity, from the vagina.
2. "Breaking of the bag of water." This rupture of the membranes may be indicated by a gush of water from the vagina or by a slow leakage.
3. Labor pains.

The first two indications are quite plain in most cases. Always call your doctor if either of them occurs. Labor contractions are harder to identify for a woman having her first baby. She is apt to be fooled by "false labor," which usually consists of contractions of the uterus at irregular intervals, with or without pain. True labor pains are

1. *Painful.* The pain may be slight, but it usually increases to a peak and then fades away, so that it can be distinguished from an ordinary

"twinge." The pain is cramplike at the beginning, when it seems to be located in the small of the back. In a few hours it moves around to the front.

2. *Regular,* or *rhythmical.* Even at the beginning, true labor pains are usually spaced quite regularly, with a pain-free period between each one.

3. *Accompanied by a contraction of the uterus.* This can be easily felt by placing the hand on the abdomen.

It is often difficult to distinguish between true and false labor contractions at first. Of course, if either of the other indications of labor appears, the question is solved. Otherwise, it is best to wait, in the case of a first baby, until the interval between the contractions has grown shorter and they have increased in intensity. The doctor has probably told you to call him if the contractions come at every fifteen or ten minutes. Even then he may want you to wait a little while so your stay at the hospital will not be so long. Don't worry if the membranes rupture before labor contractions set in. The stories you've heard about the difficulties of a "dry labor" are untrue. In fact, such labors are very often easier.

## Induced Labor

If, for some reason, the doctor feels he should start or speed up the beginning of your labor—for example, if the baby is past due and quite large—he can rupture the membranes quite easily. Labor usually occurs shortly after this.

He may also use a drug to induce labor. *Never attempt to speed up labor yourself!*

## THE STAGES OF LABOR
### The Dilation Period

The womb which holds the baby is like a large rubber bottle with a very small neck, almost closed. The neck is about a half-inch long. In order for birth to take place, the mouth of the bottle must be stretched to a diameter of about four inches to make room for the passage of the baby. The walls of the womb are little more than a powerful set of muscles. At a certain time, the muscles begin to contract and force the baby downward. Gradually the mouth of the womb, the cervix, is stretched until there is room for the baby to pass through.

While this is happening, the mother experiences labor contractions. At first, they are fairly far apart and last for a very short time. As labor progresses, they occur more often, are more intense, and last longer. At its worst, a labor contraction is an extremely intense, grinding type of pain. Fortunately its peak is short, and there is a blessed interval between contractions during which the mother can rest. Most new mothers are surprised by this interval, since pain of other kinds does not disappear so completely. Being sufficiently relaxed to take advantage of these respites makes a tremendous difference to the woman in labor.

Another reason why it is so important to be relaxed is that this encourages the cervix to dilate more rapidly. If a woman is restless during this stage of labor, it may help her to walk around a little. Sometimes breathing through the mouth, panting like a puppy, helps to relieve the tension during a contraction, and thus lessens its intensity. I feel certain that if women will give some thought, during their first, mild labor contractions, to discovering what makes *them* feel best, they will be well rewarded. At any rate, *don't* fight against the pains. Incidentally, there is nothing a woman needs to do to help during this period.

## The Expulsion Period

After the cervix is fully dilated (opened) the baby must be pushed out through this narrow and resistant birth canal. Here the mother can help by holding her breath and bearing down as though she were having a bowel movement. Even though the doctor gives her a whiff of gas to lessen the pain, which is generally intense at this time, she is usually conscious enough to bear down.

The doctor may use *instruments* to help the baby into the world. Many doctors routinely use "low forceps" at the last moment to guide the baby's head through more readily and gently than it would go otherwise. This is entirely safe for the baby.

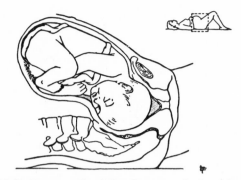

1. *Full dilation. The baby has passed through the cervix into the vagina.*

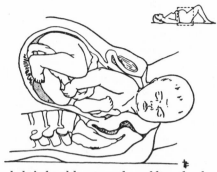

4. *The baby's head has turned, enabling the shoulders to emerge easily.*

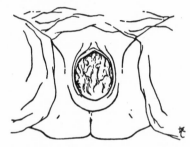

2. *The top of the baby's head has become visible.*

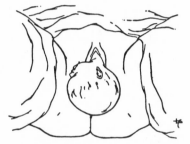

5. *The head having turned, the shoulders and body emerge easily and rapidly.*

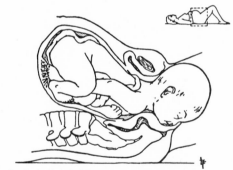

3. *The baby's head has practically emerged.*

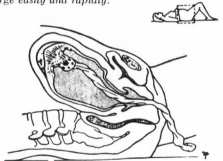

6. *The placenta (afterbirth) is tearing away from the wall of the uterus and is about to be discharged.*

*Figure 17-3. The Birth of a Baby.*

The doctor may also perform an *episiotomy*. There is a strip of tissue between the vagina and the rectum which is called the *perineum*. In the final moment of birth, the baby's head stretches this tissue, which may rip. Although the tear may be a slight one that will heal readily, many doctors prefer to prevent this from happening by cutting the tissues themselves. This makes a neat cut instead of a possibly jagged tear, and it is sewn up as soon as the baby is born. The material used for the stitches is absorbed, and therefore they do not have to be removed.

## The Afterbirth

The third stage of childbirth consists in the expulsion of the afterbirth or *placenta*. This is painless, or practically so.

## Duration of Labor

The duration of these three stages of labor varies a great deal. A woman having her first child is apt to be in labor as long as fifteen or sixteen hours, but a labor of three hours is not uncommon. For subsequent labors, eight to ten hours appears to be the average. Fortunately, long labors are usually less painful in a way. The pains are apt to be at greater intervals or of shorter duration and intensity, especially at first. The dilation period is the longest; the expulsion period usually lasts about an hour and a half for the first child, and half an hour for subsequent children. The third period lasts about fifteen minutes.

# COMPLICATIONS
# OF CHILDBIRTH

The deliveries I have discussed are considered normal. Complications of delivery consist of those in which the baby's position is not normal, or when instruments or an operation must be resorted to for some reason.

## Breech Babies

Most babies are born headfirst, which is called the *head presentation*. It is the easiest way for a baby to be born. In about four out of a hundred births, however, the child may emerge feet first, in the *breech position*. This makes little, if any, difference to the mother, but is not as easy for the baby. One baby in a hundred will lie crosswise in the womb, in the *transverse position*. In this case, the doctor prefers to reach in and turn the baby to a more favorable position.

By means of x-ray and manual examination, the doctor will know the position of the baby before birth begins, and will be prepared for the type of delivery he faces.

## Forceps (High)

In some rare instances it is necessary, for the safety of the baby or the mother, to hasten delivery before the head has appeared at the opening of the birth canal. For example, the journey may be slow because the mother is in poor condition and cannot expel the baby properly, or the baby may appear to be in danger of dying if it is not born quickly. The doctor will then reach into the birth canal and draw the baby out with forceps.

This instrument consists of two blades which are inserted separately into the vagina and the birth canal. When the doctor feels the baby's head between them, he clamps the handles of the forceps together. He then clasps the head firmly, and carefully extracts the baby in a manner simulating normal labor. The use of high forceps in delivery was dangerous in the past, and there is still some risk to the child, far more, of course, than in the use of low forceps, which simply help to lift the baby through the external opening. However, an experienced obstetrician almost never injures a baby in this way, and, because he will not use high forceps unless it is absolutely necessary, this instrument is a boon rather than a source of danger.

This procedure now has been almost entirely replaced by use of caesarean section.

## Caesarean Delivery

If, for some reason, the baby cannot be born through the vagina—because the mother is ill, or her pelvic structure is too small—the doctor can perform an operation to remove it through the abdomen. This is called a caesarean delivery, caesarean section, or caesarean operation, because Julius Caesar was supposed to have been born in this way. Women now need have little fear of such an operation. Many doctors prefer to deliver subsequent babies in this way if a woman has had one baby by caesarean section, but it is possible for her to have other babies normally in some cases. The chief danger lies in the fact that the wound from the first incision may open during a subsequent hard labor.

Although the caesarean operation is quite safe, it is still a major surgical procedure, and few doc-

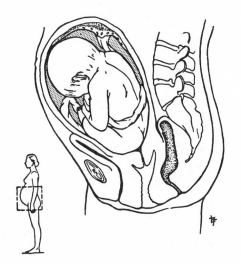

*Figure 17-4. Breech Birth. The birth process is about to begin, with the baby in the breech position.*

tors perform it without a very good reason. I would certainly not recommend it simply because it is less painful than a normal delivery.

### Difficult Labor and Precipitate Labor

Labor can be unusually difficult or prolonged if, for example, the pelvis is narrow, due perhaps to rickets. The mother may be so weak that her contractions are not sufficient to expel the baby. The obstetrician will use instruments or will operate under such circumstances. There is no reason for a mother to worry about whether her labor is unduly slow. The doctor will know and will take the necessary measures.

Precipitate labor, or spontaneous birth, is something many mothers ask about. Suppose the baby comes immediately, with little or no warning? This happens seldom, especially in the case of a first child, yet babies can, and have been, born with as little as one labor pain. To some women, this seems highly desirable, but it has definite disadvantages. The tissues may stretch so rapidly that a severe tear results; and, of course, the baby may be born before the doctor can get there. Because of the possibility of precipitate labor, we doctors urge the mother not to eat if she feels she

is starting in labor, since this could cause vomiting while she is under an anesthetic.

Any one of us may have to be an obstetrician someday. Babies have been known to arrive in taxicabs, on streetcars, and completely unexpectedly at home. For what to do in such an emergency, see page 341 in Chapter 23 on first aid.

## AFTER THE DELIVERY

As soon as the baby has been expelled, he and the mother both receive the attention of the obstetrician, who calls on his assistants if both his patients happen to need help at the same time. The doctor holds the baby upside down and removes any mucus in the respiratory tract. The baby gasps and soon cries if its breathing mechanism is in working order. (If the baby doesn't cry immediately, the doctor has many ways to help brings this about.) The doctor then clamps the umbilical cord in two places, and cuts between the two clamps. The stump of the cord, about two inches long, is bandaged. The baby's eyes are routinely treated with silver nitrate solution or an antibiotic to prevent any possibility of a gonorrheal infection. The baby is handed to a nurse who wraps him warmly and places him in a crib, while the doctor again gives his attention to the mother. Incidentally, if the membranes should happen to remain intact during the delivery, the baby will be born "wearing a caul." This was once considered to be a sign that he would be very lucky or gifted, but actually it is of no importance.

Returning to the mother, the doctor will sew any tear or the cut he made while performing the episiotomy, while he waits for the afterbirth. He can help her to expel this, if necessary. After the afterbirth has been expelled, the doctor examines it carefully to make certain none of it has remained in the uterus. If the uterus fails to contract as it should, there is danger of hemorrhage. Medicines are usually given to help the uterus contract.

Again the baby receives the obstetrician's attention. He weighs, measures, examines, and places identification marks on the infant. During the examination, he will discover any defects or abnormalities. If these are minor, they can be easily corrected at this early stage. The partial or complete correction of many others is very much facilitated if they are attended to early.

About seven births out of every hundred are premature. The degree of prematurity may be so slight that it makes very little difference. However, a baby born very prematurely requires great care if he is to survive. Fortunately, science has made it possible to reproduce very closely the conditions inside the mother's womb, providing a premature infant with the proper temperature, humidity, freedom from germs, and easily digested food. The larger the premature baby is, the better his chances. Doctors consider any baby weighing less than five and a half pounds premature. I realize that this is pretty arbitrary. To a mother who weighs less than a hundred pounds, a five and a half pound baby is quite big! However, we have to establish some figure, and it is safer for the average baby if we set it as high as five and a half pounds. So don't worry unduly if your child is regarded as premature. It just means he will get extra care!

As soon as the baby is ready, the nurse takes him to the nursery. The mother is wheeled back to her bed, when the doctor is certain she, too, is all right. If she has been lightly anesthetized, she will probably be hungry within a few hours after the delivery, and may eat a fairly substantial meal.

## Normal Convalescence

Many women say there is nothing to compare with the sense of well-being they experience after having a baby. I can remember how they used to complain about being treated like invalids, scarcely allowed to stir for several weeks.

As I explain on page 404, we have discovered that surgical patients do better if they get up soon after an operation. Gradually, we have shortened the period of invalidism after childbirth as well. Experiences during the bombings of World War II indicated that there was little, if any, harm done to mothers who had to get up out of bed almost immediately after having a baby, in order to reach a bomb shelter. Of course, no one recommends such a drastic procedure, but many doctors like to see their patients out of bed for part of the time during their first few days. They find that the bowels and bladder function better, there is less danger from infection, and the patient's strength returns more rapidly. This is a matter for the individual patient and her doctor to decide.

The mother may experience some "after-pains" during the first day or for several days after the baby is born. These are due to the contractions of the uterus, which is rapidly shrinking back to its original size. They are similar to menstrual cramps and, though usually not troublesome, can be controlled by aspirin or similar medicines.

There is a discharge from the vagina, called *lochia*, which is sometimes incorrectly referred to as menstruation. It is bright red for the first few days, then fades until it is a yellowish white on about the tenth day, occasionally blood-streaked. If it continues beyond the fourth week or recurs, the patient is probably doing too much and should see her doctor.

Occasionally a woman will have a *chill* soon after delivery. This may be a nervous or emotional reaction. It is quite likely that her nervous system is more sensitive at this time. Many doctors think this is why their patients sometimes unexpectedly burst into tears, even when they are feeling very well physically.

The mother may wonder why her baby is brought to her to *nurse* about twelve hours after he is born, before she has any milk. There are two reasons for this: the thin fluid she secretes, called colostrum, contains substances extremely valuable to the child; and both mother and child need experience in the art of nursing.

I discuss breast and bottle feeding in the next chapter (p. 260). Like most doctors, I am in favor of breast feeding. If it is at all possible, I hope you will nurse your baby, at least for a time. If your *nipples* become sore, your doctor can prescribe ointments or a nipple shield to help them.

Your intestines may be sluggish after childbirth, so your doctor will probably give you oil or a mild laxative. Your *bladder* may be sluggish, too, especially if you had a forceps or a breech delivery. If you cannot urinate, the doctor will catheterize you. This is a quite painless procedure.

It probably will make no difference to your figure whether or not your *abdomen* is bandaged. Some doctors recommend this; others do not.

Your *appetite* will probably be good, and you will be allowed a good hearty diet.

*Rest* is important. Most doctors wish visitors would stay away unless they know enough not to overtire the patient.

## YOU LEAVE THE HOSPITAL

Most mothers leave the hospital within about a week, sometimes less, after their babies are born. Even though this is half or a third the time that mothers used to stay, you may become impatient and want to go home even earlier. You may even have a spell of restlessness, and beg your doctor to let you go.

Next to the feeling you experienced after your baby was born, there is nothing so wonderful as the way you feel when you, your husband and your baby leave the hospital together. But no matter how much you long for that moment, be sure to take your doctor's advice. He knows how strong or how weak you are, and how much you are going to have to do when you get home.

Under almost any circumstances, you will probably have plenty to do when you get there. You want to do it well, so that you can give your baby a good start in life. I will tell you about that in the next chapter. In the meantime, take it easy, rest as much as you can, and be prepared for the next part of the great adventure of having a baby.

# 18
# GIVING YOUR BABY A GOOD START IN LIFE

You're home with your baby. The moment you longed for has at last arrived. And then, either gradually or in a sudden revelation, you discover it isn't the heaven you imagined it would be.

In the hospital you were waited on and cared for, the center of admiration in your pretty negligee. (You couldn't help secretly admiring yourself, with your miraculously flat abdomen.) Your only wish was that you'd be allowed to do more for yourself.

And now—now you are Cinderella after the clock struck twelve! Your back aches and your face, as you glimpse it in the mirror, is no longer blooming. There's so much to do you feel like the household slavey. Everything, from housework to family problems, has been piling up waiting only for your return to slide down and smother you under an avalanche.

As one new young mother said to me, "Don't tell *me* that the emotional upsets and depressions following childbirth are caused by glands and hormones and psychic factors! Any *man* in the pink of physical and emotional health would go right off his rocker if he had to cope with what I'm facing!"

It wasn't only that the entire household rested on her shoulders, she said, but the baby had turned into a source of constant apprehension. She was afraid to pick him up for fear he'd drop on his head; if he was quiet she was certain he had suffocated, and if he cried she knew a pin was sticking him—or worse, that he was starving because she didn't have enough milk, and she'd never learn how to make his formula. And then Aunt

Ida came by and announced that he would have to have an operation because his navel was ruptured. And then . . .

Now, in the course of this chapter I shall tell you how to care for your baby, but just in case you're worrying about any of the things this young mother mentioned, let me assure you immediately that:

There's absolutely no truth in the overwhelming majority of the stories you've heard about babies being dropped on their heads or suffocating. Of course you should be careful; but the last thing that I, as a doctor, am concerned about is the fact that you won't exercise enough ordinary common sense to avoid these *extremely* remote dangers.

There is nothing difficult about preparing a formula, despite its complicated-sounding name. It is simply milk and sugar and water, which any woman who can make a pot of tea or coffee can prepare without any trouble.

Many a healthy new baby has a protruding navel—which doctors call an umbilical hernia. After a while—perhaps days, perhaps months—the spot where he was attached to you will close and his navel will no longer bulge when he cries. But it is not at all important if it does bulge, so don't let Aunt Ida worry you. In fact, Aunt Ida should not have been allowed to visit you anyway! One of the things to settle long before you have your baby is that there will be no visitors until you have plenty of time and energy for them. How soon that will be depends on many things, but I would suggest, *no visitors for the first week at least.*

## HELP FOR THE NEW MOTHER

Personally, I think you should have help for the first month or two, and a *great deal* of help for the first and, if possible, the second week. (Double everything I say about help if you have twins!)

Some parents fail to take the question of help into consideration when they are budgeting for the baby. It is a MUST item. If relatives or friends will treat you to a diaper service, or have your other children visit them, if your husband can use some of his vacation to assist at home, or if a grandmother can take over for a while, these things enter into the matter of help. But I would like you to have a housekeeper for at least a week, preferably two. One thing you *must* insist on: anyone who is going to help you take care of the baby must be in good health.

## THE NEW MOTHER'S HEALTH

Ideally, the mother should behave as though she were convalescing from an illness for at least a week, preferably two, no matter how well she feels—and she should feel very well. Rest as much as possible. Take daytime naps. If you have no help, let heavy housework wait.

Gradually, after a week or so, increase your activities. These activities should not all be work, but should include walking outdoors for a few minutes if the weather is pleasant. By the end of the month, you should be on a practically normal schedule, except that you still need an afternoon rest and plenty of sleep. Usually it will be two months before you are completely your old self again.

You may take a shower or sponge bath as soon as you want, and a tub bath in two or three weeks after the baby was born. Ask your doctor before you take a douche. You may wash your hair whenever you feel up to it.

If the *lochia* (see page 254) continues more than four weeks, or if bleeding continues after the second week since the baby's birth, consult your doctor.

Wait at least six weeks before having sexual intercourse; at this time, the doctor will examine you to make certain your tissues have thoroughly healed. If intercourse is painful, take a hot bath first, and then use petroleum jelly or K-Y jelly to lubricate the vagina; if the pain persists, consult your doctor.

Menstruation usually returns within four to eight weeks in mothers who do not nurse their babies. The first menstrual period is almost always unusual in some way. It may be profuse, or there may be clots, or it may stop and start again. The second should be normal, or nearly normal. Menstrual periods are usually postponed if the mother nurses her baby—*but not always*. Don't count on the fact that you will not get pregnant while you are nursing. (Menstruation probably will not interfere with nursing your baby.)

You may eat anything you like, and I hope you will want to eat good, sensible meals. If you are nursing your baby, drink milk every day, and go very easy on alcoholic beverages and cigarettes. Avoid getting overweight. Remember, skim milk is just as nutritious as whole milk, and it has only about half as many calories.

It may take a while for your muscles to recover their springiness and your figure to return to normal. Whether or not to wear a girdle is up to you and your doctor. Some women feel better with one, and some without, and I have found that this usually depends on whether or not they liked wearing a girdle before they were pregnant. I think it is best not to wear one all the time, in order to let your muscles do some work themselves. Most women feel more comfortable if they wear a supporting brassiere (but not a constricting one).

The following exercises will help make you feel stronger and better. Start them about two weeks after the baby is born.

1. Lie flat on your back in bed and raise one foot slowly for a few inches, keeping your leg stiff; lower it slowly. Do the same with the other foot. Repeat about half a dozen times if you are not tired. The next day lift each leg a little higher, and so on, until by the end of a week or so you will be able to raise them until they are at right angles to your body.

2. Paddle your legs, while you are lying on your back, as though you were riding a bicycle.

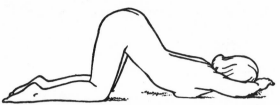

*Figure 18-1. The Knee-Chest Position. Assuming this position helps to restore the muscle tone of the uterus (womb).*

Do this until you begin to tire. Work up to about twenty-five strokes.

3. Assume the knee-chest position for about five minutes every morning and evening (see Figure 18-1). Be sure to have your knees far apart, and to *put your weight on your chest* rather than your arms or elbows.

4. Ask your doctor *if* and *when* you should begin the full set of abdomen- and back-strengthening exercises illustrated on pages 17 and 20-21.

5. Ask your doctor about the need for *breast-firming exercises,* shown in the chapter on women's problems (p. 524).

AFTER-THE-BABY BLUES. You have probably heard of the postpartum blues, the "after-the-baby blues" that strike some mothers—a period of melancholy that may come in the form of waves of sadness. In fact, such blues may well strike most mothers. What causes them is not known for certain. So far there is no proof that hormonal changes at the time of childbirth play a role, though that remains a possibility. Some have conjectured that often the blues may be a matter of "mourning for the death of the old you, the person you used to be, the happy-go-lucky career woman."

Whatever the reason for them, they tend to occur a few days, sometimes a few weeks, after the return from the hospital. There is no reason to be ashamed of them nor to be alarmed by them. They pass as you find yourself putting your baby and life now in perspective—and, as one physician has put it, as "you realize that you're basically the same person who knows how to have a good time, knows how to relate to your spouse, and you have the same ability to relate to a career if you desire."

For a time, too, many fathers feel a bit down in the dumps, partly reflecting the sadness of their wives but also grieving a bit for themselves, longing for that carefree fellow who did not have to provide for a child's future. And the blues of fathers duly pass.

For a few women, however, the postpartum blues are potentially more serious. How do you know that the sadness is normal and not some serious problem?

When the problem is serious, the depression persists for at least two weeks. It disturbs sleep. Appetite is diminished. There is a sense of hopelessness and helplessness, perhaps even a wish to die or that the child had never been born.

Such a severe reaction to childbirth almost invariably indicates that there were underlying problems before which now have been accentuated by the coming of the baby. They deserve treatment and respond to it. Talk the matter over with your doctor. He will be able to suggest what should be done and perhaps refer you to a competent therapist.

One other observation on after-the-baby blues. Some physicians have observed that, although they cannot explain why, postpartum blues seem to occur more frequently after a second child than after the first. So, if that should happen to you, don't be needlessly alarmed. And always remember that the chances are great—very great—that the melancholy will be fleeting.

## THINGS TO HAVE ON HAND FOR THE BABY

Long before the baby arrived, you undoubtedly bought the layette. But if you have been waiting to see what people would give you, or if you have not checked carefully before going to the hospital, someone should make certain you have at least the following items when you return home with the baby:

4 to 6 dozen diapers
4 shirts (long or short sleeved, according to the weather and the temperature of your house)
5 or 6 nightgowns or wrappers
2 sweaters
Hooded wrap for outdoors (how warm a wrap depends on the weather)

Your baby will also need:

## BEDDING

Bassinet, or a basket or box that can be used instead. It should be placed on a sturdy table or stand, not on the floor. *Baby should have a room of his own,* although you will want to put his bassinet in your room at night for the first few weeks.

Firm mattress for bassinet.

2 waterproof pads, 11 by 18 inches.

Waterproof case (pillowcase) for mattress—or make one out of rubber sheeting.

6 quilted pads for mattress, about 11½ by 18 (or make them from four yards of 18-inch material).

2 or 3 small pillowcases to use for sheets (muslin or cotton).

3 or more lightweight blankets, about a yard square (women's wool square scarves which are about a yard wide are cheaper and just as good). If the baby has an allergic family background, or his skin is unusually tender, he may react better to *cotton* flannel blankets.

## FURNITURE

Table to dress and "change" baby on. A good and less expensive substitute is a wide shelf that can be built against the wall. Be sure it is the *right* height, for the sake of your back!

Chest of drawers, or part of a bureau, for baby's clothes and supplies.

Playpen.

Crib, by the time baby is two or three months old. Be sure the bars are close enough so he won't catch his head between them. It should be big enough to last for at least two years, when he goes into a regular bed. If you paint it yourself, be sure to use safe nonlead paint. Ordinary paint may harm baby if he chews on the crib, as babies generally do.

Low chair and footstool to use while feeding, and a high stool to sit on while dressing baby.

## BATHING EQUIPMENT

Bathinette, or an enamel or rubber bathtub.

2-4 towels, 3 soft washcloths (old linen or soft cotton cloth, about 10 inches square, hemmed, will do for washcloths).

1 cotton bath blanket.

2 towels to use to cover bathinette or table after baby's bath.

Bath thermometer, handy if you are worried about getting the bath water too hot or cold.

Tray with supplies (tray can be homemade, from a flat baking pan, and the jars to keep things in can be food jars, cleaned and boiled, and marked with adhesive).

Supplies should include sterilized cotton; rustproof safety pins, a dozen large and a dozen small; package of toothpicks; 6 oz. plain mineral oil; "baby talcum"; any plain, unmedicated, pure soap; and a soap dish.

Rectal thermometer for taking baby's temperature (see page 287).

## FEEDING EQUIPMENT

*Note:* If you nurse your baby, you will need fewer bottles than if you know from the beginning that you will bottle-feed him. But you need some bottles and other supplies either way, for providing that "relief" bottle of milk or because you may have to stop nursing for some reason, also for water and orange juice. Some commercially prepared infant formulas are now packaged in individual, disposable bottles, ready for use without adding water. Although this makes for additional expense, there is the added advantage of convenience. If these preparations are used, some of the equipment listed below is not necessary.

Nursing bottles and nipples and covers for nipples (three 4 oz. bottles with nipples and covers is a minimum for a breast-fed baby; for others, 9 of each; although 4 oz. bottles are handy when baby is little, 8 oz. ones can always be used).

Covered saucepan large enough to boil bottles and other equipment in, with rack.

Brushes to clean bottles and nipples; covered wide-necked jar for nipples; enamel quart-size container to heat formula in; measuring cup; funnel; orange squeezer; strainer and spoon which can be sterilized; long pair of forceps (or tongs) to lift out articles.

## OTHER SUPPLIES AND EQUIPMENT

Mild soap for washing diapers.

Two covered 2-gallon rustproof diaper pails.

Mosquito netting to hang over bassinet or crib if

there are flies, mosquitoes, or other insects near the baby.

Room thermometer (the room temperature should be around 68° to 74° during the day, and may be as cool as 60° at night when the baby is covered).

Scales.

Baby carriage. You will need one soon, and it is handy to have one from the first, unless your bassinet is easy to wheel.

## DECISIONS TO MAKE IN ADVANCE

There are a number of things you can settle before the baby is born, so that you won't use up your emotional energy making decisions after you get home—when everybody gives you unsolicited advice. Of course, you will have to be flexible because circumstances may change.

### Breast versus Bottle Feeding

Like most doctors, I strongly favor breast-feeding. It has some tangible and some intangible advantages for both the baby and the mother.

Breast milk is easily digested by your baby, for whom nature especially made it. It contains practically everything he needs during the first months of life. Babies who are breast-fed seem to have a partial or temporary immunity to certain diseases. Also, the act of nursing helps to satisfy some of their emotional needs.

As far as the mother is concerned, nursing contracts the muscles of the uterus, encouraging its rapid return to normal. It makes her feel close to the baby, satisfying her emotional needs. It is less expensive, and it is not dependent on obtaining supplies. It won't ruin her figure; nursing mothers need not gain any weight even though they eat well and drink a quart of milk a day (for example, skimmed milk is far less fattening, and will do exactly as well). If the mother does not gain weight, and if she wears a good supporting brassiere, the appearance of her breasts won't be appreciably altered. Nursing does not interfere with her health. It can be compared with exercise—that is, tiring but not harmful to a healthy woman. If a nursing woman loses weight

or becomes overtired, she is undoubtedly below par in some way, perhaps emotionally, and should consult her doctor. He is very apt to have her stop nursing and curtail her activities in other ways as well. But even women who are not robust often thrive on nursing.

It is true that there are disadvantages to breast-feeding as far as the mother is concerned. Her freedom is restricted; she can't go away for days at a time. It's difficult to nurse a baby *and* go out to work, although it is possible. If, for example, she returns to her job when the baby is about two months old and on a four-hour schedule, she may be able to manage things so that she need miss only one feeding, which can be given in a bottle.

I am very much in favor of a supplementary or "relief" bottle for breast-fed babies anyway. Ask your doctor about this, since it can be a great boon to nursing mothers. He may suggest that you use your own milk at first, which you can express from the breasts by hand or by using a breast pump. (He will show you how to do this.) I think it is a good idea to use cow's milk in a formula quite early, so that the baby will get used to it. This is a great help if the mother does not have enough milk, or has to stop nursing, perhaps only for a few days, if she is not well.

The main disadvantage in nursing lies in the fact that some women really object to it. If you feel a real revulsion toward the act of nursing your baby (and *not* just an objection on the grounds that you think it will be a nuisance) don't force yourself to nurse. Or try it and stop if it disturbs you. Don't blame yourself; somebody else, not you, probably put the idea into your mind long ago, and it does not mean you are going to be an "unnatural mother." Nursing your baby is a little better than bottle-feeding him, but there is not enough difference for you to get upset. That would only spoil the very relationship which was one of my main reasons for urging you to nurse in the first place. Cuddle your baby and give him plenty of affection while you give him his bottle.

### Schedule

This is another matter you can and should decide about before your baby arrives. I hope you will choose to feed him when he wants to eat, and not follow a timetable. I am very much in favor of "demand feeding" as it is called—that is, a flexible, self-regulating schedule which the baby, rather than anyone else, works out.

A great deal has been said supporting each method. Those who favor the rigid schedule emphasize the fact that the average baby requires a sufficient amount of milk at four-hour intervals in order to satisfy his hunger and grow properly; and that this is a great convenience to the mother, who will know just when to feed him. This is true, but it fails to take into sufficient consideration the fact that all babies are not the average baby. No two children have the same appetite. Some are hungry sooner than others, or eat less at each feeding and need to be fed more often— or just because they happen to be like that. Some babies want to sleep longer at a stretch than others.

I think it is very important to satisfy a baby's hunger and thirst when they arise, and not to withhold satisfaction of this fundamental craving. It is not going to "spoil" the baby to feed him when he is hungry; on the contrary, it will make him less demanding if he is happy and satisfied. It is true that some mothers urge food—or practically force it—on babies every time they whimper; but most mothers soon learn whether the baby is crying because he is hungry or whether he would only like a little attention and stops the minute he is picked up. (Not that it will hurt him to be comforted if he is fretful.)

The thing to remember is that when you follow the self-demand method you are working *toward* a schedule. Both it and the rigid timetable system have the same objective, to give the baby enough to eat and establish a routine that helps the mother find time for everything she has to do. From my observations, they usually arrive at this end in about the same length of time! Mothers who follow a fixed schedule usually modify it sensibly, so that, in the long run, it comes fairly close to the self-demand system. For example, they feed the baby early if he is crying, rather than let him wear himself out and fall asleep exhausted. Similarly, many mothers who follow the self-demand method will awaken the baby if he happens to be sleeping about four hours after

his last feeding; they know from experience that he will be glad to eat even if he didn't "ask" for it, and that he is bound to awaken soon and want food just when his mother is busy doing something else.

So, whichever system you follow, remember that you are *working toward a goal*. Some babies do well on a four-hour schedule from the beginning, while others won't be able to wait that long, or won't be regular at all, for several months. It is wise to feed babies who weigh under seven pounds more often than once every four hours— every three hours at least.

Be very flexible about the 2:00 A.M. (or middle-of-the-night) feeding. Babies sleep through the night as soon as they are able to go that long without food, so don't deprive your baby of that feeding in the hope of speeding the time when you won't be disturbed at night. It helps to be flexible about the feeding that precedes the night one, too. That is, put it off till you go to bed if the baby is sleeping, so that he won't be apt to awaken quite as early for his next one.

## Your Baby's Doctor

Decide who is going to look after your baby's health before you leave the hospital. Will your family doctor take over, or are you going to have a "baby doctor" (a pediatrician)? Maybe you are lucky enough to live in a city that has a "Well-Baby Clinic." Your baby has had a thorough examination at the hospital; for the first six months he should be seen by a doctor regularly. Decide who that doctor will be on the basis of the suggestions I make in Chapter 26 (p. 368) and the advice of the doctor who took care of your pregnancy and childbirth. Having decided, *follow the doctor's advice*. The things I tell you in this chapter are not intended to, and cannot, take the place of your doctor!

## Circumcision

It is wise to decide ahead of time about the question of circumcision if your baby turns out to be a boy. (Although I always refer to your baby as *he*, that is only for convenience because I want to be able to say *she* when speaking of you, the mother.) Circumcision consists in cutting off the "sleeve" of skin (*foreskin*) covering the penis, because this skin may encourage the collection of a cheeselike substance (*smegma*) that can cause irritation or infection. It is a simple procedure in little babies.

You may wish to have it done for religious reasons, or you may prefer to wait and see whether or not the doctor recommends it. If your doctor thinks it should be done, by all means have it done early, as soon as he suggests; it will disturb you and the baby more later—in fact, little boys are often quite upset by having to be circumcised. Always have this minor operation performed by *a qualified person*—that is, someone of whom your doctor approves.

## CARING FOR YOUR BABY

If your baby is *premature* or delicate, your doctor will give you special instructions. Fortunately, we know enough today so that such children usually do very well, but each one is a special case in himself. In general, premature babies need to be kept warmer, requiring a very warm room, with more moisture than the air is apt to contain; they should be handled less, protected from drafts, have special diets and, in general, receive more care and attention.

If you have a "preemie" who has reached the normal birth weight of about seven pounds and requires no special care, be sure to remember that he is "younger" than the babies I am talking about. That is, if he was born at seven months, get in the habit of mentally subtracting two months from his date-of-birth age. Don't compare him with ordinary babies. It usually takes two years before he entirely "catches up" with his birth date and you can forget that he was premature. In the meantime, consider his progress by its *rate*, not by what he can do.

There have been endless debates as to which is more important in determining a child's character and nature—heredity or environment. How much can be done to shape and influence him? Is the boy next door good or bad, athletic or artistic, stolid or nervous, because of inherent qualities or because of the way he was raised?

The answer is, some of each. Babies are not alike in personality (or temperament, or inherent qualities, or whatever you want to call it) any more than they are alike in appearance. Some babies are big-boned, some are delicately built. Some are more sensitive to sound and to stimuli of various kinds. Some are lusty and some are subdued. Some eat and sleep a great deal while others may be poor eaters or sleepers regardless of the way they are handled. As they grow older, one child will have an excellent ear for music and another will have fine muscular coordination.

However, the environment—the way the baby is cared for and the surroundings in which he lives—will make a tremendous difference. Obviously, it will make a difference in his health and growth. It can also help determine, for example, whether or not a high-strung baby becomes "nervous" or a stolid one becomes lethargic, even backward. It can help determine whether or not your baby makes the best of his complicated assortment of inherent characteristics. In any normal child, this means he can become a fine person.

Your child's environment also is going to affect his intelligence. Intelligence is not a fixed quality that he is born with, but a potential that can be encouraged to grow. How you care for your baby and the stimulation you give him in those all-important first months and years of life will help determine how well he will use his mind later, and adapt to life's changing situations.

Because each baby is an individual, all babies cannot be treated exactly alike. However, all babies have the same basic emotional need for security and affection, and they all need a loving, relaxed atmosphere (as well as attention to their physical requirements) in order to develop their full potentialities.

Here are some of the things to do to help create such an atmosphere:

1. Love your baby. You may tell me with indignation that I needn't suggest such a thing—of course you love your baby! So perhaps I should say, *show* your baby that you love him, right from the beginning. Cuddling and soft words of affection will make him feel this new world is a pretty nice place to be in.

2. Enjoy your baby. Don't wait for him to do

things you can boast of with pride, but enjoy him as he is, at each stage of his development.

3. Don't worry about spoiling him. He does not need to be disciplined when he is little; in fact he will do better without it. (I discuss discipline in the next chapter; see page 279.) Comfort him when he cries. You will soon learn to tell whether he just wants attention, and when he can get along without it if you can't spare the time. The baby who gets too little attention is apt to demand more than the one who gets his share.

4. Don't attempt to train him, either. He will fall into good habits with the proper encouragement as far as eating, sleeping, and amusing himself are concerned. Don't try to toilet-train him during his first year. I discuss this subject in the next chapter, Our Children's Emotions (p. 280). Be sure to read this chapter because it contains information that will help you to give your baby a good start in life.

5. Don't worry about his being fragile. He isn't. He isn't fragile emotionally, either; that is, he won't be warped for life if you are human enough to be occasionally preoccupied or irritable or overattentive. It is his basic security that counts.

6. A baby needs a father as well as a mother. Although she is naturally the most important figure in his life, his father is also essential to him. The father should be a part of the baby's little world from the beginning, not a visitor who plays with the baby a few minutes a day and for whom the baby must be kept quiet. Too many fathers gradually assume the role of the dispenser of discipline and treats, rather than that of a parent. It may take tact and time to make the father a part of the baby's life, but it is well worth it so that their relationship will, from the beginning, be close and easy and happy. In this way the baby will have the two parents he needs, and to whom he is equally important.

7. If you should become concerned about his development, his doctor or the clinic is your best source of information. They will tell you whether your child is as big or strong as he should be at his age. It is natural to discuss such things with relatives and friends, but take their comments and opinions lightly. If you have doubts or worries about your baby, discuss them with a doctor. Be sure to tell your doctor or the clinic everything you notice about your baby, especially if it seems at all out of the ordinary.

This does not mean you should not be alert between visits for signs or symptoms that may indicate everything is not going well. I tell you how to determine whether or not your baby is ill on page 286; and I discuss minor stomach upsets in this chapter on page 272.

If your baby is sick, don't give him any medicine or "treatment." Don't try to make him eat. If he isn't vomiting or having diarrhea, let him have his milk as usual. If he is, don't offer him any food, but try to get him to take a little boiled

*Figure 18-2. Diapering a Small Baby.*

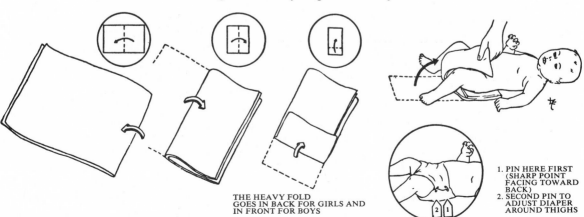

THE HEAVY FOLD
GOES IN BACK FOR GIRLS AND
IN FRONT FOR BOYS

1. PIN HERE FIRST
(SHARP POINT
FACING TOWARD
BACK)
2. SECOND PIN TO
ADJUST DIAPER
AROUND THIGHS

water frequently, unless he vomits it, in which case wait an hour or two before trying again. (See sections on vomiting, page 272, and diarrhea, page 272.) Keep him quiet and let him sleep as much as possible. Don't let him cry if something like rocking will soothe him. And, of course, call the doctor immediately.

## BABY'S DAILY CARE

A baby doesn't need to be dressed up; in fact, he will be more comfortable in his nightgown with a wrapper or sweater over it when he is out of bed. Don't bundle him up too much; his hands, for example, are usually cool. If he wears a cap, be sure it is a light knitted one so he can breathe through it if it slips down over his nose. *Don't use a pillow in his bassinet or basket.* Tuck the sheets and blankets securely under the mattress.

Let him sleep on his stomach most of the time. His head may be flattened on one side if he is accustomed to sleeping that way—but this won't be permanent. You can, however, try facing him first one way and then the other. Incidentally, if his head is egg-shaped, that won't last either. The

soft spot on the top of his head (the fontanel) is tough, so you can touch it safely. If your baby is sleeping on his stomach, be especially careful about having the bedclothes firmly tucked in, and don't leave him in that position if he has cried a great deal or "spit up."

Change his diapers when they get soiled, and when they are wet if he fusses or if you are picking him up anyway. (See illustration for ways of folding and pinning diapers.) A disposable piece of clean linen or cotton placed on the diaper to catch the stool is a convenience. Shake soiled diapers into the toilet before placing them in the (covered) pail of water. Boil, or wash them in very hot water with a plain mild soap, rinse *thoroughly*, and dry outdoors if possible. If you detect an ammonialike odor on the diapers, be sure to boil them, using a diaper bleach in the last rinsing water; this will help prevent diaper rash. If diaper rash—red, pimply rough patches—appears, your doctor will recommend an ointment and possibly other measures. You will find the two diaper pails I mentioned on page 259 useful, if you fill one with plain cold water for wet diapers and the other with soapy water for soiled diapers. Rinse a soiled diaper in the toilet before placing it in the covered pail with soapy water.

*Figure 18-3. The "Shaped" Diaper. This method of folding provides thickness without uncomfortable bulki-* *ness between the legs, and is preferable for older active babies.*

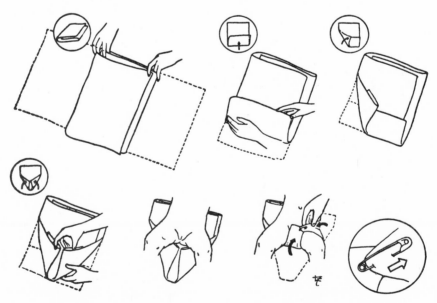

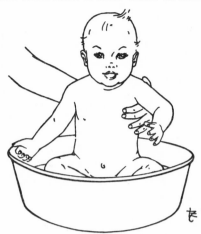

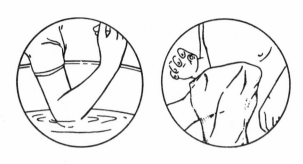

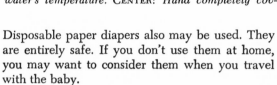

*Figure 18-4. Bathing the Baby.* Left: *Testing the water's temperature.* Center: *Hand completely cov-* *ered to protect the baby.* Right: *Method of holding the baby firmly.*

Disposable paper diapers also may be used. They are entirely safe. If you don't use them at home, you may want to consider them when you travel with the baby.

When you pick your baby up, support his body with one hand under his head and the other lower down. When you carry him, hold him on your shoulder with his head leaning over it a little so it won't bob backward. He will need support of this kind until he is about three months old.

Some fresh cool air is good for him. By the time he weighs eight pounds, he can go out when the temperature is over 60°, and by the time he weighs ten pounds he can be out for about two hours if it is above freezing and the wind is not too strong. Give him an "indoor airing" if you can't take him out. Some sun will do him good provided you keep it out of his eyes and don't let him get overheated. Avoid sunburn by starting with two minutes' exposure and gradually increasing the time. Kicking and playing naked, not even diapered, on a bed in a warm (not hot) room is good fun and exercise for him.

Every baby is bound to be exposed to some germs. But don't expose him to "new" ones. The fewer people with whom he has contact, outside of his family circle, the better. He doesn't need visitors. There should be NO kissing from visitors, and NO visitors with colds or sore throats. Be very firm about this. Aunt Grace will get over her hurt

feelings far faster than baby will get over the cold she may give him—and even if she doesn't, it is by far the lesser of two evils.

Be careful not to leave anything around that he may swallow. The main danger is that he may choke on it (see page 336). If he does swallow a small, smooth object like a button that goes down easily, tell your doctor; but this is not an emergency. Such things often pass easily through a baby. A needle or pin, however, can be quite dangerous, so get a doctor or take your baby to a hospital immediately.

## Bathing the Baby

Your doctor will tell you how soon your baby may have a real bath—probably when he is a week or two old, though some doctors prefer having the baby sponge-bathed for his first month or so. Around 9:30 A.M. is usually the most convenient time for the mother to bathe the baby, but any time that suits her is all right, provided it is before a feeding. Choose any room that is warm enough (75° to 80°) and not drafty. If you have no bathinette, put the tub on a table that is high enough for you, or sit on a stool. Be sure to wash your hands and have everything ready before you get started. Don't put too much water in the tub till you get used to bathing the baby; lining the tub with a clean diaper will prevent it from being so slippery. The temperature of the water should be about 90° to 100° on your bath thermometer, or feel comfortably warm when you dip your elbow into it.

Some mothers prefer to do most of the washing first, using the bath merely for rinsing purposes. Suit yourself about this. If you put your baby into the tub right away, be sure he isn't soiled; wipe him off with a little wet, soapy cotton first. You'll soon learn how to hold him so you will know he is secure in the tub: your left hand under his left arm, with your thumb over his shoulder and your fingers under it, so that your wrist supports his head.

Use a mild soap and a soft cloth. His eyes, ears, and nose and mouth don't need any special cleansing. If a little mucus stays in his nose, twist a bit of cotton (*don't* put it on a stick) moistened in water, and insert it in the nostril, holding onto it as you twist it so that the mucus sticks to it when you pull it out. You will want to wash his scalp once or twice a week. Apply some soap on your hands or washcloth, lather, and rinse with the cloth, being sure his head is tilted back a little so the soap won't get in his eyes. If he has any "cradle cap" ("milk crust") on his head, wash the scalp daily until it clears up. If it fails to clear, your doctor will advise you on what further to do.

Soap his body with your hands or the cloth, paying attention to the folds and creases and the genital organs (your doctor or the hospital nurse will show you what to do if the penis needs any special cleaning). Let the baby splash a little, and then lift him out, wrap a towel around him, and dry gently and thoroughly, especially in the creases. Usually nature provides sufficient oil for the baby's skin, so why add artificial oils that occasionally produce irritation or infection? Also, I see little need for talcum powders.

## Nursing the Baby

As a rule, nursing is a very simple and satisfactory way to feed a baby. You can help make it so by being relaxed about it. It is a good idea to rest first so you won't feel tense and hurried.

Your breasts require little care. Just before each feeding, wash your hands, and sponge the nipple (or nipples if you are going to use both breasts) with some sterile cotton moistened in warm water which has been sterilized by boiling. If you have a tendency to leak milk before you nurse the baby, you may find it convenient to place some pads of cotton inside your brassiere; be sure no wisps of it remain on your nipple.

You can lie on one side while you nurse, holding the baby close to you in the curve of your arm. Or you can sit in a comfortable chair with a pillow at your back and one foot on a stool so that your knee will help support the baby; your curved arm will support his back. In either case, you will probably need to hold back your breast a little between the fingers of your free hand so that his nose won't be against it, interfering with his breathing.

As a rule, babies are nursed on one breast at a feeding, alternating with each feeding. In this way the breast is emptied completely, which prevents the milk from diminishing. (Your doctor may tell you to empty the breast by hand after your baby is finished, in order to encourage the supply of milk.) Some babies nurse rapidly and some slowly. They usually get most of the milk during the first few minutes, but should be allowed to continue. The average is fifteen minutes but some babies require twice that.

Once or twice during the nursing period, and when it is over, "burp" the baby by holding him over your shoulder so any air he has swallowed will be expelled. This makes room in his stomach for more milk. Besides, an air bubble may give him a colic pain if he doesn't get rid of it. He is apt to spit up a little, so have a *clean* diaper over your shoulder. Another method of "burping" is to hold baby in your lap, letting him lean forward slightly, with your support, and rubbing or patting his back. How you help him get rid of any air he may have swallowed is strictly between you and your baby! Only results count.

I have already discussed the *schedule* of feedings. Briefly summarized: as soon as the baby is ready they should be spaced at four-hour intervals; for example, at six and ten in the morning, and at two, six, and ten P.M., with a later feeding if the baby wants it, and the ten o'clock feeding postponed until eleven or later if it is convenient for the mother and baby.

*Menstruation* usually does not interfere with

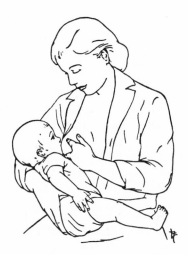

*Figure 18-5. Nursing the Baby.*

nursing. Don't take any *medicine* unless the doctor tells you to. Your baby may object to the way your milk tastes if, for example, you have been eating onions, in which case eliminate the offending item.

This is usually all there is to nursing a baby! The baby is *weighed* at least once a week. On an average he will gain:

7 ounces a week during the first three months.
4 ounces a week (less regularly) until he is six months old.
2 ounces a week (still less regularly) until he is nine months old.

Be sure to remember that *this is the average—* each baby has his own rate of growth.

If you have any nursing difficulties, consult your doctor. If your nipples become sore or your breasts tender, it may be because of an inflammation or because of the way your baby is nursing. Your doctor will discover the cause of the condition and tell you what to do about it.

If the baby fails to gain weight properly, your doctor will find out whether he is getting enough milk, probably by having you weigh him before and after each feeding. He can then determine whether something should be done to increase your milk supply. Or perhaps he will recommend

that you supplement the breast-feeding by giving your baby some formula in a bottle.

## The Bottle-Fed Baby

A formula is milk that has been modified to make it resemble mother's milk as much as possible. You can prepare a perfectly satisfactory formula at home by adding water and sugar to cow's milk (usually evaporated), and boiling the mixture to kill any germs and to make it easier to digest. You can also purchase excellent commercially prepared formulas which come in either concentrated liquid or powder form and require only water to reconstitute them. It is possible to purchase a formula in fluid form, in which the water has already been added and the food is ready to use.

The method you choose will, of course, be based on your doctor's recommendation. He will select the formula most suitable for your baby and will tell you how to prepare it.

If you will be making your own formula from milk, sugar, and water, your doctor will tell you the exact proportion of ingredients. However, just

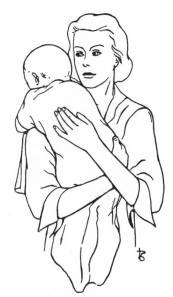

*Figure 18-6. Burping the Baby. Patting his back gently with the palm of your hand will help him expel air.*

to give you an idea of how simple it is, here is a formula which many physicians recommend:

*For a very young (seven-pound) baby*

14 ounces whole milk ⎱ or ⎰ 7 ounces evaporated milk
7 ounces water ⎰    ⎱ 14 ounces water
2 tablespoons of sugar (granulated or brown, or corn syrup)

This makes a total of 21 ounces, which are divided into five bottles, each containing a bit over 4 ounces.

*For a ten-pound baby*

20 ounces whole milk ⎱ or ⎰ 10 ounces evaporated milk
10 ounces water ⎰    ⎱ 20 ounces water
3 tablespoons of sugar (granulated or brown, or corn syrup)

This makes a total of 30 ounces, which are divided into four bottles of 7½ ounces each.

There are many ways of preparing the formula and washing and sterilizing the bottles and other equipment. They all have the same purpose: to kill any germs that may be present and prevent others from getting in the milk or on the things used in preparing and giving it to the baby. This is very important because babies are susceptible to infections from the germs which grow rapidly in milk except when it is quite cold. Naturally you cannot sterilize everything your baby touches or keep him from putting his fingers in his mouth after he touches them. Fortunately, germs do not usually live long on the things he is apt to handle, so this is not a serious problem, especially if you keep anyone with a cold or other infection away from the baby and his belongings. However, precautions must be taken with milk and water.

Unless your doctor tells you to discontinue it sooner or later than this, I suggest that you continue to sterilize things until your baby drinks only from a cup. By then it is enough to be certain the cup is really clean, the milk pasteurized, and that the baby drinks it within a short time after it is poured, so that germs won't have a chance to drop into it from the air and multiply.

Your doctor or a nurse in the hospital will show you how to prepare the formula and sterilize the bottles and nipples. However, in case you suddenly find you must do this without guidance for your own or some other baby, the following method is, I believe, the simplest. The only problem it presents lies in the fact that "skin" or "scum" often forms while milk is heated, and this may clog the holes in the nipples. This skin will not form readily if you use homogenized milk, or if the milk can be cooled quickly, which is easy if the bottles are of the unbreakable (actually, heat-resistant) type that won't crack if they are heated or cooled rapidly. I'll mention additional ways of avoiding this difficulty as I describe this method.

For it, you will need the following:

Bottles, nipples, and bottle covers, or caps.

A sterilizing pail or basin, with a cover, large enough to hold a day's supply of bottles standing upright; the ones in which the baby is given orange juice and water need not stand upright since they will be empty.

A sterilizing rack in which to stand the bottles.

A measuring cup.

2 spoons (one for measuring, one for stirring).

A funnel through which to pour the milk into the bottles.

A Mason jar in which to keep the nipples.

It is also convenient to have a pair of tongs with which to pick up bottles when they are hot, a pair of forceps or tweezers to handle the nipples without contaminating them, and a brush with which to wash the bottles.

A saucepan, with a cover, in which to mix the formula and to use for boiling the nipples, etc. The two-quart size should be large enough.

Some of these items just duplicate ordinary household equipment, but I recommend that you keep the objects you need for preparing the formula separate and use them for nothing else. You will find that your household routine runs more smoothly if you work this way.

Before starting, be sure everything you use is absolutely clean and free from soap. Regardless of the method you use, I think it is a good idea to rinse things promptly after they have been used; for example, rinse the bottle and nipple in cold water as soon as the baby is finished with a feeding. Once a day, wash everything carefully in soap and water and rinse with very hot water until you are certain there is no soap left. It is better not to dry these things; if you do, use a *freshly laundered* towel. Put everything away in a place where it won't be touched or contaminated with dust.

To prepare the formula: measure carefully the number of ounces of (cold) water called for, and put in the two-quart saucepan. Measure the exact amount of sugar, and add it to the water; stir till dissolved. (Sugar melts more rapidly in water than in milk, and it is also easier to see whether it has dissolved completely.) Measure and add the milk, and stir a few times. That is all there is to mixing the formula. Pour it through the funnel into the bottles, which are marked so that you can put the right amount in each bottle without measuring.

(If your formula calls for evaporated milk, prepare it the same way, but take precautions in regard to the can the milk comes in, because some of the milk will undoubtedly come in contact with the outside of the can as you pour it out. Wash the can with soap and water and rinse

in very hot water; sterilize the can opener or the instrument you use to punch holes in the can.)

Put the caps or bottle covers over the bottles, leaving them loose because the contents of the bottles expand with heat. If you use rubber caps that fit on snugly, put a bit of sterile cotton or gauze under one side to keep them loose. It is possible to put the nipples on at this time, but I do not recommend it as everything is going to be heated for fifteen minutes, which would cause the nipples to deteriorate rapidly, shortening their period of usefulness. Place the rack with the bottles standing upright in it in the sterilizing pail. If there is not room in the rack for the empty orange juice and water bottle, put them in the pail as best you can. Fill the pail with enough water to cover the bottles to the level of the milk, and boil for fifteen minutes, covered.

While this is boiling, wash the saucepan in which you mixed the formula, put in the nipples, the uncovered Mason jar and its cover, and the other utensils. Cover with water and boil for five

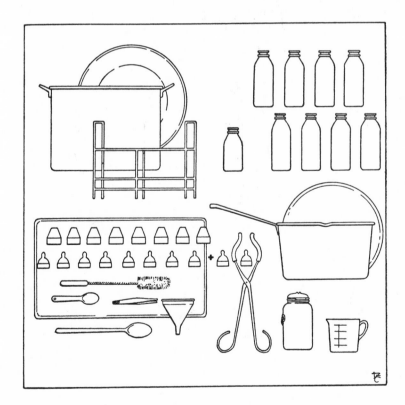

*Figure 18-7. Equipment for Formula. (See list on page 268.)*

minutes. Pour off the water carefully, fish out the tweezers and put them on the inside of the saucepan lid, or some other *clean* surface, to cool for a moment. Use them to lift out the nipples and place them in the Mason jar; cover the jar and put it away till you need the nipples. Put the other utensils away, too, handling them as little as possible.

When the water in the sterilizing pail has boiled for fifteen minutes, remove and cool the bottles as quickly as you can without cracking them. If you have unbreakable bottles, you can lift out the sterilizing rack with the tongs and place it in the sink which has cold water in it. Other bottles must be cooled more carefully, using tepid or warm water first. It will prevent skin from forming on the milk if you shake each bottle several times while it is cooling. If skin still forms, put a small piece of sterile gauze over the opening of the bottle before you put on the nipple; this will act as a strainer and prevent the nipples from clogging.

As soon as the formula is cool, put it in the refrigerator. If, in some circumstances, no refrigerator is available, or if you have any other reason to doubt that the milk has been kept cold enough to keep germs from growing, the best thing to do is to reheat each bottle before giving it to the baby. Put the bottle of formula in a saucepan containing enough water to cover the milk, and boil the water for ten minutes. Cool to body temperature before giving it to the baby.

In putting the nipple on a bottle, be sure your hands are *clean;* even so, don't touch the end of the nipple but only the part that goes over the neck of the bottle. Press the bottom of the bottle against your waist to brace it while you hold the neck of it with the nipple over it in your left hand, and pull on the nipple with the thumb and forefinger of your right hand. It may take a little practice to be able to do this easily.

If you give your baby a formula, try to make the process of feeding him as much like nursing as possible. The schedules are the same. Bottle-

*Figure 18-8. Preparing the Formula. (Described in text.)*

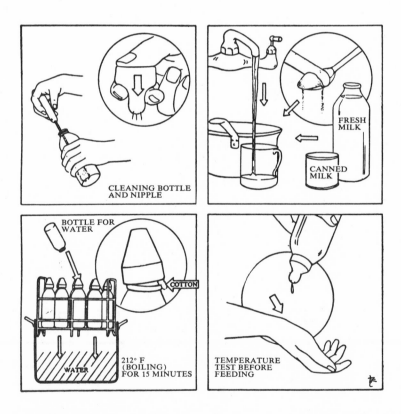

CLEANING BOTTLE AND NIPPLE

FRESH MILK

CANNED MILK

BOTTLE FOR WATER

COTTON

WATER

212° F (BOILING) FOR 15 MINUTES

TEMPERATURE TEST BEFORE FEEDING

fed babies should be "burped" in the same way as breast-fed babies.

The bottle may be warmed before the feeding, by placing it in a pan of hot water if the baby seems to prefer a warm feeding. Formula from the refrigerator may properly be offered to the baby without warming. If you do warm it, shake the bottle first, to make certain the contents are uniformly heated. Always *test* the temperature by putting some drops on your wrist; they should be comfortably warm, not hot. Hold the bottle so that its neck is always filled with milk and the baby won't be sucking in air. If it takes the baby more than twenty minutes to empty the bottle, he is probably eating too slowly because the nipple holes are too small. They can be enlarged according to directions that come with the nipples. If he takes the milk too fast, it may be because the holes are too large, and a new nipple should be prepared; or perhaps he may need to rest a minute or two while taking the bottle.

## Additional Requirements

Both breast- and bottle-fed babies need more than mother's milk or formula.

They may need *water*, depending, for example, on the amount of moisture that evaporates from their bodies. Be sure to *offer* your baby some boiled water in a sterilized bottle, but don't worry if he refuses it. This is one of the many things he knows best about. Offer it fairly frequently at first, and less often if he keeps refusing it. Don't give it before a feeding, as it may reduce his appetite.

Babies need *vitamins* (which I discuss on page 37). In order to prevent rickets, your baby should have vitamin D from the time he is about two weeks old. (Haven't you noticed how few bow-legged babies there are since they began getting vitamin D?)

In addition to vitamin D, babies require vitamins A and C. There are many excellent sources for these important nutrients. Vitamins A and D are already added to whole and evaporated milk. Vitamins A, C and D, as well as other vitamins and minerals, are usually added to the commercially prepared formulas which are in common use. Your baby's doctor may wish your child to

take vitamin supplements in the form of non-oily vitamin drop.

Orange juice is rich in vitamin C and can provide your baby with an excellent source of this vital substance. Some pediatricians prefer not to recommend orange juice for very young babies, however, because of allergic reactions that some little boys and girls develop. Your baby's doctor will guide you in this matter.

Other items of food are soon added to the baby's diet, e.g.:

| At two to four months | cereal (rice, barley, etc.), strained fruits and vegetables |
| At four to six months | soups |
| At six to seven months | egg yolk (starting with very little because some babies are allergic to it) |

After that, depending on whether or not the baby has any teeth, toast and other things to chew on are added. By the end of his first year, the baby is probably eating cereal, egg, toast, vegetable, potato, macaroni, meat, fruit and junket or other desserts—in the form of three meals a day, with additional fruit juices, crackers, and milk between meals.

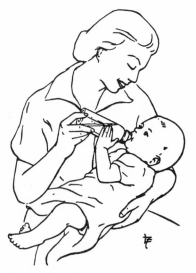

*Figure 18-9. Giving the Baby a Bottle.*

Your doctor will give you a schedule of items to add to your baby's diet. It won't matter if your baby refuses to eat them at first. In fact, the chances are that he will refuse, or throw around or spit out at least some new items. Don't get distressed. Regard these first feedings as "practice" for your baby and yourself. It is wise to introduce new foods one at a time, so that if allergic reactions develop or if the new food disagrees with your baby, you can pinpoint the cause.

## Digestive Difficulties

VOMITING. Most babies vomit (or "spit up") from time to time, usually right after being fed. In some cases the amount is enough to worry the mother, but it usually doesn't mean anything—not even if it happens daily—provided the baby is healthy and is gaining weight. As a rule, it is better to wait until the baby "asks" for food than it is to offer it to him right after he has vomited, for a surprisingly large amount usually stays down. If your baby doesn't seem well, if he vomits a large amount more often than once a day, and above all, *if he vomits with great force (projectile vomiting), be sure to consult your doctor.*

COLIC. Many babies have attacks of colic until they are about three months old. It is not always easy to tell whether a little baby has colic, although most mothers soon learn to distinguish the cry due to colic pain from one that just means the baby wants attention. A baby with colic is apt to pull up his legs and to expel gas. Putting him on his stomach and patting him may help.

Doctors do not know the exact cause of colic, but many of the things that contribute to it have been discovered. Your doctor will try to determine which of these is responsible in your baby's case, and to eliminate it. Very occasionally the baby's diet needs alteration, and often he needs more relaxation and less stimulation, as babies with a tendency to colic are often easily stimulated. Fortunately, despite his suffering (and that of his parents!) most babies, with even the most severe colic, are very healthy.

DIARRHEA. Young babies usually have between one and 10 bowel movements a day, and these are usually quite loose. This varies in different babies.

Breast-fed babies have a green-yellow stool with a bird-seed appearance. Bottle-fed babies tend to have a more pasty, moist, and yellow bowel movement. However, if the *number* of a baby's bowel movements increases a great deal and if the stools become watery and perhaps greenish, you should consult your doctor. Mild diarrhea is not serious, but it should be checked before it gets worse. (See more on diarrhea in infants and children on page 298.)

If you cannot reach your doctor, try the following:

If your baby is breast-fed, omit orange juice and other items you have added to his diet. Omit anything unusual in your own diet. Try to cut down a little on the amount he is nursing, by giving him a little boiled water just before he is put at the breast.

If your baby is bottle-fed, try one or more of the following: Dilute the formula to half its strength by adding water, or alternate formula feedings with water feedings. Brown sugar is apt to have a somewhat laxative effect, so substitute granulated white sugar if you have been using brown sugar. Omit fruit juices and other foods. In any event, if the baby continues to have diarrhea after these measures have been tried for twenty-four hours, consult your physician.

CONSTIPATION. A breast-fed baby is almost never constipated; no matter how few movements he has, they are usually soft. If he should be, it can almost always be easily corrected by giving him a *little* strained prune juice; try a teaspoonful at first, increasing the amount the next day to two teaspoonfuls if it has not been effective.

A bottle-fed baby who is really constipated (that is, whose movements are hard and not merely infrequent) should also be given prune juice. In addition, substitute brown sugar for the sugar you have been using in his formula, and avoid boiling the milk. Use a method of preparing the formula such as the one on page 269.

Don't do anything else about constipation without consulting your doctor.

## Weaning

Babies should be weaned gradually, so they won't feel that they are being deprived of anything essential. As this is easier said than done, it is important for the mother to be as calm and relaxed about the matter as she can.

Some babies are easy to wean, and will begin to drink from a cup quite happily from the time they are five to six months old. Others will want bottles until they are a year and a half old, or even older. Some babies want a bottle once a day, usually in the evening, drinking from a cup the rest of the time. Others will be weaned—and refuse to "stay weaned." *Don't* let anyone convince you that your baby is backward or stubborn because he is hard to wean. Help and encourage him as much as possible, trying to get him to take the lead. Don't force the issue or get upset by resistance and spilling. But don't be so afraid of forcing the issue that you actually encourage the baby to cling to his bottle. He will enjoy drinking from a cup, so keep at it in a calm, relaxed manner.

## Teething

On page 63 I give a schedule of the dates when a baby's teeth usually come in. In the past, any illness from which a baby suffered during the entire period that his teeth were appearing was blamed on teething. Today we know that these diseases were due to other things. Nevertheless, teething can be painful, and some babies are quite upset by it, losing their appetite or suffering from digestive disturbances. Teething may cause a slight fever, but not over 101°. You can help your baby by giving him something hard and safe to chew on—a clean rubber ring, for example (not anything that will crack or splinter, like celluloid). You can also help by comforting him if he is miserable. Your doctor will tell you if anything more can or should be done.

*Thumbsucking* and *masturbation in infants* are nothing to be disturbed about, as I explain fully on pages 281 and 282.

## YOUR BABY GROWS OLDER

The following list includes a very few of the things which the average baby does at certain ages. It is intended only to give you some idea of what you should look forward to, and for what you should be prepared.

*Sixteen weeks:* He may have begun some weeks before to smile; now the baby smiles, coos, and "plays." His eyes follow an object when it is moved in front of them.

*Twenty-eight weeks:* The baby sits up fairly well with some support. He shakes his rattle and touches it with his other hand. He rolls from his back to his stomach and moves around. He recognizes members of the family, and makes "talking" sounds.

*Forty weeks:* He sits well by himself, creeps, and often "walks" with help. He says a few "words" like "ma-ma, da-da, bye-bye."

## Accident Prevention

As soon as your baby begins to pull things and to crawl, accidents are apt to happen. I discuss them and their prevention in Chapter 22, and also on page 279. Right here I want to emphasize the fact that it is up to *you*, and not to the baby, to prevent them from happening while he is small. Be sure to "baby-proof" your house. The father should get down on the floor and look things over from the baby's angle. It is a wonderful experience in gadgeteering, I have found, to try to outwit your baby. You will soon discover where a gate should be placed to keep him out of a dangerous spot, or where a drawer containing a medicine or something else he must not put in his mouth can be shifted to a safe, high place, or a place where the paint is not safe for him to chew on, or an electric outlet must be covered so he can't play with it. Of course, keeping an eye on him is the main line of defense!

## Inoculations

On page 134 , I discuss inoculations that will prevent your baby from catching diseases that might be dangerous to him. Be sure that he has them.

Good nutrition, inoculation, the "wonder drugs" and other medicines, accident prevention—and the healthy emotional attitudes which I discuss more fully in the next chapter—make it possible today for babies to get a wonderful start in life.

## TRUST YOURSELF

Throughout this chapter I have urged you to trust your own observations and good sense, but I want to reemphasize this now.

As a new mother, you know much more than you think you do. You have probably read magazine articles on many of the aspects of bringing up baby, and maybe some books too. Your relatives and friends have been generous with advice, even when you didn't ask for it.

I know that you can take from all the articles, books, and advice what you need, and then *use it in terms of your own baby*. The loving care that you and your husband naturally give your baby is infinitely more valuable than checking the exact temperature of the bath water or knowing the "best" way to pin on a diaper. What your baby needs most of all is you. Without a mother's tender, loving care, all the right food, water, fresh air, and sunshine won't help him grow and be healthy.

Doctors can give you a lot of useful information. Only you can make it meaningful.

# 19
# OUR CHILDREN'S EMOTIONS

This chapter is not concerned solely with children. Naturally I want all children to be happy, for their own sakes. But I also want them to be happy because such children bring joy to the entire household, contributing to the happiness of all its members.

For the infant and the child himself, there is a close relationship between good health and contentment. The healthy child sleeps and eats well. That means he gets a good selection of protein, minerals, vitamins, and all the essentials to growth and development that are contained in a balanced diet. Eating and sleeping well are two "health assets" for his entire life.

The happy, well-adjusted child sticks to safety rules because he finds it easy to identify himself with his parents and other grownups. He has fewer accidents than do children whose emotional difficulties drive them to disobey rules or become daredevils.

The emotionally satisfied child is relatively free of temper tantrums, bed-wetting, stammering, tics, and other troublesome manifestations of emotional difficulties in childhood. These problems worry and upset parents, all too often resulting in a disturbed household. The resulting loss of sleep and of relaxation can decrease the father's efficency at work, or cause friction between him and the mother, or in many other ways create situations that interfere with the health and happiness of a family.

"Do our children have to become problem children in this high-tension, reckless world we live in?" *My answer is an emphatic "No."* It is true that life has become more complicated in many ways. However, it is also true that we have made great progress in learning how to bring up children.

A hundred years ago, children were regarded as inherently willful, even wicked, creatures who must be forced—by punishment, fear, and shame—into submission (and into all sorts of emotional problems at the same time). There seemed to be no alternative to this method except that of allowing children to become little tyrants, to whose whims everyone must bow.

Today we realize that children can be *guided.* This process must be a continuing one from the time the baby is born until he is ready to go out into the world. There have been tendencies, at times, to feel that some periods don't count very much in a child's emotional health, and that all one needed to do was to concentrate on the years 2 to 6, and later from 10 to 15—or on certain other periods. Such theories have been disproved. *Children, like other human beings, need love all the time.* They also need understanding during all the stages of their growth and development.

## THE "AVERAGE CHILD"

Whenever I speak about the growth and development of children, parents (especially those with a first child) ask me, "What is the average child like at this or that age? What can he do? How does he behave? How big is he, and how much does he eat and sleep?"

At *two* years of age, the average child weighs 28 pounds and is 34 to 35 inches tall. He has about 16 teeth. He sleeps about 14 to 16 hours of the 24. He has been able to walk ("holding on") since he was a year old, and by himself since he was eighteen months old; now he can run, after a fashion, as well as walk. The dozen words he could say when he was eighteen months old have increased to 200. He uses them in phrases or short sentences. He has a fair degree of bowel and bladder control in the daytime (girls do better at night than do boys).

At *three,* the child has passed through a certain amount of turmoil manifesting itself in temper tantrums, negativism, and so on, and is in a relatively stable period. He has all his "baby" teeth (20), speaks in short sentences, practically dresses and toilets himself and even "helps" around the house. His daily diet might consist of: ⅓ cup juice, ½ cup stewed or fresh fruit, ½ cup cereal, about ½ cup meat, 1 baked potato, ½ cup vegetable (cooked and raw), 1 egg, 2–3 pieces of toast, 3 teaspoonsful butter or margarine, 2 small cookies or some other dessert such as junket, and between a pint and a quart of milk.

At *five,* having passed through some additional "difficult" stages, he is in a relatively stable period. He is quite competent and independent, having reached the end of his "early childhood" and is getting ready to go out into the world of kindergarten or school. He sleeps from 11 to 12 hours a night, with a short rest or "quiet period" after lunch and occasionally a nap.

## *YOUR* CHILD

I want to make it very clear that the child I described above is "the average child." Averages are arrived at mathematically—but your child is an individual. It would be quite remarkable if he happened to be average in every detail. He's far more apt to be "above" the average in some respects, "below" it in others, and to alternate at various periods.

This may seem obvious as far as size is concerned. Everyone realizes that there are prize fighters who are perfect physical specimens in the featherweight class as well as among heavyweights. But even when it comes to size, some parents fret

because they think Sonny is too small, or Sister too big—without taking into consideration the fact that they themselves may be above or below the average in height or weight. If they themselves are of average size, they usually forget that their children have grandparents and great-grandparents, too!

It might be convenient if children followed a timetable of physical—and intellectual and emotional—development, and all parents had to do was check off the items. "Children aren't like that, and I wouldn't want them to be!" you may tell me indignantly. But do you *really* feel that way? Are you secretly a little disturbed because your child isn't "keeping up with the Jones's"? Your child will sense it if you are worrying about him.

## Growth

As far as *growth* is concerned, I think it is a good idea to record the weight and height and arrival of teeth so that your doctor will know whether the *rate* is within normal limits. Leave that up to him and don't worry about it yourself. Don't let your friends and relatives stress it unduly. Your child must not be made to feel uncomfortable about his or her physical development.

## Sleep

Provide your child with the opportunity to obtain the average amount of sleep. Of course, it won't hurt to keep him or her up once in a while on special occasions, but don't make a habit of depriving children of sleep to suit your own convenience. When I speak of giving your child the opportunity, I mean, first of all, to provide a reasonably comfortable place where he will be relatively free from being disturbed. I say *reasonably* and *relatively* because most children aren't too fussy. Your home need not be as quiet as a church; but on the other hand, few children can sleep properly if a bright light is on and if people are constantly coming in and out of their rooms or making a lot of noise. Second, and even more important, you should provide a proper *attitude* as far as sleep is concerned. How many homes do you know in which the question of getting Junior to bed is a major issue? Often getting him to bed becomes a battle, with Junior apparently determined to stay up all night, and the parents grimly or desperately struggling to win the contest.

If your child has had a good start in life, as I describe it in Chapter 18, sleep should not be a major problem, although some difficulties will undoubtedly arise at some time. If there is any trouble, don't decide your child is being bad; try to find and eliminate the cause of the difficulty. For example, your child may at some time be afraid of the dark—usually because someone, not necessarily you, has frightened him. A dim light, or the door left open just a little, "until you're old enough so you won't want it any more," will often help dispel the fear. A soft cuddly doll or teddy bear may be comforting company. Children usually go to sleep more readily if the evening meal is a simple one and they are not too stimulated at bedtime. A tapering-off period of quiet relaxation, perhaps a soothing bedtime story, is helpful. Many children like the same ritual or pattern each night. Don't put a child to bed as a punishment. Be fair and considerate; make going to bed as pleasant as possible, but also be firm about it. Some children are better "sleepers" than others; and most children sleep better at some stages than they do at others.

I remember when children's feeding problems were brought to doctors' attention more than any other. Now, sleep seems to have taken first place. Just as modern parents have learned that the child's body is a reliable self-regulator with respect to the amount of food it needs, so are they beginning to accept the fact that the amount of sleep is an individual matter. Most children go through a period of difficulty in accepting bedtime, but if you treat it calmly, as a natural and inevitable part of life, you will have gone a long way to reducing tension, and your child will be more ready to accept ending his active day.

## Eating

Similarly, eating habits often become an issue in the household. Self-regulation, which I describe on page 260, usually gets a baby off to a good start, but at some time or other most children fail to eat as well as their mothers would wish. If the mother becomes tense—sometimes even desperate

—and implores the child to eat, he may be balky in order to demonstrate his power. If she punishes him, it may make him hate the mealtime which he associates with his unhappiness. Remember, too, that your maternal urge is closely connected with the desire to feed your child. That is a good, natural—and almost overpowering—drive. But you must learn not to overdo it because then your good instinct will work harm to your child. I advise mothers to place the food before their children and remove it if they don't eat it, with the result that they are ready for it by the next meal. *But this simple method doesn't always work.* It may be necessary to use ingenuity and imagination to make certain a child is getting enough to eat.

If a child is a "poor feeder," either regularly or at certain stages of his development, the mother should calmly go about discovering the circumstances under which he eats best. Often being alone where he won't be distracted helps. Sometimes he does well with very small portions, or food that is easily chewed, or food that is easy to manipulate, or some food he likes—other foods should be gradually and tactfully added. Sometimes he prefers to be fed, even though he's old enough (by that timetable of "averages"!) to feed himself. Sometimes, especially if he is restless or overtired, it helps to read a simple story while he is eating.

In regard to eating, as well as sleeping, remember:

1. Don't worry. Children do not starve themselves. Some carefully controlled investigations have shown that even very small children who are allowed to freely choose their foods select a reasonably well balanced diet. They do not eat ice cream and candy only.

2. Feeding problems are often problems that involve something other than, or in addition to, eating. It is best to discover what they are and solve them, but if you can't, a general atmosphere of love and relaxation will help.

3. Your child is not "the average child." He may eat less or more because that is what he needs.

4. Your child grows and changes. At one time he may eat (or sleep) well; at another time, he won't. Most children eat less in hot weather, in teething periods, and during the second year of

life. During the second year there may be great variability in eating habits: some children go on "jags" and eat only meat for a week, and perhaps all potatoes the next week. Usually, their diets stay in balance if the period of the "jags" doesn't last too long.

Be sure to keep the above points in mind when you compare other phases of your child's development with those of the "average child" or of a neighbor's. Some children develop rapidly in one way, slowly in another; they may walk at the age of twelve months but say "ma-ma" quite late. They may pass through stages of slow and rapid growth. They may even develop slowly in all respects, yet "get there just the same." If you are at all concerned about your child's development, talk it over with your doctor, *not* a friend or neighbor. The doctor *knows*, the neighbor only thinks she knows.

One final note about feeding your child. If you follow the suggestions I've just given, you are likely to avoid overfeeding. Overfeeding of children, it has become apparent in recent years, causes problems. Once it was thought that chubbiness in a child was an indication of good health. But a child does not have to be chubby, and certainly not fat, in order to be healthy.

Overfeeding can lead to an obesity problem— in childhood and even later on in adulthood. Not only does overfeeding encourage a lifelong *habit* of eating too much, but there is evidence from recent studies that it causes the laying down of fat cells (adipose tissue) that remain for a lifetime. When weight is lost, the cells shrink, but still remain. At times, they may send out signals demanding to be fed. This *demand* may help explain why many people find it difficult to keep their weight down after dieting. A constant craving for food may not be wholly psychological, as many have thought; it may be at least partly based on biological demand from deprived fat cells. A lean adult may have about 27 trillion fat cells in his body; an obese person may have 77 trillion.

## Emotional Development

Studies of human emotions and how they affect our behavior have helped us doctors—and parents —understand our children's actions and attitudes better than we might have forty or fifty years ago. We know that much of what adults and children do is the result of complicated feelings, some of which we aren't even aware of. We also know enough of children's emotional growth to try to discover *why* they act in ways that seem puzzling, or inconsistent, or just plain obstinate. Since the development of reasonable behavior and good judgment comes only with growing up physically, we expect children to be governed by their feelings rather than by reason or logic. Acceptance and understanding are important aspects of *parents'* emotional development, and these are not to be confused with lack of guidance or discipline.

Glib judgments about a child's "goodness" or "badness" are useless. It is much more important to realize that a child's emotional development, along with his physical and intellectual growth, do not march smoothly down a wide highway, all in step. Quite the contrary; children are bound at times to get "ahead of themselves" in one way or another. For example, at about two and one-half they suddenly seem to become balky, contrary, tense, fearful—in short, they behave in a way that drives mother to the verge of despair. Then, perhaps quite as suddenly, they become "good" at three years old.

Of course, life is pleasanter for parents when the child is in a "good" period, but try to remember that it is pleasanter for the child, too! Periods of equilibrium are easier all around than periods of uneven development—but both are part of growth. Be sure to remember that Sally or (Sammy) is the same child at two and one-half as at three —and equally deserving of your love.

A friend of my mother's once embroidered a sampler for a daughter-in-law who was expecting her first baby. It had a border of small children in various stages of "naughtiness," and, in the middle, the words "This, too, will pass." Having brought up six fine sons and two fine daughters, it was the piece of advice she felt a young mother needed the most.

I do not want to give the impression that parents need never be concerned about their children's behavior. But I do want to emphasize the fact that difficulties are a part of growth, and that they should be regarded as a challenge to you to find ways of helping and supporting your child as he weathers the squalls. Don't be a "fair-weather" parent who loves children only when things are going well!

## Discipline

In the 1920's and 1930's, the reaction to the stern, authoritarian ways of the old European families led many American parents to an excessively permissive attitude with their children. In some homes, boys and girls were almost under no restraint at all. Now, some conscientious parents wonder if there wasn't some good in the old-fashioned tough discipline, and there are signs that the pendulum is swinging back once again.

My opinion is that neither extreme is good. Letting a child "do anything" is not good for the child. Neither should his spirit be curbed or his natural energies and curiosity squelched. Dr. Arnold Gesell, a famous specialist in children's development, calls this modern attitude *informed permissiveness.* Parents who adopt this attitude try to understand what they can reasonably expect from their children, always keeping in mind their age and basic personality. They keep their demands on their children within reason, so that they can guide them, consistently and in kindly ways, and still let them grow at their own pace and within their own limits.

I know this sounds very general, so in the following paragraphs I cite specific examples of how parents can adopt an attitude of informed permissiveness, as their children grow.

## Some Do's and Don'ts of Discipline

1. During the child's first year he is absolutely dependent for everything. I consider it unwise to put any responsibility on him for either his cleanliness or his safety. Babies and toddlers aren't willful; they're just eager to explore the world. We must help and encourage them in their courageous explorations and not frustrate them whenever they go for an appealing object. As I explain on page 273, it is up to us to protect them from danger.

2. Starting in the child's second year, he should be taught that certain things must be avoided. He must be met with a firm "No" when he plays near the stove, or climbs on a table or starts for a sharp knife. However, we must prohibit him as little as possible. In my house we did our best to move everything breakable and dangerous out of reach while our children were little. We wedged in the books, temporarily removed sharp-edged furniture, and put our one expensive lamp in the closet until company arrived! By the time the child is three, he is ready to accept a certain, definite amount of discipline as far as his own safety and that of other people—and of some objects—is concerned. He must not be permitted to run into the street, turn on the gas, pull the cloth from the table, and so on.

3. To discover whether you are demanding too much, count the number of times a day you and the other older people in the household say "No," or exert pressure in another manner. If there's a continual chorus of "No's," "Don'ts," and so on, you can be reasonably sure the discipline is too strict. Try to find ways to assume more responsibility yourself or to make it easier for your child to assume responsibility.

4. Your child doesn't "need" to be punished. When a good relationship exists between parents and children, most difficulties can be resolved without resorting to punishments. Watch how a good nursery-school teacher or camp counselor handles a number of children! The trouble is, however, that parents have other things to attend to besides their children, and a punishment is often a short-cut in their eyes. I realize that you haven't all the time in the world, and so I won't say you should never punish a child. If, for example, your firm "No" doesn't prevent him from reaching for a forbidden, dangerous object, a slap on the hand will probably stop him. In my opinion, it will in most cases cause him little more than momentary discomfort. Children have a good sense of fair play. They know when punishment has been deserved and accept it in good spirit.

Of course, you won't always do what you know you should. You will sometimes act without considering the situation carefully—perhaps because you are tired or annoyed. Don't worry about that too much. Children are resilient. Tell your child honestly that you acted unfairly because you didn't understand, and perhaps make up for it with a little treat. The child will forgive and forget the punishment.

However, punishments are usually two-edged swords, frequently causing more harm than good. It is almost impossible to find the "ideal" punishment that will accomplish what you want without causing any harm. Nagging, threatening, or shaming a child can have a very bad effect on him. Never punish him for things that are not his fault—for acting like a child instead of an adult. Most important of all, whatever disciplinary measure you take, make it clear that he has not lost your love.

## Let Children Express Their Emotions

Children express their emotions frankly, or, one might say, in undiluted fashion! They say "I love you," "I hate you," or "I'll kill him dead," when we would say, "That's nice of you," "I wish you wouldn't," or "I'd like him to go away."

Don't be shocked by this. If Johnny says "I hate you," take it in your stride, perhaps making some noncommittal remark to the effect that everyone feels like that sometimes. As soon as the child's frustration or hostility is over he will be in a loving mood again. On the other hand, if you are horrified, the child will feel guilty and repress his reactions. It is quite natural to have some feelings of hostility, even hatred. Accepting this as part of life makes it easier for children and adults to feel and express their affection and love more fully.

While children should be allowed (even encouraged) to act out and talk out their natural hostilities, they should not be allowed to hurt people physically. Children seldom know how far they should let their emotions go. We parents must show them. I think children want us to. When they go too far, they seem to welcome being restrained, perhaps by a firm word, perhaps by being removed physically from the situation.

## Toilet Training

Many parents attempt to train their children too early and too strictly—and frequently with feelings of shame and revulsion on their own part. As a result, the children may be conditioned toward being timid, unsure, worried about dirt, or ashamed of parts of their bodies. The child of a mother who takes toilet training too seriously usually discovers that he can upset or delight her by failure or success. Thus, what should be a simple physiological function to him may become a source of power or shame.

On the other hand, children who get their toilet training when they are ready for it, who are not pushed too hard, or not punished and shamed when they fail, have a better chance to realize the full potentialities of their personalities. How your child is toilet trained will not determine the kind of adult he becomes, but it may play an important part.

The most important thing to remember is that a child will, if left to himself, stop wetting and soiling when he is ready to do so. I want to urge parents to let nature take its course, with just a little guidance and encouragement. For example, the parent can make occasional suggestions about the use of the potty when the child is really ready to understand what is meant, or remind a child that it is a good idea to go to the bathroom before he becomes so engrossed in something that he won't want to take the trouble.

I disapprove of toilet training in the first year for all children, and during the second year for most children. If parents insist on attempting it early they should be prepared for many failures, especially if the child becomes ill or has an emotional upset. At such times, the parents should be completely nonchalant and willing to start over again.

We doctors often encounter parents who are so upset about the sight and smell of soiled diapers that we feel it is better if they try to train the child fairly early. But we are usually regretful, knowing that the child is being required to take on a burden the parents should be willing to carry. Talk the matter over with your doctor. If he sees that you appreciate the value of an easygoing attitude he will undoubtedly encourage it. Parents who are eager to have their children toilet trained early and perfectly, and who get tense or angry or scornful with a child who "misses" should talk to a sympathetic physician in order to discover why they take it so seriously. I predict it will do them and their children a great deal of good if they can air their own feelings. I usually find that such parents have had too strict a training themselves and, without realizing it, want to make their own youngsters submit to the same discipline.

## Thumbsucking

Thumbsucking is a perfectly harmless way in which children obtain satisfaction or reassurance. Almost all children suck their thumbs at times—when they are going to sleep, or when they are frightened or lonely. Babies also suck their thumbs (or fingers) when they are hungry and when they are teething. The best way to treat thumbsucking is to forget about it! If it is excessive—if your child sucks his thumb most of the time—*don't* start worrying about his face being distorted or his teeth and gums being injured. These things almost never happen if thumbsucking stops before the second teeth begin to appear (see page 65). But *do* think about the reasons why he requires this kind of satisfaction. A good talk with your doctor will help you discover them. Usually thumbsucking stems from the fact that the child is, in some way, being deprived of all the affection he craves—or that he needs the solace of his thumb in a situation that makes him feel tense and insecure. Babies are less likely to suck their thumb very much if they are breast-fed (which requires harder sucking than bottle-feeding), if they are bottle-fed and the holes in the nipples are not too large, if they are allowed to drink their fill, however they take their milk, and if they are allowed to grow from the breast to bottle to a cup at their own speed.

Older children who still suck their thumbs do so out of needs other than the urge to suck. They may be bored, tired, or very sleepy. They may do it when they have been scolded or are lonely or tense. Usually, children stop sucking their thumbs by the time they are four or five years old, although the habit (like many others) may persist even after the need has passed. If you are fairly certain that the habit is simply lingering on, you can generally find a way to help your child give it up. If thumbsucking is associated with twisting a blanket, you might suggest that your child cuddle a soft doll instead. But don't make an issue of it!

## Interest in Sex

Sooner or later the child will be interested in the sex organs, where babies come from, in pregnancy, and even in sexual intercourse. If his rela-tionship with his parents is a good one, he will ask questions just as freely as he asks why the grass is green. These questions may not be easy to answer, but do your best to answer them truthfully. Telling the truth is simpler in the long run. Most children don't mind having been "deceived" about Santa Claus, mainly because it was fun and because the subject was not a source of tension in their parents. Deceptions about the stork, however, are apt to create problems. It is hard for most parents to explain to a child why they told the stork story. It is much easier to answer truthfully the simple questions small children ask than it is to tackle the complicated ones they think of later on. It gets you and the child off to a good start.

Tell the truth, but not necessarily with all the details. That is usually more than the child wants or can understand. Tell it simply, without any complicated analogies about the birds and the bees.

The first thing most children want to know—often when they are as young as two years old—is where babies come from. The answer can be that they grow inside their mothers. Next, perhaps immediately but sometimes not for a while, a child is apt to ask how the baby got there. "It grew from a little seed that was there all the time," is an adequate answer. "How did the baby get out?" can be answered by, "Through a special opening that mothers have." If the child wants to know whether daddies have anything to do with it (and even if they don't ask this, it is wise to volunteer the information by the time they are three or four), say that the father's seed is needed, too.

It may be necessary to repeat all or part of this information frequently. That does not mean you should supply more facts than the child demands. Small children rarely expect any explicit information about the sexual act or the actual mechanism of birth. When they are older and do want to know, explain these matters simply and naturally in your own words. If you feel you can't do this, tell the child you will read about it to him. There are many excellent books, which your librarian will help you to locate, telling about birth in animals and human beings.

Similarly, give your child truthful answers about sex organs. Sometimes it is necessary to volunteer a little information, as children are not always able to make their curiosity or concern known to their parents. The fact that a boy has a penis and a girl does not is often a source of worry to both of them. The girl may feel deprived, and the boy may fear that something can happen to him so that he, too, will be like the girl. It often pays to take the lead and avert such problems by explaining that girls and boys are made differently because they are going to be different when they grow up—a girl is going to be a mother and a boy a father.

Although parents should avoid false modesty, most experts in child psychology advise them not to expose their naked bodies to children, even very young ones. Adults and children should not take baths together. It may disturb children to be reminded so vividly of the physical differences between themselves and their parents.

It is also important to take precautions against having children witness or hear the sexual act. Children are apt to mistake passion for violence and become frightened by seeing or listening to ardent lovemaking.

Be sure to remember that sex is *more* than reproduction. Nothing you can tell your child about the "facts of life" can be as important to him as seeing and knowing for himself what a good relationship between a man and a woman means in terms of respect, teamwork, loyalty, and tenderness.

## Masturbation

Although I speak about masturbation in various chapters of this book (see chapters on You and Your Mind, page 169, and chapter on Adolescence, page 308), I am going to discuss it here because many parents, by being upset about masturbation in small children, sow the seeds of later emotional disturbances.

Take it for granted that your child is going to masturbate. Babies play with their genitals just as they play with their toes. Unless their attention is concentrated on this area—because of an inflammation or irritation, or because of the attitude of their parents—no "bad habits" result. At various stages of their development, both boys and girls play with their own genitals, and those of other children, as a natural manifestation of curiosity. Of course, it is also a source of pleasure, but that

is no reason to worry about it. Think of it as I advised you to think of thumbsucking. When indulged in excessively, masturbation, too, indicates that the child has an emotional problem. It is a *sign*, not a *cause* of "nervousness."

I realize that it is not easy to be casual and relaxed when relatives and neighbors are horrified or upset. Just be as tactful and ingenious as you can, remembering that *your* attitude is the most important to your child. Simply ignoring masturbation if it becomes excessive is not the answer either. A child so engrossed may be having trouble making friends, or some other worries. He may also be worried about masturbating so much! If one of his parents talks it over with him openly and calmly, reassuring him that masturbation is something all children do and that in itself it is not harmful, this conversation would accomplish more than tensely ignoring the whole subject.

## Stammering, Nail Biting, Tics, and Other Habits

As I have indicated, children have periods of increased tensions in their development. These vary with the age, the home situation, and the child's temperament. They manifest themselves in various ways.

Some babies bang their heads against the crib, or rock it violently. An older child will bite his nails or make grimaces, blinking his eyes or twitching his lips. Simply trying to use the new words he is so rapidly learning may make a child stammer.

Don't increase your child's tension by nagging, scolding, or shaming him. It will simply establish the habit more firmly. Ignore these *symptoms* and try to eliminate their *cause*. Usually time will do it for you. You can help in some ways; for example, if you listen attentively to a stammering child he will relax because he doesn't have to try so hard to put his ideas across. If you play "manicuring" a child's nails you may make it easier for the biting habit to disappear. If tensions still persist, describe them fully to the child's doctor.

## The Only Child

There is no reason why an only child should be a problem unless you make him one—for example, by feeling guilty because you don't provide a little brother or sister. Be aware of the fact that children need the society of other children, and do your best to provide it as naturally and casually as possible. From the time the child is about two years old, he should occasionally have some contact with other children, if only to watch them play. As the child grows older, go to a little trouble if necessary to provide him with "part-time" brothers and sisters in the form of friends, making your house a pleasant place to visit and permitting him to visit other homes. A good nursery school can be very helpful. Make a particular effort to see to it that your child has companionship during the preadolescent period.

## Jealousy (Sibling Rivalry)

It was once assumed that having siblings—that is, sisters and brothers—automatically made every child happy. Then the pendulum went in the other direction, and we began to hear so much about sibling rivalry that it almost seemed as though every personality difficulty stemmed from the effect brothers and sisters have on one another! There is some truth in both viewpoints.

The most important thing for parents to remember is that jealousy is very painful, and that pain can have bad effects. It may take a lot of ingenuity to avoid causing any more jealousy than is necessary, but it is worth it. Of course, you can't prevent it entirely, and you certainly should not make children conceal it. But you can help your children to *overcome* it.

The first child is going to have to adjust to sharing the limelight. Make it as easy for him as you can while respecting the rights of the second child. For example, it won't hurt the new baby if you refrain from talking about him constantly in front of his older brother or sister, and it certainly won't hurt him to show you love them both.

Let your children know that they are not alike and that you would not want them to be because you love them just as they are. (This, incidentally, holds true for twins, too! I advise parents of twins not to dress them alike.) Let children know that your love is so elastic it will always "go round," with plenty of room for one more!

Love locked up in parents can't do the child much good. Both fathers and mothers should show their love. Ask yourself whether you have had time (and patience) to show your love every day. True love is realistic love, given freely without asking anything from the child. It is quite different from the kind of love which the psychiatrist Dr. John Levy calls "*smother* love." (Fathers, as well as mothers, can be guilty of smother love.) You can praise and pet a child without pampering and overprotecting him. As a doctor I prescribe *plenty* of praise, encouragement, and affection. Also, set aside a few minutes or more every day that "belong" entirely to your child, not to duties and discipline.

## The Adopted Child

An adopted child needs, even more than your own child (if that is possible), to know that you love him. Should you tell him he is adopted? By all means. I suggest that you let him know about it indirectly, by mentioning it casually and happily (but not stressing it) in his presence even before he is old enough to understand. Then, when he asks questions, answer them freely. The only difficulty I see in answering the questions of an adopted child are those concerning his real parents. Here I think it is permissible to stretch the truth a little, if necessary; for example, you can say that you are sure his own parents liked him but, for good reason (which you don't know), felt it would be better for him if they let him be your little boy—which makes you very happy.

## Special Circumstances

Children who are handicapped physically, or whose homes are upset by death or divorce, whose mother as well as father has to work, or who have illness in the family, face added difficulties. These circumstances are hard on the child—but they are also hard on the parent, and you will only make things worse if you feel guilty and apologetic about them. If you honestly feel that life is good, even though this is not the best possible situation, you will give your child an attitude that will be invaluable to him.

Be frank with your child, always remembering to keep your explanations on a level he can understand. In case of a separation, for example, you might tell a five-year-old, "We didn't get along together, so we decided to live apart. But of course we love you very much, and you'll go right on loving each of us, too, and being Daddy and Mommy's little boy." In case of death, admit frankly that you are unhappy because you miss the person who is gone, but that you have a lot to enjoy. Try to keep the child from being afraid you, too, will die—or that he will—by your matter-of-fact attitude that this is an extremely remote possibility.

Both boys and girls need a father and a mother. That doesn't mean that you should promptly remarry on that account. It does mean that you should do your best to provide a mother or father *substitute*—which can be in the form of relatives, friends, or schoolteachers, who, together, will at least partially fill the need.

### The Handicapped Child

I discuss children's diseases in Chapter 20. Here I want to speak about your attitude toward a child who is chronically ill, crippled, or physically handicapped in any way. (I discuss mental deficiency on page 199.) Such a child must not be made to feel that this handicap is everything, he is nothing. He, and his brothers and sisters, must accept it as part, but by no means the most important part, of him. Such a child should be treated naturally, without stultifying pity, anxiety, or guilt expressed by the desire to "make it all up to him." Let handicapped children know that they will be helped to help themselves, and that great progress is being made in regard to their difficulties. Adopt the attitude that there are many possibilities in life and the door is shut on only a comparatively small number of them.

Since most handicapped children will, as adults, associate with people who are not handicapped, I think it best not to "segregate" them. However, they often require different or additional schooling and special treatments, which should, in most cases, be started when they are young. Handicapped children often find encouragement in being with others like themselves for part of the time so that they don't get the feeling they are alone as far as their problems are concerned. The par-

ents of handicapped children should ask their doctor, hospital, or State Board of Education (Division of Crippled Children, Commission for the Blind, etc.) for advice and assistance. The list of organizations given on page 409 provides the names and addresses of groups devoted to various illnesses, such as epilepsy, infantile paralysis, cerebral palsy, nephrosis, and so on; they can be of invaluable assistance. Or consult the Children's Bureau, U.S. Department of Health, Education, and Welfare, Washington, D.C. 20201.

## YOUR CHILD'S EDUCATION

School plays a tremendously important part in the child's emotional as well as intellectual development. The process of growing up requires a variety of experiences that is greater than a home can provide. Adjusting to other children and to the tasks he must accomplish gives the child the practice he will need in order to live and work with others when he is adult. The very fact that he encounters children unlike himself develops his ability to discriminate. Don't worry if this ability develops slowly. At times he may adopt standards (including manners, customs, and grammar) you consider undesirable. But he has to learn how to be sociable as well as how to be himself!

A good school keeps an eye on the child's physical progress. His height and weight, general health, eyesight, and hearing are recorded, which is very useful to his regular physician. A good school is aware of the child's emotional and intellectual development, and any problems that may arise can be discovered early. The school should either supply or recommend competent assistance.

A good school is an adjunct to, not a substitute for, the home. Cooperate with your school, and with others in your community, to make it a good place for your child.

### When Should a Child Start School?

Most states provide free education for children when they are about six years old. Many of them also provide *kindergartens* which they can attend somewhat earlier.

I believe that most children between the ages of three and six will benefit from a good nursery school and kindergarten. They give children a good introduction to the world around them, and a good start in playing and being with other children and adults. They also give the mother a rest from the constant demands of her children.

It is true that children who attend nursery schools and kindergartens are apt to get more colds than if they were in contact with only one or two other children. I think that the advantages make up for this if the child is healthy, especially in the case of only children or those whose contacts would otherwise be limited.

Unfortunately there are relatively few good, inexpensive nursery schools in the country. A good nursery school is not crowded, and has a teacher who is not only well trained but whose personality is such that she can help to create a warm, loving atmosphere, with no regimentation or emphasis on "manners." If you are lucky in having a good nursery school available, by all means take advantage of it. Children as young as two and one-half to three years old can benefit from a nursery school, but they must be introduced to it tactfully and gradually. In each case, even with older children, the individual child must be considered so that he can make a satisfactory transition from home to the new world of nursery school or kindergarten.

Many mothers have formed cooperative groups and have created excellent little schools. Perhaps you can help start a good nursery school in your town or even in a rural community.

## TELEVISION

Unfortunately, it is a fact that television plays much too large a role in the lives of many children. Should children be barred from watching TV? Certainly not. There is much that is good in television programming. But a heavy diet of indiscriminate watching should be avoided. A child's emotional development, reading ability, and attention span are not helped—and there is reason to suspect they may be impaired—by long hours of passive viewing. The last thing in the world that a TV set should be allowed to become is a baby-sitter. By all means, select carefully the programs you allow your child to see and put reasonable limits on the amount of time he spends watching.

## THE ART OF PARENTHOOD

The science of child-rearing is a comparatively new one. Valuable as it is, we must never forget that being a good parent is also an art. Combine the two!

Learn as much as you can, but have confidence in yourself even if you don't know everything.

If you want further information, there are many excellent books dealing with children and their emotions. Your librarian, schoolteacher, or bookseller will have suggestions. Or you might send a card to the Children's Bureau, U.S. Department of Health, Education, and Welfare, Washington, D.C. 20201, mentioning the particular subject in which you are interested.

Don't be reluctant or ashamed to seek advice on any problem that troubles you. A talk with the schoolteacher, school physician, your own doctor, or a pediatrician may enable you to work out the difficulty almost by yourself! If not, get in touch with an expert in this field, through your doctor, school, hospital, local Child Guidance Clinic, or other community resource concerned with children.

Wise parents seek help, realizing that the majority of the problems found in their children are due to their own mistakes, or may arise merely from lack of information and confidence.

## "THE HAPPIEST TIME OF YOUR LIFE"

Don't tell children, "Childhood is the happiest time of your life." Like all the rest of us they are entitled to look forward pleasurably to all periods of life (including old age)! On the other hand don't make them feel that childhood is a painful but necessary prelude to real living. Each period of life is good in itself as well as for what it leads to.

One final bit of advice: Love your children as they are, and for what they are. They differ in temperament and abilities—and who are we to say one kind of person is better than another? Don't expect or even want them to be *different* from what they are, but help them to be the *best* of their "types." If you succeed, even partially, their childhood and their future will indeed be happy.

# 20

# FEVERS AND OTHER SICKNESSES OF INFANTS AND CHILDREN

Infants cannot tell us that they are sick. Small children younger than about three years old should not be relied on too definitely for an announcement of symptoms of illness. Even older children may become so frightened, or so drowsy from the particular illness, that they do not tell us early enough that they do not feel well. It is the responsibility of parents, and those who take care of children at school and in child care centers, to learn to recognize the sick child by certain changes in the young one's behavior and appearance.

Early recognition of the sick child means a better chance of (a) reducing the seriousness of the disease itself, (b) eliminating complications, and (c) sometimes preventing fatal consequences. For example, an infant developed a fever and ate poorly. It also had a severe cough. The mother did not realize that the child was developing a serious illness, *pneumonia*, which had already caused severe inflammation of the lungs. By the time the doctor was called several days too late, the child was almost dead of the infection in the lungs and the dehydration which had complicated the pneumonia. Fortunately, the doctor was able to save the baby by intensive treatment at a hospital. The child would have responded to treatment promptly if the mother had recognized the signs of illness early enough. And the near-fatal complications would not have set in.

*What are the signs of illness in babies and young children?* Do not rely completely on a list of symptoms and signs of disease. Get to know the child. Usually, a mother or teacher can tell as soon as a doctor that a child is not feeling right. She senses

that he is *not eating well* or is unusually *irritable*. Or she may notice that the expected spitting-up milk has turned into true *vomiting*. The mother may notice that the child is *drowsy* at a time of the day when he is usually very alert. Also, the child's mother knows his cry. There are the cries of hunger, of loneliness, and of fright from strange sounds; these are very different from the *cry that accompanies pain*. There may be some obvious explanation for the pain cry, such as an open safety pin in the diaper. It is more likely to be caused by abdominal colic, which is very frequent in infants. If the pained type of crying continues, take the child's temperature. If the temperature is elevated, notify your doctor. Even if the temperature is normal, and the crying does not subside in the next hour, it is best to tell your doctor about it.

Severe *diarrhea* is another sign of illness, as is also the appearance of *bloody or black bowel movements*.

*Unconsciousness, stiff neck,* and *convulsions* are all such important signs of potentially serious illness that your doctor should be told of them at once. If he is not available, take the child to your doctor's hospital, and have the interns or resident start the treatment until your doctor can be located.

*Cough* is more unusual in infants than adults, and therefore is an important sign of illness.

*Difficult, rapid or labored breathing* is also a potentially serious symptom.

*Hoarseness* or a hoarse quality to a baby's cry may be the sign of impending croup and should always be reported to the doctor.

When babies and small children get sick, their

286

illness usually shows itself quickly with *fever.* The best way to make sure that a child really has a fever is to take his temperature. When babies are even moderately sick, temperatures will often rise very high. A fever of 102 to 104 degrees in a child may not mean serious illness. In a sick adult such a fever would generally be much more important.

## THE THERMOMETER

There are two kinds of thermometers, the oral and the rectal. Except for the shape of the bulb there is no really important difference between them. The oral (mouth) thermometer has a long, slender bulb which can be held securely under the tongue. The rectal thermometer has a shorter and rounder bulb which will not hurt the rectum. I suggest that you purchase two rectal thermometers, as this type can be used in either the mouth or rectum and is less breakable. Keep them in separate containers marked "mouth use only" and "rectal use only."

Most thermometers for home use are in Fahrenheit degrees. These degrees are marked off in short lines and long lines. The first long line is numbered 94°. Because of lack of space every other degree is numbered, so that the numbers read 94°, 96°, 98°, 100°, 102°, 104°, 106°, 108°. Between each long degree line there are four short lines which divide the degrees into two-tenths.

The thermometer bulb is filled with mercury which spreads through the tube when the temperature rises. In reading the thermometer always hold the end opposite the bulb. Turn the glass between your fingers until you see a silvery bar that marks the top of the mercury. At whatever degree the mercury stops, that is the temperature. For example, if the mercury stops at the first short line after the degree marked 100, then the temperature reading is 100.2° because, as you remember, each short line is two-tenths.

At one place on the thermometer, a little above 98° there is an arrow which points to 98.6°. This is considered to be the "normal" temperature. The "normal" is three lines above 98 degrees. Above this point, most thermometers continue the markings in red.

## HOW TO TAKE TEMPERATURE

It is better to take a baby's temperature by rectum than by mouth because it is more accurate. Mouth temperatures are difficult to take in a baby because the mouth has to be closed for at least a minute before the mercury can register. It is very hard to keep the baby's mouth shut. Besides, he might bite the thermometer. Until the child is four to six years old it is safer and more reliable to take rectal temperatures.

If you have to report the child's temperature to the doctor, tell him whether you took a rectal or an oral reading because the rectal temperature will be slightly higher, about half a degree, or about 0.5°, and the axillary (armpit) temperature, described in the following section, correspondingly lower.

Before taking the temperature, hold the thermometer tightly on the glass end, not the silvered, and shake it with a strong twist of your wrist, until the mercury is down near the 97° mark. Shake the thermometer down over a bed or a pillow so that it won't break if it should slip from your fingers. Then cover the bulb with petroleum jelly, K-Y jelly, or cold cream so that it can be slipped in easily and painlessly.

For an infant, the best way to insert the thermometer is to place him on his abdomen across your knees. Ever so gently, push the thermometer into his rectum. Don't jab it in; go as lightly as possible. Then hold it in place between two fingers with your palm flat across the buttocks. Never let go of the thermometer. It would be best to leave the thermometer in about two minutes, but if the baby is fretful and struggles, a minute will be good enough. When the child is a little older, you can take his temperature by having him lie in bed on his side with his knees drawn up just a bit.

### Axillary Temperature

Sometimes it is too upsetting for an infant or young child to have the temperature taken by rectum. In fact, no child who is critically sick should be made to struggle unnecessarily. In such instances, rather than do the child harm, you should take the temperature by the axillary (armpit) method.

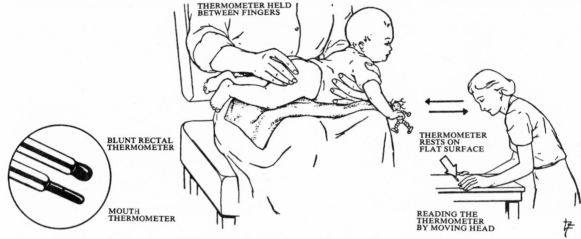

*Figure 20-1. Taking the Rectal Temperature.*

Use the thick-walled, "rectal" type thermometer. Place the silvered bulb end in the deepest part of the armpit. The armpit is then closed tightly against the chest, and kept closed over the thermometer for five minutes, as actually timed by a clock.

Be sure your doctor knows you are reporting the axillary temperature, not a rectal or mouth reading. Also, your doctor will want to know how long you kept the thermometer in the armpit.

### Mouth Temperature

When the child is ready to hold a thermometer in the mouth, take oral temperatures in preference to rectal or axillary (unless your doctor specifically requests the other method). It is important that you don't take an oral temperature right after the child has eaten or drunk anything hot or cold. Keep the thermometer in the mouth for five minutes, unless you are employing the rapid-reading type which only requires a minute. Even with the latter, it is still best to reinsert, and check the reading after another minute to make sure that the maximum temperature had been reached.

## WHAT THE CHILD'S TEMPERATURE MEANS

Don't worry if your child's temperature reading is either a little above or a little below the "normal" 98.6° marking. Even in healthy adults the temperature may vary from the "normal." Another thing to realize is that for everybody, children and adults, the temperature is lowest in the very early morning and highest in the late afternoon, so that at four in the morning the temperature reading on the thermometer will be a bit lower than it will be at four in the afternoon. Immediately after running or any violent exercise, the temperature of small children may rise even to 100° with no sign of illness. Therefore, it is best to take the temperature after the child has calmed down and rested. But if the temperature is as high as 101° even after exercise, the youngster is definitely sick and the doctor should be called.

A cold or anything more serious will cause a fever. If your baby or child has a temperature of 99° to 101° and *no other symptoms*, such as vomiting or a rash, you can wait before calling the doctor. Take the temperature every three hours. If it rises above 101°, notify the doctor. If it falls to normal, there is nothing to be concerned about. If a slight fever of 99.5° to 101° lasts more than a day, notify your doctor. Always record the temperatures and the time when taken, for your doctor.

## A WARNING ABOUT MEDICINES

In this chapter and elsewhere throughout the book I mention medicines that are helpful for various illnesses. There is a natural temptation to try penicillin or sulfa tablets, antihistamines, and other medicines which you may have available at home. Medicines may have been left over from a previous illness. Never treat your child or yourself without the doctor's advice. Even such a valuable medicine as penicillin may cause allergic reactions. Or by giving it before the doctor has seen the child, you may interfere with his diagnosis. Laxatives, cathartics, and enemas can be harmful. They too should be given only with the advice of a doctor.

## ACCIDENTS IN CHILDREN

The leading cause of death in the age group up to fourteen years is accidents. Household accidents such as burns, falls, and poisoning by common household substances head the list. Elsewhere in this book I tell in detail about accident prevention, and the first aid measures to be employed for them (see Chapters 22 and 23). Let me emphasize here that it has been estimated that two-thirds of the deaths by poisoning in children would be eliminated if *aspirin, sleeping pills,* and *kerosene* were kept in safe places (if you have children at home please check *now* with respect to these and other hazardous substances).

## COLDS

You may as well become resigned to the fact that your child will catch cold. Children are usually more susceptible to colds than adults. It isn't the cold itself that you have to worry about, but what a cold may lead to if not completely cured. Serious illnesses can start from a simple cold, and every mother should be on her guard to prevent the complications.

There are many things you can do to reduce the frequency of a child's colds. He should not be allowed to get overtired or chilled. However, you will make a mistake if you put too much clothing on him and keep him indoors in an overheated room. All children, except very young babies, should be outdoors for several hours a day in good weather so that their bodies can get used to the colder air. The room they sleep in should have a temperature of about 70°. (See page 14 on control of temperature and humidity.)

A well-balanced diet may help a child resist the complications of colds, but unfortunately, will never prevent colds. That is, a child who is poorly nourished will get sick oftener than a well-fed one, but the well-fed child will still catch colds.

Even the healthiest child will catch cold faster than a healthy adult, so try to keep him away from other people with colds. If Aunt Grace is offended because you won't let her kiss darling little Bobby while she has a cold, don't let it bother you. Aunt Grace will get over it; Bobby might not so easily.

The mother is usually in closer contact with her child than anyone else. If she has a cold or any other kind of infectious disease, she should mention it at once to the baby's doctor and ask him about the need for special precautions. Wash your hands often with soap and water and once again before handling the baby.

If your child is under two years and has a cold, make sure he is put to bed and kept warm in every part of his body. With older children it is not necessary to confine them in bed unless they are feverish. See to it that the room is free of drafts. You can get ventilation by opening the window in another room.

A most important thing you can do for your sick child with a fever is to give him adequate amounts of fluid. Encourage him to drink small quantities frequently. The reason for this is that the child loses body fluids because the fever makes him perspire. Sick children often become quite "dried out," which lowers their resistance to germs still more. To prevent dehydration give a sufficient volume of liquids so that the child will urinate normal amounts. An adequate urine output will be indicated by a light yellow color instead of a dark brownish color which usually signifies insufficient fluid. In addition to milk and water, try fruit juices and carbonated drinks; grapefruit and melons are a good source of extra fluid.

In Chapter 25, Nursing in the Home, there are many suggestions for the care of a sick child. Be sure to read that chapter if your child becomes ill.

If you think you should give your child nose

drops, ask your doctor first. Nose drops and anti-histamine pills do not cure colds, but just suppress the symptoms. Some people find antihistamine drugs less satisfactory than nose drops for ordinary colds. For allergies, however, the antihistamines are useful. But always let your doctor decide whether he wants to prescribe any medicine and what kind it should be.

There are two simple measures you can employ to relieve a mucus-plugged nose in an infant. First, loosen the mucus by putting in the nostrils a few drops of sterile saline solution (add a teaspoonful of salt to a pint of boiling water, and then cool to body temperature). Next, after a few minutes, suck out the mucus with a rubber-tipped bulb. Second, try increasing the humidity of the air that the infant breathes. An electric humidifier is a worthwhile investment, because you will certainly need it during the cold season every year for all your children. A fair substitute is to keep one or more pans of hot water on a hot radiator. Although I don't expect you to keep a humidifier running all winter long, I want to point out that very dry rooms are more conducive to colds than more humid ones.

There are no drugs that *cure* colds, although several do relieve the symptoms. Bed rest is the best way to make your child comfortable, although he will begin to rebel as soon as he feels a little better.

The most important thing to know about a cold is that its virus paves the way for other germs called "secondary invaders." These are ones like influenza viruses and pneumococcal and especially streptococcal bacteria.

## STREPTOCOCCAL INFECTIONS

The streptococcal germ can do much harm, causing sore throats, tonsillitis, sinusitis, middle ear infection, and indirectly rheumatic fever and nephritis (kidney disease). Rheumatic fever or nephritis may follow a week or so after a streptococcal infection. This does not mean that most, or even many, streptococcal infections will be followed by these illnesses. However, by guarding against streptococcal infections, the chances of getting these more serious diseases will be lessened.

The first step in protecting your child against the streptococcus is to follow the general measures already outlined for preventing colds. Also, see Chapter 7 (p. 131) on Keeping the Germs Away. Colds set the stage for streptococcal infections, which are usually spread in much the same way as colds.

A fever that develops when a cold seems to be subsiding suggests a potentially serious complication until proved otherwise by the doctor. Some of the complications are described below.

Quick treatment by the doctor will promptly suppress streptococcal infection and will almost always prevent its complications.

## SORE THROATS, SWOLLEN GLANDS IN THE NECK, TONSILLITIS, SINUSITIS, AND MIDDLE EAR INFECTIONS

These may also be caused by the streptococcus, although most sore throats, swollen glands, and severe upper respiratory infections in childhood are caused by viruses. *Tonsillitis* produces a high fever which lasts several days. The child may vomit and have headaches. His throat may become so sore that he can barely swallow. A doctor is needed to treat this sickness.

The tonsils are situated at the back of the mouth and are made up of *lymphoid tissue*. They are like the *lymph glands* and have the same purpose, to waylay and destroy germs. Yet sometimes these glands get overloaded by a heavy invasion of germs and cannot do the job properly. So instead of destroying the germs, the tonsils become overwhelmed by germs and are themselves infected.

SHOULD TONSILS BE REMOVED? In years past tonsils were removed almost routinely. Now doctors feel that they should not be taken out except when there is a good medical reason for the operation. The removal of tonsils will not decrease the frequency of respiratory infections and is not recommended for that purpose.

ADENOIDS. These may be considered to be small "tonsils" located in the part of the throat behind the nasal passages. When they enlarge they can block the outlet from the nose so much that the affected child breathes chiefly through the mouth. Also, the enlarged adenoids may block the eustachian tubes, which connect the middle part of the ears with the back of the throat. This condition may cause pain in the ears or a sense of pressure. It also can cause infections in the middle ear, and occasionally interference with hearing.

Adenoids are ordinarily removed along with enlarged tonsils. Occasionally, only the adenoids are removed.

Recurrent middle ear infections and hearing loss associated with enlarged adenoids are conditions treated by the removal of the adenoids.

MIDDLE EAR INFECTIONS. The illustration on page 111 shows the eustachian tube that leads into the middle part of the ear. Through this highway, germs can travel from colds, sore throats, infected adenoids, and tonsils. Middle ear infections are usually terribly painful, and even a young child will point with distress toward his ear as the area where he knows something is wrong. A discharge from the ear is occasionally the first sign. Fever, vomiting, headaches, and drowsiness may accompany middle ear infections. A doctor should be notified at once, or the child taken to the hospital if the doctor is not available. As you can see from the illustration (p. 111), the middle ear contains important parts of the hearing apparatus. Also, because it connects with the mastoid cells the infected middle ear can lead to the complication of *mastoid bone infection*. Also, the brain is not far from the middle ear. Neglected middle ear and mastoid infections have sometimes led to devastating infections of the brain. Before the introduction of sulfa medicines and the antibiotics, middle ear infections and their complications were very serious and frequent illnesses. Now, if a doctor is notified early enough, he can stop these infections by the use of the antibiotics. It is rare, indeed, for infected ears to require incision of the eardrum to drain the pus, an operation that at one time was one of the most frequent in pediatrics. Also, mastoid operations have become a rarity. When I was a medical student, mastoid surgery was frequent enough so that some surgeons made it their major specialty.

SINUSITIS. The sinuses are air-filled cavities in the bones around the nose. They help give our voices a pleasant resonance. Also, the sinuses make the skull weigh less by replacing bone with air. Unfortunately they are very subject to infections, although less so in children than in adults. A tiny opening connects each sinus with the inside of the nose. During a cold, the infection may spread to the sinuses which will get clogged up with pus. The pus drips out from the back of the nose into the throat, causing the "postnasal drip." This drip may cause the child to cough when he lies down. In a more severe case of sinusitis, the child will have fever and headache. Redness and swelling of the inner parts of the eyelids, the portions near the nose, may be signs of a serious form of sinusitis (ethmoiditis). There are many things the doctor can do to relieve sinusitis, such as using antibiotics and other medicines.

## SCARLET FEVER

This is a streptococcal infection in which the streptococcus happens to make a special kind of poison (scarlet fever toxin) which causes a scarlet-colored rash. In other words, not all streptococcal germs can cause scarlet fever. Not everyone is susceptible to the rash-producing poison.

This is what might happen if such a streptococcal infection occurs in a family of three children: one child may get a scarlet fever because he cannot resist the poison; a second youngster may develop only the streptococcus sore throat; and the third may carry the germ without being at all sick but may be able to pass it on to others.

At the beginning of scarlet fever, the child feels tired, restless, and irritable. Then he develops a fever and a sore throat, and begins to vomit. The skin feels hot and dry. After a day or so, bright red spots break out, starting in the body creases such as the armpits. The rash spreads to the neck, the chest, and the back. It may later cover the entire body and from a distance look like a uniform coat of redness, except for the skin around the mouth which stays pale. But the tongue will become inflamed too, a blazing bright red ("strawberry tongue"). After about two weeks, peeling of the skin

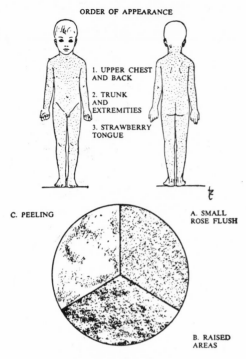

ORDER OF APPEARANCE

1. UPPER CHEST AND BACK

2. TRUNK AND EXTREMITIES

3. STRAWBERRY TONGUE

C. PEELING

A. SMALL ROSE FLUSH

B. RAISED AREAS

*Figure 20-2. Scarlet Fever.*

occurs, beginning either where the rash started or with the thinnest skin and ending in areas where the skin is thickest, like the palms of the hands or soles of the feet.

An antibiotic such as penicillin may not only shorten the course of scarlet fever but also help to prevent complications like ear infections, swollen neck glands, and nephritis. Fever can be controlled by tepid water sponge baths (aspirin for older patients). Prompt medical care can make this a benign disease.

Not only have newer treatments reduced the danger of scarlet fever but the disease itself has become less severe in recent years for reasons that scientists do not yet understand. For both these reasons, the complications that may follow scarlet fever are much less common than they used to be, and the disease no longer holds its old dread, although it is still not to be taken lightly.

## RHEUMATIC FEVER

This serious disease most often afflicts children between five and fifteen years old. It is responsible for heart disease in 2 percent of all American schoolchildren.

It should be understood that rheumatic fever is a specific disease. This is somewhat confusing to a lot of people because the word "rheumatic" has been used to describe almost any affliction of the joints in older persons as well as muscle cramps or backache.

Rheumatic fever usually follows a streptococcal infection—but not immediately. The patient has a sore throat and fever for several days, recovers, feels well for one or two weeks, then suddenly develops rheumatic fever.

It is believed that the strep germ itself does not cause the rheumatic fever. Instead, as the germ multiplies in the nose and throat, products are formed which are absorbed into the body. Some people have a reaction to these products similar to an allergy. And it is this allergic reaction which causes inflammation of the joints. The interval between the sore throat and the onset of rheumatic fever is the length of time it takes the body to develop the allergic reaction.

Rheumatic fever may produce painful, hot swelling in one or several joints; the knees, wrists, and elbows are most often involved. The attack may start in one or two joints, and then an additional joint may become involved every few days. As the new joints are affected, those that were first inflamed start to improve. For all of the joints, the pain in time will disappear.

In younger children, rheumatic fever symptoms sometimes may be deceptively mild. Instead of red, swollen painful joints, there may be only vague aching in the arms and legs.

Sometimes the sole indication of rheumatic fever is *Saint Vitus's dance*. The first sign of Saint Vitus's dance is often clumsiness; the child may spill food and drop things. When Saint Vitus's dance becomes more severe, the child may be unable to control muscles of the face, tongue, arms or legs, and may twist and jerk. But this affliction is only temporary for rheumatic fever victims.

THE HEART COMPLICATION. It has been said that rheumatic fever "licks the joints but bites the heart." Because the joint pains, involuntary movements, and other symptoms almost invariably disappear, rheumatic fever might be considered an uncomfortable but not particularly important disease—except for one thing. It can also inflame one or more valves of the heart—valves that are designed to open, let blood through, and then close to prevent backflow. Inflammation from rheumatic fever can distort a valve. Though healing follows the inflammation, the scar tissue that forms may interfere with valve function.

After a first attack of rheumatic fever, 10 to 20 percent of children have some heart-valve damage, but often it is minor. The outlook for them—and for those who escape heart damage completely—is excellent if repeated attacks are prevented, and they can be.

TREATMENT OF RHEUMATIC FEVER. Immediate bed rest and antibiotic medication are essential. So, too, a well-balanced diet. Other medications may be prescribed. Your doctor will have specific advice about how long the child should remain in bed and thereafter how progressively he may return to various activities. Some physicians now believe in allowing the child to govern the amount of activity he can safely tolerate, although it may be necessary to limit the overeager and encourage the undereager child.

PREVENTING RECURRENCES. A child who has had an episode of rheumatic fever must not be allowed to have additional streptococcal infections. After a first attack of the fever, susceptibility is increased. The younger a child when a first attack occurs, the more likely recurrences are unless precautions are taken. Without precautions, recurrences develop in as many as 90 percent of patients who have had an initial attack before the age of ten. Moreover, if the heart was not affected in the first attack, it may be in subsequent attacks; and if there was damage in the initial attack, repeated episodes may add to it. But the longer a child is well after an attack, the better his chance of avoiding a recurrence.

For these reasons, continuous preventive treatment against strep infections is vitally important. Oral penicillin, long-acting penicillin by injection, or sulfa drugs may be used. All are effective. The value of such treatment is clear. Studies have

shown that where once as many as 75 percent of rheumatic fever patients had recurrences, now, with regular preventive treatment, the recurrence rate is down to 3 percent and may go lower.

How long must prophylaxis be maintained? The risk of strep infection is present throughout life. Rheumatic fever itself tends to be more recurrent during youth, with attacks less frequent after about age thirty. But the safest procedure is to continue prophylaxis indefinitely, especially if there has been damage to the heart. Some physicians may make exceptions in adults, especially those who have no heart problem and have had no rheumatic fever recurrences for many years.

PREVENTING THE FIRST RHEUMATIC FEVER ATTACK. Streptococcal infections are common but can be treated effectively. If the strep bacteria are destroyed by antibiotic treatment before allergic reaction develops, there is little likelihood of rheumatic fever. In fact, there is evidence that even when antibiotic treatment is started as late as a week (or even a few days more) after onset of a strep infection, rheumatic fever may be prevented.

The problem is how to recognize a strep throat. Not every sore throat is a strep throat. The likelihood is that a child does not have a strep infection if his only complaint is hoarseness or a cough. However, a child can have a strep infection without having a sore throat—and that complicates the problem.

The American Heart Association recommends certain procedures for you to follow to make certain you are doing all you can to protect your child from rheumatic fever. If your child gets a sore throat and has any of the indications suggested in the following seven questions, phone your doctor at once and be ready to give him the answer to all the questions:

1. Did the sore throat come on suddenly?
2. Does your child complain that his throat hurts most when he swallows?
3. Does it hurt him under the angle of his jaw when you press gently with your fingers? And are the glands in his neck swollen?
4. Does he have a fever? How much? (Usually a strep infection brings a fever of 101° to 104°.)

5. Does your child complain of headache?
6. Is he nauseated? Has he vomited?
7. Has he been in contact with anyone who has had a sore throat or scarlet fever? (Any child who has been exposed to scarlet fever should see his doctor for preventive treatment even if he does not have a sore throat.)

Given the answers to these questions, your physician will be helped to decide if he should examine your child for a possible strep infection.

## WHOOPING COUGH

Whooping cough starts like an ordinary cold, with running nose and perhaps a little dry cough. Sometimes hours, days, or even weeks go by and nothing further seems to happen. The mother thinks her child is cured and sends him back to school. But then things begin to happen. He feels chilled; he begins to vomit; his temperature rises and the coughing spells become longer. Soon he is coughing a great deal, about eight to ten times without catching his breath. When he finally does, it is with a long noisy intake of breath, which is where the whoop comes in. If you keep in mind the important fact that *this* cough does not appear until about the second week, you won't be unduly alarmed when your child has a cough right after he catches cold.

The three main signs of whooping cough are (1) the long spells of coughing, at night as well as during the day, (2) the whoop, and (3) vomiting. The average case of whooping cough lasts for about six weeks, "two weeks coming, two weeks running, and two weeks going away." In deciding whether or not a cough which has gone on for a long time is whooping cough, the doctor may need to do some laboratory tests.

Whooping cough is a dangerous disease, especially for infants. It can be a killer because it paves the way for pneumonia.

During the first two weeks, whooping cough is very contagious. Be very careful to see that it is not spread to other children. Temporary protection to exposed children or adults in the household who have not been previously immunized against whooping cough is produced by giving a special type of gamma globulin. A booster dose of immunizing vaccine can be given to those previously immunized.

Most cases are mild enough to be cared for in the home. Severe cases, especially in infants, require hospital care. General treatment involves bed rest. The room should be well ventilated, and those conditions that provoke coughing spells, like smoke, dust, activity, or sudden changes in temperature, should be avoided. Small, frequent feedings help. Be sure to call your doctor when you suspect whooping cough, and have him follow the illness until complete recovery is assured.

Remember, whooping cough can be prevented by immunization in early infancy (see page 134).

## MEASLES (RUBEOLA)

Measles is a very contagious disease caused by a virus. The disease starts with the same symptoms as a cold—the youngster will run a fever, sneeze, and cough. His eyes are sensitive to light, become pink from inflammation. His eyes and face look puffy. All these changes give the "measly" look. After a few days a rash appears, very characteristic of measles. These spots are pink and may show up first behind the ears, on the forehead or the cheeks, and then spread downward. Usually, the spots itch when the fever is at its highest point. The rash begins to fade after two or three days. By then, the child feels much better.

Recent developments in medicine have destroyed two old ideas about measles—one, that it is a mild disease, and two, that every child should get it and be done with it. Complications such as ear infections and pneumonia are possible after measles. It can also result in permanent brain damage, and may even be fatal, although these extremes are rare. Since 1963, measles vaccine has been available, and millions of infants and children are immunized every year. The vaccine is believed to give lifelong immunity.

Ordinary measles may pave the way for an invasion by other germs. Only the minimum number of people who are required for the care of the child should be allowed in his room. Adults may infect the child with the germs of other diseases. The child with measles should be kept in bed and given plenty of fluids. If light bothers the sick child's eyes, protect them with an eye shade or visor, and, of course, avoid glare. Then sensitivity to light (photophobia) will clear up completely without any effects on the eyes.

## GERMAN MEASLES (RUBELLA)

Like ordinary measles, German measles is also caused by a virus. It begins with a slight cold, a little fever, and a sore throat. Then the rash comes in the form of rosy colored spots that quickly spread over the entire body. At first, the rash looks like a measles rash, then like scarlet fever. The lymph glands behind the ear and in the neck swell up. The rash lasts about two days.

German measles is usually a mild disease, without complications, in children. The real threat is when an adult woman catches it during the first three months of pregnancy. In such a case there is a serious danger that the child will be born deformed. If a pregnant woman—especially in the early months of pregnancy—who has not had German measles is exposed to someone who has the disease, this becomes an emergency, and she should notify her family doctor or obstetrician at once. He may advise immediate injections of gamma globulin in the hope that it might increase her resistance to the disease. The pregnant woman exposed during her first three months to German measles should consult her obstetrician and discuss the possibility of a legal abortion, if this is consistent with her religious and personal beliefs. Therefore, pregnant women who have never had the disease should avoid any contact with children who have German measles. Rubella vaccine should be given to all young girls well before childbearing age. An adult woman who receives it must wait at least two months before becoming pregnant. The vaccine is usually given to children in a combined dose with measles vaccine.

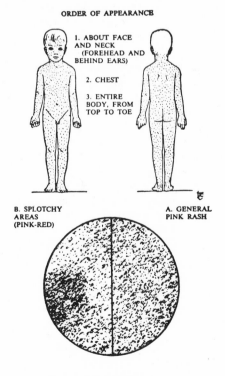

Figure 20-3. Measles.

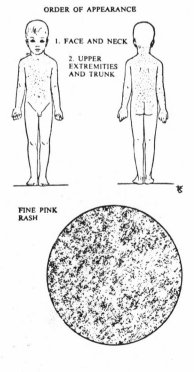

Figure 20-4. German Measles.

*Figure 20-5. Mumps.* LEFT: *Characteristic swelling due to the mumps.* RIGHT: *A healthy child, showing the location of the glands involved.*

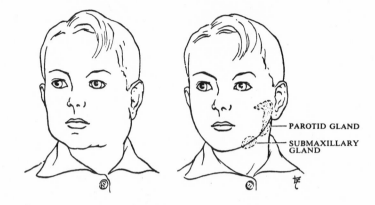

PAROTID GLAND

SUBMAXILLARY GLAND

## MUMPS

Mumps is a contagious childhood disease caused by a virus. The parotid gland beneath the ear which secretes saliva swells up, first on one side of the face and then sometimes on the other side. Less often, the virus attacks other salivary glands under the jaw. Other glands of the body are rarely infected.

In adult males, mumps can be a painful illness because it can attack the testicles. Painful though it may be, mumps involving the testicles very rarely results in sterility or impotence. The fear many people have that mumps may affect them in that way is unwarranted. Nevertheless, if the father or any other young male in the household has not had mumps, he should consult his doctor regarding protective measures. If mumps vaccine is given in time, it can usually prevent the illness. Second attacks of mumps are possible, but the first occurrence almost always gives lifelong immunity.

Call the doctor to make sure the sickness is mumps and not some other disease that may imitate it. For example, an infection of lymph glands by bacteria may look like mumps, but the treatment is quite different. Mumps is treated by rest in bed until the fever and swelling have cleared.

## CHICKENPOX

This is a virus disease. Chickenpox and measles are the most highly contagious and therefore the most common diseases of childhood.

Chickenpox is usually contracted by direct contact with someone who has it or by droplet from the nose or mouth.

First, pimples break out, usually beginning on the chest. Then the pimples become blisters which dry into scabs. The blisters come in a series of breakouts, one after another. The main danger lies in the fact that the blisters itch, and they may become infected by scratching. To ease the child's itching, place him in a cold starch bath. There should be two handfuls of starch in the tub. Because you will be unable to prevent a certain amount of scratching, keep your child's hands clean by washing them several times a day, and keep his nails cut short. The scabs are not infectious.

Call the doctor if the child appears really sick or has a fever. This is mainly a precaution to rule out smallpox or other serious diseases. Most cases of chickenpox are mild and require no special treatment except bed rest and plenty of fluids during the feverish stage. The child should stay in bed during the acute period of chickenpox and away from other children until about a week after the blisters first appear. Once the scabs are gone, it is not necessary to isolate him.

## ROSEOLA INFANTUM

Roseola infantum, or exanthem subitum, is a fairly common fever occurring in children during the first three years of their lives. It is always worth considering when the child has a fever, is irritable and drowsy, and doesn't have any other diagnostic signs such as a rash. In roseola infantum, a strange

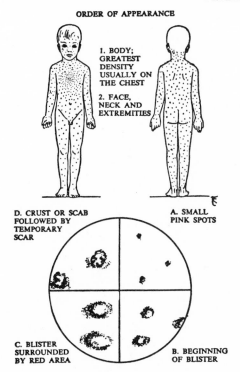

ORDER OF APPEARANCE

1. BODY; GREATEST DENSITY USUALLY ON THE CHEST

2. FACE, NECK AND EXTREMITIES

D. CRUST OR SCAB FOLLOWED BY TEMPORARY SCAR

A. SMALL PINK SPOTS

C. BLISTER SURROUNDED BY RED AREA

B. BEGINNING OF BLISTER

*Figure 20-6. Chickenpox.*

situation exists as contrasted with most childhood diseases with rashes. When the flat, reddish rash of roseola infantum finally appears after three or four days of the fever, the disease is ended, and the fever and other symptoms quickly disappear. With illnesses such as measles, scarlet fever, and chicken pox, the rash heralds the onset of the most intense phase of the illness, when the temperature is highest.

Roseola infantum yields without treatment. Its cause is not known with certainty, but it is presumed to be a virus. There is no specific treatment for the disease, which fortunately appears to confer immunity for life. If the fever is very high, sponge baths help reduce it.

# DIPHTHERIA

Fortunately, this terrible disease has been almost completely eradicated in the United States by means of immunization. Before immunization was introduced this disease killed over 25 percent of its victims. Some who recovered were incapacitated by the devastating aftereffects of diphtheria on the heart and other organs.

Every child should be immunized early and completely against diphtheria. If there is doubt about the completeness of the immunization against diphtheria, there is a check method called the Schick test which can be applied. The doctor injects a small amount of the poison excreted by the diphtheria germs into the skin. If there is sufficient antitoxin in the child's body to protect him against the disease, the Schick test will prove to be negative, and there will not be any reddened, blistered area on the skin. If the test is positive, the child must be further immunized until a negative test is obtained.

Diphtheria is caused by a bacillus type of germ. This germ usually grows on the tonsils and throat. It can infect the nose and larynx. When diphtheria develops it causes an intense reaction. The throat will be sore and swollen and there may be a grayish membrane covering the tissue. *This membrane may get so large that it, plus the swelling, can obstruct the breathing.* That is one reason why diphtheria needs immediate medical attention, usually in a specialized contagious-disease unit of a hospital. Another reason for the high fatality rate of the disease is the powerful soluble poison given off by the growing diphtheria germs. This toxic material is absorbed into the body, and affects the heart and other vital organs. It may paralyze important nerves that control swallowing or breathing.

Fortunately, a powerful antitoxin is available which can be injected to neutralize the poison produced by the diphtheria germs. However, the doctor must administer this antitoxin before the child has been sick more than three days. After that the mortality rate becomes very high despite the use of large quantities of this specific antidote.

Penicillin can eradicate the germs while the antitoxin is counteracting the unbound or loosely bound toxin.

Diphtheria usually gives plenty of warning that something serious is happening to the child. There will be fever, prostration, vomiting, as well as the sore throat. Sometimes bloody mucus appears in one or both nostrils. The doctor should be notified at once whenever diphtheria is suspected.

Recovery from diphtheria is slow. Too rapid a return to usual activity can be dangerous if the toxin has inflamed the heart muscle. Follow your doctor's advice carefully about when to let the child be active again.

## DIARRHEA IN BABIES AND YOUNG CHILDREN

Half a century ago, diarrhea was the leading cause of death in infants. There were many reasons for this, including contaminated water and milk; poor sanitation and refrigeration, which encouraged the growth of germs; and inadequate knowledge concerning infant feeding and therapy. Exposed to harmful bacteria at a time in their lives when their immunity was low, countless young children died of intestinal infections which the doctors of that period were unable to combat.

Today, this situation has been so greatly improved that we are apt to forget that diarrhea is still a serious threat to the health of babies and young children.

Fortunately, with good medical care almost. every child with diarrhea can get well. The important thing is for the parents to understand the danger signals so that treatment can be started early enough.

If a child develops severe diarhea—for example, watery stools passed more than once an hour— you should call the doctor without delay. If he cannot be reached, take the child to the hospital. Less severe diarrhea can usually be cared for at home, especially if it has been caused by foods or a formula that does not agree with the child. However, if bacterial infection is setting in, the diarrhea may progress to the point of bloody stools. This situation calls for immediate medical help.

Assuming that the diarrhea is mild, that there is no vomiting accompanying it, and that you cannot reach your doctor, this is what you should do:

1. Discontinue the usual formula or foods that the baby or child has been taking. Don't worry about his starving; he will be benefited by resting the inflamed digestive system.

2. Stop all medicines until you talk to the doctor, because paregoric, patent medicines, and many other medicines may make the children worse.

3. For infants, the usual formula may be prepared, diluted with water to one-half strength, or one-half strength diluted skim milk may be used. Prepare either of these in the usual way, taking sterile precautions, as described on page 268, and offer it to the baby in small amounts frequently.

4. For older children, a diet consisting of dilute skim milk, clear broth, ginger ale, weak tea with sugar, puddings or gelatin dessert, crackers or toast is appropriate in any mild diarrhea. But if this mild diarrhea is accompanied by vomiting and you are unable to reach your doctor, somewhat sterner measures are called for in the diet.

For babies, change to the following formula as a temporary measure: 1 quart of boiled water, 2 tablespoons of sugar or Karo syrup, and 1 level teaspoonful of salt. *Important:* use no more salt than this in preparing the formula.

Offer the same things to older children. They are apt to refuse the "formula" of water, sugar, and salt. Any clear liquid they want can be substituted for this. However, they *need* salt, which is not present in plain water or drinks such as ginger ale or very weak, sweetened tea. It should be added, in the proportion of a level teaspoonful to a quart —that is, ¼ level teaspoonful to ½ pint, which you can add to most beverages without the child's even noticing it.

Keep in mind that these very restricted diets are meant only as temporary measures, to be used until the doctor can be reached and, at any event, no longer than twenty-four hours.

## Dehydration

The greatest threat to the life of a child with severe diarrhea comes from dehydration. The loose, watery stools drain out water *plus* valuable chemicals from the body. Such substances as sodium, chloride, and potassium are essential for the regulation of the body's fluid and acid-base balances. If diarrhea continues unchecked, severe illness or even death will result from the ensuing dehydration and the acidosis that accompanies it. Dehydration may show itself by (a) decrease in the amount of urine. The urine looks dark yellow or light brown; (b) loss of the usual elastic quality of the skin; (c) sunken eyeballs; (d) rapid breathing; (e) drowsiness or even unconsciousness.

In severe cases accompanied by vomiting, the doctor will have to replace the fluid and the sodium and other chemicals by injections into the child's veins. Such injections have frequently saved the lives of desperately sick infants.

## CROUP

This condition is really a narrowing of the air passage through the larynx, the voice box in the neck where the vocal cords are located. If the narrowing is severe, the air cannot reach the lungs, and the child begins to choke. The narrowing is caused by spasm and swelling of the larynx. These may be the result of certain bacterial infections or very severe allergy, but they are most often caused by a virus, sometimes by bacteria. Fortunately, the disease is rarely fatal. But it can be terribly frightening to both the child and the parent. It usually comes in spasms. The attack is generally precipitated at night. The mild fever and the apparent healthy look of the child between the spasms—and the fact that the child has been immunized against diphtheria—usually make it certain that the illness is croup, not the onset of diphtheria of the larynx. However, always notify the doctor when the child develops a hoarse, croupy voice or cough, or seems to be having spasms of difficult breathing.

Occasionally, a severe attack of croup may represent an emergency before the doctor can be summoned. The spasm can be relieved by placing the child in a place where there is cool moist air. Hospitals are equipped with special apparatus with which to provide this cool moist air, but at home, warm, moist air can be an adequate substitute. A croup tent can be improvised by boiling water in a kettle or pan on an electric hot plate under a blanket which is placed over the child *and the parent. The parent or other adult must always sit with the child during the treatment.* The reason for this is important to know: more children have been burned to death during treatment for croup than have died of the disease itself! Keep the steam going until the spasm has been relaxed. The important thing is to allow the child to rest. Plenty of clear fluids are helpful.

If a croup tent cannot be improvised, or you cannot get a good water vaporizer rushed over from your druggist, fill the bathtub with steaming hot water, or turn the shower bath on and keep the hot water running. Keep the window and door closed so that the bathroom becomes saturated with moist air. This technique usually is as good as the above methods. Sit with the child, never taking a chance for a second that the child can be trusted not to fall into the scalding hot water. Even an older child who starts a paroxysm of croup may become so breathless and frightened that he doesn't know what he is doing.

The attacks of croup tend to repeat themselves, usually in two or three successive nights. Ask your doctor what to do to prevent further attacks. He may leave medicine that will help shorten another attack, if the spasm cannot be prevented.

*Note:* If an attack of croup doesn't respond to the above measures in twenty minutes, *or* if high fever is present, the situation is a serious emergency. If you cannot reach your doctor, rush the child to the hospital.

## MENINGITIS

Meningitis is always a serious disease because it affects the coverings of the brain and spinal cord. It may be caused by different varieties of germs, such as the dreaded meningococcus, *Hemophilus influenzae,* or pneumococcus. Other bacteria can produce the disease, too. The epidemic form is generally the result of the meningococcus.

Until the modern era of sulfa medicines and antibiotics, meningitis was one of our most fearsome diseases. Now, if treated early, it can usually be cured. Also, when epidemics threaten, we can give medicines to prevent the spread. There are no successful vaccinations against the common forms of meningitis.

The typical attack causes high fever, severe headache, convulsions, violent vomiting, and drowsiness or complete unconsciousness. There may be a skin rash. The neck and back muscles may become stiffened and painful. The brain, eyes, or ears may be permanently damaged.

A doctor should be notified at once, or the child

rushed to a hospital if your doctor cannot be reached, so that treatment can be started until he is located.

Injections of penicillin, other antibiotics, and sulfa drugs into a vein can be used to control meningitis. In a desperately ill patient, cortisone treatment may be a lifesaver.

Meningitis is highly contagious, so those who have caught the disease must be isolated. Parents who must be in contact with a child suffering this disease must be treated by their doctor. To prevent further spread, they should follow their doctor's orders carefully about cleaning the room and belongings of the meningitis patient.

## CONVULSIONS

Convulsions may signify the onset of serious diseases such as meningitis, but this is not necessarily true even when there is fever. However, the combination of convulsions and fever is so potentially ominous that medical attention must be obtained immediately. Fortunately, many of these cases turn out to be *meningismus*—false or simulated meningitis. For example, during pneumonia and other illnesses, there may be enough irritation of the brain to set off convulsions. However, as soon as the pneumonia or other infection is brought under control, the convulsions disappear.

Convulsions without fever may indicate epilepsy. This important disease of children and adults is described fully on page 465.

## WORMS

I describe worm infections (more properly called "intestinal parasites") at this point because parents so often blame them for convulsions in children. It is a safe rule that convulsions are never caused by worms.

There are three main types of worms that affect children in the United States. These are the long roundworm, *Ascaris;* the tiny, threadlike *pinworm,* which is also called the *seatworm;* and finally, the *hookworm,* which lies between these other two in size. These three worms cause many more infections than either the *tapeworm,* or the *trichina* worm which infests pork. Children are less sus-

ceptible than adults to trichinosis, but they, too, should be given pork or pork products only after these have been cooked thoroughly, as well as having been inspected by the U.S. government (see page 137).

## Roundworm Infection (Ascariasis)

These worms look like earthworms, and may sometimes be seen in the bowel movements or in the child's bed. Occasionally, one may be vomited. The worm should be saved to show to the doctor.

A child infected with roundworms may become irritable, and restless at night; he will probably develop an erratic or poor appetite. He may not gain weight or may seem to tire easily. There may be vague pains in the abdomen, abdominal swelling, and diarrhea.

Roundworms enter the body as eggs through contaminated water, food, or soil-contaminated hands. The problem lies with fecal contamination of soil.

The worms can be discharged from the intestine by special medicines which must be administered under a doctor's care. Do not try to treat worms by getting medicines at a drugstore. Children have died from overdosage of these medicines. Also, only a doctor knows how to judge when the treatment has been completely effective. Unless all the eggs and worms are killed or expelled by the treatment, the sickness will return.

## Hookworm Infections

This intestinal parasite infects children in the southern states. It enters the body through the skin, usually when children walk barefooted in infected soil. The hookworm then travels through the blood into the lungs and gets into the air passages, from which it enters the esophagus when coughing occurs. After arriving in the intestine via the esophagus and stomach after this circuitous journey, it takes up its permanent existence in the small intestines, and discharges many eggs into the feces. It breeds at a lively rate. Being parasites, the worms live off the infected person's food and body, and take valuable protein and blood-building materials from the human body. That is why anemia is one of the chief symptoms of severe hookworm infestation. The child usually looks run-down and listless.

The diagnosis of hookworm disease is made by examination of the stools for the characteristic eggs of the worms. Treatment is effective when administered by a physician or health officer. A good preventive is a pair of shoes or sneakers, but unfortunately these "medical items" are not always available in the low-income areas that constitute the so-called hookworm belt. Also, there is a problem in getting some children to give up the pleasures of walking barefoot. However, if they were educated by parents, teachers, and doctors about the dangers of hookworm disease, I believe that children would cooperate in wearing shoes—or at least compromise to the extent of wearing sneakers or sandals.

## Pinworm Infections

The pinworm is also called the seatworm and is the most common worm infection in children. The medical term for its infection is *oxyuriasis*. Pinworm infections occur in the intestine. The tiny worms measure less than a half-inch in length. They do not debilitate a child as a heavy infestation with roundworms or hookworms will. But they cause trouble by their habit of coming out around the anal region during sleep. The worms irritate the region around the anus, leading to painful scratching and restless sleep. Occasionally, a pinworm will migrate into the tiny vaginal opening in a female child where it will cause intense itching and distress. You may be able to locate it by illumination with a flashlight, and remove the worm with a swab of cotton on an applicator rod. Put the worm in a sealed bottle for the doctor to examine, or burn it if the diagnosis of pinworm infection has already been made in the child. Do not treat pinworm infections yourself. Let the doctor prescribe treatment. One very effective drug he may use is piperazine (Antepar). Or he may prefer a newer drug, pyrvinium pamoate (Povan), which can be taken in a single dose. Also, the doctor will decide what to do about the other members of the family. He will also instruct you in disinfection of the bedclothes and other materials that may be harboring the eggs of the pinworms.

## HEAD LICE

The medical name for *head lice*, or *nits*, is *pediculosis capitis*. The head louse is a tiny insect which lives on the scalp and sucks blood for its food. Almost always, the lice affect only the back portion of the scalp. The eggs of the louse are called nits. They are contained in silvery oval-shaped envelopes which are attached to the shafts of the hairs. These nits can be seen when they are plentiful, and are just large enough to be combed out by a very fine steel comb.

When the lice bite the scalp, they cause itching which leads to scratching. This, in turn, produces infections of the scalp with inflammation of the lymph glands of the neck.

The condition can be diagnosed definitely by a doctor or nurse who can recognize the characteristic nits. Schoolchildren are particularly susceptible to head lice, but anyone, rich or poor, of any age, may contract pediculosis.

In the past, many laborious treatments were used and heads were often shaved. Now, effective pesticides can be used under a doctor's supervision. Benzyl benzoate is among the preparations prescribed. The hair need not be cut or shaved as part of this newer treatment.

It is very important not to make a child with head lice feel inferior or self-conscious. Avoid making the diagnosis known to him or his playmates. It can be passed off as "dermatitis" or "infection of the scalp."

## INTUSSUSCEPTION

Intussusception (*intestinal obstruction*) is a less common illness than many mentioned in this chapter. But it does happen frequently enough for you to be on guard against it, because unless this condition is recognized within a few days of its onset a fatal result can occur. It results from the telescoping of a part of the intestine into the section ahead of it. You might imagine a smaller pipe sliding into one with just a slightly larger diameter. The smaller pipe will tend to slide down through the larger pipe, causing obstruction. Intestinal obstruction is always serious. In children it quickly leads to fatal results. Intussusception sometimes occurs when the intestines are partially filled with masses of roundworms. But usually there is no obvious cause. The child appears to be healthy. Then paroxysms of abdominal pain set in, with vomiting and restlessness. Within twelve to twenty-four hours bloody mucus is passed by rectum instead of the usual fecal matter. On the second day, fever as high as 106 to 108 degrees may appear.

Death can occur within two to four days after the onset unless the condition is relieved. The diagnosis may be confirmed by a barium test, in the form of a barium enema. This examination frequently reduces the intussusception and may completely correct the telescoping of the intestine. Treatment by surgery cures the condition completely and almost always permanently.

## POSTURAL ABNORMALITIES

A great many of the things I said about *posture* on page 21 apply to children as well as to adults. However, I feel that special attention should be given to this matter where children are concerned, because failure to attend to difficulties and defects in the posture of children can result in permanent deformity.

When I talk about poor posture in children, I don't mean that they should have the good posture characteristic of healthy adults. They are not built to stand or sit like adults. Children under nine years are not large enough or strong enough to hold in their stomachs without straining. Odd foot positions and most other postural peculiarities in children are phases of physical development and will pass as the children mature. But I am concerned about children's posture when it is unusual or poor *by childhood standards*.

The term *poor posture* is a very broad one, covering minor as well as potentially serious problems. It can be caused by weakness, disease, or deformity involving the muscles, bones, or joints. Some examples include *rickets* (p. 37), *Pott's disease* (p. 462), *congenital dislocation of the hip* (p. 462), *flat feet* (p. 116), and *scoliosis* (curvature of the spine).

Poor posture can also be due to defective vision or hearing. For example, a child who is near-sighted or hard-of-hearing is apt to thrust his head forward in order to see or hear better, and as a result his shoulders and back are thrown out of line. Clothing that is too heavy or too small may keep a child from standing straight. A bed or chair that prevents the child from lying or sitting properly can also be responsible for poor posture.

Finally, but by no means least important, emotional factors can cause postural difficulties. A shy, unhappy child who feels inferior may slump and hang his head continually. Emotional problems, especially in adolescence, have caused many cases of curvature of the spine.

I wish that I could persuade parents and teachers never to scold or nag at a child about his posture. It is obviously cruel as well as useless to tell a child with a physical weakness or disease to stand up straight and to walk properly. It is also likely to do more harm than good if the child's poor posture is due to emotional difficulties.

Regular physical examinations will determine whether or not a child's posture is poor, and will usually reveal any condition which could cause poor posture in the future. If you are concerned about your child's posture, don't wait for his regular examination to fall due, but consult a doctor as soon as possible. Taken in time, corrective measures can usually prevent difficulties and even deformities. If special exercises are needed, they should be supervised or at least initiated by a doctor or some other person with special training.

## SKIN DISEASES IN CHILDHOOD

Both the infant and young child are subject to a considerable number of minor and even serious skin diseases. Most of these, such as impetigo, scabies, and fungus infections of the skin, have been mentioned on pages 125-27 in the discussion of the care of the skin. Also, the more serious diseases such as eczema and psoriasis are taken up in separate sections because these skin conditions affect adults as well as children. Erysipelas is a streptococcal infection of the skin which also occurs in adults (p. 126).

Besides such obvious skin conditions as diaper

rashes, there is one skin disease on which children seem to have a monopoly. This is *ringworm of the scalp*. Adults very frequently are affected by fungus infections of the smooth skin; *epidermophytosis*, or athlete's foot, is a common ringworm infection between the toes. Why only children get the ringworm infection of the scalp is a strange problem. But this infection, which has the medical name of *tinea capitis*, is truly rare in adults. It is highly contagious and frequently one schoolchild infects another. Treatment is slow and difficult, and requires patience on the part of the doctor, the child, and the parent. Most of the cases occur by human infection, but it is believed that about 10 percent may be acquired from cats, dogs, and horses which harbor a form of ringworm that can affect the human scalp.

The disease is recognized chiefly by the bald patches resulting when the fungus weakens and destroys the hairs, which fall out. The itching and scratching may lead to irritations which may be confused with bacterial infections. However, if a doctor is given a chance he can make the diagnosis of the underlying ringworm of the scalp by special diagnostic methods. One of these is the use of an ultraviolet lamp which causes the fungi to fluoresce, making it possible to see them in the dark.

Local treatment of the scalp is usually ineffective, but oral doses of an antibiotic effective against fungi are curative.

### Petechial Rash

Although infants and children often have rashes that are not serious, there is one type which, though rare, is an indication of a potentially dangerous disease. This is called a *petechial rash* and is caused by bleeding under the skin. If your child has a rash, you can determine whether or not it is of this type by pressing one or more of the spots between your thumbs. If it does not blanch—that is, if the color still remains—call a doctor immediately.

Consult the Index for page references of the following, which are described in other sections of this book:

Appendicitis
Asthma
Diabetes
Dysentery and typhoid fever
Epilepsy
Head injuries
Nephritis (Bright's disease)
Pneumonia
Poliomyelitis (infantile paralysis)
Pyelitis and pyelonephritis
Tuberculosis

## CHILDHOOD CANCER

I discuss cancer in some detail later (p. 429), but a special word here about cancer in children. Although childhood cancer is not very common, it is nevertheless, next to accidents, the leading cause of death in youngsters up to age fifteen. It takes 5,000 young lives a year.

The most common types of malignancy in childhood are leukemia, Hodgkin's disease, and Wilms' tumor.

*Leukemia,* in which there is a vast overproduction of white blood cells, leads to anemia, easy bruising, fever, loss of weight and appetite, and nausea. There may also be joint pains, bleeding from the mouth, nose, kidneys, and bowels. Sometimes the disease may have a more insidious onset, with progressive weakness and pallor.

With *Hodgkin's disease,* which affects the lymph nodes (glands), a child may experience painless enlargement of the glands, usually first on one side of the neck, then the other, later under the arms and in the groin, sometimes with severe itching. As the disease progresses, there may be sweating, fever, weakness, loss of appetite and weight.

*Wilms' tumor,* which is the most common type of kidney cancer in children, actually begins in the fetus but lies dormant for a time after birth. It usually manifests itself before the fifth year. Commonly, the first indication is an abdominal mass. Pain, fever, appetite loss, nausea, vomiting, and blood in the urine follow.

I want to emphasize that many of the symptoms of these diseases are also those of other much less serious disorders, and if you notice some of them in your child, more likely than not—in fact, much more likely than not—they are not indicative of cancer. But you should report them without delay to your physician.

Even more than for some adult cancers, there have been remarkable advances in the treatment of many childhood malignancies.

At least half the children with leukemia today have a chance to survive and lead normal lives. That's true for 80 percent of those with Wilms' tumor and for 90 percent of those with Hodgkin's disease. And there is increasing hope for children with other cancers that were once, not many years ago, considered virtually hopeless.

None of this stems from miraculous new surgical techniques or the development of more mammoth x-ray machines. Instead, it results from a multimodal approach—the bringing to bear of a whole array of treatments combined skillfully to be most effective for each individual child.

Because that approach calls for the skills of many medical specialists working as a team, an individual physician or community hospital rarely, if ever, can be expected to offer optimal care.

I urge that you consult your family doctor or pediatrician at the slightest suspicion of possible cancer in your child—and without any delay. If he tells you that the child has a malignancy or if he suspects he may have, ask your doctor not about a good surgeon or radiation therapist or other specialist but rather, specifically: Where, near here, is there a team approach to treating childhood cancer? What is the closest hospital or medical center that has a pediatric cancer team—surgeon, radiation therapist, pediatrician, and other experts who work together, from the very beginning, in the treatment of childhood cancer?

## INHALED FOREIGN BODIES

When a child suddenly begins to choke and wheeze, it can be because something—a particle of food or another substance—has been inhaled into an airway.

Depending upon its size, it may cause asphyxiation or choking, gagging, and blueness. There is a risk, too, that if it remains lodged in the airway, it may cause infection.

Although the object sometimes may be expelled by coughing, more often it is not and constitutes

an emergency. The child should be examined without delay by a doctor who can locate and remove it by means of a long metal tubelike instrument, the bronchoscope.

## BRONCHITIS

The bronchi are the larger passages or tubes conveying air to and within the lungs. Bronchitis is an inflammation of the bronchi.

Acute bronchitis commonly occurs in children, although it may attack anyone of any age. In its mild form it is often referred to as a "cold on the chest." But if it progresses downward into the lungs, it can develop into a serious disease.

Symptoms of acute bronchitis include chest pain, fever, general listlessness, and considerable coughing.

When the disease is bacterial in origin, recovery may be hastened by penicillin or other antibiotics. Aspirin may be used to reduce fever, terpin hydrate to relieve a dry cough, and expectorants to loosen phlegm. The child should be kept in bed in a warm room in which the atmosphere is humidified with a vaporizer, which tends to reduce coughing. Drinking fluids should be encouraged.

## LARYNGITIS

This is an inflammation of the mucous membrane of the larynx, or voice box, affecting the voice and breathing. Symptoms include hoarseness or loss of the voice, sometimes with fever or sore throat.

Treatment requires that the child rest his voice. He should be kept in a humid atmosphere (with air kept moist by a humidifier or vaporizer). Most cases in children subside within a few days.

## PNEUMONIA

Pneumonia is an inflammation of the air cells (alveoli) of the lungs. It has many possible causes but most commonly is the result of bacterial infection in a child.

Usually, it either begins as or is preceded by an upper respiratory infection such as a cold. Symptoms may include sudden shaking chills, high fever, pain in the chest, painful cough, and rusty brown or blood-streaked sputum. The disease is serious but the outlook is excellent when the child receives early antibiotic treatment.

There are other pneumonias—"atypical" or viral—that are usually not as severe as the bacterial kind. The onset may be gradual, with mild chills, some elevation of temperature, but constant cough with much phlegm (rarely rusty or bloody). Along with bed rest, treatment may include medication for cough and inhalations of steam, as your doctor will direct.

# HEADACHES

A child will often have a headache when he has a fever, a sinus or ear infection, or a toothache. But, like adults, children can have headaches from other causes. They may, for example, suffer from tension headaches or migraine.

I discuss headaches later (page 492).

# THE HYPERACTIVE CHILD

The child—almost always a boy—may be considered the "baddest boy" in his class. He may disobey or ignore the teacher, be in constant motion, disrupt classroom activities, and, though of normal intelligence, fail to keep up with his classmates.

At home, his behavior may be unpredictable. He may be in perpetual motion and bad-tempered.

The child is an example of what has come to be known as hyperactivity or hyperkinesis, a poorly understood behavioral problem which has been variously estimated to affect from 5 to 15 percent of school-age children. The constellation of symptoms usually includes constant and often purposeless activity, distractibility, impulsiveness, restlessness, a short attention span. Sometimes there may be antisocial behavior. Often there are learning difficulties, though the intellectual level of the child may be normal or even bright.

There has been considerable controversy over hyperkinesis. In 1970, after it had been found that stimulant drugs often seemed to be effective in hyperkinetic children (almost paradoxically, the drugs that tend to make normal adults nervous, restless, and overactive had the opposite effect in the children), there was a considerable public outcry. It appeared that some public schools were prescribing the drugs for virtually every child considered "overactive" in the classroom, even though many may have been only normally exuberant and they had not been expertly diagnosed.

A few years later, public attention was again focused on hyperkinesis when one physician claimed that the condition was caused by foods and medicines containing artificial flavorings or colorings or aspirinlike compounds.

If you suspect, or have been told, that your child may be hyperkinetic, what can you do?

The American Academy of Pediatrics has given a lot of thought to this. It finds that many factors, not just true hyperkinesis, can cause a child to be overactive. They include a child's basic personality, emotional disturbances such as anxiety or depression, and seizures that may not be apparent.

So before a diagnosis can be properly made, and before treatment should begin, the child should be tested. To find specialists who can carry out the needed psychological, neurological, and psychiatric testing, your physician can call the department of pediatrics of the nearest medical school or university hospital. Or you can write to the Association for Children with Learning Disabilities at 5225 Grace Street, Pittsburgh, Pa. 15236, enclosing a stamped, self-addressed, legal-size envelope.

If your child is, in fact, hyperkinetic, drugs may be used. The most commonly employed are methylphenidate (Ritalin), pemoline (Cylert), imipramine (Tofranil, Presamine), dextroamphetamine sulfate (Dexedrine, etc.), thioridazine (Mellaril), diphenhydramine (Benadryl, etc.), and promethazine (Phenergan, etc.).

But authorities emphasize that drugs may not always be needed—and, when they are, other measures may be required as well. They suggest that both parents and teachers should be urged to set firm but consistent limits on the child's behavior, possibly by using a system of rewards and/or withholding privileges. Behavioral management of this kind may be all that is needed for children who are minimally hyperactive, and your physician may be helpful in making suggestions about such management and obtaining cooperation in school. In some children, psychotherapy may be helpful.

Drug treatment has been reported to be very successful, but authorities believe it should be used only when the child's hyperactivity is interfering significantly with his academic or social functioning. And they advise certain principles for using the drugs. Whatever drug your physician may choose to try, it should be administered in the smallest dose needed to achieve improvement in symptoms. And it should be used for as short a time as possible. For this, the child should be reevaluated as to his current need for the medication—and this can be accomplished through regularly scheduled drug-free periods, such as the Christmas holidays and the summer vacation. The child should be under close medical supervision and seen at regular intervals by the doctor, usually every two months.

Your physician may suggest a trial of eliminating foods that have been claimed to be involved in hyperkinesis—those, as already mentioned, containing artificial flavorings or colorings. He will give you directions for eliminating these from the child's diet. Recent studies indicate that the results are not as dramatic as originally claimed; some children improve while others do not.

## CRIB DEATH (SUDDEN INFANT DEATH SYNDROME)

Of all the tragedies that may strike a family, perhaps none is more distressing than the sudden, unexpected death during sleep of an apparently healthy infant.

A baby is tucked in at night, all seemingly well. Sometimes, the child has had minor sniffles or a tummy upset, but there has been nothing to make either parents or doctor think that the baby is severely ill. Sometimes, the child has appeared to be the picture of health. Yet, only a few hours later, the baby is found dead.

"Crib death"—or, as it is known medically, the sudden infant death syndrome (SIDS)—is responsible for the loss of eight to ten thousand babies a year in the United States. And while parents of victims have been distraught, many of them unable to shake off a terrible—but unjustified—feeling of having been guilty in some way, physicians have been baffled.

Many theories have been offered to try to explain the deaths. According to some, there might be an abnormal susceptibility to a virus or other infection. According to others, an overwhelming sensitivity and reaction to cow's milk might conceivably be involved. And according to still others, immaturity of the nervous system might play a part, leading to failure of breathing during sleep. But no theory has been considered adequate and none has offered any practical means of reducing the toll.

I think I should mention some recent work done. Although it does not solve the mystery of SIDS, it does suggest one factor that may enter into it—a factor about which something can be done.

In England, Dr. J. L. Emery of the Children's Hospital in Sheffield and a team of investigators have found that overconcentration of baby formulas could possibly have something to do with crib deaths. The investigators noted that many mothers, innocently believing that concentrated formulas could be healthier for their babies, were making formulas with twice the prescribed concentration so that infants were getting too much protein and salt.

The danger in excessive concentration is that it can lead to dehydration of a baby. With high concentration—too much food value in relation to the fluid content of the formula—fluid is pulled out of the baby's body.

In some highly technical work, studying tissue taken at autopsy from babies who had died suddenly, the British investigators have noted abnormalities that appear to be very much like those that could be caused by giving infants too highly concentrated formulas.

The British investigators make no claims that this is by any means the whole answer to the mystery of SIDS. And certainly I don't believe so.

But the work could be important, and it makes sense otherwise to feed a baby properly. So I would urge you to stick with a normal formula and not risk making it too concentrated. Other than perhaps any value that may have in helping to prevent crib death, there is nothing known at this time—though intensive research is going on and may soon produce important findings—about prevention.

If some family you know has lost a child in this tragic way, perhaps your reassurance that neither parents nor physician was at fault will be of some comfort.

There is now a National Foundation for Sudden Infant Death with headquarters at 310 South Michigan Avenue, Chicago, Illinois 60604, which can provide additional information, if you or a friend would like to have it.

# 21
# ADOLESCENCE

At ten years of age we are children; at twenty we have been transformed into adult men and women—perhaps even into the parents of children.

During this ten-year period we have gone from dependent childhood to independent adulthood. So gradually that the changes are scarcely perceptible, or so rapidly that they seem to occur over night, a flat-chested, chunky little girl becomes a glamorous, full-breasted woman. The small boy next door shoots up into a tall young man, the possessor of a deep voice and a beard that requires daily shaving.

This decade is also a time of great, often tempestuous emotional change. The physical changes of adolescence are easy to observe and accept compared to the development of the teen-ager's personality and changes in behavior. Attitudes and actions can change radically from one day to the next. The adolescent is trying to discover who he is and to become an independent person. Our society doesn't help him, for it flaunts the attractions of adult sex before him constantly, caters to his whims in entertainment, and then prolongs his dependence far into the teen years or even into the twenties by insisting that long and difficult years of education and training must precede his marrying and establishing a family. Teenagers have plenty to contend with, between their inner churnings and the contradictions and confusions of the world they live in!

As a doctor, I am vitally concerned with these adolescent years. Naturally, each period of life has its special health problems. Why, then, do I take this particular age so seriously? For one thing, we doctors are confronted with a new situation. At this time we cannot simply tell parents what to do for their children, or explain to responsible men and women what they should do to guard their own health. We must address both young people *and* their parents—young people who have matured in everything but experience, and parents who, while feeling responsible for their well-being, no longer can or should hold all the reins in their hands.

If the first ten years of a child's life have been good and healthy ones, the chances are excellent for a successful adolescence. But this will still be a period during which the doctor, the parents, and the maturing child must work together for that wonderful goal—a healthy, mature body and mind at eighteen to twenty-one years of age, at the time that the young person becomes a citizen and a voter, legally free to lead his or her own life.

Just because I take adolescence seriously, please don't think I'm going to join in the hue and cry against our teen-agers. Every generation gets into a lively stew about the adolescents who, in its opinion, will go to the devil at a fast rate unless they listen to their elders. Adolescents have rarely listened very much in the past, and most of them have managed to come through all right.

On the other hand, *more* of them will come through with *less* difficulty if we and they recognize the problems associated with this period—problems for the parents as well as for the younger generation. This is a time for self-examination. Parents should try to understand whether their responses to their teen-ager's behavior are justifiable, or whether they are really responding to their own anxieties. They may exert inappropriate pressures on their adolescent sons and daughters to adapt certain social customs, or to prepare for careers that the parents want for them, naturally in one of a few selected schools. It is not easy for a mother and father who have made a full-time job of caring for a child for fifteen or sixteen years suddenly to realize that their "baby" is going to leave the nest soon and become an autonomous human being. This is one reason why adolescence is such a trying time for parents too.

With understanding on both sides, controversies in the home will settle down to reasonable proportions. I am not claiming that they will be eliminated. Emotionally, the "birth" of an adult is scarcely less of an event than is the actual, physical birth of a baby. But it is just as rewarding. If parents can remember themselves as adolescents, and if children try to understand their parents' dilemmas—if they can talk freely and even joke a little about their respective problems—tensions will be greatly relieved.

## PROBLEMS OF ADOLESCENTS

Nature has a way of driving a child faster than is desirable in our complex society. Many boys and girls are sexually mature by the time they are thirteen to fifteen. Physically, they are ready for mating. *But they are not ready for marriage with all of its responsibilities, including parenthood.* Aside from the difficulties they would face in establishing and supporting a home, they are not yet adult emotionally. They want to be grown-up, yet in some ways they are still attached to childhood.

These are the two main problems adolescents face: *independence* and *sex*. They must break away from the old ways of living within a familiar framework. They must resolve the question of what to do about sexual desires; and no matter how much they are told or how much they read, they must do this themselves—or try to. In other words, what they have to arrive at is not so much a workable theory of sex, but what actually to do about the new reactions, sensations, emotions, or whatever one calls them, which are bombarding them.

As though this were not enough, a number of factors over which they and their parents have little control often complicate the picture. For example: shortly before puberty or in early adolescence, boys and girls pass through a period of preferring the members of their own sex. With varying degrees of intensity, girls avoid boys, develop "crushes," and swear eternal fidelity to some girl friend. Boys look down on girls, worship a hero, become devoted to a chum. This is a natural and valuable phase of life. It is followed by an interest in members of the opposite sex, which leads to the choosing of a mate.

However, these events don't always proceed according to a timetable. The age of children in a group, such as a school grade, varies. Those who started school early, or are unusually bright or interested in their studies, may be as much as two years younger than many of their perfectly normal classmates. A normal child may also, for any number of reasons, be older than the others in his group. Boys are usually about two years older than girls when maturity arrives. This age also varies a great deal among individuals. And, finally, physical and emotional development do not always proceed at the same pace.

All of this means that, almost inevitably, some young people will be out of step. They will be attracted to members of the opposite sex which the crowd still scorns; or they will prefer members of their own sex while their friends have gone on to dating and flirting. This is disconcerting to them. Not wanting to be on the outside, these young people will try hard to be like the majority. They will rush through, or even miss, an important phase of their emotional development; or they will be forced to remain in it too long.

Even more difficult are those situations in which companionship, when it is most needed, is impossible, and the child becomes an outsider due to isolation. This is no longer as common a situation as it was before modern transportation—and the good sense of the older people in the community—worked out means for young people in rural areas to get together not only during school but after school hours. However, it still exists. And don't forget that young people can also be cruelly isolated by the barriers of race, creed, color, or social position. Parents who exclude their own or other children for such reasons are being extremely shortsighted. Social contact is practically essential during this period, and by depriving children of companionship parents are, in effect, increasing the possibility that they will not be able to achieve independence or solve their sex problems. Obviously, this is dangerous not only to the individual child but to the community.

Achieving an equilibrium regarding sex is often no more difficult for a young person than it is to acquire a sense of balance regarding independence. At this point young people usually sum it up by saying, "Parents are the greatest problem of adolescence." In a way, this is true. Even under the best circumstances, a child seldom finds it easy to acquire a new attitude toward the man and woman he has probably regarded only as "father" and "mother" and who now must become people as well as parents to him. No wonder the adolescent swings back and forth between two extremes, which is as painful to him as it is to his parents!

## PROBLEMS OF PARENTS

Meanwhile, parents are suddenly forced to face that fact that the child is becoming an adult. This means independence—possibly leaving home for school, a job, or marriage. Particularly in small families, parents can be overwhelmed by the prospect of the loneliness they see ahead of them. How tempting it is to try to prevent the child from becoming really adult ("growing up too fast" may be the way they put it) in the hope that he or she will stay at home! It isn't easy for anyone to face the fact that middle age is here, as evidenced by the fact that the children are becoming mature, and soon there may even be grandchildren! Nor is it easy to pass the reins into another's hands gracefully and at just the right time.

Even the most mature and realistic parents face problems during this period. They know their help is still needed; their children, however intelligent and well-balanced, lack experience. Every day parents read in the newspapers, or hear from their acquaintances, about a tragic accident to a teen-ager, the ruined health of another, a marriage of necessity—even cases of homosexuality, rape, insanity! No wonder parents can't sit back and let their children court disaster. Yet if they exert undue authority, it may only cause rebellion. How much should they tell their children? Long ago, they told them the facts of life, of *normal* life and its reproduction. But how much should they tell them of life's uglier aspects now? Then, too, as a very sensible mother said to me ruefully, "Unfortunately, children don't mature in a family vacuum.

Other things keep right on happening. The baby gets sick, the grandparents need attention, Dad has to change his job. Everything seems to happen just when you know you should give your calmest consideration to this teen-ager who has become a will-o'-the-wisp and slips through your fingers just when you want to do your best."

Yes, there will always be problems and emotional stresses for both parents and children during this period. But let's not make the mistake of exaggerating them. Let's do the best we can, knowing that time and nature, which create these problems, will help to solve a great many of them.

## THE HEALTH OF ADOLESCENTS

All these problems, which I shall discuss as I go along, will be far easier to handle if the adolescent has a healthy and well-nourished body. That is why nutrition is more important than ever. The body needs a particularly good and complete diet during this period of active growth and strenuous activity. The food must be rich in protein to make new muscles and body tissue; it must contain plenty of minerals for the growth of bones; it must have vitamins for general health; and there must be ample energy-rich food to keep the fires going.

### The Right Foods for Adolescents

Teen-agers' diets tend to be poorly balanced. Youngsters go for the quick hamburger, a malted milk, and French fries. Girls especially are quick to take up food fads and to try every crash diet they read about in the Sunday supplement. Some of this behavior has to be tolerated by the wise parents. If mother provides a balanced diet at home, there may be no great harm in her adolescent children's snacking on French fries and malteds on the outside. Remember, adolescents' appetites can be enormous; they often eat more than their grown parents do.

As I explain in Chapter 2 (p. 35), humans must have proteins, minerals, and vitamins. *Protein* foods include meat, fish, eggs, and milk. They are expensive, but they are essential for growth. Two good sources of protein should be served at every meal. For example, an egg and a large glass of milk for breakfast, or bacon or a slice of ham instead of the egg. At the noonday meal, there should be meat or fish or a cheese dish plus a large glass of milk. And at the evening meal the main course should consist of fish, meat, eggs, or cheese, with another glass of milk. Between meals, milk should be taken to make a total of four glasses a day.

I emphasize milk because it not only supplies protein but is the best source of the *minerals* calcium and phosphorus, which are essential for building bones. If adolescents won't drink enough milk, it can be provided in other ways, such as in soups and desserts. It can be flavored with vanilla or chocolate. Skimmed milk (fat-free milk) is better for adolescents who are overweight, as it provides the valuable protein and minerals without the weight-adding fats.

*Vitamins* should be provided by serving fruits and vegetables; both green and yellow vegetables should be included. Liver, which is an excellent source of all the vitamin B group, should be eaten once a week. A daily addition of vitamin A and vitamin D is helpful during this period of active growth. Some margarine is fortified with vitamin A, and some milk with vitamin D. I often recommend that adolescents supplement their diets by taking one or two U.S.P. multivitamin capsules a day. Ask your doctor about this.

Extra *iron* is needed to build rich red blood for growing young people. Girls who are beginning to menstruate may require additional iron to replace that which is lost in the menstrual blood. The following foods are rich in iron. Your doctor can also prescribe supplements of iron in capsule form if necessary.

FOODS RICH IN IRON

Lean meat, especially liver, heart, kidneys
Leafy green vegetables
Egg yolk
Whole grain and enriched bread and cereal
Potatoes
Oysters
Dried fruits, peas, and beans

*Carbohydrates:* Plenty of bread and starches are also required to maintain or gain weight.

Mothers will recognize this diet suggested for adolescents as containing many of the things they were advised to eat during pregnancy. The extra proteins, minerals, and vitamins are needed for the growing adolescent just as they are for the growing fetus. The main difference between the diets is this: the adolescent needs plenty of supplementary carbohydrate and fat to provide energy for his active life, whereas during pregnancy the mother's weight gain should be kept under control.

Please read my chapter on the food you eat (p. 30). Note how to find inexpensive sources of protein, calcium, and iron if you cannot afford a diet rich in meat, eggs, and fresh milk. But do make every effort to provide these needed foods, even at a sacrifice of money that would be spent on other items in your budget. It is extremely difficult, sometimes impossible, to correct an injury to growth.

## Overweight and Underweight

Being underweight to the point of impaired physical well-being is not an important problem among American teen-agers. While many of them do tend to be thin, relatively few are so underweight that they are unusually subject to serious illness. The average, healthy teen-ager, especially when he is going through a period of rapid growth, has a rangy, spare appearance despite the fact that he is eating large quantities of wholesome food.

On the other hand, overweight is a more serious problem, both physically and emotionally, and it may have long-range consequences. The overweight adult was quite often an overweight adolescent. The potentially detrimental effects of obesity on health are becoming better known, and we doctors alert parents to the problems their children may face if they are unusually heavy in their teens. In addition, heavy boys and girls are often teased by their playmates or left out because they are unattractive. This may cause them to eat still more to console themselves, creating a vicious circle that becomes very difficult to break.

Getting young people to gain or to lose weight requires the tact of a diplomat. Here, as in so many other situations involving adolescents, each parent has to consider the individual child. However, I can make several general suggestions—which, incidentally, apply not only to matters of health but to many other situations in which the parent must exert authority.

1. Never use ridicule or let other members of the family use it if you can possibly prevent them. Ridicule is always cruel, and as adolescents are particularly sensitive, it affects them even more than it does adults.

2. Don't nag. This defeats its own purpose, especially with adolescents, who are usually impatient.

3. Give the problem serious attention, with special consideration for the particular person involved. Remember that adolescents are individuals. For example, if your child needs to gain or lose weight, consider thoughtfully which of the hints I offer in Chapter 3 (Underweight and Overweight) will work best for him or her.

4. Fall back on an authority your child will recognize. Young people are inclined to think their parents know less than they do—just as they were inclined, when they were children, to think that their parents knew everything. So the word of a doctor or health authority is useful reinforcement.

5. Many adolescents, for all their rebelliousness, accept something that is calmly and firmly presented. They respond to a certain amount of authority, to "this is how it is." So save your authority for the things that are really important.

## Skin Troubles During Adolescence

As I explain on page 122, adolescents are very apt to develop pimples, acne, boils, and other skin troubles. Be sure to read the section on *acne*, and note especially that this condition can cause problems that are more than skin-deep!

Always consult a doctor if an adolescent suffers from severe acne. He may want to refer the young person to a dermatologist (skin specialist) or the skin disease department of the nearest medical center or hospital.

Frequent *boils* may be a sign of *diabetes*. Don't forget that this disease, which you may have asso-

| TABLE 21–1 | | | | | | IDEAL WEIGHT IN BOYS AND GIRLS* | | | | | | | |

| | | | *Boys* | | | | | | | *Girls* | | | |
|---|---|---|---|---|---|---|---|---|---|---|---|---|---|
| HEIGHT | | | AGE | | | | HEIGHT | | | AGE | | | |
| INCHES | 14 | 15 | 16 | 17 | 18 | 19 | INCHES | 14 | 15 | 16 | 17 | 18 | 19 |
| 54 | 72 | | | | | | 55 | 78 | | | | | |
| 55 | 74 | | | | | | 56 | 83 | | | | | |
| 56 | 78 | 80 | | | | | 57 | 88 | 92 | | | | |
| 57 | 83 | 83 | | | | | 58 | 93 | 96 | 101 | | | |
| 58 | 86 | 87 | | | | | 59 | 96 | 100 | 103 | 104 | | |
| 59 | 90 | 90 | 90 | | | | 60 | 101 | 105 | 108 | 109 | 111 | |
| 60 | 94 | 95 | 96 | | | | 61 | 105 | 108 | 112 | 113 | 116 | |
| 61 | 99 | 100 | 103 | 106 | | | 62 | 109 | 113 | 115 | 117 | 118 | |
| 62 | 103 | 104 | 107 | 111 | 116 | | 63 | 112 | 116 | 117 | 119 | 120 | |
| 63 | 108 | 110 | 113 | 118 | 123 | 127 | 64 | 117 | 119 | 120 | 122 | 123 | |
| 64 | 113 | 115 | 117 | 121 | 126 | 130 | 65 | 121 | 122 | 123 | 125 | 126 | |
| 65 | 118 | 120 | 122 | 127 | 131 | 134 | 66 | 124 | 124 | 125 | 128 | 130 | |
| 66 | 122 | 125 | 128 | 132 | 136 | 139 | 67 | 130 | 131 | 133 | 133 | 135 | |
| 67 | 128 | 130 | 134 | 136 | 139 | 142 | 68 | 133 | 135 | 136 | 138 | 138 | |
| 68 | 134 | 134 | 137 | 141 | 143 | 147 | 69 | 135 | 137 | 138 | 140 | 142 | |
| 69 | 137 | 139 | 143 | 146 | 149 | 152 | 70 | 136 | 138 | 140 | 142 | 144 | |
| 70 | 143 | 144 | 145 | 148 | 151 | 155 | 71 | 138 | 140 | 142 | 144 | 145 | |
| 71 | 148 | 150 | 151 | 152 | 154 | 159 | | | | | | | |
| 72 | | 153 | 155 | 156 | 158 | 163 | | | | | | | |
| 73 | | 157 | 160 | 162 | 164 | 167 | | | | | | | |
| 74 | | 160 | 164 | 168 | 170 | 171 | | | | | | | |

* Taken from American Child Health Association.

ciated only with adults, frequently strikes young people, including those who are not overweight. A *carbuncle* or recurrent boils are sufficient cause to consult a physician. (See page 125.)

*Freckles* can be a source of worry to young people (see page 121). Let me remind you again that there is no way you can remove them safely at home. However, they can be prevented from getting worse by reducing exposure to the sun or by wearing protective ointments or lotions. Mothers can be helpful, when freckles are really unsightly, by providing a disguise in the form of face powder or "Covermark." Very disfiguring cases should be referred to a specialist in skin diseases who may try "peeling" therapy. Be sure to cheer up a freckler by pointing out the fact that these spots usually fade with the passing years. And, again, don't permit freckles to be made a target for family jokes.

## Awkwardness

Many young people cannot seem to handle their rapidly growing bodies. Their clumsiness is not due merely to carelessness or willfulness, as some parents seem to believe. Helping them to understand their problem, instead of complaining about it, prevents them from becoming self-conscious, which only adds to the awkwardness.

## SPECIAL PROBLEMS OF GIRLS

### Breasts

Some adolescent girls feel shy or even ashamed of their breast development. They may try to walk with their shoulders hunched over to conceal their bosoms. Mothers should encourage them to be proud of their developing womanhood. They can also be helpful in choosing clothes suitable to the girl's new figure, always making allowance for the fact that the girl's preferences are important.

Mothers not only should emphasize the fact that breast development is a normal part of puberty, but should explain that, shortly before or during menstruation, some tenderness and swelling are apt to occur and should cause no concern.

I describe the breasts and problems connected with their size and shape on page 523.

## Body Hair

The adolescent girl may develop an excess of hair over the thighs and legs or under the arms. Facial hair sometimes becomes disfiguring. Parents should take this seriously because it can be very important to a sensitive young girl. Bleaching is usually enough to keep this hair from being prominent. If neither this nor shaving seems satisfactory for unsightly facial hair, your daughter may want to have it permanently removed. This can be dangerous if it is attempted by anyone but an expert. Read my discussion of excess body hair on page 120. If an expert is not available or is too expensive, exert all your tact to convince your daughter that she should wait rather than risk infection and scars.

## Menstruation

Menstruation may precede, accompany, or follow the outward signs of a girl's maturity. It usually begins at twelve to fourteen years of age, but it may start as early as ten or as late as eighteen. Maturing early or late often runs in a family. However, if a girl's menstrual periods begin at ten or earlier, or if they have not started by the time she is seventeen, a doctor should be consulted. A doctor should also be consulted if the characteristic changes of puberty—the development of the breasts, pubic hair, and so on—occur unusually early or late. This may be due to a disorder of the endocrine glands which can be corrected, and the child usually needs help with the emotional problems that are apt to arise under such circumstances. In the average woman, menstruation occurs every twenty-eight days, but the cycle varies a great deal in different women. However, each woman has a fairly definite cycle, which should be reasonably well established by the end of the first year after the onset of menstruation or the *menarche* as this is called.

Menstruation is a normal physiological event which I describe in detail on page 84. Be sure to read that section, and also the sections on pages 514–16 in which I discuss past attitudes toward menstruation, and the various menstrual disorders. This information is essential to women of all ages. Here, I shall stress facts about menstruation in relation to the adolescent.

Many people, either consciously or unconsciously, regard menstruation as an illness, and instill fears about it into young girls. In other instances, girls reach puberty without knowing there is such a thing, so that their first menstrual period is a severe emotional shock. All girls, and boys as well, should be told about menstruation before they and their friends reach the age of puberty—preferably by their mothers.

It is not easy to say exactly how early children should be told about menstruation. As I explain on page 281, parents should not give children information which they cannot understand, or in which they are not interested. But on the other hand, children should not get the impression that menstruation is, as they often put it, "a dirty secret" which has been kept from them. The opportunities for privacy, the possibility of the child's learning about menstruation in other ways, and similar factors must help determine the age at which each child should be told about menstruation. The important thing is the mother's attitude.

Mothers should realize that menstruation is not a sickness, and it is not something to be ashamed of. It should not be called "the curse" or made to seem mysterious or shameful. Mothers should explain to their adolescent daughters that many women experience some discomfort or "cramps" in the lower abdomen, usually at the onset of a period, and that menstruation may be a "nuisance" for the first day or days, especially if the flow is profuse. However, it should cause no real difficulty. Girls should be able to go to school, take walks, dance, play ordinary games, and, if the weather is warm and the flow not profuse, go swimming. If a girl tires or chills easily, she should avoid swimming and the more strenuous sports during her menstrual period. She should not be goaded into overdoing things by a mother who is overly anxious to emphasize the fact that menstruation is normal. Girls should be told that menstrual disorders do occur, but that they are usually of a minor nature, and that a doctor can almost always cure them, or at least help them a great deal.

PAD VERSUS TAMPON. Either is safe from a health standpoint. The choice depends on the individual. If the flow is profuse, pads may be required to absorb it. Most virgins can use the small-size tampons, and mothers should not imply that a girl who uses a tampon is not "nice."

## Feminine Hygiene

Aside from ordinary washing and bathing, no "feminine hygiene" is necessary. Baths or showers may be taken during menstruation, although extremely hot or cold ones should be avoided. Women who prefer not to bathe during their periods should wash the outer genital parts with warm water and soap at least once or twice a day.

If strong odors persist, or if there is a discharge from the vaginal passage between periods, be sure to see a doctor or consult a hospital clinic. These discharges and odors usually result from an infection which should be attended to. *Douching* is seldom necessary (see page 106). Ask your doctor about it if you think that you need vaginal douches.

## SPECIAL PROBLEMS FOR BOYS

Boys arrive at puberty about two years later than do girls—that is, between the ages of fourteen and sixteen on an average, although some boys mature as early as twelve and others as late as twenty. If a boy matures at an exceptionally early age, a doctor should be consulted. I think it is particularly important to consult a doctor in the case of a boy who matures *late*. Boys are apt to be concerned about their virility if they mature late; girls are less concerned if their first periods have not arrived. There may be a glandular difficulty (see page 83) which requires treatment; but even if nothing is wrong, a doctor's reassurance may be necessary to prevent emotional problems.

Boys grow rapidly during this period, and their appetites may be enormous. Hair appears on the face and the pubic regions, the genitals are enlarged, and the boy is able to have erections and ejaculations. Nocturnal emissions ("wet dreams") start in this period.

## Nocturnal Emissions

This is nature's way of announcing the fact that a boy can become a father. It is also nature's way of relieving sexual tension.

The fluid containing *spermatozoa*, stored in the *seminal vesicles*, is discharged at night, usually accompanied by a sexual dream. This physiological event should not be, as it so often is, a cause for shame, pride, or concern. It is a natural part of adolescence, about which boys should be informed in advance. Parents should not comment upon finding seminal stains on the bedclothes or pajamas. I think it is important that girls, too, be told about nocturnal emissions so they will not be shocked by discovering their existence accidentally, or through someone who misinforms them.

## PROBLEMS FOR BOTH SEXES

### Masturbation

Of course, this is a problem for members of both sexes, although it is usually regarded as a special one where boys are concerned. I speak of it as a problem; it is one in the sense that almost every individual has been confronted with the desire to masturbate, and must work out his or her own solution to this question. It is a problem in the sense that sexual desire is not purely physical. That is, the physical aspects are, normally, closely associated with the desire for intimacy with a member of the opposite sex. This intimacy cannot exist during masturbation, except in the form of fantasy.

These are the only real problems of masturbation. The other problems have been conjured up out of whole cloth. Although they are not real, they have caused countless heartaches and even tragedies. The twin specters we have created are the devils of fear and of guilt.

Fear is unnecessary because masturbation is not harmful. *It never causes organic or mental sickness.* Guilt is unnecessary because a very large percentage of boys and girls have practiced some form of masturbation during their growing years and often into adult life. Fear and guilt cause emotional difficulties that can mar the whole future of a child. Don't inflict them on your children in order to prevent the "evil" of masturbation; there are no such evils, and you couldn't prevent them if there were.

If a boy or girl becomes addicted to masturba-

tion, practicing it, let us say, daily, the problem is an emotional one which should be discussed with a doctor or counselor (see page 183). The masturbation is a sign, not a cause, of the emotional difficulty.

### Homosexual Practices

Many boys and some girls indulge in some form of homosexual "play" with a companion or companions. Here the parents should be on the alert. Usually such practices are harmless and cease as the boy or girl matures. However, it is at this time that an older, confirmed homosexual may exert an unfortunate influence. If such a situation has arisen, the parents may need a great deal of skill and tact; in many cases they would be wise to discuss the situation with a trained person.

Such situations are less apt to arise if boys and girls know the facts about homosexuality. Most young people pick up some information on this subject. Often they pick up misinformation. This may cause them to worry needlessly about whether they themselves are "queer," or it may make a homosexual seem sophisticated and wicked—hence fascinating. Understanding what homosexuality actually is will serve as a protection for healthy adolescents.

I think every young person should know that a preference for the members of one's own sex is natural in late childhood or early adolescence, and that it may overlap—but only for a short time— the development of attraction to the opposite sex.

I do not mean that you should give your children a lecture on this subject. It is far better to make the points as the opportunities present themselves. I realize that some parents find it difficult to do this. Are you one of them? Do you feel awkward or embarrassed about discussing masturbation, nocturnal emissions, or any other subject with your children? Does your own strict early training make you act as though you thought some things were wicked when you know they really aren't? If you have any doubts, check the matter with your doctor, a marriage counselor, or someone in the field of child guidance. Such a discussion will either increase your confidence or make you decide to let the doctor or some other trained person discuss these matters with your children.

# A GOOD SEX LIFE
# FOR OUR CHILDREN

It is likely that no direct suggestions we parents offer will greatly influence what our children do about sex. However, our pattern of living, our maturity, our own example of love in the home, will undoubtedly influence our children's attitudes toward sex. I think that we parents should stand in the background, unobtrusively observing the way our children are developing so that we can, if necessary, help them so far as their attitudes and reactions are concerned.

By all means make the home a welcome, attractive place for your children's friends. By giving them freedom and privacy in and around the home, you will help them work out their normal sex urges. By restrictions and suspicions, you will simply drive them into secretive relationships which frequently end in disaster.

If your son or daughter is getting friendly with someone who is too old or too sophisticated or not the right type, don't step in and order him or her to terminate the friendship. Cultivate the friendship with invitations to dinner or a family picnic. Then when you raise questions with your child, he or she will realize that you talk from knowledge —and are not just "sounding off."

The undue influence which another person may exert on your child is best combated indirectly. If you stop to think about it, you will realize that we usually let other people do our thinking for us only when we ourselves feel insecure—when we lack information, or the stress is too great for us to cope with. Doesn't that indicate pretty clearly the line you should follow in protecting your child against being misled?

No one knows the complete answer to the difficult question about petting and sex relations for the adolescent. It depends to a great extent on the religious and cultural background of the family and the maturity and personality of the individual. My attitude is very much the same as that of psychiatrist Dr. John Levy, as given in that fine book *The Happy Family* (by John Levy, M.D., and Ruth Monroe, Ph.D.). He says:

Advising adolscents about their sex life is a highly personal and individualized problem. You cannot recommend the same behaviour for all of them indiscriminately. I rather hope that my own daughter will pet or neck, or whatever the proper term may be, preferably with boys she knows well and likes, and only with her contemporaries. Love-making of this type is a healthy preparation for marriage. I hope that she will not have intercourse or end up merely a technical virgin. Quite aside from any moral implications, such a step is risky, as I have indicated above. If she does have a complete relationship, though, I most earnestly hope that she will know what she is about, that she will not go into an affair because she happens to be tight, or thinks it's "the thing," or wants to prove that she can carry it off. These are my hopes. They are based on my observation of the kind of behaviour least likely to cause trouble in our particular social group. But she may order her life quite differently and be none the worse for it. If she is neither afraid of sex nor bamboozled by its glamour I shall be very content.

Note particularly the points Dr. Levy makes, which apply equally well to boys as to girls: (1) Adolescent lovemaking should be with friends who are approximately the same age. (2) A certain amount of petting and necking is a good thing as a preparation for the fuller, richer love of marriage. (3) If the young person prefers some other way, accept the decision with the hope that it will be a realistic one and will not cause unhappiness.

We parents should be close enough to our children so that they will know intuitively that they can turn to us for honest, sympathetic guidance and assistance, in case a catastrophe should occur —even one resulting in pregnancy or a venereal disease. If all young people could feel this way about parents—and their family doctors—how many tragedies could be avoided!

# DRUGS

As all parents know well enough, the use of drugs among adolescents has been increasing and is not confined to the ghetto.

Rehabilitation of a chronic drug user can be a long, difficult process. Prevention and intervention—turning youngsters off when they start turning themselves on—are problems of parental concern.

How can a parent begin to suspect that a child

may be taking drugs? It's important to note any unusual changes from normal behavior. If a child who has always been friendly and outgoing suddenly becomes withdrawn and hostile, something is wrong, though it may not necessarily be drug use. Some experts suggest that a youngster who keeps to himself for long periods in his room or in the bathroom, who is often on the phone and who is called by persons who will not identify themselves to parents, may be taking drugs. Other possible indications include a sharp slide in school grades, disappearance of clothing and personal belongings and thievery at home (used to pay for drugs), alienation from old friends, and taking up with strange companions.

There are physical indications. A person smoking marijuana has a strong odor of burned leaves on both his breath and his clothes which persists for hours after use of the drug. Marijuana dilates the pupils of the eyes and sometimes reddens and inflames the eyes. Other symptoms may include sleepiness, lack of coordination, wandering mind, increased appetite, and craving for sweets. There may be a tendency to laugh and giggle excessively.

If a person is high on LSD or another hallucinogen, the symptoms may be almost unmistakable: severe hallucinations, incoherent speech, cold hands and feet, strong body odor, laughing and crying jags, vomiting.

Symptoms of amphetamine usage include aggressive behavior, rapid speech, giggling and silliness, confusion of thinking, extreme fatigue, shakiness, loss of appetite. Those for barbiturates are stupor, dullness, blurred speech, drunk appearance, vomiting.

If pills are found on children who deny they are illicit drugs, the pills can be identified by a druggist or physician. If cigarette papers and possibly small seeds are found in clothing pockets, they may well indicate marijuana usage.

When a child is sniffing glue or drinking cough medicine containing narcotics for kicks, he may have a dreamy blank expression and a drunk appearance. Heroin or morphine use may be spotted by watery eyes, appetite loss, stupor, needle marks on the body.

What can be done if a child is believed to be taking drugs? Certainly, a parent has no more important function than to keep a child from harming himself. But there must be no panic and the situation must be handled with tact.

Some experts who have dealt often with the problem suggest that the parent talk quietly with the youngster, telling him that his behavior has caused concern and that the parent has wondered if he might be taking drugs and might be too frightened to say so. The parent might add that his or her prime concern is the child's health and happiness, and that while it's true that the parent is invading the youngster's privacy and the child has the right to be angry about this, the seriousness of the situation justifies the invasion. There should be an effort then to find out whether the child has only experimented briefly or is taking a drug regularly.

In discussing drugs with a child, the parent can, and should, use an intelligent, reasonable approach. It is far more likely to be successful than an authoritative pronouncement. A youngster can be reminded that hallucinogen usage is extremely dangerous risk-taking, that it has caused hundreds of victims to end up in mental institutions or to suffer injuries such as those of three University of California at Santa Barbara students when, on an LSD trip, they stared so long at the sun while holding a "religious conversation" that they never again will be able to read.

A youngster may resist any argument that marijuana is as addictive or dangerous as heroin. But a parent can remind him that marijuana can be habit-forming, cause listlessness with prolonged use, and temporarily alter vision enough to make driving extremely dangerous. And, of course, it may lead to difficulties with the police.

Barbiturates, it can be explained, can be as addictive as heroin. Strong doses of amphetamines are dangerous, too, and even hippies have been known to post signs warning that "Speed Kills."

A child tempted by drugs or already experimenting with them is not a hopeless case by any means. With wise rather than hysterical action on the part of parents, there is a good chance he may "turn off" rather than "turn on."

Where, if needed, can a parent turn for help? A good place to start is with the family physician. In most communities, help is available also through psychiatric clinics and outpatient services. Virtually every major city has a center that will refer a patient to the best agency for a particular problem. Hospitals, child-guidance centers, voluntary health and social organizations, and many law enforcement agencies (which are anxious to protect rather than prosecute, unless prosecution is absolutely essential) can tell parents what to do.

Addiction is a disease. It is not an easy one to overcome, but it is curable in many instances. In fact, as authorities point out, many addicts, when they reach the age of thirty or thirty-five, often suddenly lose the need for heroin, for example. They withdraw on their own and never go back to the habit. Why this maturing-out process, as it is known, occurs is a mystery; addicts themselves are unable to explain it. "Our problem," says one authority, "is to keep them from dying of heroin addiction before they get to be thirty or thirty-five and to replace their ten- to fifteen-year period of drug abuse with years of useful activity."

There are several major approaches to treatment in the United States. One is civil commitment, used in some states, with emphasis on education, job rehabilitation, and careful follow-up. Another is a methadone maintenance program which substitutes the milder drug methadone for heroin and includes education, job training, and other rehabilitative activities. There are also group therapy programs, typified by organizations such as Synanon and Day Top, which are regarded by many authorities as valuable.

## HOW PARENTS CAN HELP THE ADOLESCENT

To help the adolescent, we must first learn what we cannot do. There is no way of curbing the upsurge of growth and emotions and aggressions that characterize the period of puberty. One can't stop the tide. Trying to dam it will only result in intolerable pressures. However, it is possible to guide the tide into such channels that it won't wash away valuable structures.

If we are wise and learn to accept the strange new behavior of the adolescent, we will set the basis for a happy home life for the entire family. Parents who learn to "take it" from the difficult, aggressive adolescent will be rewarded in later years by love, respect, and help from the son or daughter who has been able to grow into adult life without being fought against. Parents who show sympathetic understanding for the shy, sensitive adolescent will be rewarded by the love of a mature man or woman who has been encouraged to grow up and achieve independence.

We parents should try to remember our own reactions and desires in adolescence. Recalling our own strange behavior will make us more tolerant. If we remember how we hated the authority of our parents, we will understand why our children object to strict rules. If we remember our fantasies and daydreams and grandiose plans, we will listen with tolerance, rather than derision, when our children plan to remake the world, or become poets, missionaries, or explorers when we think they should have decided to enter the family business. And we must realize, too, that our children may be quite unlike us: their adolescence may be stormy while ours was quietly miserable, or vice versa. *If we think of the adolescent as half child and half adult, we can more easily weather the storms and be gentle and firm than threatening and authoritarian.*

We adults can learn something very valuable from adolescents. Dr. Benjamin Weininger, the psychiatrist, points out that adolescents frequently have the correct attitude toward living. They are idealistic, intense about life, and hopeful that they can participate in making life better for everyone. The adolescent may not be very practical in his attempts to reach his ideals. But his way of life is worth our consideration and respect.

Our job is to help the adolescent child reach the goal of *maturity*. It is a double goal of sexual maturity and social maturity. We have already talked about how to help the child reach sexual maturity. There are a number of things we can do to help in the attainment of social maturity. Here are some practical measures:

Let the child feel he has a place in the family. Discuss or at least explain family decisions.

Give him or her the details of the family budget. Present a true picture of what things cost in terms of the parents' outlay of time and energy. Let him see that his share is a reasonable one, and not the result of an arbitrary decision.

Encourage a sense of adult responsibility about

money. Give the child a regular allowance, once a week for younger children, once a month for those sixteen or over. If it is possible, provide older children with a personal checking account, which makes them realize that they are being treated as responsible individuals.

Do everything you possibly can to enable an adolescent boy or girl (or one who is approaching adolescence) to have friends. Don't be too strict about insisting that these acquaintances be desirable. A child who has previously been well-adjusted is in less danger from "bad" companions during adolescence than he is from being kept apart from his contemporaries.

Give the adolescent a chance to leave home. If you can afford it, arrange for longer and longer visits during school vacations. Younger children can first go to camp or to visit relatives. Then let them go to visit friends. Older and more mature ones should be permitted to take jobs away from home during summer vacations. These breaks from home life give the adolescent valuable training in self-confidence. They also help reduce the tensions that adolescents generate in their rebellion against home rules and restrictions. The adolescent soon learns that there are rules anywhere he goes!

Encourage the adolescent to take his place in the adult world. For example, allow a fourteen-year-old girl or boy to drive the family car out of the garage each morning and back into the garage at night. It is against the law in most states for them to drive on the street. But they appreciate the opportunity to tell their friends that they are "driving," and that their families trust them enough to give them a task involving the car.

Let the child decide on his or her career. Show your appreciation of its importance by trying to get expert guidance for him or her. In some cities you will find specialists trained to help people find the careers for which they are best suited, as I describe on page 141. Discuss your child's aptitudes with the high school teachers. You can also help by inviting into your home friends and acquaintances who will describe their own careers in the professions, arts, or business.

If your daughter wants to enter a profession rather than marry at the same age that her mother did, let her work it out in her own way. Don't add to the social pressure that often makes a girl marry

before she is ready for it. Many girls are by no means fitted for marriage simply because they are physically mature. A girl who is shy or feels inadequate won't find her problems solved by marriage —which doesn't solve emotional problems and may only add to them. Similarly, if your son is willing to give up a lucrative family business for the lesser financial return of teaching, let him follow his own interests. If he comes back to your way of life later, it will be from a realistic desire and not with resentment at having been forced into something.

Help your children learn to know you as individuals, not just as parents—as human beings who may make mistakes but want to do the best for their children because they love them. It is better to show your love than it is to talk about it.

One way you can show your love is by remembering that the *growing egos of adolescents need psychological nourishment as much as their growing bodies need food.* But be careful not to praise your children for qualities they don't possess. They will either suspect you of being insincere or think you believe that they are better than they are, which will make them feel inadequate and insecure. Surely you can find plenty of good things you can truthfully say about your children! Just let them know that you appreciate them as they are and for what they are.

As the poet Carl Sandburg so beautifully expressed it in *The People, Yes:*

A father sees a son nearing manhood.
What shall he tell that son? . . .

Tell him too much money has killed men
and left them dead years before burial . . .

Tell him time as a stuff can be wasted.
Tell him to be a fool every so often
and to have no shame over having been a fool
yet learning something out of every folly . . .

Tell him to be alone often and get at himself
and above all tell himself no lies about himself . . .

Tell him to be different from other people
if it comes natural and easy being different.
Let him have lazy days seeking his deeper motives.
Let him seek deep for where he is a born natural.°

---

° From *The People, Yes,* by Carl Sandburg, copyright by Harcourt, Brace and Company, Inc.

# 22

# HOUSING AND YOUR HEALTH

The effect of your home and its furnishings on your safety is certain, and on your health, nearly as sure. Accidents in the home each year kill more people than tuberculosis, diphtheria, polio, syphilis, rheumatic fever, appendicitis, and murders combined. The evidence about health is a little less positive, but tuberculosis, pneumonia, colds, rheumatic fever, and other infectious diseases certainly are more common in areas where housing is of poor quality. As you would expect, under such conditions, there is also less money available for adequate diets, warm clothing, and the other essentials of good health. Medical care is obtained less frequently.

Therefore, it becomes difficult for a doctor to say *how much of a factor* housing has been when, for example, a case of tuberculosis occurs in a situation in which housing is inadequate. I would like simply to give my readers my recommendations on the subject of health and housing, and hope that you will consider them seriously. I truly believe that if your house or apartment fulfills these suggestions, you will have a greater chance of preventing sickness and injuries. Even if you have the most luxurious home, please read the section on the prevention of accidents in the home, because no home is free of hazards that can affect both adults and children.

## THE MINIMUM REQUIREMENTS OF GOOD HOUSING

1. *Enough rooms for the family*. The number of sleeping rooms is important. No child should sleep in the same room with grown people. Ideally, each child should have his own room, but two young children of nearly the same age and sex can share a room.

Children need space and privacy in the home. Too often this is overlooked. The child who has his own space for play doesn't get in the way of the adults. The child and parents are happier and more relaxed. The child develops initiative and independence at his *play*. That is the child's method of learning how to develop his brain and his muscles. He needs *undisturbed play*, and plenty of space for his blocks and toys.

Outdoor space is also necessary for children. The parents who select their houses near parks and playgrounds will be rewarded by the increased happiness of their children.

2. *Well-heated and -ventilated rooms, always free from dampness.*

3. *Enough fresh air and sunshine.*

4. *Screens kept in good order to keep out flies and mosquitoes. Screen doors that close tightly.*

5. *An inside bath and toilet; plumbing, stove, furnace, and refrigerator, all in good repair.*

6. *Roofs, ceilings, walls, and windows which are rainproof.*

7. *Rat-proofing.*

All of these requirements may not be easily met for families with very modest income. But many or all may be achieved if the desire is strong enough. The extra cost in money and effort will pay dividends in physical and mental health.

Although doctors and health officers would like

320

every family to have adequate healthful housing, how and when this will be achieved depends on the desires of our citizens to overcome the shortage of first-class housing. That part of housing and health is beyond the scope of this book. In the meantime, there is the immediate problem facing us of selecting the best possible home for *your* family.

## WHERE TO LIVE

Select your living quarters primarily for health reasons. The proper choice requires your taking a broad view of the problem. The needs of each member of the family should be considered. A worker in city industry should consider living some distance away from his work if his children need more room than he can afford close to his work. Naturally, there is a limit to the demands on time and energy that can or should be made of the parent. But it is important that all possible factors be considered.

*How much should a family spend for rent?* This depends on your income, and varies from averages of 11 percent for well-to-do families to 33 percent for the lowest income group. A quarter of the total income used to be suggested as the correct percentage for the average family to pay for housing. I advise families to spend the maximum they can afford to obtain adequately the three essentials: housing, food, and medical and hospital insurance.

## PREVENTION OF HOME ACCIDENTS

### Accident Hazards in the Approaches to and Inside the Home

A house with poor lighting will cause more accidents than one in which the entrances, staircases, and rooms are properly illuminated. There is always a direct relationship between the state of repair of stairs and railings in a house and the number of sprains or broken bones sustained by persons living there. All such danger spots should be corrected immediately. Lights in hallways and over staircases should be large enough to illuminate the entire area. Railings should be in sufficiently good repair to prevent children from falling through. Railings should also give adequate handholds for adults, especially the elderly (in whom fractured bones are very serious matters). Loose steps or slippery and worn steps should be repaired or replaced. In cold weather, icy or slippery steps should be scraped and protected, if necessary, by sprinkling with ashes or sand.

Good light inside the house is essential. The proper maintenance and prompt repair of stoves, gas pipes, electric wiring, refrigerators, and electrical appliances are as necessary as the repair of stairs and railings outside the house.

The prevention of health hazards inside the house requires more thought, more alertness, and more *family cooperation* than prevention of accidents at the approaches to the house. Everyone in a family may suffer horrible burns if just one person sets off a fire by carelessness. Each member of the family, including children, must be taught the rules. If the following rules are observed by all, the number of accidents will be reduced to a minimum.

Many families spend much of their time outside, during at least half the year. Garden tools, automobile parts and tools, toys, chairs, and other useful and enjoyable objects become dangerous when they are left in driveways or paths, on steps, or anywhere else an unwary child or adult can fall on or stumble over them. Don't litter the outside of your home! Thousands of sprains, fractures, cuts, and bruises would be prevented each year if the outside areas and the approaches to our homes were made safe.

### Fire Hazards

There are more than one thousand home fires in the United States every day. To protect your family and your property, fire prevention is vital. It requires good housekeeping and constant attention, in these major areas:

MATCHES AND SMOKING

Keep matches and lighters out of children's reach.

Place ashtrays in every room.

NEVER smoke in bed, or lying on a sofa, or reclining in a chair that invites you to go to sleep.

### ELECTRICITY

If your home has no circuit-breakers, use the right size fuse, usually 15 amperes, for your circuits. Don't use a penny for "convenience" when a fuse blows, and don't substitute a larger fuse. A fuse is a safety valve for an electrical circuit; if the fuse can't burn out when the line is overloaded, another spot will—perhaps in a wall.

Don't overload your wall outlets. If you need more places to plug in, call an electrician.

Keep an air space behind and around your television set. Don't try to repair it yourself, even if it is disconnected. A television set builds up a heavy charge of static electricity that can give you a dangerous jolt even when the plug is out.

Electrical work more complicated than replacing a wall switch or changing a fuse is not for the average do-it-yourselfer. Call a specialist who knows how to work safely and to give you good advice.

### IN THE KITCHEN

Do not light a gas stove or gas oven if there is a distinct odor of gas. Open a window. If the odor persists, call a repairman.

Never keep a coal or gas stove or a gas grate burning unless there are vents or flues to take away the gases. Keep a window partly open for fresh air. If you leave the kitchen, turn off the gas, even if this strikes you as inconvenient.

Teach children to keep away from the stove. Many burns and scalds would be prevented if children were kept out of the kitchen when hot foods were being prepared.

### CLEANING FLUIDS

If you must keep flammable liquids around the house, store them in tightly closed metal containers (never glass) in a cool, well-ventilated place away from anything else that might catch fire.

Use cleaning fluids only in a well-ventilated place, being sure there is no open flame, lighted tobacco, or electrical spark nearby.

Keep such liquids where a child can't get them.

Never use kerosene or any other cleaning fluid to start a fire in the furnace, wood stove or fireplace.

For other fire-prevention measures, see page 324.

## Hazards from Falls Inside the Home

An observant tour of your house will show you many ways of preventing falls. Keep in mind that nearly half of the 27,000 annual deaths resulting from home accidents are the result of falls. Here are a few precautions:

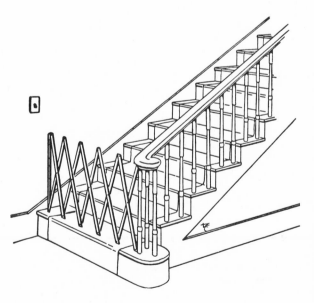

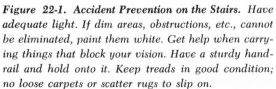

*Figure 22-1. Accident Prevention on the Stairs. Have adequate light. If dim areas, obstructions, etc., cannot be eliminated, paint them white. Get help when carrying things that block your vision. Have a sturdy handrail and hold onto it. Keep treads in good condition; no loose carpets or scatter rugs to slip on.*

*Don't leave coats, brooms or other objects on the stairs or railing. Don't let children play on the stairs. Have gates, top and bottom, for toddlers.*

Cover slippery *floors* with carpets. Anchor small rugs so that they won't slide when walked on. Be sure there are no rips to catch heels in. This is very important with the runners on stairs.

Use a rubber mat in the *bathroom* to prevent accidents caused by slipping.

Sharp-edged *furniture* should be covered or removed when children are learning how to walk. Low stools and other objects which can trip children or adults should be kept away from passageways.

Make electric light switches available for each room so that persons *walking in darkness* from one room to another will be able to light their way. It is frequently desirable for children and elderly people to keep a light on during the night, especially near the bathroom.

When children or elderly people use rooms where falls from windows would be dangerous, the lower part of the window should not be opened unless protected by heavy screens or grills. Ventilation can be obtained by opening the upper half of the window.

Stairs should be covered with carpeting or rub-

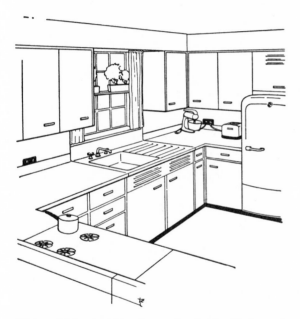

*Figure 22-2. Accident Prevention in the Kitchen. In addition to precautions listed for other rooms, be certain to: Turn off stove burners and pilot light and open window if you smell gas. Avoid spontaneous combustion by keeping oily rags in airtight tin cans only, and do not store papers, etc. Be careful with cleansing materials and other inflammables. Never start a fire with kerosene or gasoline. Stand to one side when lighting gas oven, lifting lid from boiling pot, etc.*

*Keep children away from stove; turn pot-handles in; use safety-cocks or tighten so children can't turn on gas.*

*Keep sharp objects, strong or poisonous materials out of child's reach.*

*Wipe up spilled water, grease, etc., immediately to prevent slipping.*

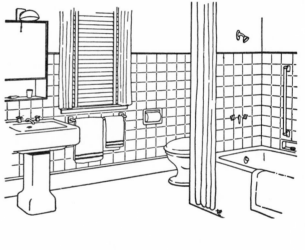

*Figure 22-3. Accident Prevention in the Bathroom. Avoid shocks; never touch a switch, wire or electrical appliance when any part of your body is even damp. Insert an insulating link or tie a string to the end of a chain pull-cord. Be especially careful with electric heaters.*

*Test hot water cautiously to avoid burns. To prevent slipping, keep floor dry, use rubber mat in tub and keep soap in dish.*

*Porcelain faucet handles crack easily; avoid cuts by substituting inexpensive metal ones. Don't leave razor blades around. Keep all medical supplies where children cannot reach them.*

ber safety treads. Also, they should be kept clear of mops, baskets, toys, and other hazards.

## Each Room Has Special Hazards

Fire and falls are the chief dangers, but as everyone knows there are countless other ones to watch for. *Each room* has its special dangers. For example:

KITCHEN. Keep sharp knives away from children. Keep lye, ammonia, acids, insect and rodent poisons, and every other caustic or poisonous substance out of children's reach. All of these, especially lye, have killed or seriously injured a great many children.

Follow the instructions already given about the danger from gas stoves and hot foods.

Keep the children out of the kitchen except when they are watched.

Adults preparing food in the kitchen need good light to prevent cuts. They need asbestos pads, tongs, and large holders for handling hot pots and pans to prevent burns and scalds.

Hot fat or grease requires special precautions. If it catches fire, *do not pour water on it* because water will spatter the fire. If you can obtain it, use sand, dirt, or ashes to put the fire out. Small fires can be extinguished by pouring salt on them, or they can be smothered with heavy wet clothes or asbestos pads. If the amount of fat is large and the flames high, pull all inflammable material away

*Figure 22-4. Accident Prevention in the Living Room. Have a screen covering entire fireplace. Fasten window curtains, etc., so they won't blow near fireplace, candles, gas or kerosene lamps. Be careful with cigarettes.*

*No slippery floors, rugs or carpets (rubber mason-jar rings sewn on under side of rugs will help to anchor them). No long electric light cords to trip over. No open sockets where young children can get at them. Don't overload sockets or tinker with TV, etc.*

*Keep furniture in repair; don't use it as a ladder.*

*Figure 22-5. Accident Prevention in the Bedroom. Observe precautions with fire and electricity already listed. Also: don't smoke in bed or sleep with heating pad turned on; put room-heater on a metal mat at a safe distance from walls, bedding, etc.; have window open while gas, oil, or coal is burning.*

*If there are young children, have bars or safety catches on windows; make certain the paint on anything they might chew is not poisonous. Prevent smothering by having baby sleep alone, with light, securely pinned bed clothes, no pillow. Keep objects baby might swallow or hurt himself with out of reach.*

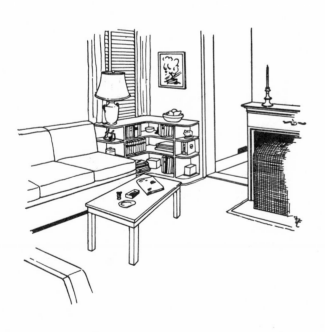

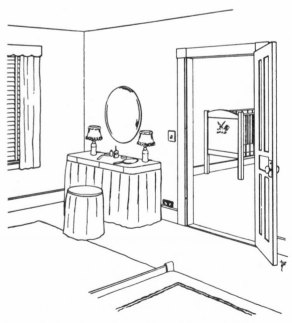

and guard against the spread of the fire by pouring water over the places the flames threaten to touch.

Have your gas range and electric refrigerator checked once a year. This service is often given free by the gas or electric company.

BATHROOM. Falls in the bathtub or shower are a frequent source of severe accidents. A rubber mat will prevent slipping in the tub. Have good lighting. Soap needs a sturdy holder.

*Never place electric equipment of any type, especially electric heaters, in the bathroom where they can fall into the tub. The safest rule is to warm the bathroom with the electric heater first, then disconnect the heater* while the baby or anyone else is in the bathtub. Don't touch an electric socket, switch, or electric appliance while standing in the water. You can be electrocuted because water helps electricity flow through your body.

Keep all medicines in a medicine chest out of the reach of children.

CELLAR. Whether you heat your home by oil, gas, electricity, or coal, have the entire system checked by a competent repairman before the cold weather. Defective heating equipment can cause serious injury or death from carbon monoxide gas as well as from fire. Flues and chimneys as well as the furnace itself should be examined to make sure they are in good condition and ready to operate properly.

If you burn coal, keep metal containers for the ashes. They stay hot longer than you might think, and they might set fire to a wooden container after you have left the cellar.

If you chop wood to start a furnace fire or to take up to your fireplace, use a good axe and be sure you know how to use it.

The cellar is often a play area, especially in winter. Try to separate the heating equipment from the children's play space. You can put up a wall easily and cheaply with a few 2 x 4 wood studs and some inexpensive pressed board partitions. Until your children are old enough to be trusted alone for an hour or more, *never* let them go to the cellar alone.

Avoid clutter. Clearly defined areas should be set aside for tools, equipment, screen, and other household paraphernalia.

The cellar, including the stairs, should be as well lighted as any other room.

Cellar stairs should be sturdy and should be kept in good condition. At least one steady railing should be provided.

The rules and precautions given here can prevent many burns, broken bones, and poisonings. Unfortunately, most of us don't like to think of accidents when all is going well. The easiest way to play safe is to organize a *home safety council* and make it a pleasant occasion and a game for the children. Once a month the family can talk safety rules and discuss any new hazards or accidents which have occurred recently.

In an article that I wrote for *McCall's* magazine on accident prevention in the home, I suggested that husbands devote themselves to the problem, too. My thought was that men know the technical side of dangerous equipment better than women. Therefore, the man in the family should take the major responsibility for checking the electrical apparatus, the furnace, the gas connections, and similar equipment. The woman could then educate the children in accident prevention.

If the children are given prizes for observing the rules, and special ones for new suggestions, plus a treat of ice cream and cake when the home "safety council" meets, they will look forward to the meetings. In this way, their interest in obeying good safety rules and making new ones will be strengthened at an early age.

# 23
# FIRST AID

This chapter on first aid contains material that may become a life and death matter for you, your family, or another fellow human being. The emergency may be such an acute, sudden one that you will not have time to consult this book. You must have the *knowledge* in advance.

In addition to knowledge, you will be a better first-aider if you also possess *experience* and *judgment.*

Let us consider this specific case: you are camping with friends when a member of the party drops an axe on his wrist and sustains a deep cut with very severe bleeding. You are twenty miles from the nearest telephone and fifty miles from a doctor. It has become obvious to all of you that a main artery has been severed because the blood is gushing out in spurts; it is bright red. Also, pressure over the wound doesn't stop the bleeding as it will do with severe cuts in veins.

Someone—perhaps you—says a tourniquet must be applied immediately or the injured person will bleed to death.

If you have the knowledge given in Figure 23-1 (p. 328), on how to stop bleeding in the arm you will be able to apply pressure with your hand over the right spot to stop the bleeding until the materials are located to make the tourniquet.

The chances are good that with this *knowledge,* you will succeed. But suppose you had previously, as a result of reading my book or attending Red Cross first aid classes, actually tested the pressure points stopping artery bleeding. How much more certain you would now be, with this previous *experience,* of success in saving the injured one's life. All you need to do in order to test the pressure points is to feel the pulse in the wrist, then apply pressure or a tourniquet in the upper arm. If you have done it right, you will feel the pulse at the wrist disappear because you have shut off the blood flow through the artery. (Figure 25-11, page 361, shows how to obtain the pulse.)

To return to our injured person: the bleeding has been stopped with an improvised tourniquet. Now the factor of *judgment* comes into the picture. Should you take him to the hospital fifty miles away, or would it be best to leave him where he is until a doctor can be brought to him some hours later? Your judgment will tell you that since a major artery has been cut, the doctor will need to sew it up in a hospital operating room. So you will vote in favor of transporting the injured one to the hospital. During the journey, your *knowledge* of first aid will save the injured person's hand from gangrene and subsequent amputation because you will remember to loosen the tourniquet every ten minutes and permit blood to flow for one minute to nourish the tissues of the hand and forearm. Your *judgment* will again be important in preventing emotional shock to the victim by making certain that he cannot see the gush of blood when the tourniquet is loosened.

What have we learned from this story (which, by the way, is based on a real incident, in which a first-aider saved her child's life)? This mother took charge because her husband was away from the camp when the axe was dropped onto her child's wrist. She didn't become panic-stricken and rush off for help which would have arrived after the child had bled to death.

Suppose this mother had not had the knowledge of first aid and had seen her child die in her presence! Do I need add anything more to convince you that the following sections on "be ready to save a life" must be studied carefully enough so that the knowledge becomes a permanent part of you?

As a minimum I would like you to learn how to handle four situations which may confront you at any time, and in which your prompt application of first aid could save a life:

SEVERE BLEEDING

POISONINGS

SUFFOCATION AND ASPHYXIA

SHOCK

Before going into the details, please learn these basic principles of first aid in serious emergencies:

1. *Never lose your head in an emergency.* This is the time quick, clear thinking and quick action are most needed. A life may depend on prompt treatment. If the sight of severe bleeding makes you too shaky, sit down in a chair for a few seconds, then go on to carry out the necessary first aid.

2. *Summon help.* Call a doctor, the police, or the nearest hospital for all possible serious cases or where there is any doubt. Do this the first chance you get *after* the first aid has been given. Better still, try to get someone to call while you are treating the injured one. If necessary, ask the telephone operator to send help.

3. *Decide about moving the victim.* You have to make this decision calmly. Persons suffering head injuries, fractures, or internal injuries must rest before being moved. Moving someone too soon, or improperly, may cause him serious harm.

## BLEEDING AND HEMORRHAGE

A severe cut or wound is dangerous because of the possibility of great blood loss.

The simplest and most effective method to stop bleeding is by direct pressure on the wound with a gauze pad or, better still, a thick compress of gauze. In an emergency any clean cloth will do.

Applying direct pressure on the wound (or *in the* wound if it is very wide) will stop nine out of ten cases of bleeding. This is important to know.

Most beginners in first aid learn complicated pressure points and the application of tourniquets. When an emergency arises they may become confused and lose precious time trying to remember complicated procedures.

The simple method of *direct pressure on and around the wound* is the fastest and the most effective.

In applying pressure it is important to keep it constant. Do not keep dabbing at the wound and lifting the gauze every few seconds to see if the bleeding has stopped. This type of treatment irritates the wound and prevents the blood from clotting. It does not give the pressure a fair chance to work properly. The only time pressure should be removed is when the blood has soaked through the gauze completely.

The dressing should be held snugly by hand against the wound for a few minutes. If no blood soaks through then the gauze or cloth should be bound firmly with tape, or next best, strips of cloth.

If the bleeding occurs in an arm or leg, raising the limb very high also helps to control bleeding, as there is less blood in an elevated limb.

Bleeding is different in arteries and veins. Bleeding from a vein comes in a steady flow. The blood is dark in color, almost a bluish red. Blood from an artery comes in spurts, caused by the heartbeat, and the color is bright red. In either type of bleeding the best treatment is direct pressure on the wound. Venous bleeding is almost always stopped successfully this way.

Direct pressure does not always stop arterial bleeding, but should be tried first. The next step is pressure by a finger or hand over the nearest pressure point shown in Figure 23-1. Another method is the *tourniquet,* a last resort.

### Applying a Tourniquet

The two places to apply a tourniquet are (a) the width of a hand below the armpit for bleeding from the arm, (b) the width of a hand below the groin for bleeding from the thigh or leg. (See Figure 23-2.)

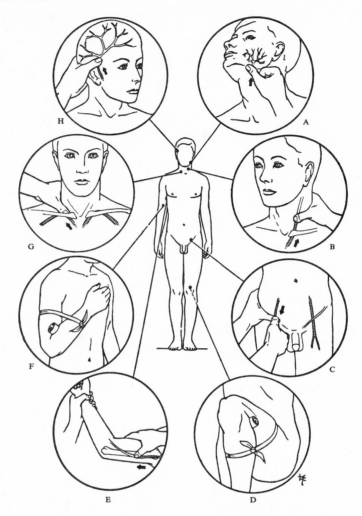

*Figure 23-1. Pressure Points on Arteries. The arrows show the direction in which the blood flows through the arteries. Pressure points are located between the wound and the heart. A. For bleeding from face. B. For bleeding from head and face. C. For bleeding from leg. (The inguinal ligament is shown as it passes over the artery.) D. For bleeding from below knee. E. For bleeding from arm. F. For bleeding from below elbow. G. For bleeding from shoulder and entire arm. H. For bleeding from scalp and upper part of head.*

1.  Use several thicknesses of gauze or cloth to make a pad.

2.  Use a wide flat strip of fabric long enough to go twice around the limb for a tourniquet (a necktie, a scarf, etc.).

3.  Wrap the tourniquet around the limb over the pad.

4.  Tie the tourniquet with a half-knot. Insert a small stick and tie again with a square knot.

5.  Tighten the tourniquet by twisting the stick. Do not twist too hard. When the tourniquet is tight enough the bleeding stops immediately like turning off a faucet.

6.  Loosen the tourniquet every ten minutes to let the blood circulate in the limb. While the tourniquet is loosened for one minute (actually timed) apply pressure by hand against the wound. If severe bleeding does not start again one minute

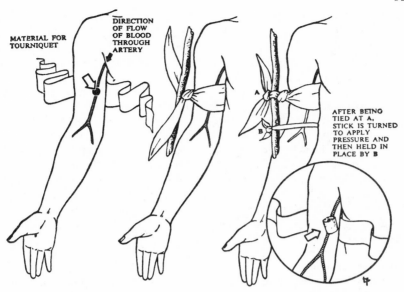

MATERIAL FOR TOURNIQUET

DIRECTION OF FLOW OF BLOOD THROUGH ARTERY

AFTER BEING TIED AT A, STICK IS TURNED TO APPLY PRESSURE AND THEN HELD IN PLACE BY B

*Figure 23-2. Applying the Tourniquet. Methods of applying a tourniquet, as described in text. Additional pressure can be created by using a bandage roll or similar object, as shown in the circle.*

after the tourniquet has been loosened, do not retighten, but leave the tourniquet in place for a while in case bleeding does recur.

Never cover the tourniquet with bandages or blankets. Leave it in the open where it can be seen by any doctor or first aid worker who arrives, and where you can get at it. If bleeding is severe, be on guard against shock (p. 334).

## POISONS

Each year now, more than one million cases of poisoning—85 percent of them among young children—occur in the United States, leading to thousands of deaths and a great deal of sickness and suffering.

Actually, the death figure given—sometimes put at 3,000 annually—is much too low, many authorities believe. Many more children may die each year because of accidental ingestion of or exposure to toxic chemicals in household agents and drugs, but the correct diagnosis may not be made because incriminating evidence is not detected or recognized. Not infrequently, for example, symptoms from irritation of the central nervous system and obvious convulsions lead to the diagnosis of viral encephalitis.

No mother, of course, deliberately goes shopping for poisons, but she buys several almost every time she goes to market. She uses them whenever she cleans house, polishes the furniture, washes dishes, paints, cleans spots off clothes. Often she may not be acutely aware of the dangers of these products for failure to pay attention to the labels. Children, naturally curious, are tempted to investigate the more than 250,000 products and myriad medicines available and often present in the home.

In a study of the precise circumstances surrounding child poisoning tragedies and near-tragedies, Children's Hospital Medical Center, Boston, made some discoveries which all parents should keep in mind:

Most poisonings involve children big enough to walk but not over three years of age.
The most dangerous time of day is during the hour just before the evening meal.
The unpleasant taste of a potential poison has little deterrent value. Toddlers will swallow virtually anything.

Parents tempt disaster when they underestimate

a young child's ingenuity or overestimate his ability to follow orders. Every day, dozens of children poison themselves by getting medicine out of bottles, even some safety-cap bottles, they are told never to touch but which are left within reach.

Reports from the nation's hundreds of poison control centers indicate that, after aspirin, the products most commonly involved in childhood poisonings are insecticides, bleaches, detergents and cleaning agents, furniture polish, kerosene, vitamin and iron pills and syrups, disinfectants, strong acids and alkalis, and laxatives.

Seventy-five percent of all poisonings in small children are with in-sight drugs or household agents, which means that three out of four poisonings are due to carelessness or negligence and could be prevented by one simple action—putting all medicines and chemical agents out of sight and reach of children.

Other measures certainly are needed. A federal law requires that hazardous household products bear information to protect users and warn against accidental ingestion by children; and vigorous enforcement and education of the public to the law's significance can help. Industry can and should develop and use increasingly effective safety closures and containers for medicines and poisonous agents, for while some children may circumvent such measures, there will be many who are unable to get a safety cap off. Any medicines administered to a child should be given on a serious basis, not as a game, and parents themselves should not take medication in the presence of small children.

## If a Poisoning Occurs

First of all, every home should have on hand two items for emergencies. One is a 1-ounce bottle of syrup of ipecac, and the other an inexpensive can of activated charcoal. The ipecac efficiently induces vomiting. The charcoal, which you can mix with water to make a souplike substance to be swallowed, absorbs any poison left in the stomach after vomiting has occurred.

Secondly, it's essential for you to know that incorrect, outdated information about antidotes and procedures is still given on many product labels as well as in many widely used first aid manuals. Although recent research has produced better knowledge of how to handle poisonings and even shown that old methods in some cases may be useless or even worse than useless, there has been delay in incorporating this information into labels and manuals.

For example, often the instructions on the labels of drain cleaners, oven cleaners, and lye products —all of which contain strong alkalis and acids— recommend drinking citrus juices or vinegar as antidotes, on the assumption that these will help by neutralizing the alkalis or acids swallowed. But experts report that the mixture of juice and alkali can generate heat and further damage internal tissue.

What can you do, then, to be certain that if your child is accidentally poisoned, your efforts to help will in fact be helpful and not useless or even harmful?

First, you can give first aid (which I will describe), and then, without delay, get expert help.

You should know that there is now a nationwide network of poison control centers. Each state has such a center. Check the front of your local telephone directory for its number. If it isn't there, ask your doctor for the number. These centers have the very latest information on what is in household products that may cause poisoning and on how best to handle a case of poisoning.

Immediately after you have given quick, simple first aid, call the poison control center or your family doctor. If you can't reach either one, call the emergency unit of the local hospital or try the police or fire department, which may have an emergency service.

Keep calm, briefly explain what has happened, what unusual symptoms the patient shows, what substance may have been involved (trade name, manufacturer, label warning).

Then follow the instructions you get—to the letter. Use the ipecac or charcoal only if told to do so.

For first aid:

*In the case of a swallowed poison:* If the child —or other person—is awake and able to swallow, give water only. Then call for help.

*In the case of a poison on the skin:* Remove any affected items of clothing, and flood the in-

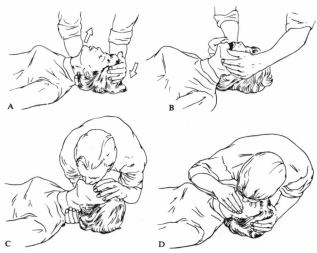

A. *Place the victim on his back and tilt his head back so that the chin points upward.*

B. *Pull or push the jaw into a jutting-out position.*

C. *Open your own mouth wide and place it tightly over the victim's, at the same time pinching his nostrils shut.*

D. *If his mouth is injured or completely clenched, place your mouth over his nose, making certain that his mouth is closed. Blow into the victim's mouth or nose. Remove your mouth and listen for the outward rush of air.*

*Figure 23–3. Mouth-to-Mouth Resuscitation.*

volved skin area with water, wash with soap and water, and rinse. Then call for help.

*In the case of a poison in the eye:* Use lukewarm, never hot, water to flood the eye, pouring it from a pitcher held three or four inches from the eye. Do this for fifteen minutes. Then call for help.

*In the case of an inhaled poison:* Immediately carry the child (or drag the adult) to fresh air. Give mouth-to-mouth resuscitation (described later) if necessary. Ventilate the area. Then call for help.

FOOD POISONING. Food poisoning is usually caused by bacterial contamination of food (p. 34 ). It can also be caused by eating toadstools or poisonous mushrooms, berries, shellfish, or other foods that are inedible or have "spoiled" or have been improperly canned. The symptoms of such poisoning are usually acute and come on soon after eating the contaminated or poison-containing food. They include pain or tenderness in the abdomen, nausea, vomiting, painful spasms, diarrhea, weakness, and in some cases, such as mushroom poisoning, dimness of vision and symptoms resembling those of alcoholic intoxication.

Waste no time in getting the victim to a doctor or hospital emergency room, especially if he has eaten toadstools, poisonous berries, or inedible shellfish. The symptoms of mushroom poisoning may not occur until some time after meal. Poison can also be caused by improperly canned food (*botulism*).

DRUG POISONING. You might not ordinarily think of *overdosage of medicine or drugs* as poisoning, but it is often treated as such. One of the problems of recognizing poisoning by an overdose of medicine is that there may be no immediate symptoms. Your suspicion may first be aroused when you notice an opened medicine container. If this happens, call the doctor immediately and tell him what the medicine is, how much was swallowed, and how much time passed since it was taken. I realize you may not know *all* these things, but anything you can tell him will help.

## ASPHYXIA (SUFFOCATION: STOPPAGE OF BREATHING)

Asphyxia is similar to being choked. Breathing is difficult, or the person does not breathe at all. However, even if breathing stops, the heart continues to beat for a few minutes. If you act quickly, you may save a life. Apply artificial respiration after electric shock, apparent drowning, or any accident that causes the breathing to stop.

Quickly explore the mouth for any obstruction —mud, sand, chewing gum, or displaced false teeth, for example—that would interfere with the passage of air. Loosen any constriction about the neck.

Continue artificial respiration for adults or children until a doctor advises you to stop. It has been found in cases of stoppage of breathing from electrical shock that victims have recovered even several hours after artificial respiration has been started. In these victims, the lungs are clear, but the respiration-control center in the brain has been paralyzed temporarily. If the first-aider can keep up the supply of air by one of the techniques described, he will save a life. In drowning accidents, the lungs may fill with water and artificial respiration should be started at once to supply air to the pulmonary circulation.

The mouth-to-mouth method is now recommended as the most effective means of artificial respiration. It is also the least complicated. Anyone accustomed to the older Nielsen or other techniques of artificial respiration should use whatever he can manage best in an emergency. Any artificial respiration method is learned best through the Red Cross or other classes.

## Mouth-to-Mouth Method

Mouth-to-mouth resuscitation (Figure 23-3) is a method of artificial respiration by which the rescuer's breath goes directly into the victim's lungs. It is the easiest, most practical and most efficient method, because the rescuer can keep the victim's air passage open, inflate the victim's lungs immediately, move more air into the lungs than with other methods, and watch the victim's chest to determine when he starts to breathe for himself.

If you use this technique, place the victim on his back and tilt his head back so that the chin points upward. Pull or push the jaw into a jutting-out position. Open your own mouth wide and place it tightly over the victim's, at the same time pinching his nostrils shut. If his mouth is injured or completely clenched, place your mouth over his nose, making certain that his mouth is closed. Blow into the victim's mouth or nose. Remove your mouth and listen for the outward rush of air, which indicates adequate air exchange. If there is no return, check for an obstruction (which may be the victim's tongue). For an adult, blow vigorously at about twelve breaths per minute. For a child, take relatively shallow breaths at about twenty per minute.

If the child is small, place your mouth over both his nose and mouth when blowing.

## Nielsen Method of Artificial Respiration

This method gives good exchange of air into the lungs. In some cases, this may mean the difference between recovery and death.

The Nielsen procedure is carried out as in Figure 23-4: Place the victim face down, with his head on his hands, and the mouth free of contact with any obstruction such as grass or clothes. (A) Kneel at victim's head. (B) Lift victim's elbow upward and outward. This will expand the lungs and cause them to fill with air. Replace the elbows in their original position. (C) Spread your fingers, place both thumbs together, and then (D) apply full pressure to the lower part of his back, so as to empty the lungs. Release the pressure smoothly, and come back to a comfortable position. Now return to the elbow lift. The two parts of the process should be completed in about five seconds (five slow counts). Keep up the process for about ten or twelve times per minute, timing yourself with a watch. Every few minutes stop to observe if the victim has started breathing by his own respiratory mechanism. If he has, then continue your Nielsen technique, synchronized so as to aid the victim's own breathing, until medical help arrives.

## Artificial Respiration for Babies

If the mouth-to-mouth technique does not work adequately, you can use the *rocking technique*, ten or twelve times a minute, lifting the baby from the horizontal to vertical position, and back again. The rocking motion, either on a board or in your arms, will pull air into the baby's lungs and expel it.

If you don't get effective results with either method, and the color is still blue, shift to the *Laborde method of artificial respiration:* Grasp the tongue, wrapping it with gauze or cloth to permit you to grip it, if you don't have forceps handy. Give the tongue a tug forward and upward every four or five seconds. Sometimes, this rhythmic action will start up the victim's own respiratory reflexes.

# CLOSED CHEST
# HEART MASSAGE

Electrical shock, immersion in water, asphyxiation, or heart attack may apparently have killed someone suddenly. Yet, the emergency procedure known as closed chest heart massage can "restore" a person whose heart has stopped briefly, or is beating irregularly and weakly. If you are sure that the victim is this seriously affected, I suggest the following emergency procedure:

Place both hands, one on top of the other, on the lower portion of the victim's chest, at the bottom of his breastbone. Apply pressure through the heel of your bottom hand and push firmly, but not more than about two inches downward. The pressure should be repeated 60 times a minute.

Since the human central nervous system and brain are permanently damaged five or six minutes after the heart has stopped beating, this last-resort technique must be started immediately after you recognize that there is no heartbeat. Although this is a first aid method that should be learned through the American Red Cross or other agency, it is important to know it so that you can attempt it if absolutely necessary, even without previous training.

If there is no response to heart massage after several minutes, try a sharp blow on the breastbone; it might get the heart started. At any rate, continue compression until professional help arrives.

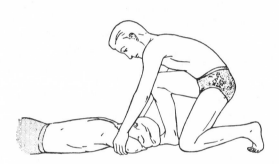

A. Preparing to raise the victim's elbows.

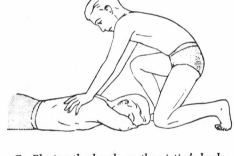

C. Placing the hands on the victim's back.

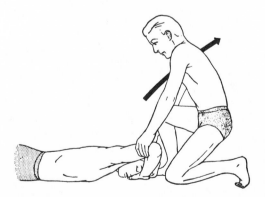

B. Raising the elbows upward and outward to expand the lungs.

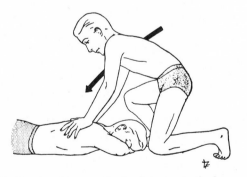

D. Pressing down on the back to empty the lungs.

Figure 23–4. Artificial Respiration. The Nielsen Method.

# COMBINED HEART-LUNG RESUSCITATION

Often a victim has an arrest of both heartbeat and breathing. Resuscitation, then, is best managed by two people—but, if necessary, you can do it alone.

If two rescuers are available, one should carry out the heart compression while the other does the mouth-to-mouth resuscitation.

If there is only one rescuer, he should carry out the breathing and massage in this ratio: After 15 chest compressions at a rate of 80 per minute, there should be 2 very quick lung inflations. With two rescuers, 5 chest compressions at a rate of 60 a minute should be carried out, then 2 lung inflations, then compressions again, repeating the cycle.

# SHOCK

Shock should not be confused with fainting. It may follow an injury (especially one involving loss of blood); an illness in which there has been prolonged vomiting or diarrhea; burns; heart attack; stroke; and poisoning by chemicals, gases, alcohol, or drugs.

When a person goes into shock he becomes pale and his skin feels cold and clammy. He breathes rapidly and his pulse beats faster and more faintly. He may become partly or completely unconscious. Severe shock may result in death. The rapid, weak pulse and cold clammy skin of the person in shock are not usually seen in people who have only fainted. To prevent shock or to speed up recovery:

1. Keep the victim lying quietly with his feet higher than his head (except in cases of head injuries). Cover him with warm blankets. Recent studies have shown that it is unnecessary to keep the patient very warm; too much heat may be harmful. If hot-water bottles are used they should be warm, not hot. Just see that he does not feel cold.

2. If he is fully conscious, give him warm drinks.

3. Remember that prolonged, severe shock may kill. Usually, the severe shock that follows a major hemorrhage, an automobile accident, or a gunshot wound, will require transfusions of blood or plasma. You can best help to prevent the fatal outcome of shock by (a) stopping bleeding if it exists; (b) relieving agonizing pains such as may be present from a severe fracture. It would be desirable to wait for a doctor to give an injection of morphine to relieve pain, before trying to transport the victim to a hospital if there is a long trip ahead for him. In the event that no pain-stopping medicine is available, talk reassuringly to the victim, and hold his hand. This may rally his vital forces enough to delay the onset of shock.

# OTHER EMERGENCIES THAT THREATEN LIFE

If you are prepared to give first aid for the severe cases of poisoning, hemorrhage, asphyxia, and shock, you will be ready to deal with almost all of the major emergencies. Here are a few more situations you may be confronted with, in which you can save a life.

## Burns

If the clothes or hair catch fire, pour water, milk, or any other noninflammable fluid on the victim if sufficient amounts are right on hand. Don't go for fluids if none are available. Take a coat, rug, blanket, or any other heavy material, cover the flames, and smother them. If you try to beat out the flames with your hands, you may injure both the burned person and yourself.

A burn is an injury to the skin, but it may also involve and even destroy the tissues under the skin. The degree of a burn depends on whether the skin is broken. In minor (first-degree) burns, the skin is red but unbroken, and there is no danger of infection. Second- and third-degree burns are much more serious. The skin is broken and blisters develop. Infection may set in through open wounds.

In minor burns apply a paste of baking soda and water, and cover the burn with sterile gauze. Your purpose is to relieve pain. You will also find helpful the analgesic ointments recommended on page 348 for your home medicine cabinet.

For minor burns, run cold water over the affected area to relieve the pain. If you have an antiseptic ointment that also has local anesthetic properties, use it. *Do not use greasy ointments on any kind of burn.*

Second-degree burns are characterized by deep reddening and blistering. Gently clean the skin if any grease or dirt is present, but *do not rub.* Soak the burned area with a solution of two heaping tablespoonfuls of baking soda (bicarbonate of soda) to a quart of water that has first been boiled, allowed to cool. Then cover the burned area with sterile gauze, wrap the victim in blankets, and take him to a hospital or to a doctor's office.

Third-degree burns involve the entire thickness of the skin. There may be some charring. Such a burn cannot heal by itself, and whatever immediate emergency care you can provide will help the doctor and hospital in their necessary long-term treatment. Some shock may be present; this should be treated by the methods I discussed on page 334. Give the victim some fluid by mouth, if he is conscious, and a sedative, such as an aspirin. Always be sure to remember any medication you give, keeping a record if possible. The burn itself should not be touched, except that any foreign matter, such as burned clothing, should be removed, without pulling at the affected area. Cover the burns with a clean cloth or sterile gauze. Keep the victim's feet raised, and keep him warm until medical help arrives.

CHEMICAL BURNS. Wash the injured area with water. Use plenty of water and use it constantly while you are waiting for the doctor to come. If chemicals get into the eyes, you can put in a few drops of pure mineral oil after the eyes have been washed several times with water.

SUNBURN. This is treated like any other burn in which the skin is reddened but not broken. Petroleum jelly or olive oil may help reduce the pain. (See also page 155.) If sunburn is severe, the victim may have shivers and a fever. Call a doctor while you keep the patient warm under blankets.

## Electric Shock

If the victim is in contact with electricity (through a wire or defective home appliance),
shut off the current or pull the appliance plug if you can do so without delay. Otherwise, because every second counts, use dry sticks, rolled-up dry newspapers, or heavy, dry gloves (rubber, if they are immediately available) to pull him away. Stand on something dry. Electricity passes easily through moist articles, and you may wind up being badly shocked yourself and not helping the victim at all if you are not careful. *Avoid touching him directly until he is away from the source of the shock.*

Severe electric shock may paralyze the respiratory center in the brain and upset the natural rhythm of the heart. Once the victim is separated from the source of electricity, use mouth-to-mouth artificial respiration to restore his breathing (see page 331). If he is breathing normally, keep him warm, quiet, and in a half-sitting position.

## Sunstroke

Overlong exposure to high temperatures, great effort in extreme heat, or lying in the sun too long can lead to sunstroke, or failure of the body's mechanism for regulating body heat. Sunstroke can be a serious threat to life when treatment is delayed.

Symptoms begin with headache, dizziness, nausea, collapse, little or no sweating, flushed, hot, dry skin, racing pulse, fast breathing, and a fever of 106 degrees or more.

The temperature must be brought down quickly to avoid shock, convulsions, delirium, coma, and death. Call a physician or ambulance at once. Meanwhile, place the patient in a tub of ice water and rub the skin until the temperature falls. Take the temperature by rectum every 10 minutes until 102 degrees is reached, then stop cooling. If temperature continues to fall, the patient now must be kept warm, and massaging must continue to prevent the blood vessels from constricting. If temperature goes up again, return the patient to the tub of cold water. With prompt and correct treatment, followed by several days of care, total recovery can be expected.

## Heat Exhaustion

Although similar to sunstroke in producing dizziness and headache, this is a relatively minor disorder—and it is unlike sunstroke in other ways.

Heat exhaustion may follow long exposure to heat or too much activity in a strong sun. The skin is clammy and cold instead of flushed and hot as in sunstroke. And sweating is profuse instead of absent, the pulse rate is not high, nor is there significant fever.

Other symptoms of heat exhaustion may include weakness and dimming or blurring of vision.

Treatment consists of lying down in a cool place with head lower than the rest of the body, slowly sipping water, and taking salt tablets to replenish lost fluids and salt.

## Snakebite

I have purposely placed snakebite close to the bottom of the list of serious emergencies to emphasize the fact that it is much less important than you have been led to believe. Snakebite accounts for only a fraction of accidental deaths compared to bleeding, poisons, and asphyxia. If people were only as cautious about their automobiles or their swimming habits as they are about stepping into ground where a poisonous snake has been seen, the national safety record would mark a real victory. (To identify poisonous snakes, see page 161.)

*Most snakebites can be prevented* by two easy precautions based on the fact that snakes bite feet and ankles, or hands. (1) In snake-infested areas, wear high shoes or heavy trousers or dungarees which are fastened to the tops of your shoes by secure ties. This will prevent bites if you accidentally step on a snake. (2) Never put your hand onto a ledge or rock unless you can see that a snake is not lying there. You should always poke ahead of your hand with a stick to frighten any snakes away. These two precautions will prevent nearly all snakebites.

TREATMENT OF POISONOUS SNAKEBITE. The bite of a poisonous snake will cause immediate swelling and discoloration near the bite.

*Step Number 1.* Apply a venous tourniquet to prevent the poison from being absorbed into the body through the veins. This tourniquet is placed *above the bite* to prevent flow of blood toward the heart. A venous tourniquet can be made with a belt, a necktie, or heavy cloth. It doesn't have to be tied as tight as an arterial tourniquet because the veins are compressed more easily.

*Step Number 2.* Decide on how to get the victim medical aid so that he can receive an injection of *antivenin*. Your judgment will be required in any individual situation as to whether the victim should be transported to the doctor, or the doctor summoned to him. Notify the doctor about the species of snake, if that is known (see Figure 9–5, page 161). If the snake can be killed safely, bring it with you to the doctor.

*Step Number 3.* Until the doctor takes over, you should start removing the snake venom from the bite. Make cuts in a crosscross fashion over the bitten area, cutting about one-quarter inch deep. Don't be frightened about the bleeding. That helps wash out the poison. Now, you can save a life by actually sucking the poison out of the place where you made the cuts. Snake poison is harmless when taken into the mouth unless you happen to have an open cut or sore. Suck out the poison and spit it out; it will not be harmful even if swallowed. (Of course, it is easier and much pleasanter to use a suction cup if there is one available in your emergency kit.)

*Step Number 4.* Do not give whiskey. Reassure the victim. Give him coffee or other warm drinks if he wishes them.

Poisonous snake venom usually travels slowly under the skin toward the heart. Except in the rare instance when the poison is inserted directly into a blood vessel, there is no fear of immediate death. However, right after someone has been bitten he may suffer severe pain and possibly shock. Keep him as quiet as possible, since exertion will hasten the passage of the venom toward his heart. Applying ice or cold compresses to the site of the injury will help relieve the pain and slow down the action of the venom.

## Choking on a Foreign Body in the Throat

This is another emergency in which you may be called upon to save a life. Perhaps no other of the major first-aid problems calls for so much coolness and judgment on your part. Suppose, for example, you have guests for dinner, and suddenly a friend, while eating his meat, swallows a large piece "the wrong way." In other words, he has lodged the meat in his glottis, the upper part of the windpipe. If he is lucky, nature will bring it up for him in a violent fit of coughing. *But* imagine the situation in which the piece of meat has lodged securely in his glottis. The person begins to choke, he makes gasping sounds, begins to turn blue. He points to his throat because his speech is cut off, begging everyone to help him. You happen to be too far away to summon a doctor, and there is no hospital near enough at hand. What do you do?

There is now a procedure—called the *Heimlich maneuver,* after the doctor who developed it— for removing an obstruction that is causing choking. In fact, there are two procedures, both simple and effective, one for when the victim is standing, the other when he is lying down.

When the victim is standing, get behind him and place your arm around his waist. Make a fist with one hand and place it, with the thumb side in, against the abdomen, below the bottom of the ribs and slightly above the navel. Grasp your fist with your other hand and press into the abdomen with a quick upward thrust. Repeat several times if necessary until the obstructing object is expelled. You can use the same procedure when the victim is sitting as you stand behind his chair.

When the victim is lying down and you can't lift him, turn him on his back and kneel astride his hips. Put one of your hands on top of the other, place the heel of the bottom hand on the abdomen, just below the ribs and a little above the navel—and, with a quick upward thrust, press into the abdomen.

If you yourself are choking and no one is present to help, you can perform the Heimlich maneuver on yourself. Press your fist, with thumb-side in, into your abdomen, below the ribs and slightly above the navel. Then drop down hard on your fist against the edge of a chair or a sink.

## FIRST AID MEASURES THAT DO NOT REQUIRE LIFE-AND-DEATH DECISIONS

### Fractures

A fracture is a broken bone. When no break in the skin occurs, it is called a simple fracture. If the broken bone pierces the skin and is exposed, it is a compound fracture. The two types are shown in Figure 23–5.

The best treatment is to keep the patient lying down quietly and to call the doctor. Never attempt to set the bone yourself unless you are a specially trained first aid worker. Often the doctor cannot determine the extent of injury without further examination and x-rays. Watch the person closely for signs of shock (p. 334).

Keep the patient lying down and warm to prevent shock. Splints should be put over the injury only if it is necessary to move him (see illustration, page 344). But if it is at all possible, it is best that he lie still. He should not be moved because if his spine is fractured, any attempt to lift or turn him may cause paralysis.

A concussion or a fractured skull may result from a severe blow on the head. Keep the victim lying quiet and warm. If he is flushed, his head should be slightly elevated; if he is pale, let his

*Figure 23-5. Main Types of Fractures.* LEFT: *The bone is broken but the ends have not separated.* CENTER: *The ends of the broken bone have separated to* some extent. RIGHT: *The end of the broken bone penetrates through the skin.*

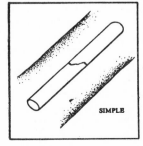
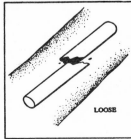
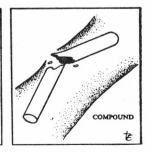

SIMPLE          LOOSE          COMPOUND

head lie on the same level with the rest of his body or slightly lower. Call the doctor.

## Head Injuries in Children

Children often bang their heads against things or bump them in falling. Usually, this causes no damage. However, to be on the safe side as far as potentially serious concussions and fractures of the skull are concerned, be sure to observe the following precautions:

If the child is knocked out, that is, if he is rendered unconscious, for even a moment, call a doctor or take the child to a hospital.

If the child is not knocked out and cries promptly, watch him for the next twelve hours. Call a doctor if the child vomits, becomes drowsy, or cannot be aroused when he is sleeping.

## Dislocations

A dislocation (Figure 23-6) is a bone out of place at the joint. Many times this is the result of a broken bone.

Send for a doctor. Never try to put the bones back into place except in a dislocation of the finger or lower jaw (and then only when medical help is not available).

*Dislocated finger:* pull the end of the finger toward you. With the thumb and forefinger gently press down on the joint until the bone slips back into place. Treat for shock if necessary. Never attempt to fix a dislocated thumb.

*Dislocated jaw:* The lower jaw hangs loose and the victim is unable to close his mouth. Wrap your thumbs in cloth to protect them against biting. Put your thumbs on the lower teeth near the gums. Press down, then back and up under the jaw with your fingers. As the jaw closes, slip your thumbs between the teeth and cheek so they will not be caught between snapping teeth as the jaw springs back into place.

## Sprains and Strains

In a strain, the muscle stretches and becomes quite painful. You can get a strain by taking a wrong step and stretching a muscle that supports the ankle. Although you may find it very painful to walk, you can still manage. Treatment consists of rest for the injured part, the gentle application of warm compresses and light massage.

A sprain occurs when a ligament connecting bone or supporting a joint is torn. In this case the pain is very severe, and if the ankle is injured, you cannot walk at all, or with great difficulty.

The injured part swells, and there is pain and discoloration of the skin which becomes red or reddish blue.

Lie down and rest the injured part on a level above the head; apply cold cloths or an ice pack to the area for ten minutes every two hours.

Sometimes what may seem to you to be a sprain is really a fracture. If a sprain is severe, it should be seen by a doctor.

## Bruises

A bruise is usually caused by a fall or a blow. The skin is not broken, but the tissues under the skin are injured, resulting in pain, swelling, and black and blue marks due to blood that has collected under the skin. A good example of a bruise is a black eye. Apply ice packs on the bruise, or a cloth dipped in cold water and wrung out. This relieves the pain. The blood that has collected is usually absorbed gradually, without causing any difficulty. If the bruise is severe and there is a great deal of swelling and pain, see the doctor.

## Cuts

For *small cuts and scratches,* cleanse the wound with sterile cotton dipped in warm, soapy water, followed by plain warm water. (Water from faucet is safe.) Then cover it with sterile gauze. If the cut is very small, a Band-Aid will do.

If the wound is very dirty, if it is a deep puncture wound or one caused by firecrackers, the patient should have an injection of tetanus antitoxin to prevent lockjaw. If he has previously been immunized with toxoid (this is true of all men in the armed forces), all he needs is a booster dose of toxoid. As a general preventive measure, everyone who has not already been immunized should have the protection of tetanus toxoid (see page 139).

Any cut that goes deeply into the skin may heal better if it is sewn together. If in doubt, let your doctor or the nearest hospital emergency room decide for you. Otherwise you may blame yourself, in later years, for an unsightly scar.

## Splinters

To remove a splinter from the skin, first sterilize a large needle by either boiling it in water or holding it in the flame of a match. Let it cool. Wash the skin with soapy water or alcohol to sterilize it, too. Press the point of the needle against the skin, scraping and digging gently until the splinter is loosened or removed. Sometimes, when the splinter is partly out, you can best remove it then with a pair of tweezers, which have also been sterilized in alcohol.

## Foreign Bodies in the Eyes

Cinders, grit, or any other foreign bodies in the eye are best removed by washing the eye liberally with clean water or sterile physiological salt solution (p. 108). Use a clean dropper. If this procedure doesn't work, then you may try direct removal if the particle is plainly visible and not imbedded in the eyeball. Make certain the light is good. Better still, if possible use a flashlight in a dark room to search for the object. You can use

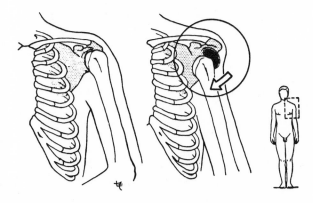

**Figure 23-6. Dislocation of the Shoulder.** LEFT: *Normal shoulder. The shaded area indicates the scapula (shoulder blade).* RIGHT: *Dislocation. The end of the humerus (upper arm bone) has completely separated from its socket (darkened area) and moved forward in the direction of the arrow.*

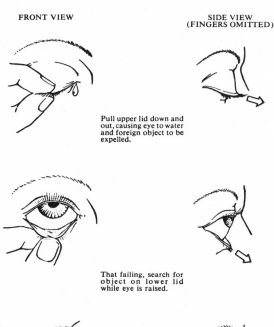

FRONT VIEW

SIDE VIEW
(FINGERS OMITTED)

Pull upper lid down and out, causing eye to water and foreign object to be expelled.

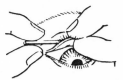

That failing, search for object on lower lid while eye is raised.

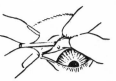

That failing, pull out and up on upper lid; place smooth match stick above margin of lid while patient is looking up; as he looks down, quickly flip lid over match stick as shown.

Foreign object is exposed and can be carefully removed with end of soft, clean handkerchief or bit of cotton on end of toothpick.

CAUTION: do not attempt to remove anything embedded *in* the eyeball.

**Figure 23-7. Removing a Foreign Object from the Eye.**

a bit of cotton wrapped around a toothpick or matchstick and dab gently over the eyelid. If the pain persists, it would be better to go to a doctor or to the nearest hospital to have the particle removed. Do not rub the eye. If the pain is severe, put a few drops of pure, plain mineral oil in the eye.

If you are far from a doctor or first aid station, and are confronted with a foreign body under the upper lid, you can invert the lid by the technique shown in Figure 23–7.

If despite all efforts you haven't succeeded, and if antibiotic *eye ointment* is available, place some of this in the painful eye until the person is brought to medical aid.

## Toothache

Toothache may be *temporarily* relieved by taking aspirin or Bufferin (see page 65), or codeine and Demerol if you have a doctor's prescription for the latter two. If the toothache is due to a cavity or the loss of a filling, put some oil of cloves on a tiny bit of cotton and pack it into the cavity. It is important to place it *in* the cavity and not just against the aching tooth. You can usually locate the hole even when it is in the inner part of an upper tooth; use a pocket mirror small enough to fit part way into the mouth, and pick up the image it reflects on a larger mirror. Pack the oil-soaked cotton firmly into the cavity with a toothpick or the sharpened end of a wooden match.

The pain of toothaches that are not due to cavities can sometimes be relieved by applying heat or cold to the outside of the jaw. (See Chapter 4, page 61, on the teeth).

## Nosebleeds

A slight nosebleed usually stops by itself. If bleeding continues or is severe, put the person in a chair and loosen clothing around the neck. Apply cold compresses to his nose and back of the neck. Because almost all nosebleeds occur in the soft part of the nose, it helps to press the nostril on the bleeding side against the bone for about five minutes. Or plug up the bleeding nostril with

sterile cotton. Keep the patient sitting, unless he feels faint. If bleeding persists, call the doctor.

## Fainting

When a person is about to faint, he becomes dizzy, turns pale, and feels weak. He may or may not become unconscious.

The best way to avoid fainting is to lower the head between the knees for about five minutes. If the person still feels dizzy, the head-lowering should be repeated.

If the victim has "passed out," loosen his clothing and see that he gets plenty of fresh, cool air. Place smelling salts or a few drops of aromatic spirits of ammonia under his nose until he revives. If he does not regain consciousness within five minutes, call a doctor.

## Frostbite

Frostbite can be dangerous since it may lead to gangrene. The most vulnerable areas are the toes, fingers, ears, and nose, which have the lowest degree of blood circulation.

Advance warning of frostbite is a tingling, numbing sensation, with the skin becoming painful and red. Burning, itching and swelling may develop. When the area loses all feeling, becoming numb and white, it is frostbitten.

Cover the frozen part with clothing or with your hands or any other part of the body. A frozen hand can be placed between the thighs or under an armpit for warmth. Do not rub with snow or anything else. Do not apply excessive heat. Place the affected part in warm water between 103 and 107 degrees Fahrenheit. Anything less will not help and anything more may do harm. Hot beverages are helpful. In severe cases, a doctor may need to administer medication to reduce the possibility of gangrene.

## Animal Bite

In all cases of animal bite, the danger of rabies exists. Rabies can be spread not only by dogs, but by the bite of foxes, cats, squirrels, coyotes, horses, cows, swine, and other warm-blooded animals. If rabies is not treated, it usually results in death.

First wash the wound under running water, scrubbing with plenty of soap. Pour warm soapy water, ten times, into every crevice of the bite. Either call or visit the doctor as soon as you can. The doctor will apply further treatment which may include the well-known Pasteur vaccine treatment, or the new serum method. If the bite was on the head or neck, the prophylactic treatment should be started at once.

The animal should be caught and examined for rabies.

## Insect Bite

For any type of insect bite, apply a paste of baking soda and cold cream, or use calamine lotion.

If stung by a bee, scrape off the "stinger" with a sterilized needle or knife, if possible, and apply washing soda or a few drops of diluted ammonia. If stung by a wasp, hornet, or "yellow jacket," use a little vinegar or rub with a piece of onion. Rubbing alcohol is helpful for wasp or ant bites. Cold compresses help to relieve the pain. Be sure to see a doctor if the sting happens to be on the tongue or any other part of the body where a swelling can be serious, or if pain and swelling persist, or if a number of stings have been inflicted.

Some people are *allergic* to the stings of wasps and bees. See a doctor immediately if there are symptoms indicating this, such as collapse or a swelling of the body. People who know they are allergic to stings, or who live in places where they are apt to be stung and where no medical help is readily available, should ask their physicians to prescribe an insect sting treatment kit, containing a syringe, epinephrine, antihistamine tablets, tourniquet, and instructions. It can be lifesaving.

The stings of scorpions, centipedes, and some spiders can be serious. Get rid of as much of the poison as possible by encouraging bleeding and by suction (see p. 336). Apply ice to slow the spread of the poison. See a doctor as soon as possible.

## Childbirth

It is extremely unlikely that you'll ever have the responsibility of helping a baby into the world, but I'm including it because people often ask about it—especially prospective fathers.

There is very little you need to, or should, do. If the baby is born so rapidly that the mother can't get medical assistance, it is almost bound to be born naturally and easily. First—the things you should not do: Don't touch the area of the mother's body around the place from which the baby emerges. Don't attempt to pull or help it out in any way. Don't attempt to pull out the afterbirth if it, too, should be expelled before the doctor arrives.

Here is what you should do: Be sure a doctor or ambulance has been summoned; the telephone operator will help if necessary—provided you are not too flustered to tell her your name and address.

Wash your hands. Touch and support only the baby during the delivery. Leave the baby between his mother's knees (which should be raised while she is giving birth), being certain his face is not in any blood or other fluid. Be sure that the cord attaching him to his mother is slack—don't stretch it. If he is not breathing, use mouth-to-mouth resuscitation (see p. 332). If the baby is gurgling or breathing with difficulty, there is probably mucus in his nose and mouth. Suck it out with a straw or something similar or wipe it out with a cloth or, if necessary, your finger. Cover the baby, all but his head, with a blanket.

Wait about an hour for the doctor. If he does not arrive you should tie the cord tightly, about six inches from the baby, with a clean piece of tape or twine; make a second tie about two inches farther away from the baby. Cut between the two tied places with a clean scissors or a sharp knife, which you have dipped for five minutes in alcohol. Put the baby in a warm place, on his side.

If the doctor still is not there, and the afterbirth should appear, don't throw it away as he will want to inspect it. After it has been completely expelled, put your hand on the mother's abdomen, just below the navel, and massage the firm lump which is the uterus. If it doesn't stay firm, cup your hands around it, and massage or knead it till it does.

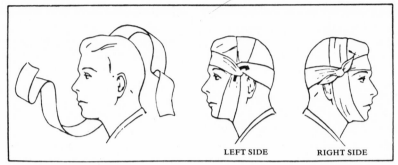

CRAVAT FOR CHEEK OR EAR

LEFT SIDE          RIGHT SIDE

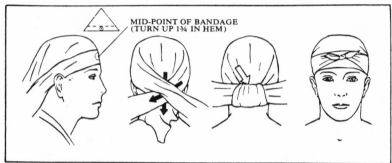

MID-POINT OF BANDAGE
(TURN UP 1¾ IN HEM)

TRIANGULAR HEAD BANDAGE

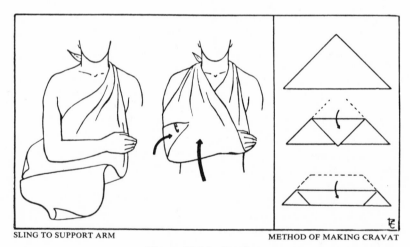

SLING TO SUPPORT ARM

METHOD OF MAKING CRAVAT

*Figure 23-8A. Bandages.*

## Other Emergencies

In various places in this book, certain emergency conditions in which you may be called upon to give first aid treatment are described. These conditions are discussed in connection with my full account of the illness in which they may occur. Some are listed below; the others you can locate quickly by reference to the Index.

CONVULSIONS IN CHILDREN (nonepileptic type), page 300
EPILEPTIC SEIZURES, page 465

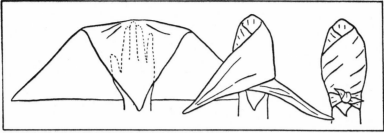

TRIANGULAR BANDAGE COVERING ENTIRE HAND OR FOOT

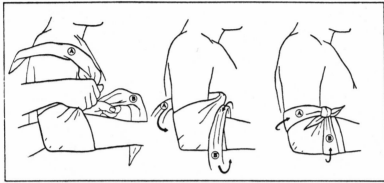

CRAVAT (WIDE) FOR ELBOW OR KNEE

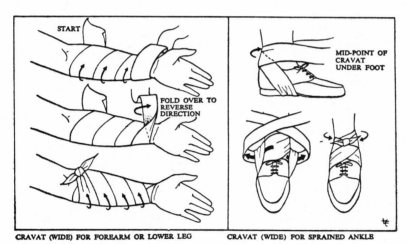

START

FOLD OVER TO REVERSE DIRECTION

MID-POINT OF CRAVAT UNDER FOOT

CRAVAT (WIDE) FOR FOREARM OR LOWER LEG     CRAVAT (WIDE) FOR SPRAINED ANKLE

*Figure 23-8B. Bandages.*

CROUP, page 299
DIABETIC ACIDOSIS AND COMA, page 78
INSULIN REACTIONS (insulin overdosage), page 78
HEART ATTACKS (coronary occlusions), page 419
STROKES (apoplexy; cerebral hemorrhage; "shock"), page 427

## BANDAGING

I have intentionally placed the section on bandaging at the very end of this chapter. In my considered opinion, it is the least important part of first aid.

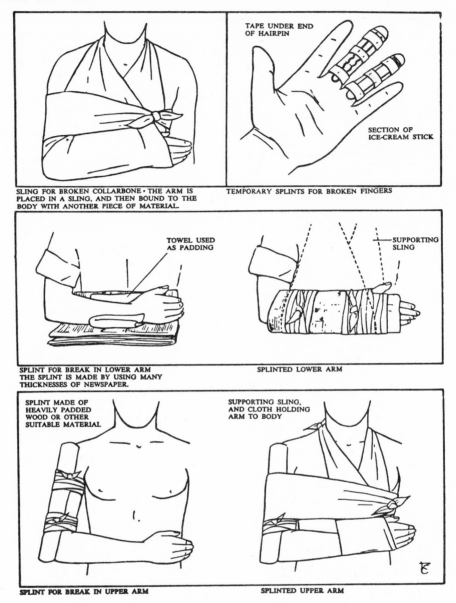

SLING FOR BROKEN COLLARBONE · THE ARM IS PLACED IN A SLING, AND THEN BOUND TO THE BODY WITH ANOTHER PIECE OF MATERIAL.

TAPE UNDER END OF HAIRPIN

SECTION OF ICE-CREAM STICK

TEMPORARY SPLINTS FOR BROKEN FINGERS

TOWEL USED AS PADDING

SPLINT FOR BREAK IN LOWER ARM THE SPLINT IS MADE BY USING MANY THICKNESSES OF NEWSPAPER.

SUPPORTING SLING

SPLINTED LOWER ARM

SPLINT MADE OF HEAVILY PADDED WOOD OR OTHER SUITABLE MATERIAL

SPLINT FOR BREAK IN UPPER ARM

SUPPORTING SLING, AND CLOTH HOLDING ARM TO BODY

SPLINTED UPPER ARM

*Figure 23-9. Splinting.*

I have become convinced, from observing as well as teaching first aid courses, and from reading books on the subject, that far too much time is usually devoted to bandaging. As a result, the first-aider tends to place undue emphasis upon it, at the cost of matters such as those I have described earlier in this chapter, which can enable him to save a life.

Emergency bandaging is simpler today than it was in the past, before Band-Aids and similar innovations of all sizes and shapes were readily available; almost everybody is familiar with them, or

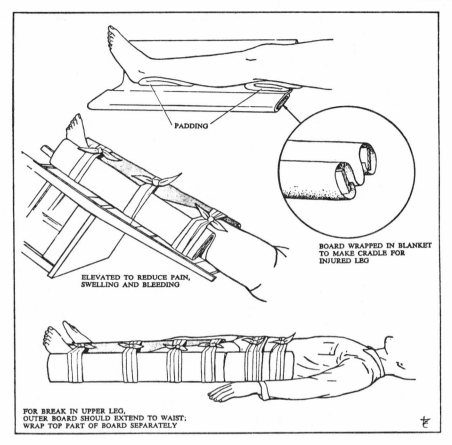

PADDING

BOARD WRAPPED IN BLANKET
TO MAKE CRADLE FOR
INJURED LEG

ELEVATED TO REDUCE PAIN,
SWELLING AND BLEEDING

FOR BREAK IN UPPER LEG,
OUTER BOARD SHOULD EXTEND TO WAIST;
WRAP TOP PART OF BOARD SEPARATELY

*Figure 23-10. Splinting Leg.*

can learn to use them with a minimum of instructions. Adhesive tape, elastic bandages, and other comparatively new products also simplify bandaging for the first-aider.

However, he may also have occasion to use the somewhat more complicated bandages shown in the illustrations. Individuals vary a great deal in their ability to make and apply these bandages. They may be clear to you after you merely glance at the pictures. If not, I suggest that you try them out as soon as possible, before an emergency arises. In case you have difficulty with any of them, ask someone to help you—a friend whose abilities lie in that direction, a first aid instructor, a nurse, or a doctor.

These are the essentials to remember when you are applying bandages: (1) in bandaging cuts, wounds, or burns, your purpose is to stop the flow of blood, or provide protection against contamination, or both. Always put a sterile pad or piece of gauze over the injured area; then put the tape or bandaging material *over that,* to hold it in place —*not* in direct contact with the wound. (2) Do not make the bandage too tight. Pressure should be applied only for the purpose of arresting the flow of blood, and should not be continued indefinitely (see page 328). If there is only a small amount of bleeding, it will stop by itself. First-aiders sometimes bandage so tightly as to interfere with the circulation; I have seen Band-Aids applied so snugly on a cut finger, for example, that its tip becomes cold and even turns blue. (3) Bandages are also used to immobilize an injured part—that is, to prevent motion which may cause further injury as well as pain. A bandage does not have to "look pretty" in order to be effective. The one you apply is usually only temporary, and will be replaced by your doctor or someone in the emergency room of a hospital. Don't be too concerned about its appearance, but concentrate on the purpose for which it is applied.

# 24

# YOUR HOME MEDICAL SUPPLIES

*First,* keep the items required for first aid in a separate container or shelf; otherwise, if they are used routinely, they may not be available when urgently needed. *Second,* take your first aid materials in a kit or box when you go for automobile or camping trips. *Third,* if you live in a rural area or any place where medical care is inaccessible, and there is no nearby pharmacy, you should arrange with your doctor to have penicillin and other antibiotics at home. (See page 162 for antibiotic first aid.) *Fourth,* keep all medicines and instruments out of reach of children. But make sure that the first aid cabinet is not locked with a key; it must be opened at once in case of an emergency. *Fifth,* all medicines should be labeled to indicate what they are, what they are to be used for, and the quantity to use, so that you will not make a mistake in an emergency. Consult the Index for uses and dosages of the medicines listed in this chapter.

## GENERAL HOUSEHOLD FIRST AID SUPPLIES

Sterile gauze pads, twelve 2 x 2 inch
Small roll of adhesive tape, ½ inch wide
A box of Band-Aids, assorted sizes
A roll of sterile absorbent cotton
A few applicator rods
A few tongue depressors
2 thermometers (see page 287)
1 flashlight
A roll of gauze bandage, 1 inch wide
A pair of scissors (bandage type preferred)

A pair of sharp-pointed tweezers
A thick, blunt needle for removing splinters
Safety pins
A tourniquet
A suitable sling to immobilize arm or shoulder in case of sprain
Elastic bandage

## GENERAL HOUSEHOLD MEDICINES

Some items that belong in the household medicine cabinet are stable for years. Others need to be replaced periodically.

The nonprescription household medicines I am listing below are useful, and you may wish to have many of them available.

One note of caution: most people keep their household medicines in the bathroom. This can be one of the worst possible places because of the moisture in the air unless the medicines are kept in completely airtight containers. Most medicines remain stable longest if they are kept away from direct sunlight, from excesses of heat and cold, and from humidity. The closet closest to your bathroom, which may be a linen closet in your home, is the best place for your medical supplies.

*Aspirin* (or Bufferin, Empirin, or other aspirin-containing tablet). Aspirin is effective in reducing fever and relieving minor pains, especially headache. For young children, flavored aspirin is available in smaller doses than the usual 5-grain tablet. Shelf life is about two years, for either kind.

*Acetaminophen,* available under many trade names, is a useful substitute for aspirin (if you do not tolerate aspirin well) for fever reduction and minor pain relief.

*Alcohol* is used for external purposes, such as rubbing or application to reduce high fever, and for sterilization of fever thermometers and other devices. Seventy percent ethyl alcohol is the most desirable and most antiseptic, as well as less irritating than greater concentrations. Shelf life is indefinite.

*Milk of magnesia* is a useful, safe, and stable laxative.

*Witch hazel* is a popular astringent (skintightener), refreshing after a shave. It is also a mild antiseptic. Shelf life is indefinite.

*Antiseptic* lotions, salves, and aerosol sprays that do not sting are available. Among them are Merthiolate and Zephiran Chloride. Aerosols are easy to apply but usually more expensive. Most antiseptics remain useful for two to three years.

*Ipecac* is a valuable emetic, or inducer of vomiting, especially useful in case of poisoning.

*Activated charcoal* is also useful in poisonings.

*Eyedrops* are soothing and generally stable for two years. *Ear drops* and *nose drops* should be used only upon a physician's specific recommendation.

*Ointments* for minor burns or insect bites are available. They include Unguentine and Calmitol. Some are also available in aerosol spray form. Stable life is two to three years.

*Antipruritics* (itch relievers), such as calamine lotion, are helpful in cases of poison ivy. They must be used frequently, preferably every two hours, and in generous quantities. They remain stable indefinitely.

*Suppositories* are two types, for relief from the itching and pain of hemorrhoids and as laxatives. They must be kept cool; in the summer, they should be refrigerated.

*Antifungal* agents include gentian violet, Desinex, Sopronol, and Tinactin. Used topically (on the skin), they help relieve the discomfort of athlete's foot and ringworm infection. Shelf life is three to five years.

# 25
# NURSING IN THE HOME

## WHEN SHOULD A PATIENT BE CARED FOR AT HOME?

Making the right decision about this is one of the most important parts of home nursing! Sometimes it is made for you: there is no choice but to care for the patient at home. If there is a choice, here are some of the points that should be taken into consideration—often they must be weighed against other factors such as expense, home conditions, and the other members of the family.

1. Remember that, once the decision has been made, it may be difficult or even impossible to change it. For example, a sick person might be terribly upset about being moved to a hospital during the course of the illness, considering it an indication that the situation had become critical or even hopeless. Don't decide impulsively. *Always talk it over thoroughly with your doctor first.*

2. In certain illnesses, a hospital is essential because of the treatment required, or the special equipment that may be needed in an emergency. Surgical operations, diabetic coma, hemorrhage from a stomach ulcer, rheumatic fever, certain cases of pneumonia, some types of heart attack, and severe strokes are in this category.

3. In general, a sick child is better off at home than in a hospital. Sick children have a great need for close contact with their parents and for their home environment. There are a few hospitals which make it possible for the mother to be with the child most of the time, and even arrange to have her sleep with the child. In this case a hospital may be best. But staying in a hospital which his mother can visit for only limited periods is apt to be a very bad experience for a child, with subsequent emotional upsets, as well as a lowering of morale. However, certain diseases such as rheumatic fever are usually handled so much better in a hospital that the scales are tipped in that direction.

4. Very old people, like children, find it difficult to adjust to a new environment. They, too, are usually better off if they are cared for at home.

5. Social conditions must outweigh the individual's needs. Patients with certain communicable diseases must often be hospitalized for the protection of others.

## NURSING IN THE HOME

Good home nursing requires more than an assortment of facts about how to make beds, take the pulse, and give medicines; it even requires more than a willingness to work hard, important as these things are. Sympathetic understanding of the patient and intelligent planning are also essential.

Sympathetic understanding is not necessarily inborn. It can be developed. If you have ever been ill or have been with a sick person, you should have some useful information to go on. Thinking about it will provide many useful clues. Also, at some time in your life you should be able to spare a few hours to visit an invalid, or help in a hospital, or devote to a church or other charitable effort in behalf of the ill. Make a point of doing this, not only as an act of kindness on your part, but for the opportunity to learn what people are like when they are ill.

Use your imagination. Ask yourself, "What would I like?" and follow it with, "But he (or she) isn't *exactly* like me, so what would he (or she) like?" The most obvious things will come to your mind first—a calm, cheerful atmosphere, efficiency, and appetizing meals. But concrete examples of things to do and not to do will occur to you from time to time if you are alert to them. Make a point of remembering them.

On some occasions, the patient will require special tests or treatments that only a trained professional nurse can administer. These may include taking blood samples, administering hypodermic injections, or giving special exercises. Your doctor can arrange for a professional nurse to come to your home when such special care is needed. Many communities have visiting nurse associations whose nurses offer part-time services. They can be called upon if special care is needed or if the home nurse must be away or decides to take a much-needed rest. The charges of visiting nurse associations are scaled to the family's ability to pay.

## Caring for a Patient at Home

Having decided to care for the patient at home, you should immediately get instructions from your doctor. These may be of a general, even casual, nature. Sometimes we doctors merely say, "Keep Johnny in bed for a few days; I'll be around to see him on Tuesday or Wednesday." In other cases, the directions may be detailed and perhaps complicated.

Always be sure you are clear about the following questions: (1) May the patient go to the bathroom, wash or bathe, sit up in bed, read and talk? (2) What, and how much, may (or should) he eat and drink? (3) What, if any, medicines should he have? (4) How often should you take his temperature (by mouth, rectum, armpit)? (5) What symptoms, if any, should you watch for; and if these appear should you call the doctor? (6) Are there any treatments you should give, such as massage or an enema? (7) Should any precautions be taken for the patient or the family?

*Write down the answers to these questions.*

## General Suggestions

Conserve your strength. A pad and pencil, if you make use of them, will be one of your greatest helps. Lists save many trips, and contribute to your confidence, so get in the habit of making them.

Plan everything ahead of time. Assemble all the things you need and keep them in a special place so they will be there when you want them. Make out a schedule of daily care, meals, and so on, based on your doctor's instructions. Before you bathe the patient, clean the room, or bring him a tray, check the supplies you may need so you won't have to go back for them.

Keep records of what you have done. A daily chart should be filled in to record the temperature, medicines, and treatments. Check this against the list of doctor's orders. This will not only make for efficiency, but will keep you from worrying that you have forgotten something.

Save your back. Watch your posture. Stand close to whatever you are doing, and don't stoop, but bend from the knees. Keep your back straight when lifting. If you are tall, sit on a high stool whenever possible instead of leaning over. Raise the bed to a convenient height by means of blocks or by putting the legs of the bed in cans filled with sand or gravel. If you are short, stand on a footstool or a box whenever you can in order to avoid having to reach for things. Wear low-heeled, comfortable shoes, and sensible clothes that won't bind you, or catch on things, or soil easily.

## Techniques of Nursing

Some of the things you may need to do in nursing your patient should be demonstrated to you—for example, giving an injection. It is also helpful to be shown how to do such things as making a bed while the patient is in it. Perhaps you can afford to engage a private nurse for a day to break you in. Or a *visiting nurse* can show you. Although there is nothing like being shown, the following procedures should be clear to you from these instructions and illustrations:

In choosing the patient's *room*, remember that you'll have to go to him often, and fixing up a room on the ground floor, for example, may save you a great many trips up and down stairs. The sickroom should be near the kitchen. If there is a downstairs toilet, that may be a great help for both you and the patient. See that the bed is placed in the best position for you and the patient —not too close to the window or radiator for his comfort, with adequate light that doesn't glare in his eyes, and near a table for your, and his, convenience. This table should be large enough to hold the things he is apt to need or want, such as tissues, a glass of water, something to read, and a bell to let you know he wants you. If you have no bell, an empty glass can be struck with a spoon.

Keep the *temperature* of the room as even as possible, around 72° to 76° in the daytime, 68° to 72° at night. A wall thermometer near the patient will help you to check this.

The sickroom should be not only clean but as free of odors as possible. If sharp-smelling antiseptics or disinfectants must be used to clean the room, their odors should be masked with a pleasant deodorant or odor-neutralizing agent. A light deodorant spray is pleasant after a bedpan has been used.

To *ventilate* the room without creating a draft, open the window from the top, or place a screen or blanket over the back of a chair, by the window. You can also open the window in the next room and leave the door between the rooms open. If the *air is too dry,* put a large, shallow pan of water on or near the radiator, or purchase a humidifier.

Bright lights and loud noises are disturbing to sick persons. All windows should have blinds, shutters, or curtains to reduce the glare of the sun, although the sickroom should not be gloomy. The house should be kept as quiet as possible, especially if the patient is napping or is ready for his night's sleep.

If you know in advance that the sick person will have to spend a long time in bed, you should consider renting, or even buying, a regular hospital bed. In many communities, hospital beds and other sickroom equipment can be borrowed from voluntary organizations at little or no cost. A hospital bed has many attachments useful in nursing, such as side rails. It can be raised or lowered at the head and feet. One great advantage is that hospital beds are higher than ordinary ones, and the

nurse can work more easily, without stooping or bending. Although I recommend the hospital bed, I know that home nursing care frequently will not include it. Therefore, the following suggestions are all applicable to the ordinary household bed.

To keep the patient from *falling out of bed,* place a kitchen chair with its back against the bed, or tie a row of chairs together and put them with their backs to the side of the bed.

You can improvise *bed tables* on which to serve meals, etc. Try setting up the ironing board so that it extends over the patient's lap when he is sitting up; or put a chair on each side of the bed and rest a board on them. You can also make a table by removing the ends and the bottom of a cardboard carton, leaving the sides and top, and setting it over his lap.

Figure 25-1 shows methods of *placing pillows* to make the patient comfortable. To help him sit up, put a card table or a board under a pillow at the head of the bed, tilted at the proper angle, to support his back. If he is lying on his side, he may find that a folded pillow at his back gives some support.

If the patient is *tall,* use a chair with a pillow on it to make an extension for the bed (see Figure 25-2).

Keep him from *sliding toward the foot* of the bed by rolling a pillow in a sheet, as in Figure 25-3.

A pillow under his legs and another at the foot of the bed will also keep him from slipping and will make his legs and feet more comfortable (see Figure 25-6).

*Figure 25-1. Pillow Arrangements.*

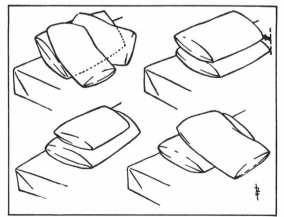

Relieve or prevent *pressure* on parts of the body such as the elbow, hip, heel, or ankle by using a "doughnut" cushion which can be purchased or made by rolling some cotton and wrapping it with a bandage as in Figure 25-4.

To help prevent bedsores, which are mainly the result of prolonged, unrelieved pressure, turn or lift the patient into a different position every two hours or so.

Figure 25-5 shows how to roll a blanket in order to *keep the patient's legs from turning out* as they often tend to do, to his discomfort.

Giving him *room to move his feet* will add to his comfort. To do this, place a pillow under the covers as in Figure 25-6. This will also prevent the weight of the covers from resting on his feet.

Figure 25-7 demonstrates how to *move* the patient toward the head of the bed if he slips down; how to move him from his back to his side; how to raise his head and shoulders; and how to help him to sit up and get up. Before the patient gets up, have him sit for a moment on the edge of the bed with his legs dangling over the side, because the change in position may make him dizzy or faint.

*Hospital beds* are made up with the following, in the order listed: mattress pad, bottom sheet, draw sheet, top sheet, blanket(s), spread, and pillowcases over the two pillows. Side rails also should be part of a hospital bed. They should be raised if there is even a slight danger of the patient falling out of bed, from weakness, lack of certainty about his surroundings, restlessness, or any other reason. I feel that, in homes, the rubber

sheet should be omitted except when it is really necessary—that is, in the case of small children or other patients who are incontinent (have no control over the bladder and bowels). I know this will sound like heresy to some members of the nursing profession, but a rubber sheet can cause a great deal of discomfort, especially in hot weather or when the bed is made by someone who is not sufficiently experienced to keep it absolutely free from wrinkles. In most cases the pad and the two sheets—the bottom sheet and the draw sheet—will protect the mattress, provided care is taken when placing on the bed a basin or anything else that might spill. A draw sheet large enough to use double will give added protection if needed.

Another thing which nurses swear by is the squared corner. This is, indeed, essential in making a bed properly. With a little practice you can learn how to make a square corner and pull the under sheet tight enough to keep it from wrinkling. Figure 25-8 will show you how to do it. Stand at the side of the bed on which you are working, facing first the top and then the foot, and complete one side before going around to the other.

*Making a bed* with someone in it seems difficult but can easily be learned. Consult Figure 25-9 and follow these directions without trying any short cuts.

Remove the spread and loosen the blanket at the foot and sides. Reach under it and remove the top sheet, leaving the blanket to cover the patient. Loosen the draw sheet, fan-folding it toward the patient so that it lies close to him, parallel with his body. Loosen the bottom sheet, which you need not remove unless it has become soiled. Smooth the mattress pad and the bottom sheet, and tuck in the bottom sheet, squaring the corners and making certain it is neat and free from crumbs. Put the clean draw sheet on the bed with its midfold in the center of the bed, tucking in the side on which you are working. Fan-fold the other half that will cover the part of the bed on which the patient is lying. Put the fan-folded part *over* the fan-folded old sheet.

Help the patient to roll toward you over the fan-folded part of the two sheets, so that he is on his side facing you (see Figure 25-9). Now go to the other side of the bed, and attend to the mattress pad and the bottom sheet as you did on the

*Figure 25-2. Bed Extender. Chair used to provide extra space for tall patient.*

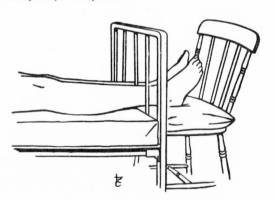

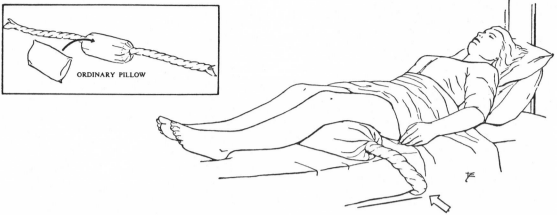

SHEET FOLDED LENGTHWISE AND TWISTED
AROUND PILLOW AND HELD IN PLACE UNDER
MATTRESS

*Figure 25-3. Support for Legs. To keep the patient comfortable and prevent sliding toward the foot of the bed.*

first side. Pull out the soiled draw sheet over which the patient has rolled, and put it aside to be washed. Next pull the clean sheet, and smooth and tuck it in. Put a clean top sheet over the blanket and remove the blanket while you tuck this sheet in at the foot of the bed and spread it over the patient. Replace the blanket, and "make" the foot and sides of the bed. Then change the pillowcases, and the bed is finished.

Keeping the patient *clean and neat* contributes to his well-being, but be guided by what the doctor suggests rather than by a fanatical desire for cleanliness. The patient's *hands and face* should be washed, and his teeth brushed, at least twice a day as a general rule. Protect the bedding with paper or a piece of rubber, and a towel while the patient attends to these things himself, if he is able. If a patient cannot wash his own hands and face, follow the suggestions I give later (p. 354) in describing bed baths.

If the patient is not able to sit up to *brush his teeth,* he may be able to do this by lying on his side with a basin close to him. Make things as easy as possible for him by handing him the toothbrush with toothpaste or toothpowder on it, holding the basin so he can expectorate into it easily, and giving him water in a glass with which to rinse his mouth. If he is not well enough to do even this much, ask your doctor or nurse whether to omit the procedure for a day, or whether to wash his mouth yourself, according to instructions which should be given to you.

The *hair* should be combed once or twice a day. If the patient is unable to do this, and if the hair is long and snarled, applying a little alcohol usually helps. Comb small strands of hair at a time, holding tight to the strand above the part being combed. Long hair should be braided.

*Rubbing his back* once or twice a day usually makes the patient feel better and is good for the skin. Use bathing lotion or talcum powder if

*Figure 25–4. Doughnut Roll. To relieve pressure and prevent bed sores.*

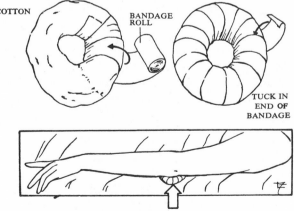

TYPICAL PLACE FOR DOUGHNUT ROLL

*Figure 25-5. Trochanter Roll. Rolled blanket support-*
*ing legs and keeping the knees from turning outward.*

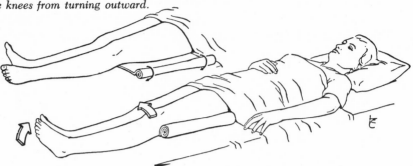

desired, and rub with long, gentle but firm strokes.

The doctor will let the patient go to the *toilet* at least once a day unless it will actually endanger his health, for doctors know that most patients find it difficult to use a bedpan. A patient who is not able to walk to the bathroom may be permitted to use a homemade toilet which you can improvise from an old kitchen chair, by cutting a hole in the seat and fastening a commode under it.

A male patient can probably use a urinal without much assistance if you place it on a towel beside him under the covers. If it is cold, warm the urinal first by putting it on or near the radiator, or by rinsing it with hot water and drying it quickly just before you bring it to him.

A *bedpan* should also be warmed in the same way. Most patients can raise themselves, or help to raise themselves, onto it by flexing their knees and pressing with their heels and the palms of their hands on the mattress. The bedpan should be placed under the patient's buttocks, the flattened end of it just below the hipbones (see Figure 25-10). Cover the patient and, unless he is very ill, leave him alone on the pan with the toilet paper within reach, but remain nearby so you can go to him when he is finished. Remove the pan, covering it immediately with a cloth. After you empty the contents into the toilet, wash the pan thoroughly and rinse in very hot water. Your hands and those of the patient should be washed right after the pan has been used. If you cannot get a bedpan, make one from an old baking tin with a board tied over it. Cutting a half-circle out of the board will make the bedpan more comfortable for the patient. Be careful to protect the patient from rough or

sharp edges by padding the board with a cloth or other padding.

If the patient is able to take a *bath* in the tub, be sure to find out how much assistance he needs. Be careful there is nothing on which he can slip or trip, and remain near by in case he needs you.

If the patient is unable to bathe in the tub, give him a *bed bath* as often as the doctor recommends. This should be given before you make or change the bed, and after he has gone to the toilet or had the bedpan. You will need a bath blanket which preferably should be a fairly small cotton one which is easy to handle and dry, two bath towels, a face towel, washcloth, soap, and a basin of warm water, and clean pajamas or nightgown. Change the water at least once, especially if it gets cool.

Remove the top bedding, cover the patient with the bath blanket, and remove nightclothes. Protect the under bedding with a towel, placing paper under the basin when you put it on the bed. Let the patient wash his own hands and face if he is able; if not, start with the face, drying it before you go on to the neck and ears, and always rinsing off the soap carefully if you use any. Next wash and dry one arm, and wash the hand in the basin. Then attend to the other arm and hand. Now wash and dry the chest and abdomen. Turn the patient on his side to wash his back and buttocks, drying thoroughly and applying bathing lotion or talcum if desired (always protect the sensitive genitals and scrotum from alcohol lotions). Turn the patient on his back again and put on clean night clothing, making certain it is folded back so it won't get wet while you wash his legs and feet. Place the basin near the foot and wash and dry one leg, starting with the groin and ending with the toes. Then wash the other leg and foot. The patient should wash the genital area if he is well enough; if not, attend to it last, and then remake the bed.

It is not very difficult to *wash short hair* without wetting the bedding. If the patient is a woman who is going to be confined to bed for some time, try to persuade her to have her hair cut short.

The secret of success in washing even long hair without wetting the bed lies in making a "trough" out of a rubber sheet, covered by a bath towel. Roll both sides and one end of the rubber, leaving the center portion flat, and the unrolled end hanging into a basin on a chair that is lower than the bed. Put a bath towel over the rubber sheet, molding it into the same form. One rolled side should be under the patient's neck and the other beyond the head, the patient lying with her face turned away from you. Give her a clean towel or cloth to protect her eyes. Wet the hair from a pitcher of quite warm water, apply liquid shampoo, rub hair and scalp with your hands, rinse, and then rinse once again. Use a towel to rub the hair dry, if a dryer is not obtainable.

There are shampoos on the market which can be used to "wash" the hair without water. However, it is risky to use one unless the patient has tried it while she was well because she may be allergic to it.

*Figure 25-6. Pillow at Feet. To support the weight of the bedcovers and prevent pressure.*

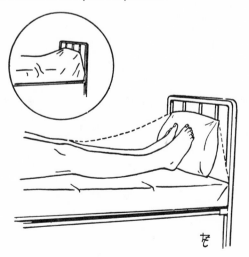

To give *water or other fluid* to a patient who is unable to sit up and drink by himself, raise his head, either by means of pillows or by slipping your left arm under the pillow and lifting it while you hold the glass in your right hand. Have the glass less than half full so it won't spill. Bent or flexible drinking tubes, which can be obtained in most drugstores, are very useful for children and patients who are too ill to drink easily. Always hold the glass and tube for the patient, and make certain that the tube is always *in* the liquid so that the patient won't suck air.

*Medicines* should be given from a spoon or glass, or in the form of pills or capsules, as directed by the doctor or the visiting nurse. Always check the bottle or container before giving the medicine and again afterward.

I describe how to take the *temperature* by mouth, rectum, and armpit, on page 287.

If the doctor wants you to take the patient's *pulse*, try to practice it on a well person, since you may require a little practice to get the knack of it. Place the tips of two or three fingers—not your thumb, because it has a pulse and you are apt to count your own pulse if you use your thumb—on the artery just inside the wrist and below the patient's thumb (see Figure 25-11). Press hard enough to feel the pulse, but don't press too hard or you won't feel anything. Count the pulse for a minute, using a watch with a second hand for accuracy. The patient's pulse should be taken when he is relaxed, and not right after he has exerted himself. Write down the number of beats you have counted, and whether the pulse seemed strong, weak, regular, or irregular.

If the doctor wants you to take the patient's *respiration*, try to do so without letting the patient know it. It is often difficult for the patient to breathe naturally if he knows he is being watched. Look at the chest for exactly a minute, counting each time you see it rise.

Don't give an *enema* (see Figure 25-12) unless the doctor tells you to. He will also tell you what to give, and other directions such as how long the enema should be retained.

Have the patient lie on his side, his back toward you, and his legs flexed—the upper one more so than the lower. Be sure the bedding is protected. Test the water with a thermometer (it should be about 105°) or by letting a little of it run on your

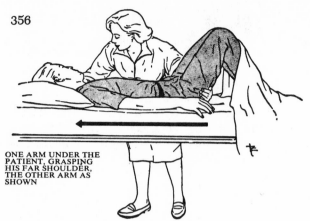

ONE ARM UNDER THE
PATIENT, GRASPING
HIS FAR SHOULDER,
THE OTHER ARM AS
SHOWN

*1. Helping the patient move toward the head of the bed.*

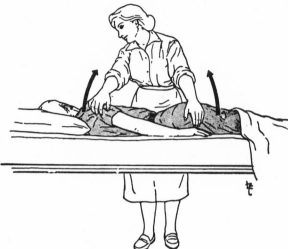

*2. Helping the patient turn from his back to his side.*

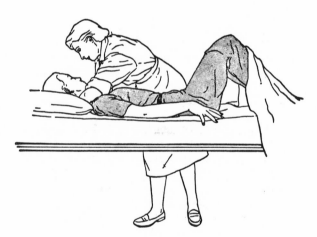

*3. Helping the patient to sit up in bed.*

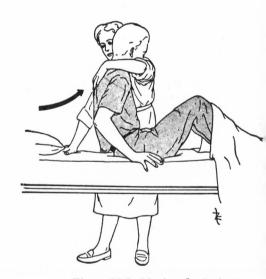

*Figure 25-7. Moving the Patient.*

*4. Helping the patient to get out of bed, or to sit up with his feet over the side.*

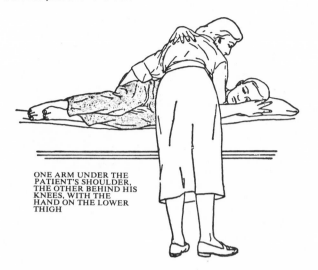

ONE ARM UNDER THE
PATIENT'S SHOULDER,
THE OTHER BEHIND HIS
KNEES, WITH THE
HAND ON THE LOWER
THIGH

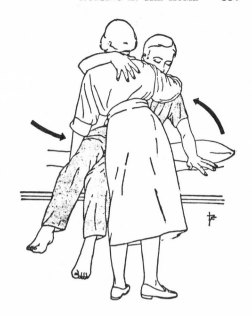

arm to make certain it is not too hot. With a piece of toilet paper, apply petroleum jelly to the rectal nozzle at the end of the tube. Open the stopcock and let some water run out into the bedpan to make certain there is no air in the tube. The patient should insert the nozzle himself if he is able. If not, insert it very slowly and gently for about two inches, pause a moment and insert another inch or two. Don't hold the bag too high—about 18 inches above the bed, as shown in the illustration. Lower it if the fluid flows too rapidly, or pinch off the tube to stop the flow if the patient complains of pain. When the bag appears empty, remove the tube carefully, and place the bedpan under the patient.

A *hot-water bag* can be used to provide heat if the patient is cold or if the doctor orders it for treatment of an affected part. Be certain the bag is in good condition; always hold it upside down for a minute after it is ready to take to the patient, to make certain it doesn't leak. Fill the bag about two-thirds full with water at 130° for adults, 120° for children. Expel the excess air before you put on the lid. Wrap in a cloth. Be sure to ask the patient whether the bag is too hot for comfort.

The doctor may order *hot moist applications* to an affected area. To keep from burning your hands while you wring out the gauze compress, put a turkish (bath) towel across a small basin, not too near the patient, and place the compress in the middle of it. Pour on very hot water. Grasp the dry ends of the bath towel and twist in opposite directions until no more water can be wrung out. Untwist the towel and lift out the gauze compress with your fingers; if you can't pick it up, it's too hot for the patient. Place on the affected area and cover with a dry towel to keep in the heat. Change when it cools, or as often as the doctor orders.

If the doctor orders an *ice bag* (or an ice "collar") to relieve pain or inflammation, be sure to check it as I described for hot-water bags, to make certain it doesn't leak. Crush the ice so there will be no sharp edges, and fill the bag no more than half full. Dry carefully and put a cover over it before applying it to the affected area. Keep the patient from getting chilled by putting an extra blanket over him, if necessary.

The procedures which I have described above will more than cover the care needed by most patients. However, the problems which patients present vary according to the kind of illness, the age of the patient, and so on. I shall describe three types of cases to serve as a general guide.

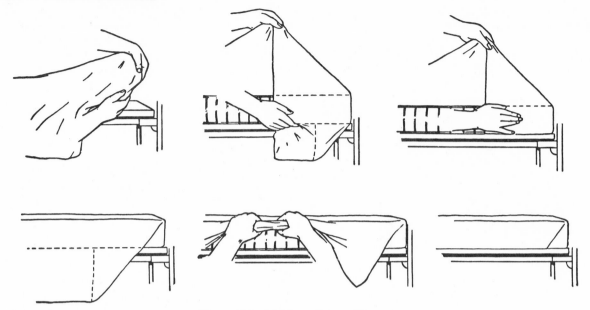

*Figure 25-8. Making a Square Corner.*

## IF YOUR CHILD HAS A COMMUNICABLE DISEASE

In caring for a child with a catching disease, you must protect others from it, including yourself unless you *know* you are immune. Even then, it is best to play safe because many immunities are not lifelong, and you want to make absolutely certain you, too, do not contract mumps, chickenpox, or some other childhood disease. Precautions vary in different diseases, and health department regulations also vary. In general, the following minimum precautions should be observed.

### Precautions

First, for your general information concerning communicable diseases, read Chapter 7, Keeping the Germs Away.

Since people, rather than things, spread most diseases, keep the patient away from others and others away from him as long as your doctor says it is necessary. If you have other children, be particularly careful not to let them go into his room. Because they were probably exposed to the disease while he was coming down with it, ask your doctor about protective "shots" (see page 134).

Many diseases are spread by the saliva, so: (1) Leave a smock or long apron in the patient's room and slip it on over your dress while you are with him. (2) Turn your face away when he coughs or sneezes. (3) Keep your hands away from your mouth. (4) Wash your hands *thoroughly* with soap and very hot water when you are through caring for him. (5) Masks over mouth and nose should be worn only at the doctor's request. Masks may frighten sick children.

If he is too sick to do it himself, place all used cleansing tissues in a paper bag, which can be pinned to the side of his mattress, and then either burn it or shake the contents into the toilet. If you must use handkerchiefs, handle them as little as possible; boil them in a pot or pail kept for that purpose before putting them in the wash. In most children's diseases, the patient's linens can be washed with those of the family, provided there is plenty of very hot water; so can his dishes.

*Special precautions are required for diphtheria, polio, scarlet fever, smallpox, typhoid fever, and dysentery, if you must care for someone with one of these diseases at home.*

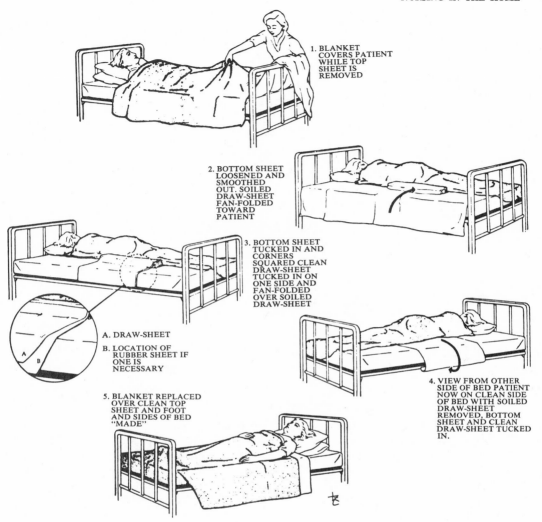

1. BLANKET COVERS PATIENT WHILE TOP SHEET IS REMOVED

2. BOTTOM SHEET LOOSENED AND SMOOTHED OUT. SOILED DRAW-SHEET FAN-FOLDED TOWARD PATIENT

3. BOTTOM SHEET TUCKED IN AND CORNERS SQUARED CLEAN DRAW-SHEET TUCKED IN ON ONE SIDE AND FAN-FOLDED OVER SOILED DRAW-SHEET

A. DRAW-SHEET

B. LOCATION OF RUBBER SHEET IF ONE IS NECESSARY

4. VIEW FROM OTHER SIDE OF BED PATIENT NOW ON CLEAN SIDE OF BED WITH SOILED DRAW-SHEET REMOVED, BOTTOM SHEET AND CLEAN DRAW-SHEET TUCKED IN.

5. BLANKET REPLACED OVER CLEAN TOP SHEET AND FOOT AND SIDES OF BED "MADE"

*Figure 25-9. Making Occupied Bed.*

After the child is well, clean the room thoroughly, air it, and put the blankets, mattress, books, and other objects in the sun for a few hours. All badly soiled articles should be cleaned or destroyed.

## Caring for Your Child

Your doctor will tell you whether he may be allowed to go to the toilet or whether he should have a bedpan. It is usually safe to carry a child to the toilet if you keep him warm.

Most children sleep a great deal and are generally "good" when they are very ill. When they begin to recover they become restless. The main problem then lies in keeping them reasonably contented without letting them overdo things. Remember that a child can use up a great deal of energy fussing and crying. Be as flexible as you can about the things that are not absolutely necessary. For example, don't make hair-brushing a painful procedure, even if it means making do with a lick and a promise or cutting out a snarl.

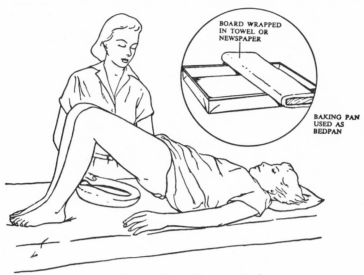

BOARD WRAPPED IN TOWEL OR NEWSPAPER

BAKING PAN USED AS BEDPAN

*Figure 25-10. Placing a Bedpan.*

The child will probably expend less energy on a favorite play toy than he would by tossing restlessly about. Why not get a box of "sick-time toys" and keep them for the illnesses that are bound to come? Keep them "special" so it will be a treat for the child to play with them. They could include a "sick" doll or teddy bear in night clothing, some toy animals to be lined up on the bed table or bed, some of mother's costume jewelry.

Put the family radio in the child's room, perhaps for part of the time, but avoid letting him listen to highly stimulating programs. Special records on your own or a borrowed record player will provide entertainment. Picture books are good when he is well enough, but don't let him tire his eyes while he is feverish. If he has measles, be especially careful to protect his eyes from glare, perhaps by means of a visor or eye shade, but don't keep his room dark. Most children like to be read to in a calm manner even if they don't always follow the story. Don't let him have any visitors who will excite or upset him.

Use your ingenuity—you'll have to, because you probably have only a limited amount of time to spend with your child. You will find that you actually spend less time with him if you go to him voluntarily than if you wait for him to call. A child often invents reasons for needing his mother simply to be reassured that he has not been deserted or forgotten. Devote some time to him, not just to caring for him. He will require less unnecessary "care" in that way. Never blame him for his illness. This is not the time to drive home any lessons about wearing his rubbers the way you told him to.

It will require a great deal of ingenuity to get most sick children to take the proper nourishment and the essential fluid. Most of them like to use straws, especially colored plastic ones, or a bent glass tube, some of which come in fancy styles for children. Keep them for illnesses and they will be a treat. Check with your doctor to learn how flexible you can be about the child's food and fluids. Your child may prefer ginger ale or fruit juice to water. Some chocolate or vanilla flavoring may make milk more acceptable. He may be delighted to be allowed to drink coffee, perhaps iced coffee. (This can be made by adding some instant *caffeine-free* coffee to milk or water.) Ice cream or sherbet goes down a sore throat easily—or a milk shake, or a soda made with flavoring, milk, and charged water to which some ice cream can be added. Custards, too, go down smoothly, supplying essential minerals and a large number of calories. Sometimes a child who feels too sick to eat, especially if his throat is very sore, will enjoy lollipops or old-fashioned rock candy, also high in calories.

Many sick children become "younger" in their taste for food while they are ill. That is, they tend to like the things they formerly enjoyed but have outgrown. They are apt to eat better if food is served in small, rather than large, quantities.

Aspirin is now put out in chewing gum and candy forms. These are more acceptable to young children (but also become an increased hazard from poisoning; be sure to keep your aspirin supply in a place where children cannot get at it). Other unpalatable pills can be ground up in a spoonful of jelly or applesauce. Giving a piece of candy immediately after the medicine will make things easier.

In Chapter 20 (p. 286) I discuss the various common fevers and illnesses of childhood, and in Chapter 19 I deal with the emotions of children. Both these chapters will be helpful to you if you have a sick child to care for.

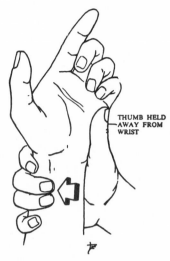

THUMB HELD AWAY FROM WRIST

*Figure 25-11. Taking the Pulse.*

## CARING FOR AN ADULT WITH A SERIOUS, NONCONTAGIOUS DISEASE

In caring for an adult with, for example, a heart condition that is expected to clear up in six to twelve weeks, you will have need of some of the more difficult (as well as the easier) nursing procedures I have described, such as giving the bedpan and changing the bed with the patient in it. As the patient recovers, you will have to help him from his bed to the chair, assist him in walking, and do many other things that present no problem in the case of a small child.

One of the prime requirements in caring for an illness of this type is to keep the patient from becoming anxious or alarmed. To do this, you will need confidence and skill in handling him. The best suggestion I can make is this: as soon as your doctor tells you what you have to do, try it out on someone other than the patient—foolish as this may make you feel! It will not only give you confidence, but it may enable you to reassure the patient by saying something to the effect that, "The doctor (or nurse) showed me how to do this, and I practiced it on Mary until everybody says I'm as good at it as any professional."

Nothing is more important than providing a calm, sympathetic, and cheerful atmosphere. Skill in handling nursing procedures will help to create this. So will a good, regular routine. Although they may not realize it themselves, most sick people benefit a great deal from having things happen according to schedule. Naturally you should try to be flexible about this routine if the patient wishes.

Be sure to keep even petty disturbances away from the patient. This may mean that you have to be rather dictatorial about visitors.

Remember that a sick adult is in many ways like a child. He, too, senses tensions and needs to feel secure, so that many of the suggestions I made in regard to caring for a sick child will apply to a sick adult. For example, look in on the patient even though he has not called you, because *loneliness* can be more tormenting than pain in long illnesses.

In serious illnesses, especially if the patient is getting along in years, his position should be changed frequently to prevent bedsores and avoid the possibility of pneumonia.

You should read about the specific disease from which your patient is suffering. (You can find it by consulting the Index.) But *don't* become an "amateur home doctor." Your patient may try to put you in this position by discussing his symptoms and asking your opinion as to whether he is better or worse. Guard against this from the very beginning because your patient may think he is worse if you stop answering questions at any point. Work out a way of coping with this from the first. Find some noncommittal but unalarming answers, such as: "The doctor asked me to write down any symptoms (or questions, or complaints) and take them up with him," or, "The doctor said that was a usual thing in this kind of illness," or "He gave me a list of things to check on, and if they're all right—which they are—he said I needn't call him," or "I have no reason for thinking this means anything, but the doctor asked me to report everything that happens so I'll tell him about it."

Above all, try to make things as pleasant as possible for the patient: his meals, his little "entertainments," and, most important, his nurse (which means you).

## CARING FOR AN ADULT WITH A CHRONIC DISEASE

Let us say, just for an example, that you must care for your mother whose severe arthritis will require her to stay in bed for six months or more. After checking with your doctor, you are apt to find that you, too, should practice some of the nursing procedures he recommends. Naturally you will need to follow some of the suggestions I made regarding the care of sick children and adults. But your main problem is a little different; it consists in finding additional ways to keep your patient from being injured physically and emotionally by her long stay in bed.

A good hospital or nurse will insist that bedsores need not occur, and that they can be cured. It is very much easier to prevent them than it is to cure them. Be sure that you: (1) See that your patient's weight is distributed as evenly as possible instead of being (for example) entirely on the buttocks. (2) Keep the bed free from wrinkles; dispense with rubber sheets if possible—and it is almost always possible. (3) Move your patient frequently. (4) Keep the skin dry and clean; use a little alcohol as a rub after bathing, and talcum; give alcohol rubs. (5) Use rolls, or ring or doughnut cushions to keep the weight off vulnerable spots such as the hip and ankle bones the minute you discover the skin is at all red. Let the air come in contact with such spots for a little while every few hours. (6) The smallest sore should not be ignored in the hope that it will go away. Get your doctor's advice and follow his directions exactly.

If the patient can do so, have her exercise her legs by bending the knees and flexing her toes. This frequent mild exercise will encourage normal circulation and help prevent blood clots from forming in the veins.

The patient's *morale* is just as susceptible to emotional bedsores. Your attitude and the atmosphere you create can be excellent preventatives. But the chronically ill patient may still be chafed by the monotony of the necessary routine.

Be sure to keep this routine from becoming depressing by varying it to make room for little treats and small surprises—perhaps by using the "company china" for Sunday dinners, or wearing a flower on your bed jacket on Saturday night, or something special in the way of food or drink. Remember that the patient who must stay in bed for a long time needs to do things, not only for his or her own entertainment, but in order to feel useful. Persuade him or her to do something as a favor to you, something that will help you, such

*Figure 25-12. Giving an Enema.*

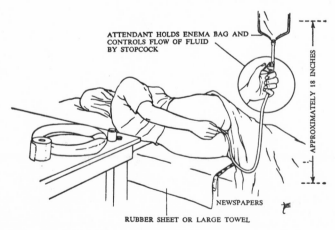

ATTENDANT HOLDS ENEMA BAG AND CONTROLS FLOW OF FLUID BY STOPCOCK

APPROXIMATELY 18 INCHES

NEWSPAPERS

RUBBER SHEET OR LARGE TOWEL

as a regular storytelling or reading period for the children, or helping with their homework, or peeling vegetables, or making something for the house or for future Christmas presents. *Never* let your patient know that it would be easier for you to do these things yourself. Even if it would, it is good for you to get some of the routine jobs off your hands. More important, it will pay off eventually, if only by giving you a happier and less demanding patient. In other words, one of the best pieces of nursing care you can give a chronically ill patient is to make a place, however small, for him or her in the home life of the family.

## HELP FROM OTHERS

In most cases of illness, you can get some help if you need it—and you often do. Find out what is available in your community through your doctor, clergyman, or social agency. You may need a visiting nurse for an hour every day or once a week, or an absolutely reliable "sitter" on certain occasions. Perhaps your patient would benefit by some of the services which various agencies offer in different kinds of illnesses, e.g., a visiting teacher or some schoolwork by mail for a partially disabled or slowly convalescing child, or training in some art or craft for a bedridden adult, or a correspondence school course in some subject you never suspected would interest your patient! Many people with long-lasting or chronic diseases have been helped to find moneymaking as well as entertaining projects.

Do not be reluctant to accept help if you cannot afford to pay for it and it is available free, or partially free. The burden of caring for a sick person is heavy enough without adding false pride to your load. It is also false economy to try to do so much yourself that you, too, become ill, or are unable to give the best care to your patient.

# PART FOUR

## You and Your Doctor

# 26
# YOUR DOCTOR

## EVERYONE NEEDS A DOCTOR

Even though you may be one of those rare and very fortunate people who can honestly say, "I've never been sick in my life," you should nevertheless have a doctor. Your perfect health is no guarantee against many contagious diseases, appendicitis, cancer, or accidents, which can cost you your life if you delay too long in getting medical assistance—as people often do when they do not have a physician to whom they can turn. Regardless of your state of health you surely don't want to gamble, either for yourself or for your family, on the chance that no emergency will ever occur. Besides, you need a doctor to help you *keep* your good health, especially as you grow older.

If, on the other hand, you are like most of us and suffer occasionally from ordinary ailments such as the "flu," there is an additional reason for you to have a doctor. His help is essential in preventing these illnesses from developing into something serious, like pneumonia. And if you are one of the less fortunate individuals who suffer from a chronic illness or general poor health, don't resign yourself to the idea that "Nothing can be done about it anyway." Tremendous advances have recently been made and are being made today, in both the prevention and cure of disease; and *everyone needs a doctor* in order to reap the full benefits of modern medical discoveries.

If you do not have a doctor, select one now. Don't wait until you or a member of your family develop appendicitis, pneumonia, or some other serious illness. Your doctor will be the central point of your health program, ready to take care of all your medical problems—including emergencies. He can handle them far better if he knows you and your physical condition beforehand.

You want to know him, too; in fact you want to know a good deal about him before you select him to be your doctor. All physicians aren't alike; in medicine, as in other professions and trades, some men have more skill and better training than others. There is a tremendous difference in the quality of medical school education and subsequent hospital experience of various doctors. It is risky to select a man for your family physician on the casual recommendation of a friend, or because his office is conveniently located in your neighborhood. Your health is too precious to trust to anyone but a very competent physician. (There are excellent women doctors today, and whether to select a man or woman is a matter to decide according to your own preference.)

## FAMILY PHYSICIAN

*The first step is to decide what type of doctor you will need.* You want someone whom you can call if illness strikes any member of your family; someone who will suggest a specialist if he himself cannot handle a condition adequately. You don't want too specialized a doctor for your family physician because he is concerned only with that branch of medicine for which he has specifically trained. An ophthalmologist, for example, would not treat your bronchitis, nor would he be expected to diagnose heart disease; he has obtained very special training to fit him for diagnosing and treating troubles of the eyes.

That is why you should choose a *general practitioner* or an *internist* for your family doctor. The *general practitioner* is trained to take care of most adult illnesses and to do a certain amount of surgery; also, he may deliver babies, take care of infants and children, and set broken limbs. The *internist* is more specialized; his field is medical diagnosis and treatment; he handles most medical conditions but does no major surgery, perhaps no surgery at all. A good internist or general practitioner will realize when his knowledge is not sufficient to cover a certain problem, and will call in a specialist or refer you to one. Although you may have needed a certain type of specialist in the past, you and your family should have *one* physician upon whom you can *all* rely; and the general practitioner or internist is best qualified for this position.

A good family doctor is not the quaint, old-fashioned character that some books and movies have portrayed him as being. On the contrary, he will always be eager to learn of new scientific developments in medical and surgical practice. This he will assuredly have the opportunity to do if he is a member of any of the medical societies, especially the American Academy of Family Physicians, which now increasingly require that members pursue continuing programs of education.

He will capably and skillfully perform periodic examinations, using all the facilities necessary to make a proper diagnosis of your condition, so that you won't discover an illness after it is too late to do anything about it. He will not hesitate to consult other physicians or to call upon a competent specialist if it is necessary, for a wise physician knows his own limitations, realizing that medical knowledge is so complex no one doctor can master it all. (By all means cooperate with your doctor if he suggests that he needs the help of a specialist or consultant, or the special facilities available at a medical center. On the other hand, you have the right to tell him you would be happier about his diagnosis or his decision to operate—or any problem that has arisen—if his opinion were seconded by a specialist. If *you* select the specialist, make certain he is acceptable to your doctor. It is proper

and sensible to discuss the specialist's fee with him directly, or through your own doctor.)

A good family doctor will be able to help you with problems of an emotional nature. If you or your family must go to a hospital he will choose one approved by the Joint Commission on Accreditation of Hospitals (see page 391). He will check up on pharmacies and suggest one where you can get your prescriptions filled safely and efficiently. He will know how to get a competent nurse and any other special type of medical service you or your family may need. And because he is a good doctor he will have a high standing in his community as a man of integrity and skill.

By now you are probably asking, "How can I ever find such a physician?" This is how I advise you to do it:

## HOW TO FIND A RELIABLE DOCTOR

1. One of the best ways to find a competent doctor is to consult a relative or close friend who is in the medical profession. He can generally suggest one or more good doctors who could serve as your family physician. Dentists, medical students, pharmacists, and medical and social workers may also be worth consulting. They have a better chance of getting accurate information for you than the average lay person has. Clergymen, lawyers, and judges may also be able to obtain this information.

2. If there is a medical school in your community you can secure a catalogue of its faculty by writing to the dean of the school. For your family doctor you will most likely want to choose someone in the Department of Medicine (the others will probably be too specialized). On page 362 of this book the names and addresses of American medical schools are listed.

3. Another way to find your family physician is to write or telephone the superintendent of a local hospital approved by the Joint Commission on Accreditation of Hospitals (see page 391). The superintendents of these hospitals will be glad to send you a list of the men on their hospital staffs. Incidentally, a physician's appointment to a hospital indicates approval of his ability, for a good

hospital will not staff a man who is not competent. Furthermore, a hospital keeps the doctor in contact with changes in medicine and with the facilities of the laboratory, modern equipment, and new ideas.

*The amount and quality of training that a doctor has had after graduation from medical school are an important indication of his ability.* Almost every physician has had at least one year's hospital training. The best doctors now take two, three, or even more years of hospital work before entering practice. If a doctor has been graduated from a good medical school and has trained at one of the good hospitals in the country, you can be quite certain he is capable of rendering the service you want.

*Make certain the doctor you choose is on the staff of a good hospital.* Many people do not realize that fully one-third of the doctors in most large cities cannot admit their patients to the best hospitals. Ask your prospective doctor what hospital he would send you to, and make sure it is a recognized, accredited institution.

4. You can obtain a list of licensed physicians from your county and state medical societies or from the American Medical Association, 535 North Dearborn Street, Chicago, Illinois 60610. The American Medical Association is a national medical society maintained to set standards for the medical profession. It also exposes impostors in the field of medicine.

The American Medical Association and the county and state medical societies require ethical conduct from the members. In addition they provide postgraduate instruction for physicians to keep them informed of new medical trends. These societies also meet from time to time to discuss developments in medicine, and they publish journals containing the latest medical information for the benefit of their members.

5. Your board of health or the county health officer can also advise you in your selection of a doctor. They might be especially helpful if you live in a rural area some distance away from a large hospital or medical school.

6. If you move from a community where you have had a physician in whom you have confidence, you can ask him to help you find a doctor in your new community. Often he can do so by communicating with physicians he knows in or near the locality to which you have moved.

Let us assume you have obtained the names of several reliable physicians by consulting one or more of the above sources. The medical societies, hospital superintendents, health officers, and medical schools obviously cannot recommend any one doctor. They will list the men who have had adequate medical training, but the final decision must be yours.

## THE FINAL CHOICE RESTS ON YOUR OWN DECISION

Your final judgment should be based on how you, personally, feel about the man. Go and talk to him—professionally, not at a social gathering. Would you find that embarrassing? Then make an appointment for a medical checkup—it is probably long overdue anyway. This won't commit you to him for life, and it will give you the opportunity to get an impression of him in the role you may want him to assume permanently. Do you think you can develop a warm, *confident* personal relationship with him? This is most important, since you must be willing to respect and follow his advice in serious decisions, perhaps even matters of life and death. Do you think you could like him? Naturally you don't expect him to resemble a Hollywood movie star, and you don't really care whether or not he voted for your choice in the elections; but you do want to feel easy and comfortable in his presence, so you can talk to him about emotional problems if they should arise. Above all, *does he inspire confidence in you?* You are not looking for the ideal man, but for a doctor you can trust.

> Honor a physician with the honor due unto him for the uses which ye may have of him.
> —Ecclesiasticus

## HOW TO DEVELOP A GOOD RELATIONSHIP WITH YOUR DOCTOR

So you have decided upon your doctor. What do you do next? First, don't wait for an emergency or serious illness before giving him the opportunity to become acquainted with *all* the members of your family—their general condition and their medical history. Arrange for a complete examination of everyone in your family. You may also want to arrange for a checkup once a year or every two or three years depending on your doctor's recommendations. The exact intervals can best be judged by him and will depend on your age and medical history.

It will do no good, I might add, to select an excellent doctor if you are not going to cooperate with him. Your part is important, too. When you are consulting him you must tell him everything, no matter how insignificant it may seem. Only in this way will he be able to determine your ailments and find the cure. In addition, always tell him what the school doctors and nurses have reported about your child's health.

When you give him information on the telephone, talk clearly. Avoid diagnosing your own illnesses and taking your own remedies—patent medicines and the like. When you are ill, call him and follow his directions exactly.

Here's a word to the wise: As a busy doctor myself I know that many physicians do not have the time to point out all the incidental pieces of information that may concern you. Furthermore, a doctor is often reluctant to advance some information himself, although he would be glad to give it if asked. So ask your doctor specific questions such as which pharmacy *he* would use to have a prescription filled, or which surgeon *he* would select if he were going to have a major operation, or whether *he* would recommend Dr. —— to deliver his own children.

## FEES

Patients are too sensitive about discussing fees with doctors. There is a financial side to the practice of medicine, and we doctors want to work it out satisfactorily for both our patients and ourselves. It is best to ask your doctor about his schedule of fees.

The first office visit, if it is part of a complete diagnostic work-up or health survey, will generally cost you considerably more than subsequent visits. Make sure you understand the charges in advance. Also inquire of the secretary or the doctor about the preferred method of payment—by cash or mailed bill.

If an operation is recommended, ask your doctor what the surgical fees will be and also ask him to obtain an estimate of all the hospital costs. Then you can find out what proportion of these costs will be covered by your Blue Cross, Blue Shield, Medicare, or other insurance plans you may belong to (see page 407). In this way you will have a realistic preview of your medical expenses.

## WHAT TO DO IN AN EMERGENCY WHEN YOUR DOCTOR IS OUT OF TOWN

Be sure you understand who covers your doctor's practice when he is away or unable to take your call. If you cannot reach him or his substitute and you need help at home urgently, telephone your local medical society or department of health, and they will recommend someone who can help you quickly. In many communities the local medical society maintains a panel of doctors who take emergency calls. If there is a situation requiring immediate attention and you cannot locate a doctor fast enough, ask the police to help you get to a hospital or to send you an ambulance.

## WHAT TO DO WHEN YOU NEED A DOCTOR AWAY FROM YOUR COMMUNITY

If you become ill when you are away from home, it is important to check before accepting medical care. Have a long distance call put through to your own doctor. Let him arrange things for you. In general, remember that many doctors keep lists of competent physicians in other communities. If they do not know a particular doctor they can locate names of qualified specialists from their national directories of specialists, or can refer you to a good local hospital. Make certain your own doctor knows about any serious illness or accident you have had while away from home, even if you have not been able to notify him immediately.

If you cannot reach your own doctor, get in touch with the superintendent of the local hospital or the county or city health officer, and ask him whom he would recommend for you. If there is a serious illness requiring surgery, do not hesitate to say, "Which doctor here would you select for yourself or your family if a serious operation had to be performed?"

If you are in a foreign country and need medical care, the United States Foreign Service will help you. Consult either the American Embassy (found in capital cities of foreign countries), the American Consulate (a smaller branch of the Embassy usually located in large cities), or the U.S. Legation (a branch of the Embassy located in smaller foreign countries).

## CAN YOU CHANGE DOCTORS?

This is not something to be done casually. If, for example, your regular doctor is not available and you call another physician, your own doctor should take over as soon as possible.

However, it is possible to change doctors at any time. *But* I would advise that you select carefully, along the lines I have indicated, so you will never have to make the painful decision to change physicians at a time of serious illness.

If you ever do wish to make such a change, you should talk things over clearly with your doctor. It is best to make sure you understand the present situation before you change doctors. If you are dissatisfied with the results of treatment, a consultation with a specialist may convince you that your own doctor has done as well as can be expected.

There may be other reasons why you wish to change and may be justified in doing so. If the doctor is always rushed during your visits, unable to devote a reasonable amount of time to you, or if he fails to tell you what is behind your symptoms, what the basic problem is, you may wish

to find another physician. You have a right also to expect him to inform you of possible alarming side effects of drugs and what to do if they occur.

## SPECIALISTS

I believe it is always desirable to make arrangements through your family doctor—or at least in conjunction with him—when you find it necessary to consult a specialist. If you do this there will always be one doctor who knows everything that has happened to you and your family.

In order to become a bona fide specialist, a doctor should be accredited by the specialty licensure board in his field. This is very important, as it indicates that he has had the extra training necessary for him to become expert in a particular branch of medicine. If he has satisfied the requirements for the specialty board, a physician undoubtedly has the proper background for his specialty. An inquiry addressed to the American Medical Association will enable you to find out whether a physician has met the requirements set for his specialty.

## DICTIONARY OF SPECIALISTS

If you are to consult specialists at some time you should know something about the principal specialists in medicine and related fields, and what they do. The following list will help you:

The *obstetrician* (ahb-stuh-tri'shun) delivers babies and takes care of the pregnant patient during the months before the birth of the baby.

The *pediatrician* (pee-di-uh-tri'shun) takes care of infants and children up to the age of twelve or fifteen. His specialty is called *pediatrics* (pee-dee-at'riks).

The *internist* (in-ter'nist) specializes in diagnosis and treatment of medical conditions of the entire body. (He is often referred to as a diagnostician or medical man, though neither of these terms defines precisely just what he specializes in.)

A *surgeon* (ser'jun) specializes in performing operations. He may be a *general surgeon* or he may confine his operations to one of the following branches of surgery:

The *gynecologist* (jin-uh-kahl'uh-jist) treats illness of the female organs; the *urologist* (yoo-rahl' uh-jist) specializes in treatment of the urinary system in women and the genitourinary system in men. For example, he would be the doctor called upon to operate on a diseased prostate.

An *orthopedist* (or-tho-pee'dist) specializes in diseases of the bones and joints.

An *otolaryngologist* (o"toh-lar-in-gahl'o-jist) deals with ailments of the ears, throat, sinuses, and nose.

The *cardiologist* (kar'de-ahl'o-jist) specializes in the treatment of heart diseases.

The *rheumatologist* (roo-mah-tahl'uh-jist) is skilled in the diagnosis and treatment of rheumatic conditions such as arthritis.

The *endocrinologist* (en'do-kree-nol'o-jist) is a specialist in problems of the thyroid and other endocrine glands.

The *hematologist* (he'mah-tol'o-jist) is a physician trained and experienced in diagnosis and treatment of blood disorders.

The *oncologist* (ong-kol'o-jist) specializes in the causes, development, and treatment of cancers and other tumors.

The *nephrologist* (ne-frol'o-jist) deals especially with the kidneys.

A *psychiatrist* (sigh-kigh'uh-trist) is a graduate medical doctor who takes care of the mind and emotions. It is important to remember that psychiatrists deal mostly with individuals who have some behavior problem or neurosis. Only a small fraction of their time is spent with the insane.

Organic diseases of the nerves and brain are treated by a *neurologist* (noo-rahl'uh-jist).

An eye specialist who has the degree of M.D. is called an *ophthalmologist* (ahf-thal-mahl'uh-jist). He is trained in surgery of the eye as well as in all its diseases.

An *optometrist* (ahp-tahm'i-trist) is not a medical doctor. He has been trained to examine the eyes for the purpose of prescribing eyeglasses. The *optician* (ahp-tish'en) is the man who fills the prescriptions made by the ophthalmologists or optometrists. He is the counterpart of the pharmacists who fill prescriptions for medicines. Neither the optometrist nor the optician is trained to treat diseases of the eye.

The *dermatologist* (derm-uh-tahl'uh-jist) specializes in the treatment of diseases of the skin, hair, and scalp.

An *allergist* (al'ler-jist) specializes in such diseases as hay fever, asthma, hives, and allergic reactions to food.

The *gastroenterologist* (gas"tro-en-ter-ahl'uh-jist) specializes in diseases of the stomach and intestines.

The *proctologist* (prahk-tahl'uh-jist) diagnoses and treats, by surgery if necessary, malfunctions and diseases of the colon, rectum, and anus.

The *radiologist* (ray-di-ahl'uh-jist) is a specialist in taking and interpreting x-rays. He uses radium, x-rays, and other radioactive substances in the treatment of cancer and other diseases.

The *pathologist* (path-ahl'uh-jist) studies changes in tissues arising from disease.

The *anesthesiologist* (an-es-thee-zi-ahl'uh-jist) specializes in administering anesthetics for surgery.

*Podiatrists* (po-digh'uh-trists) and *chiropodists* (kigh-rahp'uh-dists) are names for the experts who diagnose and treat diseases, injuries, and defects of the foot.

## SHOULD OPERATIONS BE PERFORMED BY THE GENERAL PRACTITIONER OR THE SURGICAL SPECIALISTS?

This is one of the most difficult problems facing both the patient and the medical profession. Many general practitioners are competent to handle surgery; others have not had adequate training and experience. Many operations such as removal of the gallbladder, partial removal of the thyroid gland, or stomach surgery for ulcer, require a high degree of skill and experience. Even a less drastic operation such as an appendectomy can be a very difficult procedure when it is performed on a very obese person.

What do I advise? First, talk the situation over

fully with your own doctor. If he advises a serious operation, ask him if he plans to operate himself. If not, then have him suggest the surgical specialist he would select for a member of his own family for this same type of operation. If he says that he plans to perform the operation himself—and if there is doubt in your mind about his surgical experience—you might ask three questions: (a) the number of times he has himself performed this same operation; (b) does he feel that he can do as competent a job as a specialist in surgery; (c) what are the chances of death or disability in the operation that is proposed? After you have obtained the answers to these questions, all your doubts will probably be resolved. If not, you can always go to a specialist in surgery for his opinion, or travel to the nearest medical center for an examination and recommendations. You may be told that your local doctor and hospital are equal to the task.

No family doctor can spend as much time as he would like in educating you about all matters relating to your health. Your doctor expects you to cooperate with him by reading about important subjects such as vitamins in your food, your ideal weight, prevention of tuberculosis, good posture, and the dozens of other subjects covered in this book.

## GROUP MEDICAL PRACTICE EXPLAINED

In many communities, doctors team up in group practice. Some of these groups include specialists in almost every branch of medicine; other groups may be quite small, consisting of a diagnostician, a surgeon, a pediatrician, and a laboratory specialist.

If these men live up to the standards of competence I have outlined, they will provide you with an excellent "combination" family doctor. Such a group can offer unusually good medical care because of the close cooperation between its various members. They can provide laboratory tests and the services of specialists at reasonable rates. Some groups provide service on a monthly prepayment basis for the entire family. These clinics usually provide annual medical checkups without extra charge. If you wish to learn the address of your nearest group clinic, send a postcard with your request to the U.S. Public Health Service, Washington, D.C. 20201.

## ACCREDITED MEDICAL SCHOOLS IN THE UNITED STATES

**ALABAMA**
University of Alabama School of Medicine, Birmingham 35294

University of South Alabama College of Medicine, Mobile 36688

**ARIZONA**
University of Arizona College of Medicine, Tucson 85724

**ARKANSAS**
University of Arkansas School of Medicine, Little Rock 72201

**CALIFORNIA**
University of California School of Medicine, Davis 95616

University of California College of Medicine, Irvine 92664

Loma Linda University School of Medicine, Loma Linda 92354

University of California School of Medicine, Los Angeles 90024

University of Southern California School of Medicine, Los Angeles 90037

Stanford University School of Medicine, Palo Alto 94305

(continued)

University of California School of Medicine, San Diego 92037

University of California School of Medicine, San Francisco 94143

COLORADO
University of Colorado School of Medicine, Denver 80220

CONNECTICUT
University of Connecticut School of Medicine, Farmington 06032

Yale University School of Medicine, New Haven 06510

DISTRICT OF COLUMBIA
Georgetown University School of Medicine, 20007

George Washington University School of Medicine, 20037

Howard University College of Medicine, 20059

FLORIDA
University of Florida College of Medicine, Gainesville 32610

University of Miami School of Medicine, Miami 33152

University of South Florida College of Medicine, Tampa 33620

GEORGIA
Emory University School of Medicine, Atlanta 30322

Medical College of Georgia, Augusta 30902

HAWAII
University of Hawaii School of Medicine, Honolulu 96822

ILLINOIS
Chicago Medical School University of Health Sciences, Chicago 60612

Northwestern University Medical School, Chicago 60611

Loyola University of Chicago Stritch School of Medicine, Maywood 60153

Rush Medical College, Chicago 60612

Southern Illinois University School of Medicine, Springfield 62708

University of Chicago Pritzker School of Medicine, Chicago 60637

University of Illinois College of Medicine, Chicago 60612

INDIANA
Indiana University School of Medicine, Indianapolis 46202

IOWA
University of Iowa College of Medicine, Iowa City 52242

KANSAS
University of Kansas School of Medicine, Kansas City 66103

KENTUCKY
University of Kentucky College of Medicine, Lexington 40506

University of Louisville School of Medicine, Louisville 40201

LOUISIANA
Louisiana State University School of Medicine, New Orleans 70112

Tulane University School of Medicine, New Orleans 70112

Louisiana State University School of Medicine, Shreveport 71130

MARYLAND
Johns Hopkins University School of Medicine, Baltimore 21205

University of Maryland School of Medicine, Baltimore 21201

MASSACHUSETTS
Boston University School of Medicine, Boston 02118

Harvard Medical School, Boston 02118

Tufts University School of Medicine, Boston 02111

University of Massachusetts Medical School, Worcester 01605

MICHIGAN
University of Michigan Medical School, Ann Arbor 48104

Wayne State University School of Medicine, Detroit 48201

Michigan State University College of Human Medicine, East Lansing 48824

MINNESOTA
University of Minnesota Medical School, Minneapolis 55455

Mayo Medical School, Rochester 55901

MISSISSIPPI
University of Mississippi School of Medicine, Jackson 39216

MISSOURI
University of Missouri School of Medicine, Columbia 65201

University of Missouri School of Medicine, Kansas City 64108

Saint Louis University School of Medicine, St Louis 63104

Washington University School of Medicine, St Louis 63110

NEBRASKA
Creighton University School of Medicine, Omaha 68178

University of Nebraska College of Medicine, Omaha 68105

NEW HAMPSHIRE
Dartmouth Medical School, Hanover 03755

NEW JERSEY
CMDNJ-New Jersey Medical School, Newark 07103

CMDNJ-Rutgers Medical School, Piscataway 08854

NEW MEXICO
University of New Mexico School of Medicine, Albuquerque 87131

NEW YORK
Albany Medical College of Union University, Albany 12208

State University of New York at Buffalo School of Medicine, 14214

Columbia University College of Physicians & Surgeons, New York 10032

Cornell University Medical College, New York 10021

Albert Einstein College of Medicine of Yeshiva University, New York 10461

Mount Sinai School of Medicine of the City University of New York 10029

New York Medical College, New York 10029

New York University School of Medicine, New York 10016

State University of New York College of Medicine, Brooklyn 11203

University of Rochester School of Medicine & Dentistry, Rochester 14642

State University of New York at Stony Brook School of Medicine 11794

State University of New York College of Medicine, Syracuse 13210

(continued)

NORTH CAROLINA

University of North Carolina School of Medicine, Chapel Hill 27514

Duke University School of Medicine, Durham 27710

Bowman Gray School of Medicine, Winston-Salem 27103

NORTH DAKOTA

University of North Dakota School of Medicine, Grand Forks 58202

OHIO

University of Cincinnati College of Medicine, Cincinnati 45267

Case Western Reserve University School of Medicine, Cleveland 55106

Ohio State University College of Medicine, Columbus 43210

Medical College of Ohio at Toledo 43614

OKLAHOMA

University of Oklahoma School of Medicine, Oklahoma City 73190

OREGON

University of Oregon Medical School, Portland 97201

PENNSYLVANIA

Pennsylvania State University College of Medicine, The Milton S. Hershey Medical Center, Hershey 17033

Hahnemann Medical College and Hospital, Philadelphia 19102

Jefferson Medical College of Thomas Jefferson University, Philadelphia 19107

Medical College of Pennsylvania (Formerly Women's), Philadelphia 19129

Temple University School of Medicine, Philadelphia 19140

University of Pennsylvania School of Medicine, Philadelphia 19174

University of Pittsburgh School of Medicine, Pittsburgh 15261

PUERTO RICO

University of Puerto Rico School of Medicine, San Juan 00936

RHODE ISLAND

Brown University Program in Medical Science, Providence 02912

SOUTH CAROLINA

Medical University of South Carolina College of Medicine, Charleston 29401

TENNESSEE

University of Tennessee College of Medicine, Memphis 38163

Meharry Medical College School of Medicine, Nashville 37208

Vanderbilt University School of Medicine, Nashville 37232

TEXAS

University of Texas Southwestern Medical School, Dallas 75235

University of Texas Medical Branch, Galveston 77550

Baylor College of Medicine, Houston 77025

University of Texas Medical School, Houston 77025

Texas Tech University School of Medicine, Lubbock 79409

University of Texas Medical School, San Antonio 78284

UTAH

University of Utah College of Medicine, Salt Lake City 84132

VERMONT

University of Vermont College of Medicine, Burlington 05401

VIRGINIA
University of Virginia School of Medicine,
Charlottesville 22901

Medical College of Virginia, Richmond 23298

Eastern Virginia Medical School, Norfolk 23501

WASHINGTON
University of Washington School of Medicine,
Seattle 98195

WEST VIRGINIA
West Virginia University School of Medicine,
Morgantown 26506

WISCONSIN
University of Wisconsin Medical School,
Madison 53706

Medical College of Wisconsin, Milwaukee 53233

# 27
# MEDICAL CHECKUPS

Your doctor is the key to your medical health program. You should use his services wisely and well. That means enlisting his help in the prevention of sickness, in addition to seeing him when you are actually ill.

Almost everyone says, "I think I'll get checked up by my doctor one of these days," and then waits until illness strikes, sometimes disastrously, before doing so. I do not blame patients when this happens. It is only human not to want to think about disease and medical problems when one feels in tiptop shape.

However, if we realize the great value of the periodic medical checkup, we will go through with it automatically, and regularly experience satisfaction and pleasure from knowing that everything is right with our health. When I say "we" I mean just that: doctors, too, are subject to cancer, tuberculosis, and other diseases, and need regular medical checkups *to find disease in its early, curable stage.* This, for every one of us, is the main reason for the periodic checkup—to locate the trouble before it causes damage that is serious or perhaps beyond repair.

Let me give you an example, from my own experience, of the value of the periodic checkup: a young engineer, apparently in vigorous good health, decided to have a checkup before taking a strenuous new job overseas. The x-ray of his lungs showed a small area of tuberculosis. Early tuberculosis, which often can be detected only by an x-ray, is completely curable in most instances. A year later, after treatment, the young man was healed and recovered. On the other hand, advanced tuberculosis is serious; and if he had gone

into a new and very strenuous job with this small spot in his lung, he would probably have developed really widespread tuberculosis before the disease made its presence known by such symptoms as fatigue, cough, loss of weight, fever, or hemorrhage from the lungs.

Merely for reassurance that you are not suffering any serious disease, or that you are in the earliest, curable stage of some potential threat to your health, the regular physical examination is worth the time and cost it entails. For both young and older people, it is important to catch illness early. For everyone, the knowledge that he or she is in good physical condition is a source of satisfaction and emotional security.

I find that it is difficult to convince adolescents and young adults in exuberant health that they need regular medical checkups. Yet these are essential, for disease is so terribly tragic in teenagers and young adults that every effort should be made to prevent it, or at least to find it early. Rheumatic fever occurs in young people. So, too, nephritis (sometimes called Bright's disease). Diabetes strikes at children and young adults—and usually in its severest form. Arthritis, asthma, anemias, and a surprisingly long list of sicknesses plague young people who should be going through the "best years of their lives." How tragic to find the wonderful years of marriage and parenthood marred by serious diseases that might have been minimized or cured if detected early at a regular checkup!

Therefore I prescribe regular medical examinations for *everyone*, regardless of age, sex, occupation, or physical condition.

378

Before stating the full case for periodic examinations, I want to discuss a question that people frequently ask.

## HOW OFTEN SHOULD I HAVE A PERIODIC CHECKUP?

I have already suggested that you begin your relationship with your doctor by having a complete checkup. When should the next one come? Ask him to suggest the date; it will probably be in a year, but it may be in six months, or in two or even three years. The truth of the matter is that the medical profession doesn't really know exactly how often examinations should be made. Doctors are inclined to believe that most potentially dangerous conditions will be caught early enough by an annual checkup; and they have found that most patients will accept the idea of having a yearly examination.

Some physicians believe that, after an initial examination, repeat examinations at intervals of three years or more are adequate for healthy children and for robust people in their twenties. They also feel that checkups are in order at two- or three-year intervals for healthy people in their thirties, at eighteen-month intervals for those in their forties, and yearly for people in their fifties and older. One important exception: women in the childbearing years and older should have limited examinations every year. The American Cancer Society favors annual checkups at all ages.

## CHECKUPS GIVE A CONTINUOUS RECORD OF YOUR HEALTH

The regular medical checkup pays other dividends besides its guarantee against the development of many serious diseases. It gives your doctor an invaluable record of your health. For example, if your family physician has annual records of your blood pressure going back twenty years, he isn't going to be very disturbed if a slight elevation is found on your fortieth birthday during an examination for life insurance. He may inform you that your pressure has been normal every year for twenty years, except for a few points of elevation the week before you were married, fifteen years ago. He will probably advise you to ask the insurance doctor for a repeat examination after a weekend's rest, instead of at the conclusion of an exhausting day at the office.

Blood pressure records are by no means the only important ones that accumulate as a result of regular, yearly checkups. Your doctor learns the condition of your heart, lungs, digestive apparatus, and other vital parts of your body from examining you at these periods.

If you see your doctor only when you are extremely ill, which may be at very rare intervals, you can hardly expect him to know much about your usual state of health. And then, at the age of fifty, you confront him with a question such as, "Do you think it will be safe for me to go mountain-climbing this year?" Remember that the more we physicians know about your health, year in and year out, reinforced by careful observation and laboratory examinations and tests, the better we can advise you in the crucial years of later life.

## X-RAY RECORDS

Because of the growing concern about the maximum tolerable dose of radiation over a lifetime, many physicians believe that it would be wise for everyone to have a record of all the radiation he has received during the course of diagnosis and therapy. This would include dental x-rays, fluoroscopic or x-ray examination for tuberculosis, and other work involving radiation. Another advantage of having the same doctor conduct your health checkup regularly is that he will have most of this information already, and you can tell him of any additional x-ray work.

## AN OPPORTUNITY TO DISCUSS EMOTIONAL PROBLEMS

Emotional crises and nervous breakdowns are, unfortunately, all too common. They seldom come on suddenly, but are usually the result of years of gathering tensions and problems. I believe one of the best features of the annual examination is the opportunity it gives both patient and doctor to have a heart-to-heart talk about emotional problems. You may often prefer not to discuss such matters with relatives and friends, but you can spill them to a sympathetic doctor. It is easier, too, if you have been seeing the same doctor year after year, and feel he is an understanding friend as well as a capable physician.

The checkup provides a good opportunity to work off vague fears that are troubling you. Sooner or later, most people develop a phobia, usually about cancer or high blood pressure. It has been my experience that when patients pay their hard-earned dollars for "just a checkup," they are almost always prompted by a hidden fear of some disease. Women are grateful for the assurance, upon completion of an examination, that they have no tumors of the breast or womb. Men are more likely to fear high blood pressure, a heart attack, or a stroke. When you see your doctor, bring your fears out into the open. Tell him exactly what you are worried about, including any emotional problems.

## BEST SEASON OF THE YEAR FOR A CHECKUP

Is there a good and bad time for the annual checkup? *Yes.* Remember that your doctor is a busy person, very much occupied during the fall and winter months with influenza, pneumonia, and all the other illnesses that keep him working overtime. The best time of the year for the doctor and for you, too, is the late spring or early summer. He can be leisurely then—an essential element in a good checkup. It's valuable for you to have the medical examination before your summer vacation in order to obtain your physician's advice about the amount of strenuous sports you can engage in with safety. Then, too, he will be able to check on those ten or twenty pounds you may have added during the winter months, and explain how you can remove them during the summer by sensible diet and exercise.

## PROCEDURE OF THE MEDICAL CHECKUP AND EXAMINATION

### The Medical History

The doctor or his nurse will ask a great many questions at your first checkup in order to learn every detail of your health background. In subsequent periodic checkups your doctor will want particularly to learn if any serious illness, such as cancer, tuberculosis, heart trouble, or diabetes, has shown any symptoms. This means he has to work like a detective searching for all sorts of clues. For example, itching of the genitals may sometimes be an important symptom of diabetes. Bleeding from the vagina or the rectum could lead the doctor to suspect early, curable cancer.

### The Physical Examination

The physical examination includes (1) inspection, (2) palpation, (3) percussion, and (4) auscultation.

This is the way in which these would be applied to the examination, for example, of your heart: The doctor first *inspects* the chest over the heart, looking for the heave and beat of the heart which provides a guide to its size and the way it is working. Then by *palpation*—putting his fingers and hands over the heart—he feels the way the heart beats. The normal heart feels one way, the diseased heart feels another way. For example, if a certain type of valve damage is present in the heart, the chest wall will vibrate very gently in a way that has a characteristic feel to the trained fingers. *Percussion* means striking the body with the fingers to bring out resonant sounds. Because the heart is not resonant and the adjacent lungs are, sound waves will change in pitch as soon as the doctor's fingers strike the chest over the heart. His experienced ears detect the change in note, and thus he has a guide to the precise location of the heart and its size. *Auscultation* means listening with a stethoscope. The normal heart sounds a certain way; if valve disease or some other heart trouble is present, the stethoscope picks up characteristic sounds which help in the diagnosis.

The doctor uses the same methods for examination of the lungs. In examinations of some parts of the body we find that only inspection and palpation may be useful.

No checkup is complete without an *examination of the rectum and genital organs*. These areas of the body are frequently the sites of cancers which can be terribly serious if not detected in the early, curable stage. Other diseases occur in these organs, too. The rectum and the female genital organs must be examined internally, requiring the insertion of the physician's gloved fingers. (See Figure 27-1.) In examining women he will also use a speculum, a cylindrical instrument which distends the vagina, enabling him to see the tip of the womb (cervix). It is at this time that the Pap smear is taken, as a simple check for the early development of cancer of the uterus.

## Laboratory Tests

On the basis of the patient's history and the results of the physical examination, the doctor decides which laboratory tests will be required. The blood and urine are examined and the lungs x-rayed in almost every periodic checkup. His judgment will determine whether you need one or more x-rays and laboratory tests. If he asks you to undergo any special tests, be sure you understand what they are and the directions for taking them as well as the cost involved. Frequently the doctor will send you to a laboratory, a hospital, or a radiologist's office for these tests.

# YOUR PART
# IN THE
# PHYSICAL EXAMINATION

## Fees for Periodic Checkups

Unless you belong to some prepaid or group medical care plan, such as the plans explained on page 407, you will have to pay a fee for your routine checkup. Doctors are often reluctant to suggest annual examinations, because they are sensitive about any taint of "salesmanship." It is much easier if *you* ask your doctor for an annual checkup. You might suggest, as you do with your dentist, that he have his secretary send you a reminder, mentioning a time for your appointment.

## How to Help During the Examination

You can be very helpful to your doctor during the physical examination if you will keep as relaxed as possible. It is much easier to examine the abdomen in a relaxed person than in one who

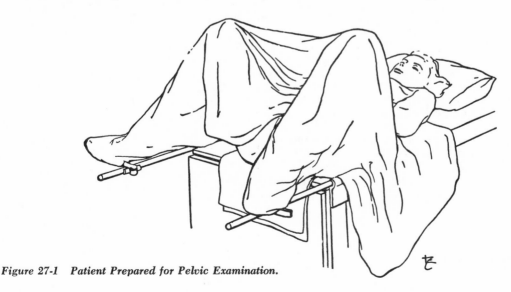

*Figure 27-1  Patient Prepared for Pelvic Examination.*

tenses all the muscles. It will frequently ease your muscles if you breathe gently with your mouth open. Usually, relaxation will result when you realize that the doctor has a reason for everything he is doing. Some of our procedures, such as asking you to say certain words like "ninety-nine," have been developed from many years of experience: the lungs vibrate best when the words "ninety-nine" are uttered.

Avoid talking or looking at your doctor when he is examining you. In order to concentrate intently on our work many of us may look grim and intense because we are focusing every bit of energy on very faint sounds in the heart and lungs. Some patients assume we are finding all sorts of serious illnesses when, in fact, we are usually only making certain that everything is working *normally!*

Women should remember that a physical examination is no occasion for false modesty. Be prepared for delicate questions, and answer them fully and completely without reticence. Cooperate with your doctor by letting him know you understand the reasons for the rectal and pelvic examinations. If he fails to make these vitally important examinations, tell him tactfully that you would like him to do so. Some doctors are reluctant to make the suggestion, and prefer to have the request come from the patient. Women should also realize that, if the doctor does not have a nurse or receptionist, he would like you to bring along a relative or friend. Unless another woman is present in the same room when he conducts a pelvic examination, his reputation may be ruined by the gossip or charges of an hysterical or malicious patient.

### Your Medical Vocabulary

It may save you some embarrassment if you learn a few medical terms for the various parts of the body. These are given in the illustrations which show you the principal parts of the body, including the genital regions. This book contains a dictionary of medical terms that will help you define and *pronounce* medical terms.

If the doctor or nurse uses a medical term you do not understand, do not hesitate to ask what it means. We doctors have a habit of forgetting that our patients usually do not know that *dyspnea* means shortness of breath, or *dysuria,* painful urination. Many others of the Greek and Latin terms have become second nature for the doctor.

However, your doctor doesn't want you to use technical words, such as "cardiac" for heart, unless you know their precise meaning. He wants, more than anything, to have you tell about your symptoms in your own way, without trying to make a diagnosis. Simply explain to him how you feel, point to where the trouble is, describe how long the symptoms have persisted, and also mention their severity. The doctor will probably take over from there and ask you questions. He may want to know if a pain is "cramplike," "burning," or "penetrating." All these differences in symptoms help him obtain a clearer picture of the cause of your illness.

### THE FINAL DISCUSSION

After the doctor has completed his examination and has obtained the results of the laboratory tests and any other required information, he will discuss these with you. He may give you the good news that you are in excellent health; or he may prescribe a diet or give you a prescription for medicine. On the other hand, if he locates or suspects some serious disease, he may refer you to a specialist for consultation.

Be sure you understand his instructions. Do not be timid; ask him any questions about your physical condition, and make sure your health is adequate for any vacation plans you anticipate or for any changes you visualize in your work schedule.

# 28

# HOW TO RECOGNIZE SICKNESS EARLY

## MAKE HEALTH INFORMATION
## A PART OF YOUR EDUCATION

After you have read this book you should never have to worry about when to call the doctor. You will act correctly and at the right time. That is one of the main reasons why this book was written for you. You will never be guilty of the type of medical ignorance which I describe in this chapter. It is intended to make people realize the importance of becoming educated about health matters. The chapter also shows how easy it is to understand many of the danger signals of illness.

### A Preventable Death

I once witnessed the tragic end of a case of medical ignorance. Visiting a great medical center some distance from my home, I was shocked to find a boy dying of diabetes. This should not have happened, not with insulin available, not in this modern era of treatment for diabetes!

I learned the sad story from the physician in charge. For a number of weeks the young boy, whose name was Freddy, had complained to his parents of feeling out of sorts. He was slowly and steadily losing weight and also appeared to be losing his strength. He spoke frequently of how thirsty he felt much of the time.

His parents were not really alarmed until they noticed one afternoon that he was unusually drowsy, almost stuporous. At that time, unfortunately several weeks too late, they telephoned the doctor. It was his busy season—flu, sore throats,

and a measles epidemic—and they had difficulty locating him. By the time the doctor heard the story and made the diagnosis of diabetes, the child was unconscious.

Freddy was rushed to one of our best medical centers. Doctors stayed with him continuously through the night injecting insulin and administering other necessary medicines. But the boy died.

We can treat diabetes today successfully, almost routinely, with insulin or other medication. Even the serious complications of acidosis and coma can be overcome if recognized early. That boy was entitled to live. The parents meant well. They were guilty only of medical ignorance.

But ignorance of the law does not provide a valid excuse in court. I believe that ignorance and neglect of the common signs of sickness are even more inexcusable, for the cost of the transgression may be death.

Many people know virtually none of the elementary facts about illness, although this information may someday represent the difference between life and death to them. Why?

### Your Doctor "Versus" You

People often assume that the doctor takes full responsibility for their health. They consult him when they become sick, and pay him for treatment and cure. But from the doctor's side of the fence we see a different situation. Often the physician is not consulted until the illness is dangerously far advanced. For example, Freddy's parents were unaware of the approaching tragedy during all those eight weeks when diabetes, untreated, was progressing toward its inevitable end. Other parents, more sensitive to medical problems, might have recognized, weeks earlier, the danger signal of excessive thirst. The problem is one of education.

Fortunately most potentially fatal diseases signal their onset with obvious symptoms. When a fever of 105 degrees and a violent chill strike, you know you need medical attention. And whether your symptoms result from pneumonia, meningitis, or malaria, your doctor can cure you.

But many serious medical conditions develop silently, without obvious warning. A woman with a cancer of the uterus (womb) may suffer no illness or pain until the growth has progressed to the stage where it may cost her life. However, it is possible to prevent serious damage from this and other insidious diseases by learning to watch for certain danger signals.

Medical alertness and knowledge can save children with diabetes and early heart trouble; adults with stomach ulcers, cancer, and many other ills.

"Hold on," you are saying. "How can you expect me to have all the specialized knowledge you doctors acquire during six to ten years of intensive training?"

That isn't necessary. The characteristic warnings of most illnesses can be recognized by all of us. A willingness to learn is the real requirement.

## THE MAIN DANGER SIGNALS

Danger signals are *warnings*. They are not a cause for panic. You don't go to pieces every time you see a sign saying "R.R. CROSSING!"

Every age and condition has its own special problems which I discuss fully in other chapters, such as those dealing with pregnancy and childbirth, mental health, first aid, sicknesses of childhood, "the killers," and so on. In this chapter, I discuss the *main general danger signals* with which everyone should be familiar.

### 1. Fever

Fever can be the signal of a serious disease or infection. Almost no one would hesitate to call the doctor when "burning up with a raging fever." But people are understandably reluctant to spend money or "bother the doctor" for the mild fever that often accompanies an uncomplicated cold or appears in some children (adults, too) when they are overexcited. In order to tell whether or not to send for the doctor, one must first *know*—not guess—whether a fever is severe or mild. Therefore you should know:

How—and When—to Use your Thermometer. There are two types of thermometers, rectal and mouth. With very young children it is usually safer to take the temperature by rectum than it is by mouth. Since rectal thermometers break less easily than mouth thermometers, it is a good idea to buy two rectal thermometers and keep one for mouth use, the other for rectal use. The temperature can also be taken in the armpit when a patient cannot, or will not, cooperate in having it taken by the usual oral or rectal method. See page 287 on how to take the axillary (armpit) temperature.

Before you take the temperature, shake the thermometer to bring down the mercury in it. Clinical thermometers, unlike those used to record the temperature of the air, don't go down by themselves; since they are "one-way" affairs, they must be shaken down before being used. Hold the thermometer tight and shake with a quick snap of the wrist; shake it over a pillow or bed so if it slips out of your hand you won't have to buy a new one. Don't run hot water over it to wash it as that may make it crack; use soap and cold water, or alcohol.

On page 287 you will find directions for reading the thermometer. It should be kept in the mouth for from one to five minutes, depending on the type of instrument you are using. Three minutes is sufficient for the average thermometer.

It is relatively easy to read modern thermometers. A little practice turning it in the light will enable you to see where the mercury ends. You will notice a little red mark to indicate "normal." The mouth temperature of the *average* person is normally 98.6°, the rectal temperature 99.6°. Remember that the temperature when taken by rectum averages nearly a degree higher than when taken by mouth, so don't be disturbed if your infant or youngster has a rectal temperature as high as 100°. Be sure to tell your doctor whether you are reporting the rectal or mouth temperature. It is not essential for him to know the temperature to a tenth of a degree. He'll be satisfied if you tell him "the thermometer read nearly a hundred degrees at eight o'clock this morning, and two hours later it had gone to a little over a hundred and two degrees."

Take the temperature every few hours, not only when you or some member of your family "feel hot and feverish" but as long as there is fatigue, nausea, vomiting, headache, or loss of appetite—the signs that generally accompany a feverish condition. Remember that aspirin and the many medicines containing it can bring down the temperature for as long as four hours, and taking the temperature during that time may give too low a reading. Therefore, it is wisest to take the temperature *before* taking aspirin. Always tell your doctor what medicines have been given.

WHEN IS FEVER DANGEROUS? If the fever is slight —under 100° by mouth or 101° by rectum—and the only other symptom is nasal congestion, a slight cough, or a scratchy throat, you can afford to wait. But record the temperature every three hours and note the severity of the other symptoms. If they become definitely worse or if the temperature rises to 101° by mouth or 102° by rectum, then it is wise to notify your doctor.

Incidentally, I am more pessimistic about sore throats and colds than many other physicians are. True, only a small percentage will be followed by severe complications such as rheumatic fever, Bright's disease, or pneumonia. But who can predict which cold or sore throat will lead to trouble? I'm for treating sore throats which are accompanied by a high fever with penicillin or other effective antibiotics at the very onset to kill any streptococci or pneumococci.

Many doctors see no justification for such caution, pointing out that even medical research workers disagree on this. Some oppose giving antibiotics on the grounds that a patient could develop a sensitivity reaction. Your own physician may be on the opposite side from me. And it may be years before the question is settled.

Meanwhile I plan to keep on going my cau-
tious way. Don't you look both ways every time you cross the street? Why? Because you know there is a slight but calculable possibility that you may be hit by a reckless driver. That is the way I feel about those streptococcal germs.

One more note of caution about the common cold and even the slightest fever: people with chronic illnesses such as rheumatic heart disease, nephritis, asthma, diabetes, or anemia should call the doctor the moment a cold or fever develops —no matter how mild.

ALWAYS NOTE THE OTHER SYMPTOMS. Any fever accompanied by a severe chill or rash should warn you that medical help is needed. A stiff neck, even if accompanied by only a slight rise in temperature, may be the first warning of polio or meningitis. A fever following an infected cut or other injury might mean blood poisoning (septicemia). Any fever with nausea and abdominal pain, especially in the lower right portion of the abdomen, *may mean appendicitis.* Appendicitis develops rapidly. It can be treated effectively in its early stages but becomes a major problem if neglected for even a few hours. Taking a cathartic can be extremely dangerous. If you cannot find your own doctor or an acceptable substitute, go to the nearest good hospital.

## 2. Pain

Pain may be a warning signal. Unfortunately, not all illnesses announce themselves with the dramatic storm warning of fever; but a great many diseases cause pain. Kidney stones and gallstones produce an acute colic as they try to force their way through narrow tubes. Certain lung diseases are accompanied by pleurisy, the pain being at its worst when you take a deep breath. Heart disease may be accompanied by a clutching pain in the chest, especially under the breastbone—angina pectoris actually means "breast pang." Some heart attacks are also accompanied by sudden weakness, profuse perspiration, paleness, and shortness of breath.

Of course, all of us occasionally have headaches and other fleeting mild aches and pains. These rarely require medical advice unless they become chronic. But if you experience any new or unusually acute pain in the chest or abdomen, notify your doctor.

## 3. Loss of Weight

What about the illnesses not characterized by fever or pain? Diabetes is one. However, it may flash the danger signals of excessive thirst and loss of weight.

Anyone who loses weight on an adequate non-reducing diet is sick. If weight loss occurs without any decrease in appetite or change in diet, it indicates inadequate utilization of food, or that the food is being burned up too fast. The doctor usually suspects diabetes or an overactive thyroid gland.

An adult scarcely needs a scale to show up marked weight loss. If your well-fitted clothes suddenly become loose, you know you have lost a significant amount of weight. Children should be weighed as often as your pediatrician or family doctor recommends. If a child loses steadily or just fails to gain at the normal rate, mention it to your doctor.

## 4. Shortness of Breath

Another important symptom is shortness of breath. Perhaps you suddenly find that climbing stairs or similar exertion leaves you puffing. This may warn you that you have merely become too obese or are leading too sedentary a life. But it may also indicate the beginning of heart trouble, anemia, or other potentially serious illnesses.

## 5. Bleeding

Always be on the alert for unexplained bleeding. When it appears without obvious cause, bleeding is usually nature's warning of trouble somewhere. It may not always look like blood. Bowel movements, for example, can be colored as black as tar by bleeding from the stomach or the upper intestines. Blood can also impart various colors to the urine, ranging from a faint pink to a mahogany brown. Blood in the stools or urine should be reported to your doctor immediately.

Coughing or vomiting of blood is equally important. Do not postpone your visit to the doctor,

promising yourself you will see him if the bleeding appears again. Nature frequently gives only one warning.

The appearance of blood is a signal for action—but not despair. If you consult your doctor immediately he can very probably cure what is wrong. Cancer is not the only illness that causes unexplained bleeding. So do stomach ulcers, hemorrhoids, and several others. Only your doctor can make the correct diagnosis—if you are alert enough to provide him with the opportunity.

All women should realize the tremendous importance of unexpected vaginal bleeding between periods or after the menopause. It may be the result of the most harmless polyp, but it may also be caused by early curable cancer.

## 6. Other Warning Signals

A *cough* which lasts more than a few weeks requires attention. *Jaundice*—yellowing of the skin and the whites of the eyes—is always a danger signal. But don't confuse a characteristically sallow complexion with jaundice. Look at the whites of the eyes; if they are distinctly yellow, it is jaundice. A marked *change in the urine*—in its volume, color, or the number of times it must be passed—should make you suspect bladder or kidney trouble. I have already mentioned *excessive thirst*. Marked *weakness* or *fatigue* can also be signals.

The warnings for cancer are: persistent unexplained hoarseness, sores that do not heal, marked change in the size and shape of moles, continued indigestion with changes in bowel habits such as diarrhea or constipation, bleeding, and a lump or growth. Women have a special problem here because of the frequency of *cancer of the breast*. They should examine their breasts regularly for a lump or other change that might indicate a tumor.

If you have seldom been bothered by headaches and then develop a *severe, persistent headache*, the *possibility* of brain tumor should be checked. Seeing *rainbows* around lights may be an indication of glaucoma, and the earlier you seek medical help the more likely your eyesight will be saved. *Cramping* of the calves of the legs may sometimes be an early sign of *diabetes*, especially if you are susceptible to the disease (were born of diabetic parents, have a thyroid condition, are a woman over forty and overweight, have given birth to babies weighing over nine pounds, or have had repeated miscarriages). Early diagnosis can minimize the disease greatly.

There you have the more important warning signs to watch for. If you are alert to them all, you will never have your own ignorance to blame for a tragedy in your family. Of course, no set of rules can cover every situation. But I do believe this chapter will enable you to recognize most illnesses early, in their most curable stage. However—one more word of caution: cancer, tuberculosis, high blood pressure, and certain other serious medical conditions notoriously give few characteristic warning signals. The best way to protect yourself and your family against them is to have the periodic medical checkups I have advised.

And finally, do remember the one cardinal golden rule which your physician will respect day and night: *when in reasonable doubt ask the doctor.*

# 29

# YOUR PERSONAL HEALTH INVENTORY

The system I have advised for you will take care of the detection and prevention of many illnesses. By regularly scheduled medical checkups you can be sure of discovering most serious illnesses before they have gone too far. By learning the danger signals you will catch many diseases before they get under way.

Unfortunately, however, some diseases do appear between checkups and may advance quite seriously. That is why I recommend a *second line of defense* in your health program: *Your Personal Home Medical Checkup.* Combined with your regular visit to the doctor, a few minutes spent once every two months on this health inventory will be an additional safeguard for your health. It is convenient to make a note on your calendar to look at this chapter on the fifteenth day of every other month.

## CHECKING UP ON YOURSELF

If the answer to any of the following questions is "yes," you should see your doctor as soon as possible at his office. If you have a perfect score of "no," the chances are reasonably good that your health is satisfactory, and that you can wait *until your next scheduled periodic health examination* —but no longer—before seeing your doctor or visiting your hospital clinic.

1. Have I noticed a sore on the skin, lips or tongue, which doesn't seem to heal over?

2. Do I get short of breath when walking on level ground, or climbing stairs, or performing types of exertion which didn't bother me in this way previously?

3. Am I troubled with indigestion, nausea, loss of appetite, abdominal pain or cramps, or the recent sudden appearance of constipation or diarrhea?

4. Have I noticed blood in the bowel movements?

5. Am I steadily losing weight? Or am I steadily gaining weight? Is my weight under or over the average weight for my height and build, given on page 45?

6. Am I getting nervous, irritable, or depressed? Have I been having crying spells? Do I have a persistent feeling that people are against me? Do I feel a nervous breakdown coming on?

7. Do I feel run down? Do I have a new persistent pain or any other new symptoms?

8. Has my skin color changed? Do I have a pallor?

9. Have I a cough that has been lasting longer than one month? Have I coughed up blood?

10. Have I had persistent hoarseness?

11. Are my hearing and eyesight as good as they ever were?

12. Have I had any dimming or fogging of vision?

13. Have I had any persistent headaches?

14. Have I felt any discomfort in my chest without obvious cause?

15. Have I noticed swelling of my feet or ankles or both?

16. Have I had any prolonged aches in my back or limbs or joints?

## SPECIAL QUESTIONS FOR WOMEN

17. Have I a noticed vaginal bleeding at unexpected times?
18. Am I troubled with hot flashes?
19. Have I felt a lump in my breast or have I been worried about cancer or tumors there or in any other part of the body?*

## SPECIAL QUESTIONS FOR MEN

20. Has my urination been abnormal recently (difficulty in starting or stopping, any dribbling, etc.)?

21. Am I ruptured, or do I think I may be?
22. Do I believe I may have contracted some illness overseas during the war?
23. Am I worried about having a venereal disease?

## IMPORTANT NOTE

These symptoms can be caused by serious, treatable diseases, BUT they can also arise from other mild conditions. As an example—shortness of breath can be caused by heart trouble or by overweight. *Let your doctor make the diagnosis for you.*

---

* I suggest that every woman reader of this book read page 433 about how to examine the breasts for cancer without becoming a victim of worry or fear.

## 30
# YOUR HOSPITAL

This chapter contains the following two sections: 1. Today's Hospitals—a description of various types of hospitals, and a guide to finding a good one. 2. When You Go to the Hospital—an explanation of what to expect when you enter a hospital as a patient.

## TODAY'S HOSPITALS

You probably have some idea of the many different kinds of hospitals there are in existence—from small ones resembling private homes and accommodating only a few patients, to tremendous, imposing structures that look as though they house an entire city. You know about hospitals that specialize in certain types of cases, and others that accept all kinds of patients.

Every hospital, however, falls into one of two groups: those that are *accredited* and those that are not. *This is the one thing you must know before you select your hospital!*

### Why Your Hospital Should Be Accredited

An accredited hospital is one which has been approved by the Joint Commission on Accreditation of Hospitals. Accreditation means that the hospital has met the following standards:

1. The physicians and surgeons are organized as a medical staff, and membership on that staff is restricted to physicians and surgeons who are graduates of American Medical Association—approved medical schools, and who are legally licensed to practice in their respective states.

2. The doctors are competent in their respective fields.

3. The medical staff has adopted rules, regulations, and policies to govern the professional workers in the hospital, and the staff meets at least once a month.

4. Members of the medical staff review and analyze their clinical experience at regular intervals.

5. A medical records department writes and keeps records on all patients.

6. Diagnostic and therapeutic facilities such as a clinical laboratory and an x-ray department, with skilled men directing them, are available in the hospital.

7. Tissue taken from a patient during surgery is checked by a pathologist to determine whether the preoperative diagnosis is confirmed by the tissue findings, and if an error was made and healthy tissue was removed without cause, the surgeon must explain his action to a tissue committee. If violations are flagrant, he may be barred from further practice at the hospital.

8. Where an operation may represent an unusual hazard to life, at least two physicians must be present, one who performs the operation and a second designated as qualified to assist.

9. Since a hospital houses patients with varied problems, infection is an ever-present possibility, and an accredited hospital must

provide a mechanism for investigating infections and finding ways to control and prevent them.

10. The hospital must be of fire-resistant construction and must use equipment as close to fireproof as possible.

An accredited hospital guards its reputation. As I mentioned in Chapter 26, it will seek out doctors of real ability for appointment to its staff. It will not permit members of its staff to perform operations for which they are not qualified. You will not find a "ghost surgeon" in an accredited hospital. (A "ghost surgeon" operates secretly and splits the fee with another physician who pretends he himself performed the operation rather than admit to the patient that there are certain major surgical procedures he cannot undertake. Of course, this reprehensible practice is forbidden by the American Medical Association.) In an accredited hospital there is no misrepresentation. The people who care for you there may not be perfect, but you can be sure they meet established standards.

Surely these things are more important to you than the fact that a nonaccredited hospital has a beautiful building or serves fancy meals! So *find out first whether or not a hospital is accredited.* I have already suggested that you ask your doctor which hospital he would send you to, and whether it is accredited. *Your doctor, or your county medical society, will give you this information.* Or send a card of inquiry to the Joint Commission on Accreditation of Hospitals, 200 East Ohio Street, Chicago, Illinois 60611. If there is no accredited hospital in your community, you will probably find one nearby; and it is well worth taking a trip to avoid taking a risk.

It is barely possible that you may have to go to a hospital that is not accredited—if there is no other place available in an emergency, or if, for example, your doctor, in whom you have confidence, assures you that the hospital has applied for accreditation and he is certain it will be granted.

## Types of Hospitals

Among the many types of hospitals in existence are *special hospitals,* which handle only particular types of illnesses, and *general hospitals,* which are organized to take care of a great variety of illnesses.

Some of the special institutions are for tuberculosis, mental illness, convalescence, orthopedics, pediatrics, maternity, and eye, ear, nose, and throat. Most people, however, are concerned with the general hospital, which has become increasingly important in recent years because it has incorporated many of the services of the special hospitals.

Another modern plan, usually found in large cities, is the *medical center,* in which specialized hospitals are grouped within the space of one or two blocks about a main general hospital.

Hospitals are financed in different ways. A small number of them are owned by private coporations, partnerships, or individuals, and are run to benefit their owners. These are *proprietary* hospitals and are often not so well equipped or staffed as other hospitals. *Government* hospitals, such as the veterans' hospitals, are built and manned and completely financed by the federal government. Many large city hospitals are supported by the municipal or county government or both; these are called *city* or *county* hospitals. Some hospitals are run by private nonprofit corporations organized for charitable purposes. These institutions are usually partially supported by endowments and gifts, and partially by community and government funds, and are called *voluntary* hospitals. Church-affiliated hospitals belong to this group.

## Functions of the Modern Hospital

Modern hospitals have many functions, in addition to being institutions to care for the sick. They are educational institutions. They provide positive preventive medical care programs for their patients as well as for the general public—instruction in ways to avoid repetition of illnesses and in ways to live with chronic ones such as diabetes, hypertension, and the like. They also help train doctors and nurses for the important job of diagnosing and treating the sick. Doctors in a hospital aid each other by exchanging the results of their research and treatment and by consulting one another about difficult cases.

## Medical Centers and Famous Clinics

I was frequently asked by patients in Boston, one of the greatest cities in the world for medical knowledge and skill, "Should I go to the Mayo Clinic for my operation?" Yet Boston has a number of medical centers and hospitals in which surgery can be obtained equal to that provided by the Mayo Clinic. Many people have heard of the Mayos, although they do not know the name of the equally excellent clinic in their own community. This is due to the fact that the Mayo brothers were pioneers, as was Dr. George Crile, who established what is now called the Cleveland Clinic, and Dr. Frank Lahey of the Lahey Clinic in Boston.

A generation or two ago, only the largest cities in this country were able to provide major surgery with adequate safety and skill. If a small city did possess a well-trained surgeon, it was apt to lack a good hospital with sufficient laboratory equipment and a competent pathologist; therefore the surgeon could not offer his patient the best possible care. The Mayo brothers established a clinic in Rochester, Minnesota, which had good diagnosticians, surgeons, and laboratories, providing everything required to guarantee good work. That was a forward step in those days, especially for the newer parts of our country.

Today, however, dozens of American cities have outstanding medical schools and centers, and hundreds have hospitals in which excellent major surgery is performed. The famous clinics have, in the main, become a part of the medical centers, and thus continue to play a vital role in the health program of the nation, especially in certain fields of medicine. For example, few cities with a population of less than 500,000 have adequate facilities for brain surgery. Diagnoses on the brain and spinal cord, which require highly complicated apparatus, can best be made at a medical center, as can diagnoses of many obscure diseases.

The medical centers *usually* offer superior medical care for the following types of surgery:

Surgery of the eye, especially cataract operations

Plastic surgery, e.g., repair of cleft palates in children

Surgery of the heart

Major surgery of the lungs, e.g., removal of parts of lungs or a whole lung for tumor or infections

Special orthopedic operations for correction of deformities of polio, arthritis, and other illnesses.

Patients in medical centers are usually referred there from smaller communities or from other hospitals. Such referrals are becoming more frequent because these large centers can best handle medical diagnosis which requires radioactive substances. In addition, the trained specialists at these medical centers are better equipped to direct the x-ray, radium, and other types of radioactive treatment for tumors, cancers, and other such conditions.

## The Important Medical Centers

Most of the leading medical centers are located in connection with a leading medical school. Many of the medical schools listed on page 373 have one or more medical centers connected with them. For example, there are the Johns Hopkins Hospital and Medical School in Baltimore, the Massachusetts General Hospital which is associated with the Harvard Medical School in Boston, and Billings Hospital and the University of Chicago Medical School in Chicago. The Mayo Clinic is now a nonprofit foundation connected with the University of Minnesota Medical School.

The famous medical school of Columbia University, The College of Physicians and Surgeons, is the focal point of a very large medical center, which many of you may have seen with its tall buildings near the Hudson River at West 168th Street in New York City. A large general hospital, the Presbyterian Hospital, is an important part of the Center, and is linked very closely, even physically, with the medical school. Other principal units are these: The Babies' Hospital (pediatrics); Sloane Hospital for Women (obstetrics and gynecology); The Squier Urological Clinic (diseases of the kidneys, prostate, bladder, etc.); The Institute of Ophthalmology (diseases of the eye); The Neurological Institute (organic diseases of the brain and nerves); The New York State Psychiatric Institute; and The New York City Delafield Cancer Hospital.

## What About Hospital Care in Rural Areas?

Unfortunately everyone in the United States does not have equal access to the valuable services of modern hospitals. People who live in rural areas are often handicapped by the inaccessibility of hospitals. Sometimes hospitals are constructed at central points in these areas in order to meet their needs; too often, however, these hospitals cannot be adequately financed or else fail to get the necessary equipment or the better doctors required to do a top job. Thus, people in rural communities often must travel to the larger cities when they are in real need of hospitalization. The problem has been somewhat alleviated by the system of sending traveling units of doctors and equipment to serve the outlying hospitals once or twice a week. Nevertheless, the major problem—how to serve the rural population effectively—still remains.

## Costs of Hospital Care

Modern hospital care is extremely expensive, and the charges vary with the kind and amount of service rendered. *Private* rooms house only one person and are therefore the most expensive accommodations; *semiprivate* facilities have beds for two to four patients in a room, and are less expensive than private rooms; *wards* take care of five or more patients, and are the least expensive.

"Patient care" is a basic charge each hospital patient must pay for room, meals, and nursing care. In addition to this, the hospital may charge extra for the use of the operating room and equipment, anesthesia materials, blood, laboratory examinations, x-ray examinations, and treatment.

There are usually three ways a patient may pay for hospital care: (1) out of his current income, (2) by a pre- or part-paid insurance plan, or (3) as a public charge in which case the government pays the bill. The expense of hospital care can best be met by adequate insurance. (See page 407 for a discussion of the Blue Cross Plan and other methods of insurance against hospital bills.)

Patients who enter on the public ward of the hospital usually cannot be treated by their own private doctors, but are placed under the care of hospital staff physicians. However, in almost every hospital the family doctor is given full reports of the diagnosis and treatment. The quality of care a patient gets on the ward depends, of course, entirely on the standards of the hospital. If the hospital's standards of medical care are high, as they are in most nonprofit hospitals, the younger physicians on the ward will be carefully supervised by experienced doctors.

If there is a choice of accredited hospitals for you to select from, your doctor will take these matters into consideration when recommending a specific one to you. Be influenced by his suggestion. Most doctors would rather work at one hospital than at another. At his own favorite hospital the doctor—or surgeon, or obstetrician—does better work because he has had more experience with the assistants and nurses who team up with him.

## Special Hospital Care

For information about what to do if you plan to travel in a foreign country see page 162. If you are a veteran or a member of the Armed Forces, be sure to learn what benefits and hospital services you may secure. Here are some medical services offered by the Veterans' Administration:

*Hospitalization* in a VA hospital or approved nursing home, with priority going to the following cases, if the hospital should be crowded: emergencies; injuries or diseases incurred or aggravated in line of duty during wartime services; nonservice-connected conditions if the veteran is unable to pay hospital charges elsewhere.

*Transportation* to and from the hospital, under circumstances similar to those listed above.

*Outpatient medical treatment* for veterans with service-connected illnesses or disabilities, in VA hospitals or clinics, or from approved private physicians.

Necessary *medicines,* either through the hospital or clinic, or from local druggists if treated by an approved private physician.

## WHEN YOU GO TO THE HOSPITAL

One out of every seven people in the United States will go to a hospital this year. Don't be alarmed at the possibility that you may be one of them. Today's hospital is not just a place for someone who is seriously ill or requires a major operation; the one-in-seven group includes maternity cases, people who are having their tonsils removed, and cases admitted for observation or special diagnostic tests.

Some people fear hospitals because their parents did, or because of stories that have been handed down to them. Although there was justification for being afraid of hospitals in the old days, there is no resemblance between the modern hospital and the "pesthouse" of the past. The tremendous progress of medical science is nowhere exhibited to a greater degree than it is in the change that has taken place in hospitals. For example: one hundred years ago (even less, in many places) doctors did not know that germs had anything to do with diseases or wound infections, and consequently they didn't even wash their hands before performing an operation or delivering a baby. The very idea of *trained* nurses was so new that few people had even heard of it; the first nurses' training school in the United States was established in 1872. Once, hospitals were primarily for people who were too poor to be cared for in their homes; but now no one is too wealthy to go to a hospital.

Hospitalizing children and old people presents some special problems which I discuss on page 349.

Let us assume that you are going to the hospital for special diagnostic tests, that you have had symptoms of hyperthyroidism, but your doctor cannot be sure of this diagnosis without making use of the equipment and facilities the hospital affords.

## How a Patient Is Admitted to the Hospital

Your physician calls the hospital with which he is affiliated and arranges for you to stay there, telling the hospital officials the time of arrival and the type of accommodations you will want. (As I mentioned previously, it is important to choose a doctor who has access to the facilities of an accredited hospital, because hospital staffs are so arranged that a doctor cannot treat you there unless he belongs to the staff of that particular hospital.)

You arrive at the appointed time with a few personal effects such as pajamas, slippers, robe, and toilet articles. The receptionist at the desk greets you, and asks your name and the name of your doctor. Then she leads or directs you to the admitting office. Here the admitting officer, if she thinks you are well enough, takes time to tell you the hospital rules and to ask you a few questions so she may complete her hospital records. She will also discuss your plans for paying the hospital bill. After that she will call a student nurse or an orderly to take you to your room or ward, and will also notify the switchboard and the information desk and the attending hospital physician that *you* have arrived.

You may have seen nurses in different kinds of uniforms. You may see *probationers* who are in the early months of their training and who perform routine hospital tasks as part of their preparation for becoming nurses. After passing an examination a probationer becomes a *student nurse* for the remainder of her course, which usually takes three years. After graduating she becomes a *trained nurse* or *graduate nurse*, and after she passes a state examination she becomes a *registered nurse*, or "R.N." Many nurses take special courses in addition to those that are required, in order to fit themselves for nursing specialties.

## Hospital Life and Activities

The supervising nurse on your floor greets you and helps you change into hospital bed clothing. Probably your own doctor will be responsible for your care; if so, he has left detailed instructions concerning the examinations and tests you will need.

First on your schedule is *hospital routine*. The attending nurse checks your weight, temperature, pulse, and respiration, and records them on your bed chart. She also orders your diet, according to your doctor's instructions.

A nurse will answer your call if there is anything you need, and a circulating library service is usually at your disposal if you feel like reading. (In many hospitals, attendants distribute games to children, or may even have story hours for them.) You can probably have a radio in your room, and television sets are available for rent in most hospitals. Under-the-pillow receivers are available so that you will not disturb any other patients in your room.

The hospital, you soon discover, is a busy place. From the managing board to the janitors, the hospital crew is working around the clock. Here is what goes on behind the scenes:

## The Staff Doctors Assist Your Doctor

Staff physicians and young doctors rounding out their medical education are continually making rounds of the wards, observing changes in the condition of the various patients and administering prescribed treatments to them.

Do not assume that every young doctor who lives in the hospital is an intern. Today, in the larger hospitals, doctors frequently spend three to five years in training after they are graduated from medical school. For one or perhaps two years they are called interns; then they become assistant resident doctors, and finally in their third, fourth, or fifth years, chief or senior resident physicians. The chief resident has had seven to nine years of training from the time he entered medical school; that is why your own doctor has great confidence in him. If it becomes necessary, the chief resident will always call the family doctor to the hospital outside of his regular hours there.

Most doctors visit their hospital patients once or twice each day. Naturally, your doctor keeps these visits on a regular timetable so that he can meet his office appointments and his schedule of home calls. Do not expect him to spend more time with you than is necessary, or ask him to see you outside his regular visits unless there is a real emergency that cannot be handled by the staff doctors.

## Other Staff Members

Not far from patient rooms are the clinical and pathology laboratories where trained people are helping to diagnose ailments by performing the proper tests on patient specimens. Here a *pathologist* and his staff of technicians use modern scientific instruments and chemicals that enable them to determine patient progress, to diagnose disease, and to discover new means of combating disease.

In these laboratories, with the aid of radioactive iodine and other tests, your doctor will obtain valuable help in determining whether you are really suffering from hyperthyroidism (our hypothetical diagnosis).

The hospital may also have a department for *physical* and *occupational therapy*. The directors of this department will have been graduated from physical or occupational therapy schools approved by the Council on Medical Education and Hospitals of the American Medical Association. Physical therapists render massage treatment and the like to persons crippled or suffering physical defects or ailments. Occupational therapists train disabled persons for new skills and jobs that are compatible with their disabilities; occupational therapy also includes crafts and other work to help patient morale.

In another part of the hospital are the *dietitians*. They prepare nutritious meals and at the same time consider the needs of individual patients.

In another department licensed *pharmacists* are filling prescriptions for the drugs and medicines staff physicians will use to treat patients.

The x-ray department is another busy section of the hospital. Here a physician, specializing in this type of work (a *radiologist*), is taking x-rays and reading them for diagnosis. He may also give x-ray treatment for many types of disease.

If your hospital is a large and modern one, it will probably also have a dental clinic. Here there are *dentists* to take care of emergency dental trouble and make oral examinations of entering patients.

A vital part of the hospital is the *blood bank*. Here many pints of blood are stored, ready for those who may need it—accident victims, patients undergoing operation, or those suffering from such diseases as leukemia (see page 431) and other conditions which require blood transfusions.

Large quantities of *medical equipment* such as oxygen tents, portable mechanical "lungs," and infant incubators are kept in the hospital for anyone who might need them.

The hospital is a closely integrated unit. Unseen workers such as housekeepers, carpenters, engineers, electricians, plumbers, bookkeepers, and secretaries perform the necessary duties that maintain the hospital.

## The Outpatient Department

We have not yet mentioned a vital part of the behind-the-scene ways your hospital serves you, the patient. You may not see it this visit; you may never see it at all; but it is there, and many people come into contact with it every day. This is the *outpatient department,* the part of the hospital giving medical care to ambulatory patients, and often offering help and guidance to patients who have been dismissed from the hospital.

Doctors in the outpatient department treat accident and emergency cases which come in during all hours of the day and night; in addition they diagnose and treat almost every type of disease which entering patients may have. The outpatient department is often arranged according to the specialties of medicine, with divisions for heart disease, cancer, and other illnesses, as well as for prenatal, baby, and child care. In these clinics patients can secure the valuable services of specialists they probably could not afford in private practice.

People use the outpatient clinics not only when they cannot afford a doctor in private practice, but also as an addition to the medical care they are obtaining from a private physician.

Patients entering here first have a preliminary examination in which trained men diagnose their ailments and, if necessary, send them to the specialists they may need for treatment.

Some patients go directly to the specialists, when they are referred by their own family doctor. Treatment in these clinics is by appointment.

It is important to realize that there is no stigma attached to using a hospital clinic. It doesn't imply that you are penniless or unable to pay for part of your medical care. The diagnostic techniques required in some illnesses have become so technical, or the treatment so specialized and extensive, that hardly any but a very well-to-do person can be expected to assume the entire cost.

The outpatient department may also sponsor educational programs to teach the public preventive medicine.

## Social Service

Another special part of the hospital is the *medical social-service* department. Here patients are helped to solve their personal problems, such as home conflicts that interfere with recovery, or worries regarding convalescent care and treatment, or the fear of being unable to secure a job after discharge from the hospital. Medical social-service workers are concerned with restoring the patient to a functional place in the community after he leaves the hospital.

## The Hospital Director

All the many activities of the hospital are coordinated by the director. In some hospitals he is called the supervisor or manager, and some Catholic hospitals are supervised by a nun who is called the administrator.

If you have any questions about hospital charges, if you want to know about insurance company charges or about Blue Cross, Blue Shield, or Medicare payments, the director's office will help you.

If you have complaints about the care you receive, first bring them to the attention of your doctor or the head nurse in charge of your floor. Then if you feel further discussion is warranted, request an interview with someone in the director's office.

## The Hospital Ombudsman: Patient's Friend

A common criticism about hospitals, particularly large ones, is that they seem indifferent to patients' individual personal problems. Now, in many hospitals, if you have a complaint, you can get someone to listen—someone, in fact, appointed for the specific purpose of hearing complaints and adjusting them whenever possible. That person may be called an ombudsman or patient representative, and may be either a man or woman, sometimes an experienced former nurse, with broad understanding of hospital procedures and with authority to investigate and when necessary to do something about a patient's complaints.

Some complaints stem from misunderstandings. A patient, unfamiliar with hospital activities, may not realize that a nurse who seems brusque and has no time to chat may have a dozen more blood pressures or temperatures to take within a specified period.

But some complaints—about doctors, nurses, or other hospital personnel—are justified. Hospital personnel may sometimes forget how upset a patient is by his illness, worries about his work, his children, his bills. He needs someone to listen and explain things to him. Often a complaint can be resolved by a representative's chat with nurses or doctors.

Whether or not there is a patient representative, you have the right—and, in fact, even a duty—to report any incompetence to the nursing supervisor, hospital administrator, or your physician.

It's important to understand a basic fact: that if a nurse or someone else in the hospital seems unobliging, it often is because of restrictions put upon them by your physician's instructions. A nurse, for example, can't accommodate with an unauthorized sleeping pill or an addition to a restricted diet. You have to take up such matters with your physician.

## A "Patient's Bill of Rights"

In 1973, the American Hospital Association issued a twelve-point Bill of Rights for patients and urged hospitals to distribute copies to incoming patients. The rights are really reaffirmations of long-established principles known to health professionals but not to many patients.

Knowing about these rights may be of great value to you.

As a patient, you have the right:

1. To considerate and respectful care.
2. To obtain from the physician complete current information about diagnosis, treatment, and prognosis, in terms you can understand.
3. To obtain from the physician information necessary for informed consent before any procedure or treatment is begun; to information on significant alternatives; and to know the name of the person responsible for the treatment.
4. To refuse treatment to the extent permitted by law and to be informed of the medical consequences of refusal.
5. To every consideration of your privacy concerning your own medical care; persons not directly involved in your care must have your permission to be present at case discussion, consultation, examination, and treatment.
6. To confidentiality of all communications and records pertaining to you.
7. To expect that within its capacity a hospital make a reasonable response to your request for service and not transfer you to another institution except after you have been given reasons why.
8. To obtain information concerning any relationship of your hospital to other health services so far as your care is concerned, and concerning the existence of any professional relationships among individuals who are treating you.
9. To be advised if the hospital proposes to engage in human experimentation affecting your care and to refuse to participate in such research.
10. To reasonable continuity of care, including postdischarge follow-up.
11. To examine and receive an explanation of your bill no matter who pays it.
12. To know what hospital rules and regulations apply to your conduct as a patient.

## If You Need Surgery

Let us assume that three days have passed and the hospital tests have substantiated your doctor's suspicions that you have hyperthyroidism. Your doctor feels your type of overactive thyroid gland can best be treated by surgical removal of most of this enlarged gland. He explains why he believes surgical treatment is better in this case than medical treatment, and suggests that you be examined by a surgeon who has had considerable experience with operations on the thyroid gland.

If you like the surgeon he suggests, and the surgeon also confirms the diagnosis, your doctor will arrange for your operation. (See Chapter 31 on surgical operations.)

After you have recovered sufficiently from your operation, your doctor will arrange for you to leave the hospital, possibly to a *convalescent home* for a week or two before returning to your home. Such a place should be licensed, which means it is inspected and fulfills medical and nursing requirements as well as those regarding fire hazards, cleanliness, adequate meals, and so on. The board of health can help you and your doctor answer questions about convalescent or nursing homes.

Even if you have seen only part of the hospital and its amazing departments, you will still leave knowing that it is a place where modern facilities and well-trained people take good care of the sick.

I must confess I have described the best type of hospital. Unfortunately there are a number of hospitals in which the medical standards are high but the spirit of humanity seems to be lacking. I have crusaded for a better appreciation of the needs of the patients in hospitals, as have other doctors and writers in recent years. From my own observations and from letters I have received from readers throughout the country, I find that most hospitals are becoming far more understanding toward the personal needs of their patients.

# 31
# WHAT YOU NEED TO KNOW ABOUT SURGICAL OPERATIONS

What happens when someone needs an operation? Let us assume that after the completion of the tests during the hospital stay described in the last chapter, the doctor decided that an operation was necessary to remove most of the enlarged thyroid gland. He would proceed to explain the pros and cons of medical versus surgical treatment for hyperthyroidism, giving his reasons for suggesting the latter. Then he would probably arrange for an examination by a surgeon who had had considerable experience with operations on the thyroid gland. The family doctor would explain that he himself would not attempt such an operation since he was a general practitioner who had chosen to limit his practice almost entirely to diagnosis and treatment of medical conditions. (See page 372 for discussion of operations by a general practitioner versus a specialist.)

Assume that the surgeon agrees with the family doctor's diagnosis and recommends an operation. It is agreed by all concerned that the operation be performed as soon as the necessary preparations are made.

## PREPARATION FOR A SURGICAL OPERATION

Before an operation is undertaken the patient is carefully examined to make certain he is in sufficiently good condition to undergo it. X-rays will be taken and other tests made after he has gone to the hospital, to be certain he does not have tuberculosis, diabetes, nephritis, or some other serious illnesses. How good the patient's health should be varies with the type of operation he is facing. Modern surgical methods have made it possible to operate successfully on many patients who are not in good health, but such a procedure is undertaken only when it will subject the patient to less serious risks than those involved in failing to operate. The doctor carefully weighs all the factors.

In addition to the tests already mentioned, blood tests would be made to make certain the patient's blood clots normally and to determine his blood type in case he should need a transfusion. A nurse or attendant shaves and thoroughly washes the part of the body to be operated upon; and, after a good night's sleep, the patient is ready for surgery.

By this time the doctor has undoubtedly explained precisely what he plans to accomplish by the operation. He should be willing to discuss any danger that might be involved, and how he hopes to avoid it. No good surgeon will oversell himself or the operation. You, the patient, should ask anything you want to know about the operation at least a day before it is scheduled, as the chances are you won't see the surgeon on that day. Don't be alarmed if you don't see him; he will be busy with preparations while you are being taken to the operating floor of the hospital. Usually the anesthetist and your own family doctor will be present and will tell you how to make the experience of taking an anesthetic an easy one—by not fighting against it, for example, so that before you know it you are breathing deeply, and sleep has come.

There are three types of drugs that may be used before surgery. Sedatives, such as a barbiturate, may be given to help you relax and rest. A good night's sleep prior to surgery is helpful and a sedative may help you sleep well despite normal anxiety about the operation.

Another type of agent that may be used is a drug such as atropine or scopolamine to decrease mucus secretion in the mouth and throat.

A little before you go up to surgery, you may receive a drug such as morphine or Demerol or a tranquilizer to help promote relaxation and also enhance the effects of the anesthetic.

Usually, it's possible to let you know the day before surgery the exact time at which it will be done. Depending upon a particular hospital's rules, your family may or may not be able to see you off to the operating room. In most hospitals, there is a waiting room not far from the operating suite, and as soon as the operation is finished, your family may meet the surgeon and talk with him there.

## ANESTHETICS

The operation will be painless because of anesthetics—drugs that induce sleep or otherwise cause loss of feeling. In the little more than the century since the discovery of ether, anesthesia has become a complex science requiring highly specialized knowledge. Leading medical schools now have departments of anesthesia, with well-trained specialists in charge, and there are many anesthetics to choose from, some affecting the whole body (general) and some only part of it (local).

### General Anesthetics

These put the patient to sleep. *Ether,* which is administered through a cone or mask, is a general anesthetic, and causes the patient to sleep throughout even a long operation. *Nitrous oxide* ("laughing gas"), which is also inhaled, is sometimes given for short procedures or before the patient is given ether, since it induces sleep more pleasantly. Although *chloroform,* once used as a general anesthetic, is now considered dangerous because it may damage the liver, a relative and a safe inhalant is *halothane.* This related anesthetic is used with special caution, because in certain cases it also may cause liver damage. Several other commonly used inhalants produce light or deep sleep—*ethylene* is one of the lighter anesthetics.

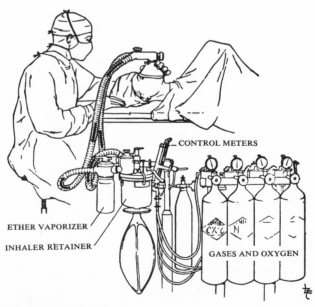

CONTROL METERS

ETHER VAPORIZER

INHALER RETAINER

GASES AND OXYGEN

*Figure 31-1. General Anesthesia (Ether, Gas).*

*Cyclopropane* is another of the inhalation anesthetics.

## Intravenous Anesthetics

Drugs that can be dripped into a vein in the arm or leg at a controlled rate to induce sleep very quickly, often within seconds, are in increasing use. They include pentothal, which is often used, too, in dental surgery.

For some short, relatively minor operations, an intravenous anesthetic may be the only one needed. Intravenous anesthetics are often used as an aid in regional or local anesthesia, permitting a light sleep while pain is prevented by the regional or local agent. Sometimes, in what is called *balanced anesthesia,* an intravenous agent may be combined with a spinal or local as well as a gas.

## Spinal Anesthesia

This can be used to completely anesthetize a specific part of the body. A needle is inserted between the vertebrae in the back, and regulated doses of an anesthetic such as Novocain are injected into the spinal fluid. The injection may be administered high in the back for surgery on upper or midabdominal organs, lower down for lower abdominal organs.

With spinal anesthesia, the patient, no longer sensitive to pain at the operative site, can remain fully conscious. There is a side effect—headache that may persist for several days to a week or more—in about 5 percent of patients receiving spinal anesthesia.

When a patient prefers not to remain conscious, he can be put to sleep during spinal anesthesia (or any of the other regional or local methods) by injection of a barbiturate into a vein.

## Epidural and Caudal Anesthesia

Somewhat like spinal anesthesia, these are variations in which the anesthetic agent is injected outside the spinal canal. More of the drug is needed and it takes somewhat longer for full effect to be obtained, but epidural and caudal methods avoid the possibility of later headache.

## Regional (local) Anesthesia

Much as a dentist can inject an agent such as Novocain to deaden pain in a specific area when a tooth is to be extracted or extensive drilling done, so the anesthesiologist can inject an anesthetic at a specific site, temporarily blocking or deadening specific nerves that carry pain impulses from that site. The neck, the side of the face, a hand or an arm, for example, can be anesthetized when surgery is to be confined to the area. With such regional or localized anesthesia, there is no effect on heart, lungs, and general condition, which may be especially valuable for high-risk patients.

## Topical Anesthesia

Painting or spraying an anesthetic on mucous membranes is useful for some procedures, particularly those involving eye, nose, and throat. Topical anesthesia in some cases may be used to produce superficial deadening of pain and may then be followed by injection of a local anesthetic.

*Figure 31-2. Spinal Anesthesia.*

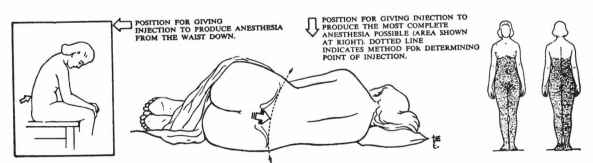

POSITION FOR GIVING INJECTION TO PRODUCE ANESTHESIA FROM THE WAIST DOWN.

POSITION FOR GIVING INJECTION TO PRODUCE THE MOST COMPLETE ANESTHESIA POSSIBLE (AREA SHOWN AT RIGHT). DOTTED LINE INDICATES METHOD FOR DETERMINING POINT OF INJECTION.

## Choosing the Type of Anesthetic

As you see, there are numerous methods of anesthesia, and often there is a choice of suitable methods for a particular operation.

For tonsil removal, for example, either a general or local may be used. For major breast surgery, a general is often employed, but for a minor breast procedure either a local or general may be used. For abdominal surgery, a general or spinal may be employed. For prostate, bladder, and kidney operations, spinal, epidural, or general may be used.

It is the surgeon's responsibility to select, often in consultation with the anesthesiologist, a good anesthetic. The better hospitals all have good departments of anesthesia.

I advise patients to leave the choice of an anesthetic to the surgeon. However, if he says that he can do an equally good job with either a spinal or a general, you might ask your family doctor to help you make the decision. He should know your particular personality better than the surgeon. (This is very likely your first acquaintance with the surgeon.)

As I look back on my choices when I have been operated upon, I wish that I had always selected "going to sleep" when there was an equal choice between a general and a local or spinal. Local anesthesia does not always render the operative site 100 percent free from all types of pain sensation during the entire course of the operation. On the other hand, some people who have tried both prefer a certain amount of discomfort to losing consciousness.

## STERILIZATION AND ASEPSIS

While you have been sleeping, the surgeon has scrubbed his hands for a full ten minutes to rid them of dirt and germs, perhaps also using an antiseptic solution. The surgeon is meticulous about washing his hands because the gloves might break or might already have an invisible hole through which germs could enter the operative area.

The surgeon and his whole team aim to prevent any germs from entering the part of the body on which the operation is performed. Everything that touches the operative area is sterilized. Every doctor and nurse who assists goes through the same routine of scrubbing and putting on sterile clothes. All the instruments have been freed of germs by treatment with heat or chemicals. Each person in the operating room wears a cap over the hair and a mask over the mouth and nose to prevent germs from entering the air.

Before the surgeon incises the skin, he sponges it carefully with disinfectant such as iodine, alcohol, or other powerful germ killers. Then he takes his position at the operating table along with his assistants and prepares the operative field.

## THE OPERATION

The surgeon or an assistant covers the body with sterile sheets. He encircles the area upon which he will work with towels and special cloths. When he is ready to begin, only the operating area is exposed.

The surgeon cuts the skin with a special type of knife called a scalpel. He pulls back the edges of the skin with retractors. Then he methodically works to the area where he will find the thyroid gland or whatever structure he is working on. If there is bleeding as he cuts through the tissues, he clamps off the bleeding vessels with special forceps called hemostats.

The next stage in the procedure will depend on the type of operation he is performing. For example, he may remove the appendix, a tumor, or part of a gland; or he may repair a hernia, a perforated intestine, or a severed blood vessel. In any event he will work deftly, handling the tissues and organs as little and as gently as possible to avoid bruising them or shocking the patient. Even though the case may be a simple one—a clear-cut case of appendicitis, for which he has operated countless times—he is always on the alert. There *could* be something different about this patient; he *could* be suffering from something in addition to appendicitis. The surgeon concentrates upon the specific task he is performing, yet he never forgets the general condition of the patient.

## THE OPERATING TEAM

Of course, the surgeon is not working alone. An operation involves the teamwork of several highly skilled people. The chief surgeon has the big job of planning the incision, opening the operative area, finding the trouble, and repairing it. In an extensive operation the surgeon may be assisted by an experienced doctor (perhaps the head resident physician in surgery). The surgeon may need other doctors to help with various maneuvers during the operation and to keep the opening the right size with retractors. There is the anesthetist to administer anesthesia, and usually two nurses to hand instruments to the surgeon and perform the other incidental jobs necessary in an operation.

In many good operating teams the assistants and nurses are so attuned to the chief surgeon's needs that he hardly has to ask for an instrument. They frequently anticipate his requests and have the proper needle, clamp, or other instruments ready for him.

## COMPLETION OF AN OPERATION

When the surgeon has completed his job, he ties or cauterizes bleeding vessels. He uses several different types of thread and catgut sutures for these procedures. He wants to make certain there will be no bleeding after the operation. This is tremendously important in internal operations involving the cutting of large arteries. For example, the removal of a kidney necessitates the severance of the main renal artery. If this vessel were to open and start bleeding after the operation, a serious internal hemorrhage would develop that could threaten the life of the patient. Surgeons anticipate such dangers and prevent them by tying important arteries twice.

After a careful check to make sure that no sponges or instruments have been left in the operative site, there comes the final step in the operation, the closing of the incision. This may be done with thread sutures or, sometimes, with metal clips. If the incision is in the neck (as it would be for a thyroid operation) the surgeon makes the incision in one of the natural folds of the skin; he will use clips or other materials for closing the incision so that the minimum scar will appear.

In some operations a drainage tube may be led out from the area of operation through part of the incision. This drainage tube may be needed to help siphon off pus, or excess fluid, or may drain the bile temporarily in operations on the gallbladder. The tube is usually removed in a few days.

## EFFICIENCY, NOT MELODRAMA, CHARACTERIZES OPERATIONS

The most noticeable thing about an operation is the smooth, methodical, and cooperative manner in which it takes place.

A lawyer friend, watching an operation with me not long ago, commented, "I was struck with how impersonal it all seemed."

He was right; it was impersonal, and in such an atmosphere the surgeon and his assistants work most efficiently. The attention of the operating team is concentrated to a remarkable degree upon the task being undertaken. Each knows his job and does it competently, almost automatically. If the surgeon or his assistant should become emotional about an amputation or the discovery of a cancer, he might not work at his best; for this reason doctors usually do not operate on members of their own families.

## IS SPEED IN SURGERY DESIRABLE?

Not so many years ago surgeons prided themselves on the speed with which they could perform an operation. The modern surgeon, however, is not pressed for time, because pain has been controlled by good anesthesia, and shock can be prevented by transfusions of blood made available by modern blood banks. In addition, the antibiotic and nutritive fluids prepare the patient so well for the operation that the surgeon can be relaxed and sure of the situation.

Speed is still desirable under certain circumstances, such as accidents involving severe hemorrhage. But in the main, it is less important than it is for the surgeon to take time enough to handle the tissues very carefully, and thus avoid injuring them, which was one of the main causes of danger and difficulty of surgical operations in the past.

## THE PATIENT'S PART IN RECOVERY FROM AN OPERATION

After the operation has been completed, you will awaken in another room, either your own or one on the operating floor. Do not be alarmed if you find yourself in an oxygen tent or receiving fluid by means of a tube inserted into a blood vessel. Such techniques were once a last resource, but are used widely today to contribute to the patient's comfort and speed his recovery. Nurses should not be asked, by either you or your family, what these procedures are for. It is generally regarded as inadvisable for a nurse to explain the doctor's orders. There are many reasons for this, including the fact that a nurse may care for a number of patients and will not know enough about the case, including the personality of the patient, to answer questions in the best way.

You and the doctors and nurses now have work to do *to prevent complications*. Major complications can develop following an operation, but owing to the care taken by doctors they are usually prevented. In fact, most of the terrible things you have heard about complications following surgery belong to the past. Modern surgery has made phenomenal advances in the past few decades, including the prevention of the troubles that followed operations.

There is little likelihood that you will develop a blood clot in the lungs, collapse of the lungs, or infections if you cooperate with your doctors and nurses. It has been found that moving the legs helps prevent the formation of blood clots in the veins of the lower part of the body. These clots are dangerous because parts of them may break off and travel to the lungs where they can block a major blood vessel, and cause serious trouble. This complication is prevented by the exercises that you perform. The practice of getting patients out of bed, and having them walk even the first or second day after a major operation, helps prevent these and other complications. This technique is called *early ambulation*. After some types of operation it is necessary to breathe deeply and to cough. This helps expand collapsed portions of the lungs and wards off pneumonia; it may be painful when the patient has a large incision or one that moves with coughing.

These postoperative methods, plus other improved techniques such as the use of intravenous fluids, pay good dividends in getting patients out of the hospital in remarkably brief periods of time compared to previous decades. Today's patients feel much stronger after major surgery, too.

## WHAT IS ELECTIVE SURGERY?

Many operations, such as those for acute appendicitis or for perforation of the stomach by an ulcer, compound fracture, or bullet wounds, are performed on an emergency basis where every minute or hour is important.

Other operations do not need to be performed the moment the diagnosis is made, but can wait. If there is no hurry, the surgery is called *elective surgery*. Such operations can be put off until a time when things are apt to be under less pressure as far as the patient, the doctor, and the hospital are concerned. Among the operations that come under this category are repair of hernias, hemorrhoids, varicose veins, plastic surgery, and many cases of enlarged tonsils.

Other operations may fall in between the emergency and the elective. For example, if a tumor of the breast has been diagnosed, the doctor will worry about cancer. He does not need to operate that day, but he does not want weeks or months to elapse, because in the interim a small, curable cancer might enlarge to a dangerous stage.

Have confidence in your doctor. If he advises an operation, consider it seriously.

In some conditions diagnosis is difficult because it cannot be checked by x-rays or other positive tests, and the doctor must rely on his judgment, based on his experience and ability. Among these conditions are tumors of the breast, tumors of the uterus (sometimes called fibroids), enlarged prostate gland, and gallbladder disease. Your doctor will probably welcome the suggestion that a specialist be called in or, if you live in a rural district, that you go to the nearest medical center for examination. In cases of major surgery or when there is any doubt in your mind, ask for an examination by a qualified specialist in the field.

## IS YOUR OPERATION NECESSARY?

The great majority of the approximately fifteen million operations performed annually in the United States are undoubtedly honestly advised and skillfully performed. Most patients need have no worry when faced with need for emergency surgery or for other obviously desirable non-emergency surgery.

But it is also true that some operations not really needed are performed. In surgery, as in all professions and occupations, there are a few "bad apples," charlatans performing needless operations simply for the fees and even, in a few cases, because of an egotistical need to have full operating schedules. And there are some surgeons who may perform operations because they may know no better, having failed to keep up to date on possible alternatives, on newer, nonsurgical methods of treatment.

Sometimes the patient, even if unknowingly, may encourage needless surgery. When they cannot judge the needs or quality of care, some people may consider that more care is better care.

Moreover, the failure of many patients to investigate the competence and background of a surgeon and their failure to use their right to question and explore a recommendation for surgery, just trusting to blind faith, may allow some surgeons, so inclined, to get away with needless surgery.

There are controls over unnecessary operations. As we've seen earlier, accredited hospitals must have tissue committees to review tissue specimens taken from patients undergoing surgery as a check on whether operations performed are necessary. A surgeon who does needless surgery is likely to be given, very quickly, a stiff warning.

Today, about 5,000 of the 7,000 hospitals in the country are accredited. In the remaining hospitals, there may or may not be procedures for trying to eliminate unnecessary operations.

## What You Can Do to Help Make Certain

Except perhaps in a serious emergency, don't be rushed—or rush yourself—into an operation.

When possible, see your family physician first rather than decide you may need surgery and go directly to a surgeon. The family physician can use his professional judgment and, if he believes surgery may be needed, can send you to a surgeon.

When you visit the surgeon, don't fail to ask him to outline what alternatives there may be to an operation and the possible benefits and complications of the procedure. Be wary if a surgeon seems to want to rush you into an operation when clearly there is no emergency—and wary too if he is too busy to give you enough time to answer questions.

Much public attention has been paid recently to certain classes of operations—hysterectomies, hemorrhoidectomies, and tonsillectomies—which may be performed too routinely. Others sometimes mentioned include removal of symptomless varicose veins, thyroid surgery, and spinal disk surgery. If yours is to be one of these, you may want to be especially convinced that it's really needed and that the gain is very likely to outweigh whatever risk may be involved.

If you have any doubts remaining about the need for an operation that is not an emergency one, don't hesitate to get a second opinion. A second surgeon—suggested by the first surgeon or your family doctor—may see your problem in a different light and perhaps capable of being solved by nonsurgical treatment. If he, like the first surgeon, considers operation advisable, you can prepare for surgery more confidently.

You *do* have a right to a second opinion. "Patients should realize," says Dr. William R. Barclay, a top official of the American Medical Association, "that they're the boss, since they are purchasing a service. If the patient wants to get another doctor's opinion, he should feel no embarrassment about it."

# 32
# HEALTH INSURANCE AND COMMUNITY SERVICES

At one time, people used to say with considerable justification that only the very rich and the very poor could obtain adequate medical care. The rich could pay for it and the poor could get it free in clinics or hospitals, where

Today, most people with moderate incomes have *insurance* covering most of the costs of medical care. In addition, old-fashioned charity is being replaced by *community services*, to which everyone is entitled.

## INSURANCE

Americans spend more than 3 percent of their disposable income for health insurance premiums. The basic types of insurance are the following:

*Hospital Expense Insurance.* This pays all or part of the cost of hospital room, board, x-rays, medicines, and other expenses. Some plans reimburse the patient. Others, notably Blue Cross, reimburse the hospital directly.

*Surgical Expense Insurance.* This pays part or all of the cost of an operation. The amount paid depends on the nature of the operation. Under some plans (Blue Shield, for example), if a patient's income is below a certain level, the surgeon usually agrees to accept the fee listed in the policy in full payment. Patients whose incomes are higher than a given amount pay the surgeon something above the stated amount.

*Medical Expense Insurance.* Under this plan,

visits to a doctor's office or his house calls are reimbursed, in an amount and with a limit set in the policy.

*Major Medical Expense Insurance.* This insurance plan helps to pay the cost of extended sickness or injury. These policies generally have a deductible clause: typically, the patient pays the first $100 or $200 himself, then the plan pays 80 percent of the balance, up to some limit, perhaps $25,000. There are many variations on this type of policy, the coverage naturally varying with the amount of premiums.

*Loss-of-Income Insurance.* This insurance, also called *Disability Income Insurance*, pays benefits when the insured person is unable to work because of illness or injury.

Blue Cross and Blue Shield are the best-known plans. Blue Cross is designed to pay all or part of hospital bills, and Blue Shield to pay those of the doctor. It is possible to subscribe to either one or both of these plans.

Commercial insurance companies offer many kinds of health and accident insurance policies. It is usually possible to find one that meets the needs of the individual. They are particularly valuable for those not eligible for the "Blue" plans or who want additional protection.

Patients over 65 may be covered by Medicare, the government health insurance plan, which has two parts—hospital insurance and medical insurance. Every person over 65 registered for Medicare has the hospital insurance coverage, but only those who have requested and paid for medical insurance are covered for doctors' services as well.

## IMPORTANT FREE MEDICAL SERVICES

In recent years public health groups have gone more and more into the field of personal health services for general health maintenance and for certain special diseases. Public health departments and voluntary health agencies offer many *personal, free services* that may be worth hundreds of dollars to you or, even more important, provide you with some vital medical assistance you would otherwise be unable to afford.

These free personal health services are not "charity." They are an essential part of the country's overall health program, as necessary in their way as free vaccination or the elimination of malaria by mosquito control. You have a right to and *should* use these services if you need help in your own fight against our common enemy, ill health and disease. It is important that you learn the types of services your particular health department provides. They may be of tremendous value if chronic illness should strike you or your family, or if you have young children who need frequent dental and pediatric care.

Free services are made available by the health departments in many cities for the following important medical problems:

Alcoholism
Cancer detection
Dental diagnosis and care for school children
Diabetes
Infant care and well-baby clinics
Mental-health clinics
Narcotics addiction and curbs on smoking
Nutrition instruction
Nutritious lunches for school children
Physical examination of school children
Prenatal care for the pregnant mother
Tuberculosis
Venereal disease clinics

Under certain circumstances almost any family would need one or more of these services. A patient with a chronic disease such as mild or recovering tuberculosis may be able to finance the cost of seeing the doctor but not the additional burden of frequent x-rays or the laboratory tests on the sputum. The public health department will frequently provide these essential x-ray and laboratory tests free.

As is pointed out in the chapter on teeth, many large families need to obtain part of the dental care required on a free or reduced-cost basis. In such cases, your health department may provide the dental service you need, or can suggest adequate clinics.

People can often handle the expenses involved in an occasional trip to the doctor and the purchase of a few medicines. But when some severe and long-lasting illness occurs, they find the burden of paying for adequate medical care too heavy for them to carry.

Your doctor understands better than you may imagine the tremendous financial burdens imposed on a family by heart disease, nervous breakdowns, or other severe disabling sickness. He will be very willing to cooperate with the health department in having his services supplemented by the public health nurse, the public health nutritionist, or whatever auxiliary care the public health department gives.

## VOLUNTARY HEALTH AGENCIES

In addition to the health facilities offered by tax-supported agencies such as the local health department, your state health organization, and the United States Public Health Service, there are many organizations that offer valuable health services. They are supported by contributions from individuals, foundations, corporations, trade unions, and the like. We all know about the National Foundation (formerly National Foundation for Infantile Paralysis), the American Cancer Society, and several other of the large and long-established ones. However, it is good to scan the following list and see how many organizations exist, and what varied areas of illness they cover.

If you, a member of your family, or a neighbor has a continuing problem with rheumatic heart trouble, arthritis, deafness, diabetes—to list but a few examples—you should communicate with these organizations to learn precisely what services they render. Many of them are able to help finance special problems connected with rehabilitation and the long pull of nursing care required by chronic illness. For example, a child with nephrosis (kidney disease) may recover after as long as ten years of disability, during which period he might require almost continual nursing care. Surely any parent faced with such a difficult problem would want to communicate periodically with the American Nephrosis Foundation and learn about special clinics where the child may receive the benefit of new treatments and special nursing.

## Health and Welfare Organizations

*Accident Prevention*

National Safety Council, 425 North Michigan Avenue, Chicago, Ill. 60611. Gathers and distributes information about accidents and their causes, and ways to prevent them. Statistical, library, and information services.

*Alcoholism*

Al-Anon Family Group Headquarters, 125 East 23d Street, New York, N.Y. 10010.

Alcoholics Anonymous (National), Box 459, Grand Central Annex, New York, N.Y. 10017.

National Committee on Alcoholism, 2 East 103d Street, New York, N.Y. 10029.

National Institute of Mental Health, Public Health Service, Department of Health, Education, and Welfare, Bethesda, Md. 20014.

Salvation Army: some branches have special workers in this field.

Local clinics and welfare agencies in many large cities.

*Arthritis and Rheumatism*

The Arthritis Foundation, 3400 Peachtree Road, Atlanta, Ga. 30326. Information on the rheumatic diseases and aid for those afflicted.

*Blindness*

American Foundation for the Blind, 15 West 16th Street, New York, N.Y. 10011. Information on all aspects of blindness.

Braille Institute of America, Inc., 741 North Vermont Avenue, Los Angeles, Calif. 90029. Information, casework, books in braille and of other types for the blind at cost; lending library service.

Eye Bank for Sight Restoration, Inc., 210 East 64th Street, New York, N.Y. 10021. Arranges for the donation of eyes for corneal transplants. (There are eye banks in other large American cities.)

National Council to Combat Blindness, Inc., 41 West 57th Street, New York, N.Y. 10019.

National Industries for the Blind, 1120 Avenue of the Americas, New York, N.Y. 10036. Rehabilitation of the blind.

National Society for the Prevention of Blindness, Inc., 79 Madison Avenue, New York, N.Y. 10016.

Research to Prevent Blindness, 598 Madison Avenue, New York, N.Y. 10022.

The Seeing-Eye, Inc., Morristown, New Jersey. Raises and trains Seeing-Eye dogs. Trains blind persons in proper care and handling of the dogs.

*Cancer*

American Cancer Society, Inc., 777 Third Avenue, New York, N.Y. 10017. Information on diagnosis and treatment of cancer. Aid to patients, as needed.

National Cancer Institute of the National Institutes of Health, U.S. Public Health Service, Bethesda, Md. 20014.

*Cerebral Palsy*

American Academy for Cerebral Palsy, 1520 Louisiana Avenue, New Orleans, La. 70115.

United Cerebral Palsy Associations, Inc., 66 East 34th Street, New York, N.Y. 10016. Provides information on cerebral palsy and the possibilities for those affected.

*Chronic and Crippling Diseases*

Disabled American Veterans, P.O. Box 14301, Cincinnati, Ohio 45214. Aids disabled veterans in hospitals, insurance, employment, and similar matters.

Goodwill Industries of America, 1913 N Street N.W., Washington, D.C. 20006. Provides employment for handicapped persons in a suitable environment.

Institute for the Crippled and Disabled, 400 First Avenue, New York, N.Y. 10010. Gives educational and vocational treatment and advice for rehabilitation. Services cripples, mutes, hard of hearing, and certain types of heart cases.

National Amputation Foundation, 12-45 150th Street, Whitestone, N.Y. 11357.

National Society for Crippled Children and Adults, 2023 West Ogden Avenue, Chicago, Ill. 60640. Provides information on all types of crippling conditions. Local units have professional consultants and provide employment service. Operates Easter Seal Research Foundation.

### Cleft Palate

American Cleft Palate Association, Parker Hall, University of Missouri, Columbia, Mo. 65202.

### Deaf and Hard of Hearing

American Hearing Society, 919 18th Street, N.W., Washington, D.C. 20006. Provides information and maintains local chapters handling such projects as lip-reading classes.

National Association of the Deaf, 814 Thayer Avenue, Silver Spring, Md. 20910. Seeks to improve the employability and status of the deaf.

Alexander Graham Bell Association for the Deaf, 3417 Volta Place, NW, Washington, D.C. 20007.

### Diabetes

American Diabetes Association, Inc., 1 West 46th Street, New York, N.Y. 10036. Information on diagnosis and treatment of diabetes. Encourages establishment of summer camps for diabetic children.

### Epilepsy

Epilepsy Foundation of America, 1828 L Street, NW, Washington, D.C. 20036.

### Heart Disease

American Heart Association, 7320 Greenville Avenue, Dallas, Texas 75231. Provides information relating to the prevention and care of heart disease. Includes rheumatic fever.

### Kidney Disease

The National Kidney Foundation, Inc., 116 East 27th Street, New York, N.Y. 10016.

### Lung Disease

American Lung Association, 1740 Broadway, New York, N.Y. 10019.

### Maternity

Maternity Center Association, 48 East 92nd Street, New York, N.Y. 10028. Publishes pamphlets and conducts classes to instruct expectant mothers and fathers.

### Mentally Ill or Retarded

Association for Children with Retarded Mental Development, 902 Broadway, New York, N.Y. 10010.

Association for Help of Retarded Children, 208 East 16th Street, New York, N.Y. 10003.

Association for Mentally Ill Children, 12 West 12th Street, New York, N.Y. 10011.

National Association for Mental Health, Inc., 1800 North Kent Street, Arlington, Va. 22209.

### Multiple Sclerosis

National Multiple Sclerosis Society, 205 East 42nd Street, New York, N.Y. 10017.

### Muscular Dystrophy

Muscular Dystrophy Association of America, Inc., 810 Seventh Avenue, New York, N.Y. 10019.

### Myasthenia Gravis

Myasthenia Gravis Foundation, 230 Park Avenue, New York, N.Y. 10017.

### Rehabilitation

Audiology and Speech Correction Center at Walter Reed Army Hospital, Washington, D.C. 20012.

Department of Defense, Washington, D.C. 20301. Employs disabled civilians and rehabilitates disabled servicemen and women.

National Rehabilitation Association, 1522 K Street, NW, Washington, D.C. 20005. Rehabilitates the mentally and physically handicapped.

New York University-Bellevue Medical Center, Institute of Physical Medicine and Rehabilitation, 400 East 34th Street, New York, N.Y. 10016. Also the Disabled Home Makers' Program, at this address.

Office of Vocational Rehabilitation of FSA, Washington, D.C. 20201. Administers the Federal-State program for rehabilitating handicapped persons.

Veterans Administration, Washington, D.C. 20420. Rehabilitates disabled veterans.

State rehabilitation programs, usually administered through the Department of Education or through a special board.

*Sterility*

Planned Parenthood–World Population, 810 Seventh Avenue, New York, N.Y. 10019. Gives information to childless couples, birth control information to doctors; publications on marriage and parenthood.

Many local sterility clinics associated with hospitals and Planned Parenthood Leagues.

*Tuberculosis*

American Lung Association, 1740 Broadway, New York, N.Y. 10019. Provides information on all aspects of tuberculosis, and sponsors diagnostic services.

State and local health departments provide for treatment of tuberculosis patients, and state agencies aid in rehabilitation after recovery.

*Unmarried Mothers*

The Children's Bureau, Social Security Administration, Department of Health, Education, and Welfare, Washington, D.C. 20201.

Florence Crittenton Homes Association, Inc., 608 South Dearborn Street, Chicago, Ill. 60605. Has branches in many cities.

The American Red Cross, The Salvation Army, and other service groups give aid and assistance to married and unmarried mothers.

# PART FIVE

## You and Your Special Problems

# 33
# THE KILLERS
## AND HOW TO OUTWIT THEM

I am purposely calling the diseases I discuss in this chapter the Killers, in order to drive home your need to be on guard against them. In time of war, every soldier on active duty knows that failure to be aware of the existence of danger may cause him to walk into an ambush. We must all recognize the danger of our worst enemies, the killing diseases.

My choice of a subtitle, How to Outwit Them, is equally deliberate. These enemies are powerful. But they are not *all-powerful*. Medical science can, with your help, prevent, control, or cure them. We are no longer at the mercy of those age-old murderers, pneumonia, tuberculosis, and appendicitis. Even cancer can often be prevented or cured. Modern methods of treatment enable many people with high blood pressure, heart disease, diabetes, and hardening of the liver (cirrhosis) to live out their *normal life expectancy*.

Surgical operations that were not even dreamed of when I was in medical school are performed every day in large medical centers, saving the lives of thousands and making normal living possible for thousands more.

"Hold on, doctor!" you are probably saying. "Take a look at the statistics. Aren't heart disease, cancer, and the other diseases you mention, the chief causes of death?"

They are, it is true. But my point is: they can often be outwitted. And even when we can't be victorious, we can force these enemies into an advantageous truce. Take the case of a man who, according to the records, has died of cancer of the prostate. *But,* by proper treatment, the disease was controlled for a considerable number of years, so that he led a fairly active, good life until he was seventy-three. We have to admit that cancer won the battle—but under those circumstances, it was far from being an "unconditional surrender."

## OUR MAIN ENEMIES

Early this century, pneumonia, tuberculosis, and inflammations of the intestines (diarrhea and enteritis) were the three leading killers. Today, pneumonia and tuberculosis are much less dangerous than they used to be, while diarrhea and enteritis are no longer entitled to a place among the top killers.

Cancer and diseases of the heart are now at the head of the list. Look at the following table showing the killers of yesterday and today, so that you will know your worst enemies.

### TABLE 33–1
#### LEADING CAUSES OF DEATH

| 1900 | Today |
|---|---|
| 1. Pneumonia | 1. Heart disease |
| 2. Tuberculosis | 2. Cancer |
| 3. Diarrhea and enteritis | 3. Diabetes |
| 4. Nephritis | 4. Stroke |
| 5. Heart disease | 5. Accidents |

## PREPAREDNESS

Here are some *general* rules to follow in order to minimize the danger of attack and increase your chances of victory. This is a checklist; I discuss these points in detail elsewhere in this book.

1. Have periodic medical checkups (see page 378).

2. Recognize, and report promptly, all "warning signals" that occur between checkups (see page 384).

3. Keep your weight normal, or slightly below normal, after you reach middle age (see page 45).

4. If you have, or are threatened by, a disease, study the information about it given in this book. Do this so that you can be a *good patient,* but *NOT in order to treat yourself.* Trust your doctor, and cooperate with him. Follow his instructions. Let *him* do your worrying for you.

5. Keep in touch with your doctor, and when this is impossible, get another doctor. Medical science is continually developing new medicines and treatments for diseases, including the Killers. You probably won't learn about them unless you have a doctor. Only too often, people are told that no treatment can help them, and then decide "There's no use seeing a doctor when nothing can be done for my disease." Meanwhile, for example, a new operation may be developed which could relieve the heart condition from which they are suffering.

6. Keep away from quacks, faith healers, and advertised "cures." Shun them as *allies* of the Killers. Adopting a "Why not try them and see?" attitude may prove *fatal.*

## HEART DISEASES AND OTHER DISEASES OF THE BLOOD VESSELS

It may seem strange to you that I include diabetes and kidney diseases such as nephritis in this section. I do so because the worst effects of these diseases are frequently seen in the heart or the vascular system. Doctors usually regard the diseases I discuss here as belonging to one "family" of ailments—the *cardiovascular-renal.* I take up the subjects in the following order:

Symptoms of heart disease
Congenital heart disease
Syphilitic heart disease
Rheumatic heart disease
Bacterial endocarditis
Coronary heart disease
Hypertension (high blood pressure)
Diseases of the kidneys
Diabetes
Hardening of the arteries
Strokes (also called "apoplexy" and "shocks")

I am dealing with strokes last because they can result from high blood pressure, nephritis, diabetes, and many forms of heart trouble.

The main job of the heart is to circulate the blood through the body (see page 92). The healthy heart can do this tremendous task without difficulty. But there are many diseases, some simple, others complicated, which can injure this wonderful piece of machinery.

Heart disease leads the list of Killers today by a considerable margin. We must not overlook the fact that this is due at least in part to the years that have been added to our lives. People who might formerly have died of pneumonia or some other infectious disease while they were in their forties, now survive to be sixty-five or more; and heart disease is more common in older than it is in young people. But we must also not overlook the fact that heart disease is the leading Killer, and it is well worthwhile to learn how it can be outwitted.

### Symptoms of Heart Disease

There are certain general symptoms that may indicate there is something wrong with the heart. They do not definitely *prove* the existence of heart disease. But they are sufficiently important so that you should see a doctor if you discover any of them. By doing so promptly, you will either avoid needless worry or be in a favorable position to cope with the enemy before it becomes firmly entrenched.

Your doctor will examine your heart and perform certain tests to determine what the symptom means. He may find it necessary to refer you to a heart specialist who is trained to make further tests such as an electrocardiogram in order to make certain whether or not your heart is sound, and if not, the nature and extent of the difficulty.

1. *Increasing dyspnea (shortness of breath) on exertion.* Almost everyone normally becomes short of breath or even gasps for air after rushing to catch a bus or climbing a number of stairs. Breathlessness is also apt to occur, to a slight extent, as people get older, especially if they are overweight. But if activity you formerly were able to carry out without trouble begins to leave you quite breathless, be sure to consult your doctor. It may indicate heart trouble, though it is not an absolute sign. For example, nervous tension causes some people to feel as though they can't draw a deep breath when they need one, or makes them sigh frequently in a breathless manner.

2. *Nocturnal dyspnea (shortness of breath at night).* Be sure to see a doctor if you awaken from sleep at night with a choking sensation or a feeling of suffocation. Some people with heart trouble find they require a number of pillows to prop them up in order to make breathing easier.

3. *Edema (swelling) of the ankles.* If your ankles swell at the end of the day, consult your doctor. It may be due to poor circulation. Women and sometimes men find their ankles have a tendency to become puffy if they have to stand a great deal, especially in the summer. In some women, puffiness occurs before menstrual periods. People with varicose veins may also find their ankles swell a little. These conditions are nothing to worry about. I am concerned about a swelling that differs from the one to which you are accustomed, especially if it interferes with putting on your shoes, or if you can make a deep mark in it by pressing with a finger. *If in doubt, ask your doctor.*

4. *Angina pectoris (pain over the heart or in the middle of the chest).* This may be a very important clue to the fact that something is wrong with your heart. The sensation may be described as feeling as though a rock has been placed on the chest or over the heart. It may be a sharp pain, or a "tight" feeling, as though one were wearing a vest that should be unbuttoned. It usually follows exercise or excitement, and sometimes a heavy meal. Ordinarily it lasts only a minute or two, and is relieved by remaining motionless.

If you experience such a sensation, especially if you are over forty, be sure to tell your doctor. It may only be a gas pain or indigestion. But on the other hand, a serious heart condition may reveal itself by no sign except "heaviness" or pain. Don't try to determine which it is. Many people mistake gas pains for heart trouble, or wrongly diagnose a real heart condition as indigestion. A competent physician will not make this mistake. However, he may have to see you a number of times; and tests, such as the electrocardiogram, may be required before he can be certain.

5. *Other symptoms.* Fortunately, *dizziness, fainting spells, blue lips,* attacks resembling *asthma,* and *extreme fatigue* usually distress people sufficiently to make them consult a doctor. They should be regarded as warning signals. Spitting or coughing up *blood,* or a *cough* that persists in spite of treatment, can also indicate heart disease.

*Palpitation (fluttering of the heart)* is NOT in itself a danger signal. Many healthy people have "extra beats" of the heart, or feel as though it had "flopped over" or stopped for a moment. It may occur when they get excited or overtired, or have been drinking too much coffee or smoking too much. It does not indicate anything harmful. People with heart disease may also experience palpitation, but they will usually have other symptoms as well.

*Paroxysmal tachycardia* is the medical term for a certain type of palpitation. It starts suddenly and ends abruptly, with the heart beating furiously; sometimes it lasts for hours or even for days. This, of course, is not the same as the normal speeding up of the heart due to exercise or excitement. It is usually not serious and may not be related to any organic heart disease. People who are nervous or worried may have frequent attacks of paroxysmal tachycardia and live to a ripe old age without developing heart disease. It is a functional, not an organic, ailment in the majority of instances.

*Functional heart disease,* also called "*nervous heart,*" may bring about many symptoms of organic heart disease. However, there is no change in the organs to account for this. "Nerves" or emotional tensions are usually responsible (see Chapter 12).

## Congenital Heart Disease

This means heart trouble which is present at birth. One example you may have heard of is a "blue baby." In these babies, born with a fortunately rare abnormality, the blood does not flow properly from the heart to the lungs. Some congenital abnormalities do not reveal themselves until later in life.

Care of the pregnant mother has helped to reduce congenital heart trouble. For example, since the discovery that an unborn baby's heart *may* be injured if the expectant mother has German measles at a certain period of the embryo's development, pregnant women are careful to avoid this otherwise harmless disease.

Great progress has been made in correcting or improving congenital heart conditions, and much more progress is certain to come. Less often than ever need doctors say, "Nothing can be done." Surgery that seemed visionary only a decade or two ago is almost commonplace today. For example, thousands of men and women whose hearts were damaged by rheumatic fever when they were children can look forward to living full and active lives because specialists in heart surgery can repair or replace their damaged heart valves. The so-called blue babies—infants born with serious defects of the heart or circulatory system—can be saved and restored to normal, healthy living through open-heart surgery.

Your doctor, or a heart specialist he may refer you to, can tell when a congenital heart condition exists and how it can best be studied and possibly corrected. An exact diagnosis requires elaborate equipment and tests. Only a highly skilled surgeon can perform the necessary operation. If you live in the average small community, you will have to travel to a large medical center for this very special diagnosis and surgery.

## Syphilitic Heart Disease

Syphilis can damage the circulatory system, most often by injuring the aorta, the main artery leading from the heart. It is especially dangerous when it damages the aortic heart valve which separates the heart from this great blood vessel.

The germs of syphilis invade the wall of the aorta and the aortic heart valve, causing weakness and scarring. The valve may leak, so that some of the blood pours backward into the left ventricle instead of forward from the heart. Then the heart has to do the extra work of trying to force the blood out again.

Impairment of the heart by syphilis is far less common than it used to be, thanks to the widespread attack on this dangerous disease. When the day finally comes—as it can and must—that syphilis is wiped out completely, syphilitic heart disease will also be eliminated. (See page 447 for a discussion of the prevention of syphilis, and other aspects of this disease.)

## Rheumatic Heart Disease

Rheumatic fever is decreasing, but it is still a frequent cause of heart disease. Early diagnosis and effective treatment are helping to reduce the incidence of this serious disease. Children and young adults are most often the victims, but many adults suffer heart injury because of rheumatic fever. Sometimes its signs do not appear until the person has reached middle age. (See page 292 for a full description of rheumatic fever.)

Rheumatic fever may injure the covering of the heart, the heart muscle, the lining of the heart, and the valves. Damage to the valves creates serious mechanical hindrances to the proper functioning of the heart—pumping the blood. The valves may leak, as in syphilitic heart disease, or the opening of the valve may shrink so that it is not wide enough to permit the blood to flow through as it should. Surgery now can provide relief for many patients.

## Bacterial Endocarditis

This serious disease was formerly invariably fatal, but can now often be cured with penicillin and other antibiotics. It is separate and distinct from rheumatic fever, but I mention it here because it most commonly occurs in people whose heart valves have already been affected by rheumatic fever. It also occurs in people who have congenital abnormalities of the heart valves. Bacteria, carried by the blood stream, infect these areas.

Bacteria sometimes invade the blood stream for a short period after an operation on the mouth, nose, throat, intestines, or female genital tract. This is most apt to happen in operations of the mouth and throat, such as a tooth extraction or the removal of tonsils. Bacteria, including a type of germ called the green or *viridans* streptococcus, live in everyone's nose and throat. They are harmless to people in good health. But the operation opens a passageway into the tissues, giving the germs an entrance into the blood stream. If these germs reach heart valves that have been damaged, they can cause a dangerous illness. Therefore, people who have had rheumatic fever or who have congenital heart trouble (including congenital narrowing or *coarctation of the aorta*)—no matter how slightly the valves may have been damaged—*must take sulfa drugs or penicillin before certain operations* or tooth extractions in order to be on the safe side. Your physician will advise on this.

## CORONARY HEART DISEASE
(Disease of the Coronary Arteries—the Vital Blood Vessels of the Heart)

Arteriosclerosis, or "hardening," of the coronary arteries impairs the heart because it affects the arteries which supply blood to the heart muscle. It narrows their diameter, making it difficult for the blood to flow through. It also causes irregularities in the otherwise smooth lining of the arteries. When the flow of blood has been slowed down, and there are tiny grooves in its channel, blood is apt to settle in these places and form clots. (See arteriosclerosis, page 427.)

Arteriosclerosis of the coronary arteries can cause pain over the heart, *angina pectoris,* which is one of the symptoms I described above. These brief attacks of pain are caused by the fact that the heart muscle is not getting enough oxygen from the blood. For angina, the doctor may prescribe nitroglycerin tablets to be taken not only when an attack develops but also beforehand, in anticipation, when a patient engages in activities known to produce angina.

### Heart Attack

In a heart attack, an already narrowed coronary artery or one of its branches becomes closed off, usually because of a clot that forms and blocks the vessel. Because blood cannot get through, the part of the heart muscle served by that vessel is affected.

With a heart attack, there is usually chest pain, similar to that of angina pectoris, but now the pain does not disappear with rest and is not helped by nitroglycerin. Commonly accompanying the pain is a feeling of great anxiety. The face may turn ashen gray and there may be a cold sweat. Often there are retching, belching of gas, and vomiting. Shortness of breath is common.

*Figure 33-1. Coronary Thrombosis.* LEFT: *At time of attack. The flow of blood through part of the left coronary artery is blocked (shown in inset), cutting off the circulation in the shaded area.* RIGHT: *Re-* *covery from attack. Scar tissue has built up. Blood vessels of the right coronary artery (indicated by arrow) now supply the affected area.*

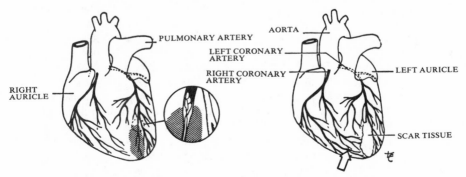

PULMONARY ARTERY

AORTA

LEFT CORONARY ARTERY

RIGHT CORONARY ARTERY

RIGHT AURICLE

LEFT AURICLE

SCAR TISSUE

A heart attack can be massive, producing almost immediate death, because blood flow to a major part of the heart muscle is cut off and the area dies. But far more often, only a relatively small area of the muscle is affected. Still, too many people with the latter kind of heart attack—and with hearts still "too good to die"—succumb for lack of quick action, delay in getting help.

A major danger after a heart attack, even a relatively minor attack, is heart rhythm abnormality. That abnormality may progress to the point where the heart fibrillates (just quivers uselessly), no longer pumping blood. Death soon follows.

Today, however, if a patient suffering a heart attack gets to a hospital, it is highly likely that serious rhythm abnormalities can be overcome and even prevented from occurring. It's essential for anyone experiencing a heart attack—or any symptoms even suggesting the possibility—to get to a hospital emergency room without delay and, once there, to say, "I think I may be having a heart attack." That will get him immediate attention and quick measures to guard against serious rhythm abnormalities.

*What future is there for a person who has recovered from a heart attack?* Years ago it was thought that any such attack, if not immediately fatal, would lead to death within a very few years. Now we know this is not true. There are scores and scores of thousands of cases of complete recovery.

It is not true that once a heart attack, invariably there must be another.

With newer knowledge of the factors involved in coronary heart disease, measures can be used to help combat the disease, to help prevent recurrences, and to help prevent first attacks.

## Preventive Measures

Doctors speak of risk factors in coronary heart disease. They mean that in addition to any possible basic risk which may stem from heredity, a given individual can add to the risk of developing the disease by (1) wrong diet, (2) obesity, (3) smoking of cigarettes, (4) lack of adequate exercise or physical activity, (5) poor control of diabetes if present, (6) high levels of cholesterol and blood fats, (7) uncontrolled high blood pressure, (8) poor control of gout if present, and (9) possibly excessive emotional stress.

It is highly unlikely that all of these factors would be present for any one individual, but if they should be, he would have twenty-five or more times the likelihood of getting a heart attack than a person with none of the factors. Even if only a few factors are present, the risk gets high. Hypertension (high blood pressure) alone, for example, may increase the risk as much as threefold.

Just think of this: something can be done about almost every one of these factors. They don't have to inevitably add to risk. Blood fats, when elevated, can be brought down to normal by proper diet, weight control, and, if necessary, medication. See the sections on high blood pressure and gout for information about how these diseases can be controlled.

Diabetes is an important problem in itself and a contributor to heart disease risk. But if a patient eliminates other high-risk factors, he should have a good chance of escaping a heart attack, especially with good control of the diabetes.

Anyone can stop smoking if he has the motivation. I have offered advice earlier on breaking the habit. Surely, a habit that brings risk of heart attack, cancer, and emphysema deserves to be eliminated. Similarly, it is possible to bring weight down to proper levels.

Stress is part of life and unavoidable. But what appears to count far more than stress itself is the individual reaction to stress. Some people even impose stress upon themselves. These are the people with what are called Type A personalities—those who must constantly meet deadlines, often self-imposed ones, who chronically struggle to get an unlimited number of things (often poorly defined) done in the shortest period of time. They have excessive drive and aggressiveness. They must be motivated to slow down at least a little, to put things in perspective.

Getting adequate exercise is valuable. It helps to make the heart work more efficiently, and it may aid in the development of new blood vessels (collaterals) to feed the heart muscle. Many physicians now put patients recovering from heart attacks on a carefully regulated program of exercise—as an aid in full recovery, prevention of recurrences, and even overcoming any persistent angina pectoris.

Today, too, when angina reaches the point of causing incapacity, there is the possibility of surgery. Many operations have been developed and performed successfully. In some, arteries from areas near the heart are brought over and attached to the heart muscle to increase blood supply. In other procedures, a vein graft may be used to bypass obstruction in a coronary artery.

# HYPERTENSION
## (High Blood Pressure)

Hypertension is a disease that greatly increases the tendency toward heart attacks and toward such other diseases as stroke and kidney failure as well.

We know now that elevated blood pressure affects more than twenty million Americans—and that it is a very subtle, stealthy disease. Many who have it don't know it because the elevated pressure can be present for many years, doing damage, without producing any symptoms. Almost invariably, hypertension is discovered not because of such symptoms as headache, dizziness, fatigue, or weakness—which it may produce when well advanced and which even then may be mistaken for other problems. Rather, it is discovered when a physician—during a routine check, during an insurance examination, or for other reason—measures the pressure.

As you know, the heart pumps blood into the arteries, which distribute it throughout the body. As the blood is forced through the arteries it presses against the walls of these strong, elastic tubes. The pressure is highest when the blood is being forced ahead by the pump (this is the *systolic* pressure) and the lowest between beats, when the heart relaxes (the *diastolic* pressure). These pressures are measured when the doctor puts the blood pressure cuff around the arm. In typical normal children, the systolic pressure, which is the one people usually have in mind when they think about blood pressure, is from 75 to 100. Young adults range from 100 to 120, and older people from 120 to 140. There is no truth to the old saying that blood pressure should be one's age, plus 100.

These preceding figures are only *averages*. However, when the systolic pressure tends to be higher than the average, and the diastolic pressure above 90, hypertension may be present. Sometimes, it's a temporary matter. Sometimes, pressure readings are elevated simply because of nervousness. But when repeated measurements show that the blood pressure consistently is above 140/90, the patient is considered to have hypertension.

Hypertension is a serious problem for many reasons. For one thing, excessive pressure burdens the heart, which must pump harder because of the pressure elevation. To accommodate to the task, the heart may enlarge. Eventually, an enlarged heart may weaken. Each year about 50,000 Americans have been dying of such hypertensive heart disease.

Moreover, just as excessive water pressure in a garden hose may damage the hose after a time, so excessive pressure in the coronary arteries may damage the internal walls, providing nesting places for excessive fats in the blood. Some investigators believe that high pressure may even help force the fats into the walls to start the buildup of artery-narrowing deposits.

## Causes

In only about 10 percent of people with hypertension can some definite physical cause be found. It may be a narrowing (*coarctation*) of the aorta, the great artery emerging from the heart; this type is curable by an operation that eliminates the narrowing.

An adrenal gland tumor, called a *pheochromocytoma*, is usually benign but produces large amounts of hormones that elevate pressure; it, too, is curable by surgery. Obstruction to normal blood flow in a kidney artery may lead to high blood pressure, and this type of hypertension can be cured by bypassing or otherwise correcting the obstruction surgically.

In the remaining 90 percent of cases, hypertension is classified as essential, meaning that the basic cause remains unknown.

## Treatment

Essential hypertension can be treated effectively in almost every case. Sometimes, it yields remarkably well to weight reduction. In people who may be taking excessive salt in the diet, moderation of salt intake alone, or in combination with medication, brings pressure back toward normal.

When drugs are needed, the physician now has available a wide variety. He can choose a medication likely to be suitable for the individual patient, combine it with another if necessary, and adjust dosage until a treatment is arrived at that controls pressure effectively and produces minimal or no undesirable side effects.

The ideal is to bring pressure to normal and keep it there. Many physicians now find that a big help in this is to have patients take their own blood pressure readings at home. Such readings may provide a truer picture of the blood pressure than measurements in the doctor's office, which sometimes tend to make the patient anxious. And home readings may simplify treatment, making fewer visits to the physician necessary.

## The Value of Treatment

Much evidence now has accumulated to show the value of treating hypertension and bringing elevated blood pressure levels down to normal. Perhaps the most famous studies are those that were done by the Veterans Administration Cooperative Study Group in eighteen VA hospitals across the country.

In the first of the VA studies, the patients ranged upward in age from thirty and had diastolic pressure of 115 to 129, at least 25 points above the 90 considered normal. Some received active treatment with antihypertensive medication; others, for comparison, received placebo (inactive) pills. There were no deaths over the next several years in the actively treated group, 4 in the other group. There were 27 serious events—heart attacks, strokes, heart failure—among the placebo patients, only 2 among the treated. The study was stopped much earlier than planned so the placebo group could be switched to active treatment to reduce their risk.

In another VA study, the patients had only mild hypertension—diastolic pressure of 90 to 114, just above the 90 considered top normal. Again there were two groups, actively treated and placebo. The study showed a two-thirds reduction among the treated group of the risk of developing a heart attack or stroke. Even within the five-year period of the study, more than 10 percent of the patients in the placebo group went on to develop severe hypertension; no patient in the treated group did.

## DISEASES OF THE KIDNEYS

The work of the kidneys in purifying the blood and regulating body water and salt content has been explained earlier. Serious damage to these important organs can endanger life. When kidney function is seriously impaired, uremia (which means "urine in the blood") sets in as a potentially fatal end result.

After the kidneys produce urine, they must pass it through two sets of tubes: the ureters leading to the urinary bladder, and the urethra leading from the bladder to the exterior. Anything that prevents normal flow through these tubes can produce back pressure which may seriously affect kidney function; usually such back pressure is also accompanied by infection. Such a situation can stem, for example, from an untreated enlarged prostate gland in a man.

Blood purification in the kidney is carried out by two million delicate filters which must be free of disease to function properly. Also, blood vessels designed to feed into the filters must be healthy, for the filters cannot thoroughly purify if inadequate amounts of blood reach them.

Not only may the kidneys be damaged by diseases of their own, but others may affect them. For example, high blood pressure may injure kidney blood vessels, so prevention or control of high blood pressure is an important measure for prevention of kidney disease. This is also true for artery disease, atherosclerosis, which can affect the kidney arteries. Diabetes, too, may damage the kidneys. So control of both atherosclerosis and diabetes is important for kidney health.

Other diseases, less common, can seriously affect the kidneys if uncontrolled. They include overactivity of the parathyroid glands (hyperparathyroidism), subacute bacterial endocarditis, gout, disseminated lupus erythematosus, and sarcoidosis. Excessive intake of vitamin D may also affect the kidneys adversely.

You may be surprised that I have not thus far used the term *Bright's disease,* which to many people is synonymous with kidney disease. I have done this to indicate that much has been learned about the varieties of kidney disease and damage since the time of Dr. Richard Bright, more than a century ago.

The term *Bright's disease* is no longer adequate. Physicians now use more specific terms—such as glomerulonephritis, nephrosis, and pyelonephritis —instead. These three major diseases affecting the kidneys will be described separately. It should be mentioned that these diseases, as well as some others, reveal their presence by certain changes in the urine. That is why a careful doctor always includes a complete urine study as part of his examination. He may also want to culture the urine for bacteria to make certain that no silent infection of the kidneys or passages leading from them will escape attention.

I want to impress on you that if your doctor wishes consultation with specialists in both internal medicine and urology when the diagnosis of kidney disease is not absolutely clear, he is justified even if it means sending you to a distant medical center. Effective treatment, based on clear diagnosis of any kidney disorder, is worth a great deal to you.

## Glomerulonephritis

Acute glomerulonephritis can occur at any age but is mainly a disease of children and young adults. It almost always follows a streptococcal infection, usually a strep sore throat, developing ten to fourteen days afterward.

In a typical attack, the patient's face and eyelids become puffy. Urine may be scant and may appear bloody, brown, or have the look of coffee with cream. There may be headache, fever, shortness of breath, and tenderness in the flanks. The doctor usually finds some increase in blood pressure. He also makes the diagnosis by characteristic findings in urine and blood.

Most patients recover in a matter of weeks or months. Treatment may include antibiotics, diuretic drugs, and other measures.

Most of the 5 percent or fewer patients who do not recover completely will go into a latent or subacute phase of the disease. They will have no symptoms when the disease is latent but will show changes in urine and may eventually develop chronic nephritis and uremia. The latent period may last for months or years.

In the subacute stage, the patient may have all or many of the symptoms of nephrosis (to be described), and this state is often called the *nephrotic stage* of glomerulonephritis. Eventually, the patient enters the advanced stage of chronic nephritis.

Patients with latent or chronic nephritis pass albumin in their urine. That is why a test for albumin is carried out at medical checkups. In the latent and chronic phases, there may be no symptoms, so diagnosis has to be made by careful examination of the urine for albumin and for red blood cells and casts (cylinders that take the form of kidney tubules and indicate kidney disease to the trained eye).

Eventually, most people with latent nephritis move into the chronic phase and slowly over months and even many years toward the serious uremic stage. During the chronic phase, there may be headaches, weakness from anemia, some shortness of breath, intermittent swelling of the ankles —or there may be no symptoms at all. During this stage, the doctor relies mostly on laboratory tests to tell him the degree of function of the kidneys. He knows that when function falls to about 10 percent of normal, uremia may soon follow.

The key to prevention of glomerulonephritis lies in avoiding strep sore throats—avoiding people who have them as much as possible. If you develop a sore throat and fever, the doctor should be notified immediately. Prompt eradication of strep sore throat by appropriate antibiotic treatment may decrease the risk of subsequent nephritis.

## Nephrosis

Nephrosis may be a disease by itself or it may be a stage of glomerulonephritis. The type called *true, lipoid nephrosis* occurs almost entirely in children. It is characterized by edema, or waterlogging, so pronounced that the child seems swollen like a balloon. The accumulation of water under the skin is painless. Fluid also may accumulate in the abdomen, which appears distended.

In contrast to chronic glomerulonephritis, nephrosis does not permanently damage the kidneys. Before modern treatment became available, children with nephrosis were often disabled for periods of up to ten years, lying in bed with their huge swellings. They were prone to infections.

Today, the outlook is far more pleasant for the patient with true nephrosis. Infections can be controlled by antibiotics and edema by steroid hormones. It does, however, take special skill to regulate steroid dosage, and it may be desirable to have the child treated at first at a medical center that has a specialist in this disease.

In adults, there are occasional cases of true nephrosis which clear completely without damage to the kidneys. But most adult nephrotics are undergoing a stage of glomerulonephritis and may eventually experience decreased kidney function.

## Pyelitis and Pyelonephritis

Pyelitis is an infection of the part of the kidney that collects the urine after it has been discharged from the special filtering units, the *nephrons*. Pyelonephritis indicates that infection has affected the nephrons as well. Because it is difficult if not impossible to have a kidney infection without some invasion of the nephrons, the more modern approach is to classify the kidney infections as *acute* and *chronic pyelonephritis*.

An acute attack begins suddenly with fever and chills. Frequently, headache, nausea, and vomiting appear. There is pain in the kidneys that can spread to the lower abdomen and groin. Urination is frequent, urgent, burningly painful.

Usually acute pyelonephritis can be terminated within a week or two with antibiotics and other medicine now available. Bed rest is the rule. The physician will make sure that fluid balance of the body is maintained and urinary output increased.

The outlook is very favorable if there is no anatomical abnormality that interferes with the free passage of urine. But the physician knows how easy it is to mistake apparent cure for complete cure. If cure is not complete, infection may hide in the kidneys and lead to chronic pyelonephritis.

To try to make sure that an acute attack clears completely, the patient, no matter how well he or she may feel, may be asked to return for examinations and urine cultures and perhaps remain on antibacterial medication for some weeks or months. Also, since the doctor knows that kidney infections frequently are associated with anatomical abnormalities in the pathways for urine excretion, he may want special x-rays or urological examinations of bladder, ureters, and kidney to detect any abnormalities which may require surgical remedy.

Young women are particularly susceptible to kidney infections, especially if they have any gynecological disorder. Pregnancy, too, may foster development of acute pyelonephritis because the enlarging uterus may press on the ureters leading from the kidneys. Knowing this, doctors watch the urine during pregnancy for any evidence of infection.

Older men, too, are often prone to this disease when the prostate becomes enlarged, thus interfering with urine flow.

Chronic pyelonephritis is usually a continuation of the acute infection which has defied treatment or not been properly treated. It can run a course of many years with repeated attacks, during which symptoms are similar to those of the acute form.

Antibiotics and other bacteria-killing agents are used in treatment. Sometimes, a badly diseased kidney may have to be removed.

## Cystitis

This is an infection of the urinary bladder. Since the bladder is so closely related to the kidneys, cystitis is considered here.

The characteristic symptom is urgent, painful urination. The need to urinate is frequent but the output is scanty. There may also be pain and tenderness low in the abdomen.

It is essential to eradicate cystitis completely because there is danger of infection spreading to the kidneys.

Antibiotics, sulfa drugs, or other antibacterial agents will clear up cystitis. Immediate relief of symptoms does not mean full cure. Drugs should be continued for the full period prescribed by the physician to avoid chronic cystitis. Commonly, with effective treatment, cystitis will clear completely within about two weeks. The chronic kind needs much more treatment for a far longer period.

## Kidney Stones

Stones (calculi) are a fairly common problem. They are deposits of mineral or organic substances which may vary in size from tiny pebbles to a *staghorn stone* which may be large enough to fill the entire pelvis of a kidney.

Kidney stones usually develop when too much of a substance formed in the kidney appears in the urine or when the urine is too acid or too alkaline to hold some substance in solution. Infection, too, may act as a focus around which material can precipitate (or fall out) of solution to form a stone.

Thus, one important preventive measure is to keep the kidneys free of infection. Another is to keep the urine dilute by drinking adequate amounts of fluid, especially during hot weather or when engaging in work or sports that lead to heavy sweating.

Some disorders are sometimes accompanied by kidney stone formation. Thus, gout may lead to the deposition of uric acid stones in the kidneys, and overactivity of the parathyroid glands may cause so much calcium and phosphorus to appear in the urine that they settle out and form stones. It is important that such disorders be treated with-

out delay as a means of preventing stone damage to the kidneys.

Some kidney stones may remain silent for years and may in fact never cause symptoms or trouble. Others start to pass out of the kidneys and, in doing so, cause severe pain and tenderness over the kidney area, frequent and painful urination, blood in the urine, fever, chills, and prostration. Small stones may get through and be eliminated in the urine. Larger ones, however, may become impacted in the kidney, ureter, or bladder and may have to be removed surgically.

I want to note here that when a patient must be kept recumbent for an extended period—because of a major fracture, for example—there is some risk that the bones will give off extra mineral which may form kidney stones. The alert physician, realizing this, can do much to prevent stone formation by increasing fluid intake and the flow of dilute urine, reducing mineral content of the diet, and using certain medications to reduce absorption of minerals from the intestine.

Because of the many ways kidney stones may

*Figure 33-2. Removing a stone from the right ureter by means of a cystoscope and catheter.*

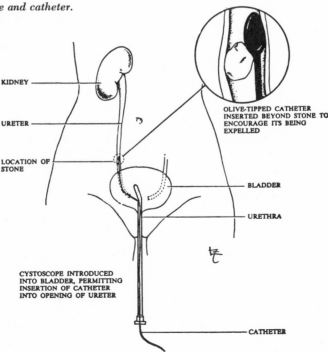

KIDNEY

URETER

LOCATION OF STONE

OLIVE-TIPPED CATHETER INSERTED BEYOND STONE TO ENCOURAGE ITS BEING EXPELLED

BLADDER

URETHRA

CYSTOSCOPE INTRODUCED INTO BLADDER, PERMITTING INSERTION OF CATHETER INTO OPENING OF URETER

CATHETER

form and their potential for trouble, they call for special blood and urine studies and x-ray and urological examination. Once the nature of the stones is clarified, it may be possible to prevent further formation by use of special diets or medicines. Anyone who has experienced renal colic—one of the worst of pains—or who has undergone kidney surgery would agree on the importance of prevention.

Although there has been no means of dissolving stones once they have formed, promising experimental work is now going on with a chemical that may be helpful in many cases.

## Stones in the Bladder

Occasionally a stone may either form in the bladder or pass into the bladder and remain there. The symptoms may include urinary frequency, blood, pus, and albumin in the urine, and painful urination. Most stones pass eventually into the urethra and out of the body. In stubborn cases, however, the physician may use a cystoscope, an instrument that is passed through the urethra into the bladder, to remove the stone.

## Uremia

Uremia is a toxic state of the body. It occurs when waste material normally excreted by the kidneys is retained in the blood, as the result of poorly functioning kidneys.

We have already noted some causes of kidney malfunction. Others include bad reactions to blood transfusions, severe shock, extensive burns, trauma, vitamin D overdosage, diabetes, and congestive heart failure. Poisons, too, are important causes, and they include carbon tetrachloride, mercury compounds, cantharides (Spanish fly), bismuth, wood alcohol, and occasionally even some otherwise useful sulfa drugs.

When uremia appears, fatigue, malaise, and nausea may be among the manifestations. There may be need to pass urine during the night. There may be pallor, and the skin may take on a slightly lemon color. As uremia deepens, there may be vomiting, itching, an odor of urine on the breath. In addition, there may be signs and symptoms of failing heart or high blood pressure. Toward the end, black and blue spots and a whitish deposit of urea may appear on the skin. Coma follows; then, death.

Until the advent of dialysis and kidney transplantation, all the doctor could do was to treat symptoms and modify diet to try to slow down the relentless course of chronic uremia. Now many lives can be saved.

Dialysis purifies the blood of the toxic materials that the diseased kidneys cannot excrete. This is achieved by passing the patient's blood through a machine which allows the poisonous substances to wash out. Currently, about 32,000 Americans are on dialysis, usually treated by machine about three times a week. Once dialysis machines were available only in hospitals. Now they are increasingly available in special facilities where the cost is less than in hospitals. And increasingly, too, machines for home use are available.

Dialysis has some limitations. Considerable time must be devoted to it. Diets must be restricted because the automatic adjustment of the natural kidney is gone. And there may be anemia for lack of adequate amounts of a kidney hormone that plays a role in the production of red blood cells.

Almost certainly improvements are coming. Now on trial is an experimental dialysis machine, a plastic body vest which can be worn anywhere —in the office, at the movies, during travel—and which, like the natural kidney, can work continuously rather than intermittently to cleanse the blood more thoroughly. Scientists are also seeking hormonal replacements for the secretions of the normal kidney.

Kidney transplants are increasingly successful. Of all organ transplants, they have the best record. When a transplant comes from an identical twin, the success rate can exceed 90 percent. When it's from a close relative—a brother or sister, for example—chances of success are 80 percent. And for donor kidneys from unrelated cadavers, the chances are about 50 percent.

Despite a common impression to the contrary, older people receiving transplants do fully as well as younger. And a 19-year-long study by Harvard physicians of 300 donors, aged 12 to 80, has established that life expectancy with one kidney is not reduced and donors lead healthy lives with little if any change in life-style.

What's needed is greater availability of donor kidneys, especially from cadavers. But they must be removed without delay if they are to be useful. Helpful for that would be wider use by healthy people of donor cards or other documents willing their kidneys, and other organs, for further use after their death.

## DIABETES

You may be surprised that I mention diabetes as a factor in heart disease. But a high incidence of atherosclerosis is associated with diabetes. The artery disease appears to develop much more often, at an earlier age, and in more severe form in diabetic persons than in the general population.

Determining the exact role of diabetes in artery disease is complicated because there is a high incidence of high blood pressure and obesity among diabetics—and both of these of themselves are factors in atherosclerosis. It is known, however, that changes in lipid metabolism—the way the body handles fats—occur when a diabetic passes from good control of his disease to inadequate control.

So it is vital, if you have diabetes, to maintain good control and to have periodic checks to make certain that the control is good.

See Chapter 5 (p. 74 ) for the complete description of diabetes.

## HARDENING OF THE ARTERIES
(Arteriosclerosis, Atherosclerosis)

We have previously discussed hardening of the arteries in connection with coronary heart disease.

As you know, *arteriosclerosis* means artery hardening. Actually, today, the preferred word for such artery disease is *atherosclerosis*. *Athero* means "soft swelling." So atherosclerosis is a more accurate term because the artery disease starts with a soft swelling and progresses to hardening.

When atherosclerosis begins to develop, the first visible indication may be a fatty streak in the inside lining of an artery—a thin, yellowish, slightly raised line. It may be no more than half an inch long and an eighth of an inch wide.

As atherosclerosis progresses, the streak increases in size and becomes the typical *plaque* of the disease, which you may have heard about. A plaque is filled with fatty material. The plaque grows in size, and with time, calcium may be deposited in it, making it hard.

As plaques enlarge, they begin to stick out into the channel of the artery, much as do scales forming within a corroding pipe. As this happens, the vessel's ability to carry blood is diminished.

It is this process that goes on in coronary heart disease. It can also affect a kidney artery and be responsible for kidney disease. It can affect a brain artery and be responsible for stroke. And it can affect arteries elsewhere in the body—in the legs, for example, where it produces cramping pain.

Much remains to be learned about atherosclerosis. Much is being learned. There is a constantly growing body of new knowledge. Because of the constant and rapid growth of that knowledge, your doctor is the best source of information about the problem and its treatment and prevention.

Some things do seem clear. There are sensible measures you can take that reasonably can be expected to help prevent atherosclerosis or retard its development. Being checked for high blood pressure and bringing it under control if it is present is certainly one.

Moderation in diet appears to be another. That means moderation in eating foods high in cholesterol and fatty foods. Not only may that help to keep blood fat levels low—high levels, as you know, are associated with atherosclerosis—but it also can help to keep your weight down. And obesity is a factor in atherosclerosis, diabetes, hypertension, and other problems. It is a well-known fact that the thin person has a longer life expectancy than the obese person. Virtually all doctors will agree that after the age of thirty-five, it is better to be slightly underweight than overweight.

Like most physicians, I strongly advise men and women with atherosclerosis to stop smoking or at least to smoke as little as possible.

## STROKE

*Stroke,* also known as *apoplexy* and *cerebrovascular accident* (*CVA*), involves injury to the brain. It may be followed by such serious consequences as paralysis of one side of the body, loss of speech, impairment of memory, and even death. Until quite recently, strokes were regarded with such fatalism by physicians as well as laymen that little was done to prevent them or prevent their end results. Now, fortunately, strokes are better understood.

A stroke is the damage to an area of the brain that results when the area is deprived of oxygen and other nutrients. In 60 percent of cases blood flow is blocked by a local clot, in another 20 percent by a clot coming from another part of the body and lodging in an artery feeding the brain, and in the remaining 20 percent the problem lies with a leaking or burst artery, that is, hemorrhage.

In almost every instance of blood clot blockage, the underlying cause is atherosclerosis or dis-ease of the artery wall; and in hemorrhage the underlying cause is atherosclerosis or a combination of atherosclerosis and high blood pressure.

Because a stroke may result from an accident to an artery, large or small, anywhere in the brain or leading to the brain, the consequences can be quite varied. A stroke may block out a tiny area of the memory center, or it may deprive a large section of the brain of oxygen, producing unconsciousness, paralysis, labored breathing.

One of the major developments in recent years has been the finding that a significant number of strokes arise from damage to arteries outside the brain itself—often in vessels in the neck leading to the brain. These vessels are accessible to surgical repair.

Another significant development is the recognition that while a major stroke may seem to come

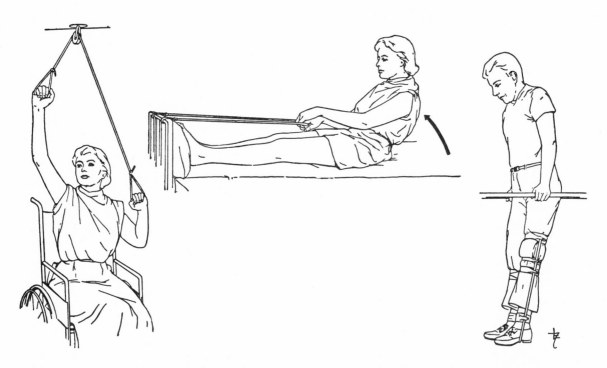

*Figure 33-3. Home Methods for Rehabilitation Following a Stroke.* UPPER: *Bedridden patient exercising arms, back, and legs. The stronger hand is placed over the weakened one.* LOWER LEFT: *Wheelchair patient using stronger arm to help exercise weakened one.* LOWER RIGHT: *Arms having been strengthened, patient helps support himself on rails or chair backs; leg braces (one short and one long) give additional support for walking.*

on suddenly, the stroke process is not necessarily sudden and may even provide early warnings.

Such warnings may include one or more of the following, all lasting only a few moments: fainting, stumbling, numbness or paralysis of the fingers of one hand, blurring of vision, seeing bright lights, loss of speech or memory.

Unfortunately, too often people, after recovering from a brief episode of these warning signals, do not recognize what they might be and pass them off as the results of fatigue, worry, or some other minor cause. Thus the opportunity to prevent the approaching stroke may be lost.

Any one or a combination of such symptoms should be the signal to notify your doctor or, if he is not available, to go to a hospital. Special x-rays of the arteries leading to the brain or other tests can be performed. If the cause of the symptoms appears to be a clot in an artery of the neck or other accessible spot, it may be decided to remove the clot; or if the artery has become very narrowed by disease, the deposits may be reamed out or the artery section bypassed with a new channel.

It has been learned that vigorous rehabilitation efforts can do much to overcome paralysis and speech impairment when a major stroke has occurred. Now, within two or three days after a stroke, or as soon as the patient is conscious, a program of exercises is started in bed, to be followed by out-of-bed and later out-of-hospital exercises. Special braces for the leg may be helpful, and slings for a paralyzed arm. Speech therapy, if needed, is started early.

## PHLEBITIS AND THROMBOPHLEBITIS

Phlebitis means an inflammation of the wall of a vein. In thrombophlebitis, the inflammation is accompanied by the formation of a blood clot in the vein.

A favorite site is a leg vein, and the symptoms include leg swelling, heaviness, and aching pain.

Thrombophlebitis has sometimes been called *milk leg* because occasionally it follows birth of a baby, occurring at about the time lactation begins.

But thrombophlebitis can develop under many other circumstances—when a vein is injured by accident or by infection, and when blood tends to "pool" or accumulate in the legs. Such pooling may occur with inactivity or bed rest, heart disease, obesity, varicose veins, fractures, and after surgery. Recently, too, some women using oral contraceptives have been found to have increased tendency to vein clot formation.

Thrombophlebitis has also been called the *chair disease* because it is a potential threat to anyone who spends much of his life sitting.

Thrombophlebitis can sometimes be a serious matter if it occurs in a deep vein of a leg—for there is some risk that the clot may break loose and travel to the lung, becoming a pulmonary embolism.

Doctors now use a variety of methods to deal with thrombophlebitis. They may use a drug, heparin, which acts to prevent clot formation, in people who may be prone to the problem because they are undergoing major surgery or require prolonged bed rest. The same drug may be used, too, in treating thrombophlebitis when it has occurred.

Under ordinary circumstances, you can go a long way toward protecting yourself against thrombophlebitis by avoiding sitting or standing still for long periods, which encourages blood pooling in the legs. If your job requires a lot of standing, move about as often as you can, and occasionally get up on your toes. If you must sit for extended periods—at work or in traveling—make it a point to contract your calf muscles and move your feet about frequently. It helps, too, to elevate your legs horizontally every once in a while and to get up and walk around, even just briefly, from time to time.

## CANCER

There is no reason to run away from the idea of cancer. Face it squarely. You will see that it can be actually far less terrible than most people imagine.

Cancer can be treated successfully. In many instances it can be completely cured. Countless people who have been treated for cancer have lived long, healthy lives, with no sign or symptom of the disease. Examinations made throughout their lifetime and after their deaths revealed no trace of it. *Cancer is definitely curable.* I repeat and underline this *fact* because it is so important for you to believe it.

The very word cancer is horrible to most people. The fear of this disease casts a shadow on lives which cancer itself will never touch. Those on whom it does lay a hand often become so terror-stricken they are unable to fight back. I know a lovely woman, previously well-balanced, who was emotionally paralyzed by the appearance of a lump in her breast. She did absolutely nothing about it until her friends could actually notice the change in her bosom—and by that time it was too late.

## Why Are People So Afraid of Cancer?

The reasons vary, but they usually include some, or all, of the following:

1. Despite the progress that has been made in regard to this disease, old attitudes persist. In the *past,* there was little if anything that could be done about it. Many years ago, Dr. Oliver Wendell Holmes discovered that the noted author, Nathaniel Hawthorne, had cancer. The way Dr. Holmes thought of it was: "the shark's tooth is upon him." In those days, to have a cancer was like falling prey to a shark.

2. Even today, cancer is the second greatest killer among diseases.

3. It can attack people of all ages—men, women, and children. It can affect almost any part of the body. Therefore no one, at any time, feels completely safe.

4. It seldom issues clear and obvious warnings. There is no simple test that can definitely rule out all possibility of cancer, nothing, for example, to compare with the blood test for syphilis or urinalysis for diabetes.

5. The cause of cancer is not known, and we tend to feel helpless when facing a mysterious adversary.

These are, indeed, reasons for regarding cancer as a serious enemy. But they are not reasons for becoming panicky. Quite the contrary. Even though the enemy has not been wiped out, medical science is winning many battles. The Killer

has not been caught and destroyed, but he is being cornered. In such a situation people must be alert. They cannot rely for their protection entirely on the authorities, that is, on the doctors, but must cooperate with them. Panic is not compatible with intelligent cooperation!

In my opinion, too much emphasis has been given to cancer as an enigma. It is true that we do not know all about it. But we know a great deal. We know enough to win countless victories. Our knowledge provides us with weapons to win even more, if everyone uses this knowledge.

## Cancer Explained

The tissues of our bodies grow by the division of cells. A cell is the earliest and simplest form of life. It is a single unit, like a building block. One cell divides to make two cells. These two new cells divide to make four, and so on. New cells are smaller, but otherwise exactly like the parent cells. They grow until they reach their normal size.

When the body reaches maturity, it stops growing and settles down to the size it will maintain for the rest of its existence. A certain number of new cells keep forming—for example, to repair damage. When you cut yourself, the wound heals by the formation of new tissue. When a certain point is reached in this process, nature normally cries, "Halt!"

It is still a mystery why cells divide until they have made just enough new tissue to replace the injured parts, and then stop.

We also do not understand why cells sometimes go on multiplying until there is too much tissue. That is what a tumor is—a lump or mass produced by the unchecked growth of cells in some part of the body.

Tumors are either *benign* or *malignant.* A benign tumor may be large or small. It may stop growing when it is no more than an inoffensive little lump with a thin membrane around it. It may become so large that it causes trouble because it occupies too much space. *But it does not spread* as a malignant tumor does. An example of a benign tumor is the *lipoma*—a fatty tumor or soft lump of the skin which you may have seen. Another example is the fibroid tumor of the uterus.

A *cancer* is a *malignant* tumor—a shapeless mass

which *keeps on growing in a disorderly fashion.* Some cancers grow rapidly, some slowly. But they do not stop, nor do they remain confined to a small area. This is what makes them dangerous and is the reason why we cannot afford delay in the treatment or removal of a cancer.

If not checked, cancers grow until the enlarging tissue crowds and presses on other organs of the body. The cancer prevents the organs from doing their proper work, and also robs the healthy cells of their food and blood supply. Some cancers spread like wildfire, destroying the organs around them. Pieces of cancer tissue may break off and, carried by the blood or the lymph, start growing in a new and perhaps distant part of the body. An untreated cancer in its late stages can be compared with a fire which has started in the basement and sends a spark up the stairway to the attic to set off another fire there.

> I want to insert a note of warning here: *Only a doctor can tell whether a tumor is malignant or benign.* Usually, he has to examine a bit of the growth under a microscope in order to know whether or not it is a cancer. Never decide for yourself "It's only a harmless growth." Once a cancer begins to spread, the chances of a cure diminish rapidly.

## Different Types of Cancer

Most cancers occur in people who are over forty, but cancer can appear at any age. It even afflicts children. There are many varieties of cancer, some of which are common while others are quite rare.

Cancers are divided into two large groups: *sarcomas* and *carcinomas*. Sarcomas usually affect the bones and muscles, and are apt to grow rapidly and be very destructive. The carcinomas make up the great majority of the cancers of the breast, stomach, lungs, womb, skin, and tongue.

Fortunately, most cancers grow, at first, only in the site where they originated. Even then, the cancer may invade the neighboring cells and tissues, and perhaps destroy valuable structures. However, it becomes far more dangerous when it spreads, or sets up new growths, in other parts of the body. The new cancer is called a *metastasis* or

*metastatic lesion.* A cancer can spread from the kidney to the bones, or from the lungs to the brain, apparently by way of the blood stream.

When cancer enters this stage, it becomes very difficult to cure. Yet, in some instances, it can still be held in check. For example, widespread metastases from a cancer of the prostate gland have been cleared up and kept under control for many years by surgery and hormones.

Obviously, the time when cancer can best be cured is in the *early period* of its growth, before it destroys neighboring tissues or spreads to other parts of the body.

PRECANCERS. These, in themselves, are harmless changes in the tissues of the body. Their danger lies in the fact that they have a *tendency to become cancerous.* They include *leukoplakia* of the mouth and tongue, thickened white patches (*not* ordinary canker sores); some *moles;* any *chronically irritated spot* on the skin or the mucous membranes of the mouth and tongue; *polyps,* such as those of the large intestine which, although harmless, can become cancerous; some forms of lymph gland tumors such as the slowly growing follicular type of *lymphoma.*

It is most important to know about precancers, so that they can be removed or destroyed in time to prevent the possible development of a potentially serious cancer.

HODGKIN'S DISEASE. We are not certain whether or not this disease is cancer. It usually afflicts young people, causing a progressive enlargement of the lymphatic glands (see page 115) throughout the body. In most cases, it starts in lymph glands located in the neck, the groin, the armpit, or even internally in the chest or abdomen. Because it can become widespread, invasive, and destructive like a cancer, and because it responds to treatments in the same way that cancers do, it is commonly classed as a type of cancer tumor.

LEUKEMIAS. In most forms of this disease, the number of white blood corpuscles increases tremendously—nature again failing to call "Halt!" They respond to cancer treatments. Therefore, doctors agree that the leukemias should be grouped with other cancer diseases at the present time.

## Cancer Is Not Contagious or Communicable

Fortunately, cancer is not contagious. No cancer has ever been transmitted from one patient to another. In the laboratory, scientists have succeeded in transmitting *animal* tumors and cancers. However, doctors, pathologists, nurses, and others who handle human cancer daily have never "caught" the disease. It is therefore perfectly safe to visit, associate with, or care for anyone who is sick, or even dying, from cancer.

## WARNING SIGNALS OF CANCER

Cancers cause different symptoms according to their location, state of development, and so on. In a moment, I shall tell you more about cancers in specific parts of the body. Be sure to read the sections that apply especially to you: for example, cancer of the prostate gland if you are a man, and cancer of the breast and of the uterus if you are a woman.

Here I shall list the main warnings which cancer gives. I have written about them before (see page 386), but they are important enough to be repeated. *Everyone should be familiar with all of them.* It can mean a great deal to you—or to your dear ones who may not know these signals.

### THE EARLY DANGER SIGNS OF CANCER

1. Any lump or thickening, especially in the breast, lip, or tongue.
2. Any irregular or unexplained bleeding. Blood in the urine or bowel movements. Blood or bloody discharge from the nipple or any body opening. Unexplained vaginal bleeding or discharge, or any bleeding after the menopause.
3. A sore that does not heal, particularly around the mouth, tongue, or lips, or anywhere on the skin.
4. Noticeable changes in the color or size of a wart, mole, or birthmark.
5. Loss of appetite or continual indigestion.
6. Persistent hoarseness, cough, or difficulty in swallowing.
7. Persistent change in normal elimination (bowel habits).

### Special Note: Pain Is Not Usually an Early Sign of Cancer

None of the above signs *necessarily* means cancer. The *only way* to discover whether or not they mean cancer is by a complete examination. If any of these signs apply to you, go at once to your doctor, to a cancer detection clinic, or the clinic of a reputable hospital.

## SIGNS AND SYMPTOMS OF CANCER IN VARIOUS PARTS OF THE BODY

### Stomach Cancer

(This is a common type of cancer, especially in men.)
1. Continued lack of appetite.
2. Continued indigestion not due to faulty habits of diet.
3. Pain after eating.
4. Loss of weight.
5. Anemia.

### Cancer of the Colon and Rectum

1. Periods of constipation which mark a change from usual bowel habits, sometimes followed by episodes of more frequent elimination, or diarrhea.
2. Cramps in the abdomen and a sensation of incomplete elimination, or a feeling that there is a lump in the rectum.
3. Rectal pain, and rectal bleeding, e.g., blood spots on the toilet tissue or in the bowel movements.
4. Cancer of the rectum is often confused with hemorrhoids, or piles, and therefore may not be recognized in the early stage. A thorough physical examination by a doctor should determine whether the condition is piles or cancer. Sometimes piles appear suddenly, due to a cancer higher up in the rec-

tum. Do not neglect hemorrhoids (see page 509).

## Cancer of the Uterus

1. Increased or irregular vaginal discharges.
2. Return of vaginal bleeding after the menopause.

## Cancer of the Breast

(This is the most common malignancy among women.)

1. Painless lumps in the breast.
2. Bleeding or discharge from the nipple.

Cancer of the breast is most frequently found in women over the age of forty. Only one woman in a hundred develops cancer. And these cases can be cured if detected early. Women can train themselves to find early, curable tumors by self-examination of their breasts. It is not necessary to perform the following steps more than once a month:

a. Immediately after the menstruation period has ended, when the breasts are normally soft, look into a mirror and raise both arms over your head so that the sides of the breasts are visible. Study your breasts carefully, noting whether one breast looks higher than the other or whether one breast seems larger than it was the previous month. Also check on any slight depressions or dimpling of the skin over the breast.

b. Using the right hand on the left breast and vice versa, push the breast back gently against your chest and feel for any small lumps.

c. Feel the armpits for any swelling.

The best time to make this examination is in the morning. If you decide that something may be wrong, you have all day to reach your doctor, if only to get his reassurance. *Not every lump* in the breast means cancer. Many are harmless formations due to glandular functioning. Let your doctor decide. Fortunately, he can now avail himself of a special type of x-ray study for breast cancer, a technique called *mammography*.

Remember the motto: do not be alarmed, but be on the alert. Between the monthly checkups, *do not think about tumors, cysts, and cancer.* If you can't do this, and there are women who can't

dismiss it from their minds, read page 549 for my advice.

## Skin Cancer

(This is the easiest type to detect and cure.)

1. Sores and ulcers which do not heal.
2. Moles, warts, blemishes, scars, or birthmarks that suddenly change in color, size, or texture.
3. Growths constantly exposed to irritations, as, for example, from brassieres or from shaving.

For your own protection, don't use razor blade surgery or other home treatment on moles and warts.

## Lung Cancer

This form of cancer has been on the increase in recent decades. Most medical authorities attribute this to increased smoking. Lung cancer is prevalent among heavy smokers, who use more than a package of cigarettes a day, but it can also strike nonsmokers. Chain smoking of cigarettes, pipes, or cigars is a medically risky habit, as well as expensive. (See my comments on the calculated risk in health, page 547).

1. A cough which does not let up after two weeks, or a change in an old "cigarette cough." Wheezing or other noises in the chest.
2. Coughing up blood or bloody sputum. Any sputum which looks rusty, pink, or blood-streaked.
3. Shortness of breath without a good cause like running or climbing steps.
4. Chest ache or pain.

Many of the symptoms of cancer of the lung are like those of tuberculosis. Unfortunately, the early curable stages of both sicknesses do not produce any symptoms. For double protection, get an immediate and thorough examination, including an x-ray, to protect yourself against the development of either cancer or tuberculosis. And then have an x-ray of your lungs taken each year. Not even a lung specialist can detect the *earliest* stages of tuberculosis or cancer by means of the stethoscope alone.

## Cancer of the Mouth, Tongue, and Lips

This is found more often in people who neglect their teeth, have ill-fitting dentures, or have not paid attention to persistent sores or other abnormalities in the mouth. Tongue cancer may be encouraged by prolonged smoking of a pipe or cigar which is held in the same position in the mouth, for example, in the man who always lets his pipe hang from one side of his mouth so that the smoke hits the same spot on the tongue. Watch for:

1. Any sore which does not heal.
2. Any white patch replacing the normal pink color of the tongue or the inside of the mouth.

Avoid irritation of the tongue or inner cheek surface by prompt repair of jagged teeth or poorly fitted dental plates.

## Kidney, Bladder, and Prostate Cancers

Some of the following signs more often mean prostate enlargement (see page 481), which is not cancer, than actual cancer of this gland:

1. Blood in the urine, or reddish or pink urine.
2. Difficulty in starting urination.
3. Increasing frequency of arising at night to pass urine.
4. Burning sensation during urination.

## Brain Tumors and Cancers

Benign and malignant growths can affect the brain. Even a benign tumor of the brain may become serious because, as it grows, it cannot expand readily. The bony skullcase confines it. The pressure exerted by the tumor on the brain can damage or destroy parts of this vital organ. Brain tumors may cause:

1. Headaches
2. Disturbances of vision
3. Dizziness
4. Nausea and vomiting
5. Paralysis

## HOW CANCER IS DETECTED

I have mentioned some of the ways a cancer indicates its existence, pointing out that a thorough examination by a doctor is necessary to determine the real significance of these signs.

### The Medical Examination

A checkup for cancer requires a *thorough* examination. This must include the skin, the breasts, the genital organs, and the internal organs of the chest and abdomen. A vaginal examination is essential for women, and a rectal examination for both sexes. As I point out on page 382, no woman should gamble with her health, and perhaps her life, because of false modesty. Tell your doctor you desire a *complete* physical checkup.

Everyone should have routine examinations periodically, the frequency depending on one's age and other considerations (see page 379). After forty, a yearly checkup is advisable. When there is a danger signal, or any doubt concerning a possible danger signal, be sure to have an immediate examination.

### Additional Tests for Cancer

Do not be alarmed if your doctor suggests tests in addition to the routine examination. He may simply feel, as you do, that it is wise to take all precautions.

X-RAYS. A routine chest x-ray can be taken in conjunction with a physical checkup, or it can be performed independently. In many cities, free chest x-rays are made available. It is advisable to have one made every year, since early lung cancers, as well as tuberculosis and some diseases of the heart, can sometimes be detected in this way.

The free x-rays are usually small snapshots or microfilms. Your doctor may want to make a full-sized film of your chest. He may also want to take x-rays of other parts of the body.

For examination of the stomach and intestines, the x-ray involves special techniques which may seem fairly complicated, including the use of barium sulfate which is either swallowed or inserted through the rectum. When barium, in the form of a milky drink or enema, is in the stomach or large intestine, the organ is revealed as a silhouette on the x-ray film. In some instances, even this does not give the desired information, and still further examinations are needed.

SPECIAL EXAMINATIONS. Your doctor has available highly specialized instruments that are extremely valuable in studying the internal organs and locating small cancers in their early, curable stages. These instruments work on the principle of a periscope. A slender, usually flexible, tube is inserted into the region to be studied. A tiny bulb at the end lights up the area of the body which is being examined. Looking through the other end, the doctor can see this either directly or by a system of lenses or mirrors. Some of these methods, which I list below, require the services of a specialist.

Bronchoscopy: for the bronchi, the tubes leading to the lungs
Esophagoscopy: for the esophagus, the tube which leads from the throat to the stomach
Proctoscopy: for the rectum
Gastroscopy: for the stomach
Cystoscopy: for the bladder
Laryngoscopy: for the larynx, or voice box

RADIOISOTOPES are now used widely in diagnosing cancer in certain organs, such as the thyroid gland and liver. Radioactive forms of iodine, phosphorus, gold, iron, or cobalt tend to concentrate in certain organs, making it easier for doctors to diagnose the state of that part of the body.

## Biopsy

This is *the* definite way of determining whether or not even a tiny growth is cancerous or precancerous. A bit of tissue is removed and examined under the microscope. This examination is made by a *pathologist,* a doctor who specializes in determining from the appearance of the tissue whether it is normal or shows signs of a tumor or other disease.

The material for examination is obtained in different ways depending on the tissue or organ involved. It may be a very simple procedure which can be done in the doctor's office, or it may require an operation. Biopsies of some tumors are taken through the endoscopic examining instruments I listed above. Thus, growths in the rectum are biopsied through the proctoscope, and those in the lungs are often biopsied through the bronchoscope.

Sometimes it is not possible to perform a biopsy until the time of actual operation on a tumor, especially if it is located internally or deep in the breast. In such a case, a small piece of tissue is removed during the operation and given to the waiting pathologist, who freezes it immediately, examines it under the microscope, and gives the report to the surgeon. This procedure is called the "frozen section technique." The findings of the pathologist enable the surgeon to know how to proceed with the operation. If the tissue is not cancerous or precancerous, he may remove very little—in certain circumstances, nothing at all. If it is cancerous, he will remove a far larger amount of tissue. Even though a doctor may be fairly certain in advance that a growth is benign or that it is malignant (cancerous), the biopsy provides practically 100 percent proof.

A biopsy is a valuable method of diagnosing diseases other than cancer, including some mild but troublesome ailments such as chronic skin condition. Do not be frightened if your doctor suggests a biopsy. Let him make the decision.

## The Papanicolaou ("Pap") Smear Test

This simple test is used in detecting cancers of the lung, of the stomach, and particularly of the cervix, the mouth of the womb. A bit of fluid obtained from these parts of the body is put on a glass slide and placed under the microscope. Many cancers have been detected in this way when they were still so small that they caused no symptoms, did no damage, and were completely curable.

## Blood Test

It would be wonderful if we could take a sample of blood and, by studying it, determine whether or not a cancer was present in any part of the body. Medical science has not yet advanced this far. The blood is tested chemically for cancer of the prostate and for a rare malignancy of the bone marrow called *multiple myeloma*. A blood smear and blood count help in the diagnosis of *leukemias,* but this is not a chemical test. As yet there is no general blood test which will indicate whether a cancer of any type is growing somewhere in the body. Reports of such tests raise our hopes, but so far none of them has proved to be completely accurate. Perhaps a dependable blood test will be developed. Do not depend on such a test, or any other "new test for cancer" you may hear about, without first checking with your doctor.

## THE TREATMENT OF CANCER

The aim of cancer treatment is the *complete* removal or destruction of all cancerous tissue. Once this has been accomplished, the cancer is gone just as surely as a fire that has been extinguished. In many cases, this can be done before the cancer has caused any damage.

### Surgery

The principle of cancer surgery is the total *removal* of *all* of the cancer. The surgeon cuts away some of the normal tissue as well, so that he can be certain of getting all the cancer cells. If a cancer is large or internally situated, this is a major surgical procedure. It must always be undertaken by a qualified specialist in a good hospital. (See page 371 on how to locate a qualified specialist in surgery. He will operate only in an accredited hospital.)

### X-ray, Radium, and Cobalt

The principle of x-ray, radium, and cobalt treatments for cancer is total *destruction* of *all* the cancer. They give off penetrating radiation which damages tissue, especially tissue that is growing. Since cancer tissue grows rapidly, it is destroyed

more rapidly than the normal body tissue. Some types of malignant growths are affected more quickly than others by radium, x-ray, or cobalt.

These treatments must be administered by specialists. *Excess* radiation can be very harmful, since it will destroy normal as well as cancerous tissue. Your family doctor may be able to recommend a competent *roentgenologist* (radiologist). Or follow the suggestions on page 371 which describe how to locate a specialist. If you cannot afford his services, be sure to follow the suggestions on page 408 regarding clinics, medical centers, and so on. This is no time for halfway measures of false pride!

Surgery, x-ray, radium, or radioactive cobalt may be used singly or in conjunction with one another.

### Medicines and Chemicals

Certain substances are helpful in the treatment of certain cancers. Some chemical compounds *retard* the growth of cancer. *Nitrogen mustard,* for example, has been used for leukemias and Hodgkin's disease.

More recently, a whole series of *anticancer chemicals* have been developed and doctors have been arriving at methods of making the best possible use of them, sometimes singly, sometimes in various combinations, to combat more and more types of cancer. Additionally, certain materials have been found helpful in stimulating the body's immune, or defense, system so that it helps to wipe out cancerous cells. Commonly now, *chemotherapy* (use of anticancer chemicals) and *immunotherapy* (use of agents to stimulate the immune system) are combined with surgery or radiation for more effective treatment.

Certain cancers respond to treatment with *hormones,* such as stilbestrol, a female hormone, which is given for cancer of the prostate, and certain of the male hormones which are used in treating cancer of the breast.

*Radioactive isotopes* have been helpful in diagnosing and treating certain cancers, notably *radioactive iodine* for cancer of the thyroid, which is quite rare. The isotope is taken by mouth in water. *Radioactive phosphorus* is being used in some diseases of the blood-forming organs, especially in *polycythema vera,* also called *erythremia,* a rare disease in which too many red blood cells are produced.

## CONQUERING CANCER

Think of cancer as a powerful enemy. Think of yourself as equally powerful, possessing great allies in your doctor, the discoveries of medical science, and your own intelligence.

Cancer may never come near you. But do not count on that. Take steps to outwit, avoid, and fight cancer as you would any other danger that was lurking about.

1. The most important step is the regular physical checkup. Half of all cancers occur in parts of the body which the doctor can readily examine. The American Cancer Society estimates that 70,000 people in this country are saved every year by *early* treatment of cancer. Unfortunately, it also estimates that *another 70,000 could be saved*—but are not.

2. Avoid irritations and repeated injuries to your tissues that may pave the way for cancer. For example:

    a. Irritations of the tongue and inner cheek surfaces by jagged teeth or dental plates that do not fit properly.

    b. A black or hairy mole that is constantly being rubbed by clothing.

    c. Tears or scars of the womb, following childbirth, that have not been repaired.

    d. Dry or scaly patches on the neck or face that are constantly scraped raw by shaving.

    e. Exposure to cancer-causing substances such as coal tars, lubricating oils, paraffin, and arsenic. Always take proper precautions if you work with or handle these substances.

3. Keep your skin, mouth, and teeth clean. Visit your dentist, as well as your doctor, regularly.

4. If you are a woman, examine your breasts once a month by the method I described on page 433.

5. Don't discuss your symptoms with people outside the medical profession, and don't accept or give any advice except "SEE YOUR DOCTOR." There is not time to "try the medicine that absolutely cured Mrs. Smith whose condition was just like yours." And there is no need for the worry that well-meaning people often cause. Let your doctor or a cancer clinic decide for you.

6. Beware of "sure cures" for cancer. They are promised by quacks, either deliberate fakers or self-deceived crackpots. Some innocent people advocate a "cancer cure" because they believe it actually worked on them. The fact is that they did not have cancer in the first place. No matter what the "cure" consists of—ointments, salves, herbs, lotions, medicines, mysterious "rays," or vapors—it is a fraud and a menace to your health. It will not only take the money you need for proper treatment, but cause you to lose valuable, often critical, time which you should be spending under a doctor's care. Some "cures" actually cause a cancer to grow more rapidly. Only a reputable doctor or clinic can make use of surgery, x-ray, radium, and other reliable methods of curing or treating cancer.

7. Learn the danger signals on page 432. I repeat this once again because it is so important. If you have, or suspect you have, any of them, go to a reputable physician or clinic *at once.* Time is cancer's greatest ally.

8. Get the best possible treatment if cancer strikes. Increasingly now, such treatment is combination therapy. It calls for a concerted attack. For that, a team of specialists—in surgery, radiation, chemotherapy, immunotherapy—may be required. Such treatment may not always be available in small community hospitals. If your physician advices treatment at a major medical center, where the best approach to therapy can be expected, it is wise to follow his advice, even if it means that you have to travel some distance.

Great strides are being made in conquering cancer. Never before in the history of medicine have so much money, effort, and intelligence been mobilized to combat this powerful foe. We are still far from our ultimate goal of finding the cause and cure of every type of cancer. But the death rate for many types of cancer has been greatly reduced in recent years. Thousands of lives have been saved and are being saved every year from death due to this Killer.

Let me give you just a few examples. Little more than a decade ago, childhood leukemia was almost uniformly fatal. Today the cure rate is well over 50 percent and mounting rapidly. At one time, Hodgkin's disease was 75 percent fatal; today, more than 80 percent of patients are being cured. The cure rate for Wilms' tumor—a kidney cancer and one of the most common malignancies of childhood—now is topping 80 percent. Recently, newer methods of treating lung cancer have begun to change the once almost hopeless picture for that malignancy. Cure rates, too, are moving upward with encouraging rapidity for other cancers, including those of the colon and rectum.

But medical science alone cannot conquer cancer. You must play your part calmly, alertly, and intelligently in order that *you* will be victorious in the fight against cancer.

# ACCIDENTS

Accidents are a leading cause of death and disability. They occur mainly in the home, on the streets and highways, and on the job.

I have discussed accidents and their prevention in the home and on the job on pages 321 and 142. Now I want to say something about accidents on the highways in order to help eliminate this frightful menace.

Being a parent, I share the terrible anxiety of most parents regarding highway accidents to children. As a physician, I see what the average person, perhaps unfortunately, does not see: the mangled bodies which arrive at the hospital after the accidents. For every death, there are usually several people who are injured. Some of them are permanently crippled or disfigured, or they never recover full use of their brain.

Highway accidents kill many *young people* who are just on the threshold of life. The death and disability rate among teen-agers in automobile accidents is horrifying.

What can parents and doctors do about the deaths from highway accidents? First, we must

*set an example* for our children by being safe drivers ourselves. This means following the rules for good driving set down by the National Safety Council and other experts in accident prevention. And we must stick to these rules at all times. How can we expect teen-age children who are just beginning to handle cars to become safe drivers when they hear their parents or parents' friends *boasting* of the high speed of the new car, or the way they "got away" with a bit of recklessness on the road, or, worst of all, how they made it home from a party after too many drinks.

## Prevention of Accidents

1. THE EQUIPMENT FACTOR. Automobile accidents can be reduced by keeping your car in the best possible shape. That means having good brakes, good windshield wipers, nonglaring lights. Right and left turn indicators are helpful. An extra rear-view mirror should be installed on the driver's side. I use blowout-proof tires, and feel much happier about driving, having once had a tire fail on a mountain road. And, equally important, is the periodic checkup of the car's equipment. Find the equipment defects before they cause trouble.

Safety belts are standard equipment on new cars. Safety harnesses, which come over the shoulder and attach to a belt around the waist, offer even greater protection against injury in accidents. Headrests for the front-seat passengers can ward off the serious effects of whiplash injury to the neck.

2. THE PERSONAL FACTOR. The personal equation, the human factor, is a big one in accidents. Most of us love high speed. We even like danger. But when high speed leads to death and disability, it just doesn't pay. Highway accidents would be greatly reduced if everyone observed the legal speed limits. It is amazing how much more you enjoy driving when you decide in advance that you will reach your destination at safe rates of speed. You even remember the scenery. You can enjoy talking to whomever accompanies you. And you keep out of hospital accident wards!

Young people who are "speed crazy," and who won't change their habits after discussions with parents, should be required to discuss this with the family doctor. He will tell them what lies ahead from accidents. Also, he will try to explain and channel the tensions of youth that are behind the need for "daredevil" driving. The worst offenders should consult a psychiatrist before they kill not only themselves but a carload of their teen-age classmates.

People should not drive who have been drinking whiskey, wine, or beer. Is there a safe amount? That depends entirely on the individual. It is best to let the nondrinker in the group do the driving, or to take a taxi. (Alcoholic beverages are discussed on page 22.)

3. THE HEALTH FACTOR. Every driver should have good vision, good hearing, and be in good health. If there is any question about this, let your doctor help you overcome the physical defect before you have an accident. There are amazingly few diseases which are an absolute bar to driving. Usually, it depends on the severity of the illness. Everyone with a definitely diagnosed chronic illness that affects the nerves, brain, heart, muscles, etc., should discuss hazards in driving with his doctor.

## What to Do When an Accident Occurs on the Highway

I have covered most of what needs to be done in the first aid chapter, in the section on fractures and under such titles as shock, hemorrhage, etc.

Always stop severe bleeding first. Then treat shock. Set up roadblocks, flashlights, or flares to prevent the injured (and yourself) from being hit by other cars.

Remember that emergency ambulances take the injured to the nearest hospital or doctor. Its facilities may not be adequate for serious injuries. Have your own doctor notified at once, even if you are many miles away. Your doctor may want to call in a brain surgeon or an orthopedic specialist to help the local doctor in the event of severe concussions or a broken back or neck.

If you decide on local medical care for severe injuries, it is best to rely on the hospital superintendent. Ask him to call the Chief of the Surgical Service. This physician will either take over or, after surveying the situation, assign a competent brain, orthopedic, or reconstructive surgeon as the

findings demand. In some severe injuries from highway accidents, several surgeons will be required for the different types of injuries.

A last word: the most careful automobile driver I have met is a busy plastic and reconstructive surgeon who specializes in automobile accident cases!

## THE LUNGS

Everyone knows that we must have lungs in order to breathe the air we need to sustain life itself. I have described the lungs and the essential work they do on page 94. Fortunately, like the kidneys, they have a tremendous reserve capacity. It is possible to live comfortably even if one lung has been completely destroyed or removed. But we must have a definite amount of healthy lung tissue in order to breathe adequately. If too much of it becomes infected or destroyed, we eventually succumb because of lack of oxygen. In severe infections of the lungs, such as pneumonia and tuberculosis, the patient faces an additional danger from the toxins, or poisons, of the germs causing these diseases.

The lungs can also be destroyed in other ways. For example, silica and asbestos, if inhaled for a long time, turn the delicate, porous lungs into tough fibrous masses. Air cannot get through the fibrous lungs, and the patient faces suffocation. Industrial workers should guard against the dangers of silica and other irritants (see my chapter on your job and your health, especially page 141).

In middle-aged and older people, the lungs sometimes lose their elastic, porous quality. The millions of tiny air sacs begin to break down and the lungs lose some of their ability to absorb oxygen from the air and give off the body's waste carbon dioxide. This disease, known as *emphysema*, affects large numbers of people, many of whom suffer without knowing exactly why. This disease may claim as many as 50,000 lives annually. Studies have shown that about 90 percent of all emphysema sufferers are heavy smokers—another urgent reason you should cut down or cut out smoking.

Some other less common, but potentially serious, lung diseases include lung *abscesses, bronchiectasis,* a chronic infection of the air tubes, *sarcoid-*

*osis, cystic disease,* and *fungus* infections such as coccidioidomycosis (San Joaquin Valley fever), actinomycosis, and blastomycosis. I have described cancer of the lung on page 433.

Fortunately, almost every Killer disease of the lungs can be prevented, cured, or alleviated—IF the advice given in this book is followed, and the doctor is given a chance to treat the disease in its early stages.


## CHRONIC BRONCHITIS AND EMPHYSEMA

Most people are aware of the serious problem of lung cancer. But the major single cause of disability of lung origin in the United States is emphysema rather than lung cancer. It causes a significant number of deaths each year in itself and in addition is often a contributing factor to deaths from surgery, heart disease, other lung diseases, and many other disorders.

Many factors are known to predispose to emphysema. Chief among them is cigarette smoking. Rarely is someone who has never smoked affected by the disorder. And often severity is directly related to the number of cigarettes smoked.

Air pollution and exposure to industrial fumes of some types increase the severity of respiratory symptoms. Recently, an inherited defect in the production of a certain enzyme has been detected in some patients with emphysema. It seems to be particularly common among those seriously affected at a younger age than most.

Detection of emphysema and chronic bronchitis —and I will shortly discuss how one compares with the other—is complicated by their insidious nature. They may take a long time to produce symptoms and by then may have caused considerable damage.

Certain clues, however, can make a physician suspicious that a patient may be showing early signs of chronic bronchitis or emphysema. One is a history of chronic "cigarette cough," usually worse in the morning on arising and frequently productive of sputum. Another is a history of frequent respiratory infections which are severe and take long to resolve. There are other possible clues: on physical examination, the physician may detect some wheezing after forced expiration or may find an increase in chest diameter ("barrel chest").

Not everyone with such symptoms and signs necessarily has emphysema or chronic bronchitis, but the physician may suspect this is the likely diagnosis if there is no past history of asthma, other lung or heart disease, and if there is a smoking history of some duration. By making use of certain simple lung function tests (spirography), the physician can confirm the diagnosis.

The regular medical checkup is the time for detection of symptoms and signs that indicate that emphysema may be present—and with early detection, appropriate measures can be taken to prevent worsening. All too often it is severe shortness of breath or severe respiratory infection that brings the emphysema patient to the doctor for the first time—at a point when much damage may already have been done.

Are chronic bronchitis and emphysema different diseases? When lung tissue is examined under the microscope, a distinction can be made. But during life the distinction is hazy because the two problems often coexist. For this reason, they are frequently described together under the name of *chronic obstructive lung disease (COLD)* or *chronic obstructive pulmonary emphysema (COPE).* The word *obstructive* refers to the changes in the air passages which conduct air to the lungs.

The air passages, called *bronchi* and *bronchioles,* have cells that destroy invading organisms. They have other cells that produce mucus to trap foreign material. The mucus is washed up to the throat, where it is swallowed or eliminated through the mouth and nose. Cigarette smoke impairs these mechanisms and particularly hampers proper elimination of mucus. As a result, chronic infection sets in, destroying or weakening and narrowing the bronchioles. Retained mucus acts to narrow the air passages, too, making cough less efficient and leading to further retention of mucus and narrowing of the bronchioles.

As a result of the obstruction and distortion of lung architecture, a greater force is needed to expel air. This puts abnormal strain on the walls of the *alveoli.* These are the little sacs in the lungs where oxygen and carbon dioxide are exchanged. With abnormally high and prolonged pressure, the alveoli become overdistended and disrupted.

The stage of mucus collection and chronic inflammation is called chronic bronchitis; the stage in which the alveoli are destroyed is called emphysema. During the chronic bronchitis phase, the patient may have persistent cough and sputum production; it is when the alveoli become compromised that shortness of breath sets in.

In the beginning of obstructive lung disease, there may be persistent cough and repeated respiratory infections. Gradually infections become more severe and disabling for longer periods. Shortness of breath and wheezing will sooner or later become evident, progressively limiting activity. But these indications may take as few as five years or as many as thirty years to appear.

The earlier treatment begins, the better. Among the most important measures are elimination of cigarette smoking and avoidance of irritating fumes (perhaps requiring use of air filtering devices in the home). Colds and minor respiratory infections will be treated vigorously to try to avoid serious lung infection. In some instances, antibiotic treatment may be needed continuously.

Exercises may be prescribed for developing muscles ordinarily not used for breathing. These muscles can help increase breathing effectiveness.

Methods of promoting drainage of mucus through positioning of the body are of value. Medications to help liquefy thick secretions or help keep bronchioles open are often used. In some cases, periodic treatment with a machine that pushes air into the lungs (*intermittent positive-pressure breathing,* or *IPPB*) to help open collapsed areas in order to drain mucus collections or prevent their formation is valuable.

Milder forms of chronic bronchitis and emphysema can be handled by the family doctor. More advanced cases require the care of specialists.

## TUBERCULOSIS

The *tubercle bacillus,* the germ causing tuberculosis, usually attacks the lungs, although it sometimes invades other parts of the body such as the kidneys, lymph nodes, skin, larynx, bones, joints, intestines, and certain portions of the male and female sexual organs. It only rarely attacks the heart, liver, or brain.

Tuberculosis germs work slowly as compared with many other disease germs. That gives us valuable time to fight the disease before it does any permanent damage. But while it takes a long time for tuberculosis to develop, it may take even longer to cure it.

### How Tuberculosis Is Contracted

A certain number of cases of tuberculosis are caused by *unpasteurized milk* and other dairy products which may contain tuberculosis germs. Tuberculosis of the lungs, however, is caused by germs which are transferred to healthy people from the lungs of a sick person in sputum which he coughs up. Tuberculosis germs can live for months in dried sputum.

Patients with known cases of tuberculosis are taught to protect others by covering every cough or sneeze with a handkerchief or cleansing tissue. However, there are believed to be 300,000 people in this country who have been infected with tuberculosis and do not know it. Some of them have reached the stage where they can infect others. Most people, particularly city dwellers, will be exposed to these germs sooner or later. Fortunately, this does not mean that they will all contract tuberculosis.

When tuberculosis germs reach the lungs and begin to multiply there, the body rushes its defenses to the infected area. The body is almost always victorious in this *first* skirmish. It kills some of the germs and covers the remainder with tough scar tissue. Although the imprisoned germs stay alive, they are rendered powerless. This first infection usually causes no symptoms. However, it is important to know about it in order to take precautions to keep the germs localized.

A simple skin test enables the doctor to find out whether or not tubercle bacilli have ever entered the body. If this *tuberculin test* is positive, the doctor will then proceed to discover whether the germs are safely imprisoned or whether they are active and causing disease. The *only sure way* of doing this is by an x-ray photograph.

Today, having chest x-rays taken is far simpler and easier than posing for ordinary photographs. They are available at little or no cost, through hospital clinics, factories, or mobile community x-ray units. Through the countless numbers of these x-ray pictures that have been made, it has been clearly shown that many people who have had an infection do not develop *active* tuberculosis. This indicates nature's capacity to fight tuberculosis germs. But these x-ray pictures perform the far more valuable service of detecting active tuberculosis in its very early stages, before it has done any real damage and can most easily be cured.

## Symptoms of Tuberculosis

A child or very young person with active tuberculosis will usually suffer from one or more of the following: loss of pep, poor appetite, loss of weight, and fever. Even though these symptoms may be caused by something other than tuberculosis, they must be regarded as warning signals. The tuberculin test is very helpful in diagnosis where young children are concerned.

In older people, listlessness and vague pains in the chest may go unnoticed as they are often not severe enough to attract attention. Unfortunately, the symptoms which most people associate with tuberculosis—cough, sputum raising, fever, loss of weight, and hemorrhage from the lungs—do not appear when the disease is still in its early, most easily curable stage. Often these symptoms do not occur until a year or more after the germs have started their attack. In aged people, the symptoms are apt to be very mild (see page 534). In its early stages, the disease can usually be detected *only* by an x-ray of the lungs.

## The Treatment and Cure of Tuberculosis

Long periods of rest in sanatoria, usually placed in the fresh surroundings of countryside or mountainous areas, were once commonly prescribed for tuberculosis sufferers. Major chest surgery was frequently resorted to. Now, powerful medicines have been developed for the treatment of tuberculosis. These include *isoniazid, streptomycin,* and *para-aminosalicylic acid* (PAS), sometimes used in combination. Other effective agents also are available and may be used. They include *ethambutol, rifampin,* and *viomycin.* Bed rest and a relaxing atmosphere still are recommended, along with the new medications, although the period of rest is not nearly so long as it once was. All the sanatoria have not been shut down, but home care, under a doctor's watchful eye, is much more frequent than it was only a decade ago.

TREATMENT OF OTHER TYPES OF TUBERCULOSIS. Tuberculosis of the lymph glands, the kidneys, genitals, etc., is usually treated in much the same way as lung tuberculosis. Whether rest, medicines, or surgery—or a combination—should be employed will generally require a consultation between the family doctor and a specialist in tuberculosis.

## How to Prevent Tuberculosis

Tuberculosis is one of the most easily avoided of all the Killers. The best precautions are (1) keeping in good condition, (2) avoiding unnecessary exposure to tuberculosis germs, and (3) detecting tuberculosis in its earliest stages. A burning match may go out by itself, but it *may also cause a fire.* Why not put it out when it can easily be extinguished?

Here are some rules to follow:

1. Have a medical checkup every year (see page 379). Be sure it includes a tuberculin test or an x-ray picture of the chest. The stethoscope alone cannot detect *early tuberculosis.*

2. Go to a doctor or hospital clinic for an x-ray and examination if you have a cough, cold, or bronchitis that does not clear up in two or three weeks, if you are tired and listless, lose weight, have pains in your chest, "night sweats," a fever, or cough up blood or blood-streaked sputum.

3. Keep your resistance to tuberculosis high by regular and sufficient sleep, meals, and relaxation. Be sure your diet is properly balanced, your work not too exhausting, and your home and place of work comfortably warm and free from dampness. (See Chapters 1, 2, 8 and 22.)

4. Use pasteurized milk only. The tuberculosis germs in cattle may be transmitted through unpasteurized milk, causing tuberculosis of the bones, joints, and lymph nodes, especially in children. See page 137 for directions on home

pasteurization of milk if you cannot buy it in your community.

5. Keep a good distance from people, inside your home and outside, who cough, especially if they do not cover their mouths with a handkerchief or tissue. Make "covering a cough" a habit in your family.

6. Wash your hands before meals or after you have touched articles which are apt to be contaminated—for example, a subway strap.

7. If you have a family history of tuberculosis, tell your doctor, and be especially careful about following these rules. Although tuberculosis is not inherited, it does tend to appear more frequently in some families than in others.

8. If someone with whom you or any member of your household is in contact develops tuberculosis, be sure to have a checkup and x-ray immediately, and again in six months. Don't get panicky about this. Being exposed certainly does not mean that you have been infected. But do not ignore the possibility of danger. Why wait until you smell smoke before you discover whether or not the match is burning?

Since the beginning of this century, tuberculosis has dropped from Number One to Number Thirteen in the list of Killers. This has not happened by accident! Our knowledge of this disease should make it possible to remove it from the list entirely, to force this enemy into unconditional surrender. With your help, and that of others, tuberculosis can be rendered powerless.

# PNEUMONIA

Pneumonia, an infection of the lungs, can be caused by (1) the *pneumococcus* or certain other bacteria or (2) *viruses*. Both types are infectious and can spread from person to person. Most people carry the pneumococcus and other pneumonia-causing germs in their throats at all times, but when they are well and strong, the germs do no harm. When the body is weakened, resistance to the pneumonia germs is lowered, and the body cannot successfully fight against them. The time to be most on guard is just after an ordinary cold begins, especially the third and fourth day, and during and after an attack of influenza, whooping cough, or measles. Overexposure to cold after a great deal of sweating, and insufficient rest, also create conditions favorable for an attack of pneumonia.

If the disease affects one or more lobes of the lung, it is called *lobar* pneumonia. When both lungs are affected, the lay person usually calls it "double pneumonia." The doctor terms it *bilateral*. *Bronchopneumonia* refers to pneumonia that is localized chiefly in or around the bronchial tubes. It is usually, but not necessarily, milder than lobar pneumonia.

## First Signs of Pneumonia

The symptoms are easily recognized except in aged people (see page 534). They are: a cough, sharp chest pains, blood-streaked sputum, and a high fever which generally starts with a shaking chill. Anyone with these danger signals should get into bed immediately and remain there. The doctor should be called promptly. This is an emergency disease. Every moment counts in curing it. If treatment is started at once, the chances for recovery are excellent.

## Pneumonia Caused by Bacteria

Most people who speak of pneumonia refer to this type. If the germs happen to be the pneumococcal variety, the chest pain, cough, bloody sputum, and fever usually start suddenly. With some other bacteria, the symptoms appear more gradually. This form of pneumonia occurs most frequently in the late winter and early spring.

Bacterial pneumonia was one of the leading Killers a generation ago. Today, thanks to medicines such as penicillin and other antibiotics and the sulfa compounds, the danger to the patient's life has been practically eliminated—*provided that treatment is started in time*. The new drugs, miraculous as they are, can do little good if this Killer disease has made too much headway.

## Viral Pneumonia (Primary Atypical Pneumonia)

This form of pneumonia is called atypical because it was previously far less common than the bacterial variety. However, now that pneumonias due to bacteria have been greatly reduced, the atypical type is more prevalent. It is rarely fatal except in patients with complicating illnesses. Actually, atypical pneumonia may be more often caused by organisms called *Mycoplasma*, which are a kind of bacteria, rather than by viruses. If the causative organisms are *Mycoplasma*, the disease will respond to antibiotics.

## Prevention

Because the new medicines have rapidly cured so many cases of pneumonia, some people are beginning to forget that it is still a potentially serious disease. Don't make that mistake. It is well worth your while to guard against pneumonia.

The best prevention is good general health. Get plenty of rest and nourishing meals. Avoid overexposure and take immediate care of a cold. Avoid contact with others who have colds. Most of us carry around many germs which do not harm us because our bodies have built up a resistance to them. But we may be powerless before an invasion of "foreign" germs from another individual.

For some people—such as those in older age groups and those with chronic diseases such as diabetes and heart, liver, and kidney disease, who may be particularly susceptible—a new vaccine is 90 percent effective in immunizing against pneumococcal pneumonia.

# DISEASES OF THE LIVER AND GALLBLADDER

In the chapter on everyday care of the parts of the body, I told you some important things about the liver and gallbladder. If you turn to page 102 and review them, it will help you to a better understanding of the diseases of these organs.

There is only one *liver* in our bodies. It is an absolutely indispensable organ. Complete removal or destruction is followed by death in a very short time. Fortunately for all of us, nature has given us a tremendous amount of reserve liver tissue. It has been estimated that more than 80 percent of the liver cells can be damaged or destroyed before symptoms of liver insufficiency will appear. Another very fortunate fact about the liver is its great capacity for regeneration and rebuilding itself after disease has injured the cells or even destroyed large numbers of them.

As with the kidneys and lungs, if too much of the liver is destroyed by disease, a condition of insufficiency sets in. If this is not corrected early enough, disability and eventual death will occur.

The *gallbladder*, on the other hand, can be removed completely without harm to the body. It appears to be a quite unnecessary organ.

When the gallbladder is removed, the *bile* flows directly into the intestines. Even though the gallbladder may not be essential, the *bile* is needed to help in the digestion of food. Furthermore, the liver removes some of the waste products from the blood stream and disposes of them in the bile. These waste products are then eliminated in the feces. The brown color of bowel movements is due to bile. If the liver becomes diseased, the bile may not be disposed of properly. It may then pile up in the blood stream, causing the eyes and skin to become yellow. This yellowing is termed *jaundice*. It is most easily observed in the eyes. However, it may come on so gradually that it is not immediately noticed by those who are in daily contact with the jaundiced person.

Jaundice is often an indication of a disease of the liver, although it can be due to other things. For example, if the tube leading from the liver and the gallbladder to the intestine is blocked by a stone loosened from the gallbladder, the bile will accumulate and get into the blood stream, causing jaundice. Certain diseases of the blood, such as *hemolytic anemia,* increase the amount of the yellow pigment of the bile. This, too, will cause jaundice.

A particular type of liver disease that also causes jaundice is *hepatitis*. Hepatitis is an inflammation of the liver that produces other symptoms such as appetite loss, nausea, fever, tenderness in the region of the liver, and liver enlargement. Hepatitis sometimes may stem from another disorder such as cirrhosis of the liver or infectious mononucleosis. It may be caused by alcoholism without cirrhosis, toxic materials such as carbon tetrachloride, phosphorus, some anesthetic agents, antibiotics and other medications. It also may be a viral infection. The virus may be transmitted through contaminated foods or liquids or by transfusion of infected blood. There is no specific drug treatment for hepatitis. Once, strict bed rest and a low-fat, high-carbohydrate diet were considered essential but no longer are, and diet and activity may be adapted to the individual patient's condition. In very severe cases, prednisone and growth hormone have been used, although their value is uncertain. Exchange blood transfusion is credited with enabling some severely afflicted patients to recover. When hepatitis is due to a toxic material, the material must be removed.

Because jaundice can be caused in many ways, and because each condition requires different treatment, it is extremely important to see a doctor at the first sign of jaundice. He will determine its cause and prescribe proper treatment. Although it may not mean anything serious, jaundice must always be regarded as a danger signal.

## Other Important Danger Signals

Another symptom of liver disease may be a gradual, unexplained enlargement of the abdomen, with or without swelling of the ankles. Vomiting blood or passing bloody or black, tarlike stools are also symptoms of liver disease or other potentially serious disorders requiring immediate medical attention. Some symptoms of liver disease are not readily identified as such because they are often indications of other diseases. These include fatigue, loss of weight, nausea and poor appetite, anemia, and hemorrhoids. They, too, are warnings that should send you to the doctor for an examination.

Unfortunately, many people disregard jaundice and other symptoms that may indicate a liver disease. This is particularly sad, for although modern medicine can sometimes cure advanced cases of liver disease, the greatest progress has been made in curing it in its early stages.

## Cirrhosis of the Liver

Cirrhosis is a chronic disease in which liver cells degenerate and surrounding tissue thickens and scars. It is most likely to affect a middle-aged man with a history of chronic alcoholism. Cirrhosis also may have other causes such as severe hepatitis, malnutrition, and congestive heart failure.

The symptoms include fatigue, weight loss, low resistance to infections, and gastrointestinal disturbances. As the disease progresses, other symptoms may include jaundice, vomiting of blood, loss of libido and, in a woman, absence of menstruation.

Because of poor circulation of the blood through liver blood vessels, a backup of pressure may lead to *varices*, or swollen veins, in the esophagus which may rupture and drain blood into the stomach. In the latter case, surgery may be required to overcome the pressure backup.

Treatment for cirrhosis includes a nutritious high-protein diet, strict ban on alcohol, and often the use of vitamin supplements. A corticosteroid drug such as prednisone may be used in some cases. Distention of the abdomen with fluids may require fluid and salt restriction and use of a diuretic drug to help increase fluid elimination.

## Diseases of the Gallbladder

You may wonder why I include gallbladder diseases among the Killers when you may have known people who have suffered from them and considered them little more than a nuisance. I do so because I feel people are inclined to minimize these diseases, particularly women who are very apt to have mild gallbladder disturbances. They tend to take a casual attitude toward what *can be a Killer*, but need not be if taken seriously.

ACUTE INFLAMMATION OF THE GALLBLADDER (Acute Cholecystitis). When the gallbladder is acutely inflamed, the symptoms are generally extremely severe. There are acute pain and tenderness in the right upper part of the abdomen in the region of the gallbladder, accompanied by fever, nausea, vomiting, and prostration. Such a condition requires immediate attention, preferably in a hospital, because if the inflammation does not subside quickly, the gallbladder must be removed before it becomes gangrenous and ruptures. This complication is apt to be fatal. If the operation is performed early by a skilled surgeon, the chances of complete recovery are excellent. The operation for removal of the gallbladder is called *cholecystectomy*. Sometimes the patient is so sick, or the gallbladder area so inflamed, that the surgeon cannot operate to remove the organ. He then does a less demanding operation in which a drain is placed in the gallbladder. This procedure has the medical name of *cholecystostomy*.

GALLSTONES. We do not understand why stones form in the gallbladder. They are definitely associated with obesity and pregnancy. Women are more apt to be troubled by gallstones than are men. Gallstones may be present for years without ever causing trouble. All too frequently, patients are operated upon for gallstones when the problem is actually in the nearby stomach, duodenum, pancreas, liver, or kidney. That is why a serious operation such as the removal of gallstones should be undertaken only after your doctor has had plenty of time to study the situation. Also, he may very justifiably suggest a consultation with an internist or surgeon who specializes in diseases of the gallbladder.

Gallstones do cause real mischief, though much less than is usually attributed to them. The stones can move from the gallbladder along the tube leading into the intestines (the *common bile duct*,

*Figure 33-4. The Gallbladder.*

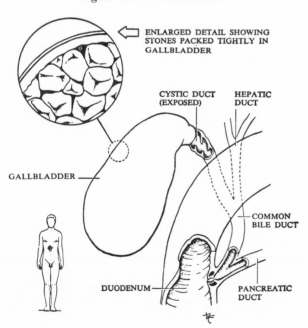

ENLARGED DETAIL SHOWING STONES PACKED TIGHTLY IN GALLBLADDER

CYSTIC DUCT (EXPOSED)  
HEPATIC DUCT

GALLBLADDER

COMMON BILE DUCT

DUODENUM

PANCREATIC DUCT

see Figure 33-4). On its way, the stone may cause severe pain which has a cramping, colicky quality and is one of the worst pains known. Such an attack of *gallbladder colic* may subside, or the stone may lodge in the main bile duct, causing obstruction of bile flow, and jaundice. This will require surgical removal. It is a very serious operation, especially if delayed to the point of extreme jaundice and impaired liver function. It should be performed only by a very experienced and skilled surgeon.

Usually, gallstones cause difficulty of a more chronic nature. They lead to symptoms of vague discomfort and pain in the upper abdomen. There may be dyspepsia, nausea, and an intolerance to fatty foods. Slight jaundice may be present. The existence of gallstones can be discovered by x-ray and other tests. If there is persistent trouble from stones, it is best to have them removed before one becomes lodged in the common bile duct. The operation, when performed under ideal conditions, is 99 percent safe. When removing the stones, most surgeons remove the entire gallbladder so that no stones can form later on. Gallstones are given the medical name *cholelithiasis*. Usually, some chronic infection or inflammation of the gallbladder accompanies the gallstones. This is named *chronic cholecystitis*. Sometimes, there is chronic inflammation of the gallbladder without any stones. The symptoms and treatment are much the same as for chronic gallstones.

## Other Potentially Serious Diseases of the Liver and Gallbladder

In addition to the diseases just described, there are others which can impair or destroy the liver. Infections such as abscesses may form in or around the liver. These may be caused by bacteria such as the staphylococcus or the colon bacillus. Also, the organism that causes *amebic dysentery* has a special predilection for the liver. Many patients with this type of dysentery develop liver abscess, which, fortunately, can be successfully treated. But it is best to get at the disease early enough so that it will not spread to the liver. Sheepherders in some foreign countries are frequently infected with a parasitic worm from their dogs. This condition may lead to a large *echinococcus cyst* of the liver which can be treated by surgery.

Cancer may arise as a primary neoplasm in the liver, or it may develop there as a secondary metastasis from a cancer of the stomach or some other part of the body. The gallbladder is subject to primary cancer. Syphilis may affect the liver.

# SYPHILIS

Penicillin and other medicines have revolutionized the treatment of this serious disease. However, this does *not* mean it is no longer a Killer. But it is tremendously reassuring to know that syphilis can be readily and *completely* cured. There is no longer any truth to the old saying "once a syphilitic, always a syphilitic." Fear and shame have been the greatest allies of this potentially terrible disease. Today, this fear is absolutely groundless. There is no need for shame. From the doctor's viewpoint, syphilis is a preventable and curable disease, not a punishment for sin.

Ironically, the fact that syphilis is curable seems to have made many people careless. The number of cases of syphilis is rising throughout the world, including the United States. I want to emphasize again and again that this is a serious disease and that it can harm the body beyond repair. As I discuss on page 105, the surest method of prevention is to avoid sexual intercourse with an infected person. If there is any doubt about the partner's health, a condom should be worn during intercourse, and the entire genital area scrubbed with soap and water afterward.

Syphilis is the correct medical name for this disease which is also called "the pox," "siff," "lues," "bad blood," and "haircut." In the main, it is transmitted through sexual contact. Infection can also occur through kissing. In extremely rare instances, it has been contracted by drinking from a glass previously used by a syphilitic person. It is not caught from contact with toilet seats.

The spiral-shaped germ of syphilis is called *Spirochaeta pallida* or *Treponema pallidum*. It is quite different from the germ causing gonorrhea, which is an entirely separate venereal disease (described on page 485). Both gonorrhea and syphilis may, however, be contracted together.

## Primary Syphilis

After the syphilis germs have entered the body, there is no sign of infection for a period which averages about three weeks, although it may range from ten days to three months. The first sign is a sore, or *chancre*, which usually appears on the spot where the germs have entered the body. A chancre can resemble a pimple, blister, or open sore. It is generally firm or hard, and accompanied by little or no pain. It is most frequently located on the sex organs, but may be on the lips or fingers. In men the sore is generally on the penis, although it may be on the skin nearby, including the thighs. Two or three chancres may be present simultaneously. In women, a chancre is sometimes concealed in the inner sex parts where it may not be seen or felt.

It is foolhardy to make guesses about sores on the sex organs. Even competent physicians often cannot tell whether or not a sore is a syphilitic chancre until they conduct special tests. By examining material from the sore under the microscope, they can see whether the germs of syphilis are present. *Any* sore on the sex organs should be examined and tested by a physician immediately. If it is not syphilis, a great deal of needless worry will be avoided. If it is syphilis, treatment can be started at once with assurance of a *prompt cure*.

Not all people infected with syphilis develop chancres.

The Wassermann and other blood tests for syphilis will usually fail to detect the disease at this early stage.

The chancre heals of its own accord without treatment, and is usually gone before the blood test is "positive"—that is, indicates the existence of syphilis. For this reason, people have been lulled into a false sense of security or have dropped treatment before they were cured.

## Secondary Syphilis

The second stage of the disease occurs about nine weeks after infection. A rash may appear, often covering the entire skin, including the palms of the hands and the soles of the feet. The rashes of secondary syphilis may resemble anything from measles to *psoriasis* (see page 506), so that even experienced doctors cannot be sure without a Wassermann test, which will be positive by this time. Sores of various kinds may appear in the lining of the mouth and throat and around the genitals and rectum. There may be pain in the bones and joints, often a fever, headache, and feelings of general illness. The eyes may become affected and, occasionally, the membranes of the nervous system. The secondary stage of syphilis disappears by itself, but the symptoms may return because the germs are still present. This second stage is highly contagious.

These stages of syphilis—the *primary* (chancre) and the *secondary*—are together called *early syphilis*. Strangely enough, during early syphilis the disease is most dangerous to others and least dangerous to the person who has it. It is in *late syphilis*, which may occur five, ten, or more years after the disease has been contracted, that the order is reversed, with the disease becoming less infectious to others and extremely dangerous to the victim.

## Late Syphilis

If undiscovered and untreated, syphilis may continue for many years before there is obvious harm to the body. If treatment is inadequate in the early stages, the blood test may become negative, but the person is still infected and vulnerable to the late, fatal stages.

Late syphilis may cause blindness or severe disease of the bones and joints, the skin, or the internal organs, since the unchecked spirochetes can invade every cell of the body. The forms of syphilis most often resulting in death are those that damage the nervous system and the heart.

Syphilis may attack the heart or the aortic valve and the main blood vessel leaving the heart, called the aorta. This causes disability or death from heart failure or from rupture of the weakened aorta (aneurysm).

The most serious form of syphilis of the nervous system is *paresis*, a severe disorder of the functions of the mind. If untreated, paresis will cause complete insanity and death. Another nervous disorder is *tabes dorsalis,* or *locomotor ataxia,* with loss of sensation of position. The person does not know where his legs are and loses his balance in the dark.

## Congenital Syphilis

One especially tragic form of this venereal disease is *congenital syphilis,* in which the germ is transmitted from the mother to the unborn infant. This may happen when there is no visible sign of illness in the mother. Such babies may be born dead or are later seriously handicapped with deformities such as blindness or deafness. *All* pregnant women owe it to their future children to have a routine blood test for syphilis in the first months of pregnancy. Early treatment will always prevent infection of the unborn child.

## Detection of Syphilis

Syphilis is very variable and may not show all, or even *any*, of the usual early symptoms. Detection requires routine testing for syphilis. This is done on admission to all good clinics and hospitals. Testing should also be included in every medical examination and should be conducted routinely and periodically, like free chest x-rays. These precautions are widely used at present, but they should be extended to include *everybody*.

## Prevention

The surest method of prevention is avoiding sexual intercourse with infected persons. Syphilis is not confined to prostitutes. It is impossible to tell by a person's appearance or social status whether he or she has syphilis. The condom or rubber sheath prevents the passage of the spirochetes during intercourse. However, the neighboring skin and thighs may become infected afterward. The minimum precaution includes thorough soap and water washing of exposed areas of the skin in addition to the use of a condom. Although "sanitubes" are of some value, the fact that they are used after coitus may not ensure *prevention* of infection if the condom has not been used. A condom plus soap and water washing should never be omitted. If any sore appears on the sex organs, a competent physician should be consulted at once. Any of the other symptoms described should take you to the doctor without fail.

*Syphilis can be eliminated completely in our country if we all recognize that this sinister Killer breeds on shame and ignorance.* It becomes a personal and social duty for all of us to expose the disease, wherever it may lurk. The health and happiness of too many families have been destroyed by false modesty and neglect.

Remember, your doctor does not sit in moral judgment on venereal diseases. He is interested only in prevention and cure.

## APPENDICITIS

Although appendicitis is not among the leading killers, it still claims some lives needlessly. It is more prevalent between the ages of ten and thirty, but there is no age that is immune.

When the appendix becomes inflamed and infected, the process can spread so fast that gangrene and rupture may set in within a matter of hours. Rupture of the appendix leads to peritonitis, one of the most serious of all diseases.

On page 102 in the chapter on the parts of the body, I describe the appendix, its location, and its apparent uselessness to the body.

### Cause of Appendicitis

The appendix is a hollow tube. If the end of this tube becomes plugged by a hard bit of fecal matter, intestinal worms, or other material, the normal drainage from the tubelike appendix cannot take place (see Figure 33-5). The appendix then becomes susceptible to bacterial infection. Streptococci, staphylococci, colon bacilli, and other types of germs find this a fertile soil for their activities. The germs multiply and cause inflammation. Visualize the situation as a sort of boil which will rupture into the peritoneal cavity unless (1) the body's defenses overcome the infection or (2) the surgeon removes the infected appendix before the "boil" breaks and discharges the pus.

### Symptoms of Appendicitis

Typically, at the beginning, there may be pain in the umbilical or navel area of the abdomen. Loss of appetite, nausea, and vomiting may follow. Although constipation is usual, about 10 percent of patients have diarrhea instead. After several hours, the pain usually shifts to the lower right abdomen over the appendix, is continuous, and may be dull or severe. Usually the pain is sharpened by movement, coughing or sneezing. There may be mild fever (up to 102°) in adults, sometimes high fever in children.

Because the tip of the appendix in some cases may be located other than where it is expected to

*Figure 33-5. Appendicitis and Ruptured Appendix.*

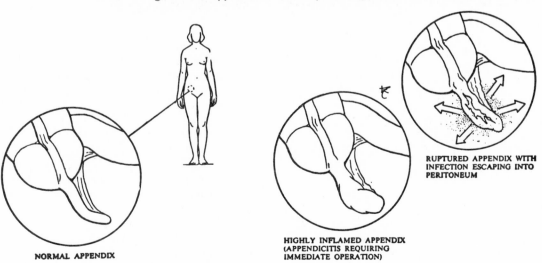

NORMAL APPENDIX

HIGHLY INFLAMED APPENDIX
(APPENDICITIS REQUIRING
IMMEDIATE OPERATION)

RUPTURED APPENDIX WITH
INFECTION ESCAPING INTO
PERITONEUM

be in the lower right part of the abdomen, symptoms may vary. The tip may sometimes be on the left side, producing pain there.

## Diagnosis

In addition to these symptoms, the doctor looks for positive evidence of an inflamed appendix. There may be tenderness over the appendix when pressure is exerted there. Somtimes pain is experienced in the region of the appendix during the examination through the rectum, or through the vagina in the female patient. A laboratory test, the white blood count, is also helpful in making the diagnosis. The doctor always searches for other diseases which are sometimes mistaken for appendicitis—e.g., gallbladder attacks, kidney stone or kidney infection on the right side, even the onset of pneumonia, rheumatic fever, or diabetic coma. In women, there is the possibility of a ruptured ectopic pregnancy, a twisted ovarian cyst, or a hemorrhaging egg follicle at the middle of the menstrual cycle.

It should be apparent that great skill is required in making the diagnosis in certain cases when the symptoms and findings are not exactly typical. In such a situation your doctor may wish to have a consultation with a specialist. No reputable physician wishes to remove an appendix unnecessarily. However, one of the greatest tragedies of all is to see a patient who is disabled, or even dies, because of too great a delay in diagnosing a case of appendicitis which did not present typical symptoms. As the old medical saying puts it, "Better a live patient without an appendix than a dead one with his appendix in place." If two doctors agree that there is a real possibility of appendicitis, even though they are not completely certain of the diagnosis, my advice is: by all means have your appendix removed. The operation, when performed by a skilled operator in a good hospital, has a very low mortality rate. Healthy young people usually leave the hospital in less than a week after the appendix has been removed.

## Complications

If the appendicitis goes on to the serious complication of peritonitis or to form a large abscess, the patient will require expert medical and surgical skills, found only in a good hospital, to save his life. Fortunately, the situation is better than it was a few decades ago, because of the antibiotics. But never minimize the seriousness of an infection spreading from the appendix.

## How You Can Save a Life

It isn't often that one can do something that will save a life, but appendicitis is very apt to present such an opportunity.

Statistics show that when a person with appendicitis takes a laxative, his chance of dying is three times as great as it would be if no laxative had been taken. With more than one dose of a laxative, the possibility of dying is seven times as great. This is due to the fact that laxatives or cathartics increase action in the intestine, and may also increase the pressure within the little sac. The more the pressure, the more likelihood that the sac will burst. The same is true for enemas. It has also been shown that a delay in operating lessens the chance of a cure. So many people have died as a result of taking "a good physic" when they were developing appendicitis that I am inclined to call laxatives the "first assistant" of this Killer.

Here are the rules to follow in order to save a life—your own, or another's—when appendicitis gives its warning signals. First of all, be sure to remember that ANY ABDOMINAL PAIN LASTING FOR MORE THAN THREE OR FOUR HOURS MAY BE APPENDICITIS.

1. *Call your doctor immediately.* If you have no doctor, you can obtain a thorough examination for appendicitis in the emergency room of any reliable general hospital. You should be taken there by auto or taxi, if possible.
2. *Remain as quiet as possible.* Do not massage the abdomen.
3. *Take NOTHING by mouth—no food, water, or medicines. Especially avoid taking any cathartic or laxative.*
4. *Do not take an enema.*
5. *Do not use a hot-water bottle.* If the pain becomes very severe, an icepack may be applied.

# 34
# THE DISABLING DISEASES

In this chapter, I discuss the major disabling diseases. The reasons I have chosen some of them will be obvious to you. For example, I believe you will agree that diseases such as arthritis, asthma, and multiple sclerosis belong in this category, because they frequently disable but rarely kill. Many other illnesses, however, are more difficult to classify. For example, polio, or infantile paralysis, is a major disabler, but can also be a frightfully dangerous killer. A stomach ulcer may grumble along for years causing a limited amount of disability, and then may erupt as a fatal hemorrhage or perforation.

I have selected for this chapter the diseases in which disability, either total or recurrent, is a *chief feature*. I consider this important, because people suffering from these diseases are apt to become the forgotten souls in modern medical care. This is particularly unfortunate because, as I plan to show you, something can be done to make life easier and better for patients with even the most severe disabling diseases.

Even though great progress has been made and is continually being made in preventing and curing the disabling effects of the diseases I discuss in this chapter, I think you would find it depressing to read about them all at once. Therefore I am listing them below, so you can choose the ones of most interest to you or your family, and read them first.

Peptic ulcer (including gastric and duodenal ulcer)
Asthma

Arthritis (including rheumatoid and osteo-arthritis, ankylosing spondylitis, gout, juvenile rheumatoid arthritis)
Backache
Bursitis
Other disabling diseases of the bones and joints (including osteomyelitis, tuberculosis of the bones and joints, congenital dislocation of the hip, clubfoot, frozen shoulder, and fractures)
Poliomyelitis
Multiple sclerosis
Epilepsy
Parkinsonism
Neuritis and neuralgia (including Bell's palsy, sciatica, shingles, intercostal neuralgia or neuritis, and cervical rib syndrome)
Alcoholism
Cerebral palsy
Disabling diseases of the muscles (including muscular dystrophy, myasthenia gravis, and familial periodic paralysis)
Loss of eyesight
Diseases of the ear and labyrinth
Low blood pressure (hypotension)
Influenza
The anemias
Ulcerative colitis
Enlarged prostate gland
Hernias
Infectious mononucleosis
Gonorrhea and other venereal diseases
Brucellosis (undulant fever)
Leprosy (Hansen's disease)

451

Tropical diseases
Malaria
Amebiasis (amebic dysentery)
Sarcoidosis (Boeck's sarcoid)

There are many other disabling diseases which I have dealt with elsewhere in this book. These include the disabling mental illnesses such as schizophrenia, and almost all the "killer" diseases such as heart disease, tuberculosis, etc., which frequently go through "disabler" phases.

## PEPTIC ULCER

(Gastric Ulcer and Duodenal Ulcer)

An ulcer is simply an open sore. Doctors use the term *peptic ulcer* (*peptic* is derived from the Greek word for digestion) to indicate that the sore is in the stomach or the duodenum, the first part of the intestines which connect with the stomach.

Peptic ulcer is an extremely prevalent problem, affecting an estimated ten million people in this country alone. Although recently it has been declining a little in the population as a whole, it appears to be increasing somewhat among women. It still remains more common, however, among men. It may occur at any age, although it is rare in very young children.

The cause of ulcers is not yet fully understood, but it is definitely associated with the presence of an excessive amount of acid gastric juice. This gastric juice, which is secreted by the stomach, is needed for digestion. In people with ulcers, there is excessive secretion, not only after eating, but also between meals and at night during sleep. Some people secrete larger quantities of this gastric juice than do others. We know that worry and anxiety can increase the secretion. For this reason, ulcers are considered to be a *psychosomatic disease*, which I discuss on page **182**. Although we do not know exactly how ulcers are caused, we know that the excess secretion of gastric juice is bad for the ulcer and prevents it from healing.

### Symptoms

The most common symptom of an ulcer is a burning sensation or discomfort in the upper abdomen, usually felt about two or three hours after meals or in the middle of the night, although the distress may occur sooner after meals. The pain generally subsides promptly upon eating, drinking milk, or taking an antacid. Nausea and vomiting can also occur.

Sometimes complications may produce other signs and symptoms. If an ulcer should erode a nearby blood vessel, bleeding may follow. There may be slow seeping of blood, resulting in anemia and the associated loss of health and strength.

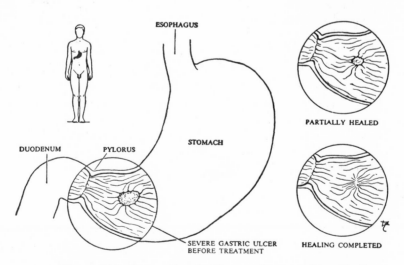

ESOPHAGUS

DUODENUM     PYLORUS     STOMACH

SEVERE GASTRIC ULCER
BEFORE TREATMENT

PARTIALLY HEALED

HEALING COMPLETED

*Figure 34-1. Severe Gastric Ulcer, Before and After Healing.*

The bleeding may be in the form of a sudden hemorrhage, which threatens life itself. Blood is sometimes vomited and appears brownish because of the effect of the stomach acid. Blood in the bowel movements may be responsible for black or tarry stools. In the case of a massive hemorrhage, the patient becomes weak, faint, and thirsty. He requires immediate medical attention and hospitalization.

An ulcer may perforate through the wall of the stomach or duodenum. This causes excruciating pain in the upper abdomen. Patients describe it as "the worst pain of my life." They must be rushed to the hospital and operated upon immediately to prevent a fatal outcome.

## Diagnosis

A peptic ulcer can be diagnosed by x-ray and fluoroscopic studies of the stomach and duodenum after barium has been swallowed. The barium helps to visualize the ulcer. In some instances, a special lighted tube, a *gastroscope*, may be inserted to permit observation of the ulcerated area. Removal of gastric juice for analysis may also be used for diagnosis. In most ulcer patients, gastric juice flow is increased and the fluid has more than the usual acidity.

Some people have an ulcer without realizing it. This disease may continue unsuspected for years, the symptoms vanishing for longer or shorter periods of time, so that the patient attributes them to "indigestion" or constipation. The latter frequently accompanies ulcers.

Anyone with symptoms *suggesting* a peptic ulcer should see a doctor promptly. There are a number of reasons for this. In the first place, there is no need to endure the discomfort or pain which sooner or later becomes disabling, if only in the sense that the victim, sometimes so gradually he scarcely realizes what is happening, is no longer able to enjoy life fully. In the second place, an ulcer which has caused only mild discomfort can suddenly threaten life. And, finally, there are other potentially dangerous diseases which can resemble a gastric ulcer, some of which require immediate treatment. They include the following:

1. *Cancer of the stomach.* Although a true peptic ulcer probably never develops into a cancer, it is often difficult to distinguish between the two. Gastroscopic examinations help to determine this. If the disease is an ulcer, it will respond and heal with medical treatment, whereas cancer of the stomach does not disappear with such treatment. However, if there is doubt, an operation must be performed.

2. *Chronic gastritis.* The lining of the stomach may undergo changes which can cause symptoms similar to those of an ulcer, including pain, burning, "indigestion" and even bleeding. These changes of the stomach lining, called chronic gastritis, can be distinguished from an ulcer by means of x-rays and the gastroscope.

3. *Chronic alcoholism.* This may cause varicose veins of the stomach or the nearby esophagus, which may imitate some parts of the ulcer picture (see page 470).

4. *Hiatus hernia.* This is the name for a condition which sometimes occurs when there is an enlarged opening in the diaphragm muscle, through which the stomach pushes, or "herniates." It can produce symptoms of an ulcer. Such herniation can be diagnosed by an x-ray, and, if necessary, treated by operation.

5. *Diseases of the gallbladder, liver, large intestine, and right kidney.* These organs are situated close to the stomach and duodenum, and may cause symptoms that are mistaken for an ulcer. X-rays and other tests are necessary to make the correct diagnosis and provide proper treatment.

Never attempt to make the diagnosis of ulcers yourself. A competent doctor will not rely on symptoms alone, but will make the diagnosis only after the most searching tests.

## Treatment

For most ulcer patients, medical treatment can be effective. Medication and diet give the body a chance to heal the ulcer much as it would heal an open sore elsewhere, provided there is no continued irritation. The aim of medical treatment is to reduce or eliminate the irritation by reducing the amount of acid formed, neutralizing already present acid, and calming the patient if necessary. Antacids may be employed to neutralize excess acids. Certain drugs may be used to partially block nerve stimulation of stomach secretions. A newer drug, cimetidine, which promises to be helpful in healing ulcers, is the first to act directly on the cells in the stomach that secrete acid, working to markedly reduce their output.

Once, special "bland" diets were almost universally accepted by physicians as being of prime importance. But their necessity is no longer taken for granted. The American Heart Association has pointed out that diets rich in cream and milk may be potentially harmful over prolonged periods because they may possibly raise blood fat levels and influence development of atherosclerosis, in which clogging deposits build up in arteries. More and more physicians now advise ulcer patients that eating regular meals to help buffer or neutralize stomach acids is probably more important than the contents of the meals.

Frequently, with such treatment, symptoms may disappear within a week or so. But to ensure complete healing of an ulcer, the treatment should be continued for four or five weeks.

Surgery may sometimes be needed. For one thing, some ulcers refuse to heal and continue to cause pain. If a resistant, nonhealing ulcer is in the stomach rather than in the duodenum, there is an added possible reason for surgery. What appears to be an ulcer may be a cancer masquerading as an ulcer. While medical tests may often distinguish ulcer from cancer, sometimes accurate diagnosis can be made only by examination of the area through surgery. Duodenal ulcers are almost never malignant. Surgery also is needed for ulcer complications—bleeding and perforation. Another possible complication that may require corrective surgery is obstruction that may result when, sometimes, an ulcer produces inflammation or scarring at the outlet of the stomach or in the duodenum. With obstruction, there may be such symptoms as vomiting of food and foul, gaseous belching.

## Advice to Ulcer Patients

There are three main reasons why ulcers cause so much pain and disability. I wish to emphasize again the two that I have already mentioned. First, patients tend to ignore the symptoms, feeling that they are not important or can be endured, and try to alleviate them with cathartics and other useless medicines. Second, individuals who develop ulcers are frequently tense, inclined to drive themselves and to dislike taking things easy.

The third reason is that ulcer symptoms usually vanish with treatment long before the ulcer itself has healed. Doctors find that most difficulties occur in patients who do not stick to the treatment. Having abided by the rules for a time, they become neglectful and gradually forget them entirely.

You need not be disabled by an ulcer if

1. You consult a doctor as soon as you observe any of its symptoms.
2. You learn, with the help of a psychiatrist, if necessary, how to minimize tensions.
3. You cooperate with your doctor until he, *not you*, decides your ulcer is healed.

## ASTHMA

Asthma, technically called *bronchial asthma*, is a disease of the bronchial tubes which lead from the windpipe, or *trachea*, into the lungs. It will help you to understand this distressing and often disabling disease if you turn to page 94, on which I explain the nature and functions of the lungs and of these tubes.

The bronchial tubes ordinarily do not furnish any marked resistance to the entrance or exit of air, so that we are not even conscious of the fact that we continually inhale and exhale, at the rate of about sixteen times each minute. However, in asthmatic attacks the bronchial tubes tend to close down, causing asthmatic wheezing. If the attack is severe, the sufferer seems almost to be suffocating. He apparently uses all his strength, just trying to breathe. He becomes pale and bluish and usually perspires. This spasm of the bronchial tubes can usually be relieved quickly by an injection of adrenaline. Fortunately, most attacks are mild and do not last long. Many of them can be prevented or stopped by modern medical treatments.

Bronchial asthma is a chronic kind of illness, marked by these attacks. In severe cases, the bronchial tubes become swollen and offer greater resistance to treatment. Plugs of clinging mucus may form in the tubes and cause chronic irritation and coughing. They are dislodged and brought up as sputum. If the attacks are frequent, prolonged, and severe, the lung tissue is damaged. This puts a strain on the heart. Eventually, heart strain can result from severe, chronic asthma.

The average case of asthma is mild and is more of a recurrent nuisance than a threat to health. Nevertheless, there is a small percentage of cases in which asthma is not only a disabler but can even be a killer. It is always essential to get, and follow, competent medical advice, especially in the case of young patients, before asthma can damage the heart or lungs.

## Causes of Asthma

Bronchial asthma can be caused in several, quite different ways. That is one reason you should consult a doctor promptly, and never make your own decisions on the basis of some treatment which helped another asthmatic patient.

ALLERGIES. One type of bronchial asthma is definitely allergic. An individual may have hay fever and asthma simultaneously during the ragweed season or may experience attacks of asthma only at this time. Other pollens may be responsible, including animal fur or feathers, face powder, certain foods, in fact, any number of *allergens* (see page 499).

A person with asthma should, therefore, be tested for allergic sensitivity. Discovering the responsible substance or substances may require a great many tests and the efforts of a specialist in allergy and asthma. The patient, too, should become a "medical detective" and try to furnish the doctor with clues. A laboratory worker I know eventually tracked down the cause of his asthma, and it was confirmed by his doctor with tests. He could handle any animals except rabbits. Whenever he touched them or cleaned their cages, he developed an asthmatic attack. In this case, the cure was obvious: a change of job.

INFECTIONS. Many cases of bronchial asthma are associated with bacterial infections, especially of the sinuses, throat, and nose. Sometimes these improve very markedly if the infection clears up. Of course, it is important for such people to avoid colds, sinusitis, and infections of the nose, throat, and respiratory passages.

EMOTIONS. There is also a type of asthma which seems to be entirely emotional. Yet, many allergists believe that in such cases there is a basic sensitivity to some allergen such as house dust and that emotional tensions act as a trigger or intensifier of symptoms.

## Diagnosis

Other diseases can cause wheezy, asthmaticlike breathing. Heart disease, obstructions in the bronchial tubes, and several other conditions can mimic bronchial asthma. Be sure to have an accurate diagnosis made by a competent physician. Cooperate in every way in helping the doctor discover the cause of your asthma. This may require the combined efforts of an allergy specialist, a specialist in internal medicine, and a nose and throat specialist. It is well worthwhile in order to avoid the years of suffering and disability that may result if the asthma causes permanent damage.

## Treatment

Physicians today have available a growing armamentarium of drugs that can be used to relieve asthma attacks when they occur and to reduce their frequency and severity.

Older and still useful agents include ephedrine and aminophylline. Corticosteroids or cortisone-like drugs have been used in severe cases in the past. A newer corticosteroid drug, beclomethasone, has the advantage that it is administered in spray form and has a local effective action without causing systemic side effects, such as easy bruising and "moon" face. Its value has been established in many studies.

Another newer agent is cromolyn sodium. It is administered with a special inhaler and has even been helpful in allowing many asthma patients to take part in sports and recreational activities without suffering attacks.

In some cases, it appears, asthma may be related to chronic sinusitis, and medical management of the sinus condition or, sometimes, surgical drainage of the sinuses may be helpful.

Recent developments offer a far better outlook now for asthma patients.

# ARTHRITIS

The correct definition of arthritis is an *inflammation of a joint*. However, the term is widely misused and is frequently applied to vague aches in almost any part of the body. You cannot have arthritis in a part of the body such as the middle of the thigh, for example, because it has no joint. Joints of the body are found at the knees, wrists, elbows, fingers, and toes, and also the hips and shoulders. The neck and back have joints between the bones of the spine. Even if you do feel a pain in a joint, it may not always be due to arthritis, because there are many other parts that comprise the joint structure. These include ligaments, tendons, muscles, cartilage, and bursae.

*Symptoms of chronic arthritis are pain, swelling, stiffness, and deformity in one or more joints.* They may appear suddenly or come on gradually. The aches and pains are not always the same. Some people feel a sharp, burning, or grinding pain. Others liken it to a toothache. Moving the joint usually hurts, although sometimes it is merely stiff.

*Is rheumatism the same as arthritis?* Rheumatism has come to mean so many things to so many people that it is almost impossible to define the word. Therefore, doctors like to use more specific words for diseases of the joints, muscles, ligaments, and bursae. That is why I am not grouping these illnesses under the title "rheumatism," but instead describe them as arthritis, gout, bursitis, etc.

*Infectious arthritis* is a bacterial infection inside a joint. This can develop from a wound that damages the joint. Also, bacteria may get into a joint from the blood stream. An example of such a disease would be arthritis due to gonorrhea, in which the germs are carried from the infected, pus-containing genital organs through the blood to the joints. Infectious diseases such as tuberculosis, brucellosis, or undulant fever may attack the joints. The infected joint is painful and may become swollen.

See your doctor if any joint hurts or becomes hot, swollen, or reddened. Treatment is very successful with the aid of penicillin and other modern medicines, but must be started promptly. Joints are precious. Treat them promptly.

*Osteoarthritis* is a most common joint disorder in people getting into old age. It rarely develops before a person is forty years old. This disease is due to wear and tear of the joint tissues and the growth of bony bumps which appear at the joints and interfere with ordinary movements. Some pain is felt but it is not severe. Any disablement is usually minor. Most people so affected need not fear serious crippling. Measures of relief from discomfort are provided for by doctors. Sometimes, an orthopedic specialist will be needed to decide if severe osteoarthritis needs special braces, exercises, or even surgical help.

*Rheumatoid arthritis* is the most serious form of arthritis. Its cause is unknown. It is common among young adults, usually starting before the age of forty. Individuals with mild cases need not fear that deformities of the joints *necessarily* lie in store for them. But they should be under the *regular care* of a physician to make sure the disease does not get worse. Acute attacks of rheumatoid arthritis can be followed by permanent changes in the joints, leaving them stiff and deformed. This disease differs from an attack of rheumatic fever, in which the joints always return to normal. Severe arthritis, like rheumatic fever, can produce many symptoms, such as a rundown feeling, poor appetite, anemia, fever, pleurisy.

## Treatment

It is most important that patients with arthritis be seen regularly by a physician. Many doctors do not wish to undertake, or are not experienced in, the care of arthritis. Patients may often have to be referred to specialists—rheumatologists—or to major medical centers.

The mainstay of treatment in rheumatoid arthritis remains aspirin. It is a very valuable agent—when used properly. In small doses, aspirin relieves mild to moderate pain and lowers fever. In rheumatoid arthritis, however, inflammation as well as pain must be combated. Aspirin has the ability to work against inflammation when it is used in sufficiently large doses. A few tablets will not do this. Substantial amounts of aspirin are required. And when aspirin is prescribed in the right amounts for the individual patient, it is often helpful.

Some patients do not tolerate aspirin well. For them, newer drugs may be helpful. One such drug is Motrin; others are being made available.

Today, too, gold salts—newer preparations of them and better knowledge of their use—are often effective. They are given by injection, commonly once a week until the total needed therapeutic dose has been given. After that, they may be administered at intervals of three or four weeks.

When aspirin and other similar treatment, or gold therapy, fails to provide adequate relief, other methods may be tried. They include antimalarial compounds and corticosteroid drugs.

In very severe cases of rheumatoid arthritis and osteoarthritis, with unyielding pain and crippling, surgery now is often possible. *Synovectomy,* an operation in which excess membrane is removed from a joint, may be indicated in some cases. In others, to overcome pain and deformity, a joint may be fused in a neutral position.

A dramatic development in the 1960's was a workable artificial hip. Hip replacement surgery today is frequently performed for severely afflicted arthritic patients unresponsive to medical management.

And now, too, prostheses (replacements) for many other joints are available. There are now prostheses or implants for knees, ankles, toes, fingers, and knuckles; most recently, new shoulder and elbow joints have been developed. With such prostheses, pain may be overcome, deformities surmounted, and normal or near-normal motion restored.

I should like to emphasize that not by any means is surgery an inevitable need. Medical care, provided it is expert care, is very often all that is needed. It may be coupled with application of heat, other physical therapy, and rehabilitative exercises.

It is when good medical care is not successful that the new surgical developments permit reconstruction of more and more joints, making possible rehabilitation for many patients who might once have been considered virtually hopeless.

## Ankylosing Spondylitis

This special form of arthritis affects the small joints of the spine. There is stiffening of the joints and ligaments so that movement may become increasingly painful and difficult. The disease has been referred to as "poker spine." The stiffening may sometimes extend to the ribs, limiting the flexibility of the rib cage, so that breathing is impaired.

Ankylosing spondylitis most often affects young adults. It used to be thought to be about ten times as common in men as in women, but recent studies suggest that it may afflict women as often as men. In women, it may sometimes be thought to be rheumatoid arthritis. And some women may think their nagging back pain symptoms are due to menstrual cramps.

Ankylosing spondylitis is chronic. But if pain can be relieved so as to permit posture-maintaining exercises, it is possible to avoid crippling and achieve a fully productive life.

Gold therapy has been ineffective, and corticosteroid drugs have not proved particularly useful. However, two drugs—phenylbutazone and indomethacin—have been found to help about 90 percent of patients. The drugs may sometimes produce side effects which can be eliminated when they are withdrawn. A recent study also indicates that aspirin may be effective for some patients and should be given a trial before resort to the other drugs.

## Gout

Gouty arthritis is the one form of arthritis which can be most effectively attacked.

Gout is an inherited ailment related to abnormal metabolism, or body handling, of certain important compounds, called *purines,* in foods. As a result of the faulty metabolism of purines, an increased level of a breakdown product of purines, called *uric acid,* builds up in blood and body tissues.

When excess uric acid is deposited in joints, it can cause an inflammatory reaction by the joint tissues, leading to severe pain, swelling, and stiffness. The joints usually affected are those of the lower extremities, particularly the great toe, but any other joint in the body can be involved. The arthritis of gout can be severe and disabling if untreated and may lead to permanent deformity. In addition to damage to joints, uncontrolled gout can injure the kidneys.

Gout is much more common in men than in women.

Excellent medicines are available not only to

relieve the agony of gouty arthritis once an attack has begun but also to prevent attacks.

Colchicine can stop an attack, usually within twenty-four hours. Phenylbutazone is another agent that may be used once an attack has started.

For prevention, one long-used drug is probenecid. It acts to promote excretion of uric acid via the kidneys, thus reducing the amount in blood and tissues. It is taken regularly.

Another agent, allopurinol, also is preventive, acting in a different way. Allopurinol blocks the enzyme that converts materials into uric acid, so that uric acid is not formed. The drug also stimulates the breakdown and excretion of uric acid deposits that may already have accumulated in the body.

Certain foods may precipitate gout attacks. In most cases, however, it is no longer considered necessary to ban many "rich" foods from the diet (those with high purine content), with the possible exception of such items as anchovies, sweetbreads, liver, and kidney.

### Juvenile Rheumatoid Arthritis

Although rheumatoid arthritis is not nearly as common in children as in adults, it does affect an estimated 200,000 American youngsters.

Juvenile rheumatoid arthritis (JRA) can sometimes begin, much like adult arthritis, with swellings of many joints. But it is now known that it can take other forms as well. It may sometimes begin with pain and swelling of a few joints or even a single joint, which may mistakenly be attributed to a fall or other injury. And sometimes it may begin with a spiking fever, fleeting nonitching rash, and occasionally abdominal pain, before obvious signs of arthritis appear weeks or months later.

JRA is a difficult disease but far from a hopeless one. With early diagnosis and effective treatment, a relatively normal childhood can be preserved for most youngsters, excellent functional status can eventually be regained in at least 80 percent, and remission (or disappearance of the disease) occurs in about two thirds.

Optimal treatment is many-sided. Drugs are used—starting, as in adult rheumatoid arthritis, with aspirin. If aspirin is not adequate, gold salts or antimalarial drugs may be employed.

But a child with JRA needs more. An exercise program tailored to the child's needs is at least as important as medication in maintaining joint function and muscle strength. For this, help from an expert physical therapist is needed. Most parents, with instruction from a therapist, become very competent cotherapists.

Many physicians have no experience in treating JRA. If your child has the problem, your physician may be able to recommend a specialist, or you may inquire at the nearest major medical center which may have such a specialist on its staff.

## BACKACHES

The backbone, or spine, is a column made up of many small bones which are held together by tissues called *ligaments*. Between each layer of bone lie *disks* made of *cartilage*. The disks act as cushions for the bones. Through the spinal column runs a tube which contains the *spinal cord*. Many of the main nerves of the body extend from the spinal cord. Because of the way the bones and disks are loosely strung together, the backbone is very flexible and allows for bending and other kinds of body movements.

There are many common misconceptions about backaches. A major one is that a backache is usually due to a "slipped disk." Far more often than not, a backache has nothing to do with a disk problem—or other organic disorder. Recent studies have shown that more than three fourths of people who suffer from backaches can be assured that they have no disk or organic problem of any kind and that their pain can be relieved without resort to surgery. Recurrences can be reduced in frequency or severity or both, and may even be eliminated, by relatively simple measures.

Let's consider first the "slipped disk" problem (see Figure 34-2). Actually a spinal disk does not slip. What happens in the case of a so-called slipped disk is that the rim of the disk weakens and tears, and part of the soft gelatinous center of the disk becomes extruded. The extruded, or herniated, portion then may press on sensitive nerve roots, producing pain, sometimes so great as to be disabling.

Most often, the disk involved is low in the spine

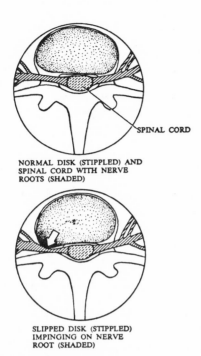

NORMAL DISK (STIPPLED) AND
SPINAL CORD WITH NERVE
ROOTS (SHADED)

SLIPPED DISK (STIPPLED)
IMPINGING ON NERVE
ROOT (SHADED)

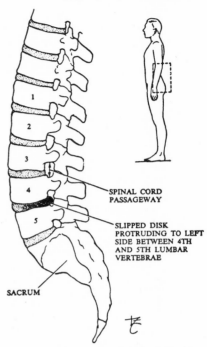

SPINAL CORD
PASSAGEWAY

SLIPPED DISK
PROTRUDING TO LEFT
SIDE BETWEEN 4TH
AND 5TH LUMBAR
VERTEBRAE

SACRUM

*Figure 34-2. Slipped Intervertebral Disk.* LEFT: *Cross sections of vertebra and disk as viewed from above.*

RIGHT: *Lower spine as viewed from left side; nerve roots omitted.*

and may press on the root (in the spine) of the sciatic nerve, which runs down the thigh and into the side of the foot. Pain then may be felt all along the course of the nerve. Usually the leg pain comes first; then may come low back pain and muscle spasm.

Actually, even when there is pain in the sciatic nerve, called *sciatica,* it may not be from the pressure of a disk. Sciatica also can arise when a muscle goes into spasm, contracts abnormally, and puts pressure on the nerve.

When a herniated disk *is* pressing and causing trouble, it is sometimes possible to relieve the pressure by heavy pelvic traction. By no means is surgery routinely needed for a disk problem.

Backache sometimes can result from arthritic changes in the spine. Occasionally backache is associated with a congenital abnormality. The pain is not due to the abnormality itself but rather due to unusual stresses imposed by the abnormality on surrounding structures, especially the muscles. In such cases, surgery may be required to correct

the abnormality, but often, without recourse to surgery, braces and corsets may be helpful. And frequently exercises are helpful to strengthen particular muscles that can be used to counter the pain-producing effects of the unusual stress.

Slight variation in length of the legs is not unusual. In most cases, a difference of as much as half an inch causes no problems. But a greater difference, and on occasion even a lesser one, may be a contributing factor in back pain. In such cases, a shoe lift may be prescribed.

Back pain sometimes can stem from conditions that have nothing to do with the back itself. Heart disease sometimes may produce back pain. So may other diseases—of the lungs, abdomen, kidney, uterus, ovaries, fallopian tubes, or prostate. Women sometimes have pain referred to the back because of menstrual disturbances, pregnancy, pelvic congestion, and even because of ill-fitting diaphragms.

But it has become apparent in recent years that the problem in the great majority of backaches lies with muscles, muscles in the abdomen as well as in the back itself, muscles that are weak, unable to perform properly, and easily subject to injury.

In his excellent book, *Freedom from Backaches* (Simon and Schuster), in which he goes thoroughly into the various causes of backache and the various measures that can be used, short of surgery, to provide relief and prevent recurrences, Dr. Lawrence W. Friedmann has this to say about the muscle problem in backaches:

Consider a tree or a telephone pole held erect by four guy wires so it is stable even in high winds. If one of the wires is cut, the tree or pole may fall, and it will fall in the direction of an uncut wire.

That situation is only partially analogous to what happens in a human with weak stomach muscles. In theory, perhaps, such a person's back should fall backward, since there is no guying or support from in front. But this does not happen because we have a sense of balance which assures that we will maintain our center of gravity above our feet. So, to compensate for weak abdominal muscles, we shift weight, leaning slightly forward, hanging on our back muscles since they are the stronger guy wires.

But this has a deleterious effect, placing continuous excess strain on the back muscles. After a time, they fatigue and hurt. And in our society, weakness of abdominal muscles is one of the most common causes of back pain. . . . Sprains and strains are common when tired or weak muscles are called upon suddenly to do more than they are capable of doing. Nor is this a matter only of unusual exertion such as shoveling snow or lifting a very heavy load; even a sudden coughing spell may be enough to produce damage.

The immediate cause of acute pain in most backaches is spasm, involuntary contraction of muscles. If a muscle is injured or under excessive strain, it may go into spasm, and other nearby muscles may do the same in an effort to splint or protect the strained muscle and prevent further damage.

But spasm can be very painful. When a muscle is in continuous contraction, small blood vessels are squeezed shut, blood flow is impaired, oxygen is in short supply, and waste products accumulate and produce pain.

What can you do if you are a victim of chronic backaches? By all means, ask your physician to recommend an expert. Let him check you thoroughly. Chances are, he can eliminate the possibility of any organic problems (if these do exist, you can get treatment for them). If there are no organic problems, the likelihood is great that you can be helped by a program of exercises designed specifically to strengthen weak musculature or by other relatively simple measures.

You don't have to accept chronic backache as a permanent problem. Nor do you have to fear that the only relief is to be found in surgery.

Certain factors sometimes enter into backaches and are correctible on your own:

1. Your mattress may be soft and sagging, thus curving your spine when you sleep. You may find it advisable to try a bedboard between mattress and springs. At first, it may be more difficult to fall asleep on this harder-than-usual surface, but after a few nights most people become accustomed to it and would miss it if it were removed.

2. Your posture may be at fault. A good test of posture is to stand with your back against a wall, your weight resting easily and evenly on your feet. Your shoulder blades and buttocks should touch the wall. If only your shoulders touch, you are round-shouldered; if only the middle of your back touches, your spine is curved too much. If you stand up straight, you will find that automatically your abdomen is held in also, a good way to help prevent sagging abdominal muscles.

3. You may be carrying too much at one time, for instance, a heavy shopping bag in one hand. This tends to curve your spine either to the right or to the left, causing the back muscles and ligaments to become strained.

4. Your work habits may be at fault. If you must sit at a typewriter or desk all day, don't slump, but sit upright. It does seem easier to let your head drop forward and your chest fall in, but good posture will repay you in greater energy and a pain-free back.

For the occasional, mild backache, simple home treatment may help greatly. In addition to taking two aspirins every four hours and resting on a hard mattress, I have found that moist heat, *at temperatures only slightly above body temperature,* has given me great relief. I like to place a dispensable wooden or plastic chair in the shower and sit there relaxed and supported with a lukewarm trickle of water keeping a towel moist on my back.

# BURSITIS

This is an inflammation of the lubricating parts around joints. In the illustration, you can see how a normal bursa helps a joint work smoothly. Also, you will see an inflamed bursa containing a deposit of calcium material.

Our joints would creak and wear out if there were no efficient "oiling system." Nature has provided this in the smooth surfaces inside the joints, and the bursae around the joints. Sometimes these smoothly working bursae become inflamed. When they do, there is severe pain, which makes it impossible to move the adjacent joint.

Bursitis may manifest itself in an acute or a chronic form. The *acute* form comes on suddenly. Sometimes, chilling or a draft on the joint may set it off. Or excessive use of the joint, for example, in typing or piano playing or athletics, may inflame the bursa. Usually the shoulder is affected, but almost any joint in the body can be the site of bursitis. The acute attack is very disabling because of the intense pain. The inflamed bursa can sometimes be felt as a tender swelling near the shoulder or whichever joint is affected. Sometimes nature will heal the acute attack by permitting the inflamed spot to rupture and drain itself. This will be helped by resting the joint in a sling or by going to bed. Moist heat frequently helps, whereas dry heat or diathermy may cause more pain (see page 357 for method of applying moist heat).

Other patients find that cold applications are more effective. Usually, a short period of experimentation will tell what will best relieve the pain. If aspirin, Bufferin, or Empirin does not reduce the pain, then your doctor may have to prescribe Demerol or codeine for a few days.

If nature does not relieve the attack, a skilled doctor can usually help by inserting a needle into the inflamed area and draining out the fluid and calcium salts. At the same time, he may puncture the bursa in several places to prevent reaccumulation of the fluid and calcium salts. The doctor will generally instill a small amount of Novocaine, Darvon, or other local anesthetic to relieve the pain. Usually, if the needle finds the right area, an acute attack of bursitis is quickly relieved. Many patients often get prompt relief from an injection into the bursa of cortisone or hydrocortisone, together with small oral doses of hydrocortisone.

*Chronic bursitis* may follow the acute attack. There is continued pain and limitation of motion around the joint. In the shoulder, an x-ray will usually reveal calcium salts, which have been deposited in one of the important bursae around the joint. If rest, heat, and medicines do not relieve the condition, surgery may be required to remove the deposits of calcium salts or free the area of chronic inflammation. Such an operation generally requires the skill of a specialist in orthopedic surgery. Sometimes chronic bursitis consists of a painless swelling of the bursa around a main joint. "Housemaid's knee," "tennis elbow," and "typist's shoulder" indicate occupations that may keep a bursa acutely or chronically painful or swollen.

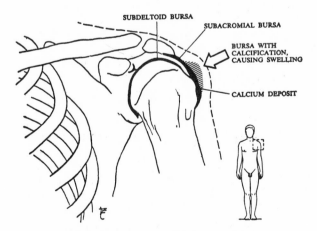

*Figure 34-3. Bursitis with Calcification.*

# OTHER DISABLING CONDITIONS OF JOINTS AND BONES

## Disabling Infections of the Bones

Until the introduction of medicines which can destroy staphylococci and streptococci, prolonged disability frequently resulted from bone infections caused by these germs. They may cause an acute infection of the bone, similar to a small boil in the skin. This is called *acute osteomyelitis*, which is indeed serious because the germs can invade the whole body and, if they do not kill, can lead to severe chronic bone disease. This infection, which causes acute pain and fever, generally strikes at the long bones of the arms and legs. Children and young adults are most often affected. *Prompt treatment* with penicillin and other antibiotics will usually eradicate the infection. If not, surgery will be required to drain the affected area. The acute attack is an emergency. If your doctor is not available, go to the nearest general hospital or, if the patient is a child, to a hospital that has a children's department.

CHRONIC OSTEOMYELITIS. Thanks to the new antibiotics, there has been a great decrease in this terribly disabling bone disease. Formerly in patients afflicted with osteomyelitis, the shinbone, for example, might continue to drain pus for years, despite surgery and the best medical treatment available. Now even the chronic cases can be greatly helped because the antibiotics aid the surgeon in performing operations to remove the dead, infected pieces of bone and let fresh bone grow.

TUBERCULOSIS OF THE BONES AND JOINTS. Most of you have seen individuals with disabling hunchback, which is caused by the erosive action of tuberculosis on the bones of the spine. This is *Pott's disease,* fortunately now rare in the United States. Tuberculosis can affect almost every bone, as well as the hip joint and other joints. This form of tuberculosis is sometimes due to a specific strain of the tuberculosis germ from infected cows. The bovine strain is communicated through *unpasteurized* milk obtained from tuberculous cows. The conclusion is inescapable—there is no better argument for pasteurization of all milk and milk products than the assurance it gives that tuberculosis germs will not be ingested.

## Miscellaneous Disabilities

There are many congenital and acquired disabling conditions that affect the joints and bones in addition to those already described. I want to mention a few common ones, especially those that can be helped.

CONGENITAL DISLOCATION OF THE HIP. This condition is present at birth, more frequently in female than male children. However, it may not be evident until the child starts to walk. Then it will be noticed that the gait is not symmetrical. It is extremely important to diagnose this condition before the child does much walking with the weakened hip joint. At this time, proper treatment can cure the condition without surgical operation. If the condition is neglected, even for a year or two, surgery will be needed to reconstruct the hip joint. Such surgery will require a specialist in orthopedics. If necessary, the child should be taken to the nearest medical center that specializes in children's surgery. Sometimes, for people living in isolated areas, this means an expensive journey of hundreds of miles. But the child will bless you for it in later life when he learns that he can walk normally and not be handicapped with the limp and waddling gait that accompany congenital dislocation of the hip. Also, a neglected dislocated hip joint can wear out so badly in later life that major reconstructive surgery will be required to prevent total incapacitation.

CLUBFOOT. This is another congenital condition which seriously affects the foot. It can be corrected by early treatment. Sometimes only strapping or casts are required. Serious cases will need expert orthopedic surgery as advised above for congenital hip disease.

FROZEN SHOULDER. This very disabling limitation of motion of the important shoulder joint can develop after bursitis. The condition, which results from bands of adhesions around the joint, can also be due to other causes. If exercises, rest, and medicines do not help you, then a doctor who has had experience in the technique may free the adhesions by manipulation of the shoulder. This is done under anesthesia, and must be performed expertly to avoid tearing or breaking important structures in and around the joint.

RECONSTRUCTIVE SURGERY OF JOINTS. Regardless of the origin of the joint trouble, there is usually something that can be done to improve the joint's function. I have mentioned the help that arthritic patients can obtain (see page 456). Joints may be injured in accidents. Sometimes such joints may require special orthopedic operations to reconstruct them. New joints may be fashioned out of plastic or metal. Such surgery can be performed

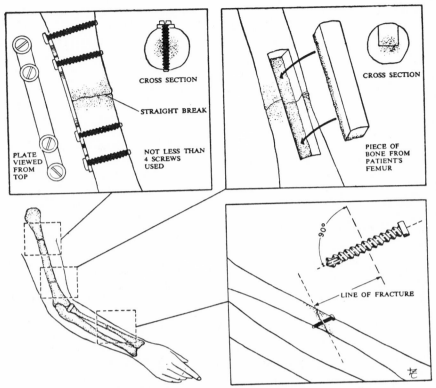

CROSS SECTION

STRAIGHT BREAK

PLATE VIEWED FROM TOP

NOT LESS THAN 4 SCREWS USED

CROSS SECTION

PIECE OF BONE FROM PATIENT'S FEMUR

90°

LINE OF FRACTURE

*Figure 34-4. Surgical Repair of Fractures. Main Methods of Helping Bone to Knit Properly.* LOWER LEFT: *Diagram showing possible locations for surgical repair in arm.* UPPER LEFT: *Metal (vitallium) plate and* *screws, especially for large bones.* UPPER RIGHT: *Bone graft; section of bone transplanted from patient.* LOWER RIGHT: *Vitallium screw holding small bone together.*

only by surgeons who are very skilled in this highly specialized field of reconstructive orthopedics.

## Fractures

Fractures usually cause only temporary disability. However, if the bone does not heal properly, there may be disability for life. Fractures in elderly people tend to knit poorly, and may need special attention. Also, in the growing child, fractures must be set correctly so that there is no interference with growth. I have described the common types of fractures and how to apply first aid for them on page 337. Also, in the section on accidents (p. 321), I have stressed the need for prevention. How-

ever, fractures do occur more and more frequently in our high-speed age. Some of the worst result from automobile accidents.

There is a tremendous difference in fractures and in the time and skill required to treat them. A noncomplicated fracture usually requires only a plaster cast, which can be applied by the family doctor, and heals over in several weeks. However, a double break of the forearm presents a serious problem. A specialist in orthopedic surgery may have to carry out the difficult procedure of inserting a metal pin in one bone and fastening a plate on the other. It is well worth the effort involved, as it will result in a strong, normal arm. Fractures of the long bones, especially of the thigh, usually require special apparatus and cannot be treated successfully by casts. Always ask your doctor,

"What can be done to bring about the *best* healing?" It is worth a considerable investment in time and money to prevent a shortened bone or impaired movement of a joint.


# POLIOMYELITIS
(Infantile Paralysis)


Polio, short for *poliomyelitis,* has ranked high among the disabling diseases. For that reason, everyone rejoiced to hear that vaccines had been found to prevent polio.

Vaccination is based on the principle of *immunity,* which I describe fully on page 134. Briefly, it is effective because our bodies can create an immunity to some diseases when we are given preparations of the proper germs, which are either dead or so weakened that they are no longer dangerous.

Polio is an infection of the central nervous system which attacks the cells of nerves that control the muscles. It may destroy or weaken them, causing paralysis. Most commonly, it affects the arms and legs. Less frequently, it paralyzes the muscles of breathing or swallowing. Actually, it can affect any muscle. *It does not affect the mind.*

Most cases that are reported occur in young children but polio attacks people of all ages. Although it may strike at any time of the year, the majority of cases are in the summer.

Before going any further, I want to remind you that this disease is not often a killer. In addition, the majority of those who have it do not suffer from paralysis or weakened muscles. Of those whose muscles are weakened, many are never paralyzed; and those whose muscles are paralyzed, more than half recover without serious aftereffects. I emphasize this because I want you to realize that there is no reason to become panicky about polio, even though I urge you not to ignore it until it has been completely eliminated.

Polio is caused by a virus (see page 132). Actually, there are at least three types of polio viruses, causing different kinds of poliomyelitis. Small as this organism is, scientists have been able to isolate and study it and have learned many of its habits. It has been found in the nose and mouth, and also in excreta from the intestines.

It has been found not only in polio patients but in people who do not appear to have the disease. There is proof that a great many people have been infected by polio without being sick at all, or else they were so slightly indisposed that they thought they had a cold or the "flu." These individuals are lucky because even this slight infection enabled them to build up some immunity to the disease. Older people are more likely than younger ones to have developed an immunity against polio by repeated mild exposures to it. This probably accounts for the fact that relatively few people contract polio when they are exposed to it, and for the fact that the majority of victims are children or young adults.

## Vaccination Against Polio

The first effective vaccine was developed under the direction of Dr. Jonas E. Salk, and the vaccine is commonly referred to by his name (but Dr. Salk would be the first to admit that many others helped in the long chain of experiments that led to the development of an effective vaccine). The Salk method requires three injections in order to provide an adequate immunity, and a booster shot is given once each year thereafter.

The next vaccine against polio was the oral type in which harmless, weakened strains of polio can be swallowed in a pleasant-tasting liquid. A number of scientists were responsible for the development of this type of very convenient vaccination, but the preparation of choice appears to be the one developed by Dr. Albert B. Sabin. His triple vaccine is given in one dose between the ages of six and nine months.

Every baby, child, and young adult should be vaccinated against this fearful malady. All adults regardless of age should consult their physicians and let them decide on the need for vaccination against polio.

## Symptoms

The early symptoms of polio include fever, headache, vomiting, fretfulness, drowsiness, sore throat, change in bowel habits, stiffness and pain in the back and neck. These do not necessarily mean polio. *But don't ignore them.* It is true that many diseases of childhood start in this way, but they, too, can be serious, and it is best not to dismiss them as "just a cold" or "upset stomach." Call your doctor promptly, for early good treatment can prevent not only death but the disabling effects of this disease.

# MULTIPLE SCLEROSIS

Multiple sclerosis is one of the most common diseases of the nervous system in the United States. However, it is by no means well known to the public. In the first place, it is not a killer, and in the second, it does not usually strike dramatically. Periods of improvement usually alternate with periods of symptoms.

But multiple sclerosis can be extremely disabling. Although patients may recover almost completely from severely paralyzing attacks of this disease, medical science has not as yet discovered any way of halting it. In recent years, it has received more attention from the public, and increased research will undoubtedly eventually uncover its cause and cure.

In multiple sclerosis, hardened patches due to inflammation are scattered at random throughout the brain and spinal cord, interfering with the nerves in these areas. Therefore, the disease is also called *disseminated sclerosis*. Why these patches become inflamed and hardened is still unknown. They usually occur in young adults.

The hard patches come and go. The symptoms depend on the portion of the nervous system that is affected. Since the location, extent, and duration of the injuries vary, it is difficult to describe a *typical* case of multiple sclerosis.

## Symptoms and Effects of Multiple Sclerosis

The most common of these include:

1. A tremor or shaking of the limbs, often making the patient weak and interfering with fine movements such as sewing or writing. Speech may become slow and monotonous.

2. Unsteadiness in walking, and an inability to maintain balance.

3. Stiffness in walking, the knees failing to bend.

4. Difficulties in vision. The patient may "see double" or lose part of the visual field. For example, he may be unable to see toward the upper left with either eye.

5. Paralysis, which may occur in any part of the body.

## Treatment

Good general care is necessary to keep up the body's health and resistance to disease, as multiple sclerosis is apt to grow worse following any illness. Expert nursing care may be required. Physiotherapy, including massage and exercise, will prevent the affected muscles from becoming unnecessarily weakened or paralyzed. Because this disease frequently grows worse when there are emotional disturbances, and because patients who are disabled by it may become depressed, a psychiatrist or psychotherapist (see page 182) may be helpful.

Patients with multiple sclerosis can often lead long, useful lives, as did Dr. Norman Goldsmith, who practiced medicine despite severe multiple sclerosis, as described in a book that I co-edited, *When Doctors Are Patients*. The National Multiple Sclerosis Society, 205 East 42nd Street, New York, N.Y. 10017, provides information and assistance concerning all phases of this disease, including rehabilitation.

# EPILEPSY

In recent years the public has been adopting a sensibly frank and open attitude toward many illnesses, including tuberculosis and venereal disease. However, for some reason, a "hush-hush" policy regarding epilepsy still prevails.

In the past, epilepsy was looked upon as a disgrace. People who suffered from it were shunned, regarded as insane or, at the least, "peculiar." Parents would try to hide the fact that a child had epilepsy. Consequently, people with epilepsy had to endure not only the disease but humiliation and a sense of inferiority that set them apart from others. Naturally, this often actually made them feel "peculiar." In addition, the fact that so many cases of epilepsy were concealed hampered medical research.

Even so, medical science has made great progress in understanding and treating epilepsy. We know now that it is *not* a kind of insanity. Epileptics are *not* "inferior." Nor are they superior, even though a number of exceptional people have had epilepsy, including Julius Caesar, Peter the Great, Lord Byron, Dostoevski, and Flaubert. Brain damage or mental deterioration occurs in only a very small percentage of certain types of epilepsy, or in cases which have been grossly neglected over a long period of years. In the overwhelming majority of cases medical treatment can, to a great extent, prevent disability.

## Symptoms of Epilepsy

The word epilepsy means a seizure. It is specifically applied to a certain type of seizure characterized by a loss of consciousness, momentary or more prolonged, and involuntary convulsive movements. Some lay people call this a "fit."

In minor seizures, or *petit mal*, the loss of consciousness is momentary. Although there is often a twitching about the eyes or mouth, there is no change of posture. The epileptic remains seated or standing and appears to have had no more than a lapse of attention or a moment of absent-mindedness.

In *psychomotor* epilepsy, there is very brief clouding of consciousness with some repeated purposeless movement such as hand clapping, followed by brief periods of forgetfulness.

In major seizures, or *grand mal*, the victim falls to the floor unconscious, often foaming at the mouth, biting, and shaking his limbs violently. Involuntary bowel movements or the passage of urine may occur. The patient may hurt himself during such a seizure. The observer may mistake it for fainting, "blacking out," or even a "stroke," although the convulsive movements should indicate that it is an attack of epilepsy. Fortunately, people with epilepsy frequently experience a warning called the *aura*, before a major attack occurs, and this enables them to lie down and avoid falls.

*What to Do if Someone Has an Epileptic Seizure*

1. At the beginning of the attack, lower him to the floor. Remove any hard objects he may strike.

2. Put an object between the back teeth on one side of his mouth. Make sure it is too big to swallow. A folded handkerchief or a roll of paper will do. The purpose is to prevent him from biting his tongue or breaking his front teeth. Do not try to force the mouth open, but wait for it to relax momentarily. Keep your fingers out of his mouth or you may be badly bitten.

3. Do not try to force any liquids down his throat or to move him during a convulsion. When the attack is over, make sure he rests quietly until he regains consciousness fully. Do not rush him to a hospital unless he has a series of seizures.

An epileptic seizure is the result of a temporary disturbance of the brain impulses, an abnormal electrical discharge, so to speak. It might be compared to the static you get on your radio. Medically, it is called *cerebral dysrhythmia*, meaning a disturbance of the brain's normal rhythm. Apart from the temporary disturbance, there is nothing wrong with the brain as far as intelligence and emotions are concerned.

## Diagnosis

Anyone who has fainting spells, fleeting unconsciousness, convulsions, or fits of any sort should be studied by a competent doctor. They may be due to a disease other than epilepsy—for example, diseases of the heart or arteries, nervous reflex disorders, and psychoneuroses. In order to make a diagnosis of epilepsy, a number of tests may be required. An *electroencephalograph* record is helpful. This is made by a machine with electrodes, which are placed on the head to record the brain waves, showing the electrical activity of the brain. Some individuals who are entirely well, however, have brain waves like those seen in epilepsy. X-rays of the skull, and perhaps air injections into the ventricles of the brain in order to permit special x-rays, may be necessary.

If these tests reveal that the patient has epilepsy, the services of a specialist will probably be required. It is essential to discover what type of epilepsy it is, since the treatment varies considerably.

## Cause and Treatment

In *acquired epilepsy*, the cause is physical, such as a brain tumor or a wound or blow on the head. These injuries irritate the brain and set off the abnormal electrical discharge. A cure may be achieved by an operation to remove the tumor or repair the injury.

*Ordinary epilepsy* is also called *genuine epilepsy* or *idiopathic epilepsy*, which means cause unknown. This is the most common type, and it is what most people have in mind when they speak of epilepsy. It usually begins early in life. This type of epilepsy is not directly inherited, although it is generally believed that a predisposition or tendency to it may run in families. While the cause is still unknown, a great deal is known about it, especially in regard to treatment.

There are now several very effective medicines which entirely eliminate or greatly reduce the seizures. These include phenobarbital, Dilantin, Tridione, and others. They must be administered *only* by a competent physician. Individual cases vary a great deal and continuous care is essential, especially during the early stages of treatment, to determine the most effective medicine and dosage. After the patient's convulsions are under control, he may need to see the doctor only infrequently.

However, it is vitally important for every patient to visit his doctor at intervals, and continue taking the medicines unless he is instructed to stop. Patients who stop medication without such instructions from their physicians may suffer a recurrence of their attacks, which must then be brought under control all over again. After there have been no attacks for a sufficient period of time, the doctor may gradually cut down the medication. But this should never be undertaken by the patient.

These new medicines can usually prevent the disabling effects of epilepsy. Individuals with epilepsy can now hold responsible positions and lead practically normal lives, with few restrictions beyond those imposed in having to take medicine and consult their doctors. Psychiatric help (see page 183) is valuable in some cases, especially with patients who are emotionally disturbed for any reason. Organizations such as the Epilepsy Foundation of America, 1828 L Street NW, Washington, D.C. 20036 provide helpful information for epileptics and their families.

# PARKINSONISM

*Parkinsonism* is a disease of the nervous system which is characterized by stiffness of muscles and tremors. It has been called *paralysis agitans*. At first the patient may be troubled by mild tremors of the hands and nodding of the head. Then it is seen that his face does not have its usual mobility. For instance, the capacity to smile may have disappeared. This is called the "masklike" face of parkinsonism. As the disease advances, the shaking tremors of the muscles progress and may involve the entire body. The back tends to become bent forward. Yet the mind is unaffected. If the patient is fortunate enough to have a job that requires chiefly mental effort, he can frequently continue working for many years.

Parkinsonism occurs in later life. In some cases, it may result from viral infection or carbon monoxide poisoning, but usually the cause is unknown.

## Treatment

Several medications are now available to help patients with parkinsonism. A drug called levodopa is often effective. Another helpful agent is amantadine. Also valuable, sometimes in combination with levodopa, are trihexyphenidyl, benztropine mesylate, and antihistamines such as diphenhydramine.

Some surgical procedures, involving destruction of a small area in the brain, have helped many sufferers.

# NEURITIS AND NEURALGIA

When pain accompanies an illness, it is usually because the disease has inflamed an organ and irritated the ends of the *pain nerves*, or pain fibers. Thus, an infection of the skin such as a boil is terribly painful because there are many pain nerves in the skin. These become irritated by the stretching of the boil and the toxic action of the pus and bacteria. However, there are conditions in which the nerves *themselves* become inflamed. Such nerve inflammation is called *neuritis*. If the irritation affects a nerve which carries pain fibers, there will be severe pain perceived by the brain, which is the central receiving station for all pain nerve fibers. We usually speak of this pain as neuralgia. When nerves that do not carry pain fibers, such as the *motor nerves* to muscles, are destroyed by the polio virus, there may be total paralysis without any pain. It may seem strange to you that large areas of the brain substance itself may be cut without any pain sensation. This is due to the fact that pain nerves go to only special areas of the brain.

Diseases such as multiple sclerosis, polio, and parkinsonism affect the brain and/or spinal cord. Other maladies affect the *peripheral nerves* which connect the brain and spinal cord with the muscles, organs, skin, eyes, etc. The many peripheral nerves may be affected by a variety of diseases and injuries. When a peripheral nerve is involved, the condition is called *neuritis* or *neuralgia*.

The peripheral nerves usually contain both pain and motor fibers. Thus a disease which affects the peripheral nerves would be expected to, and usually does, cause painful symptoms plus some paralysis of muscle power.

## Generalized Neuritis

Certain toxic substances such as lead, arsenic, and mercury may produce a generalized poisoning of the peripheral nerves, with paralysis of the limbs, and also pain and tenderness. There are many other causes of generalized neuritis, including alcoholism, vitamin deficiencies such as pellagra and beriberi, some types of allergy, diabetes, severe vomiting of pregnancy, thallium toxicity, and some virus and bacterial infections.

Some attacks of generalized neuritis begin with fever and other symptoms of an acute illness. On the other hand, neuritis caused by lead and alcohol toxicity comes on very slowly over the course of weeks or months.

TREATMENT AND PREVENTION. In most instances, the attack will subside by itself or when the toxic substance is eliminated. Rest and a good diet containing extra vitamins, especially of the B group (see page 37), are helpful. Physiotherapy may relieve the pain or the paralysis. Prevention of generalized neuritis is based on the knowledge of the dangers of poor nutrition (p. 39), industrial hazards (p. 145), chronic alcoholism (p. 470), and infections.

## Special Types of Neuritis and Neuralgia

Frequently, instead of a generalized irritation of the nerves, only one nerve is afflicted. For example, a person may be sleeping in a cold draft which blows on the left side of the face. The next morning, the side of the face which is "powered" by muscles controlled through the facial nerve may be temporarily paralyzed. This type of paralysis is called *facial palsy* or *Bell's palsy*. When caused by drafts and infections, the paralysis clears up after some days or weeks. Sometimes, a tumor will press on the nerve and cause facial palsy, or the nerve may be injured by a blow, a cut, or a bullet. In that event, the results of treatment will depend on the success in treating the tumor or injury. If the cause of facial palsy is not apparent, or the condition does not improve, your doctor is justified in sending you to a neurologist for the opinion of a specialist.

## Sciatica

Consult the illustration on page 469, showing how the sciatic nerve traverses the long distance from the spinal column to the legs. The sciatic nerve is the widest nerve in the body, as well as being of great length. It is exposed to many different kinds of injury in the back, in the pelvis, and even along its course in the lower extremity.

SYMPTOMS AND CAUSES. Injury or inflammation of the sciatic nerve causes pain which travels down the leg from the thigh or back into the feet and toes. Certain muscles of the leg may be partly or completely paralyzed, making it difficult to move the thigh and leg. When this occurs, the doctor makes a careful search for the origin of the sciatica. He knows that this will generally reveal some definite reason for the neuralgic pain. There may be a back injury (see page 459), or irritation from arthritis of the spine, or pressure on the nerve which occurs during some types of work. Also, certain diseases such as diabetes or gout may be the inciting factor. It is true that some cases of sciatica will turn out to be the idiopathic variety, that is, without known cause. However, because of the long and painful and disabling course of severe sciatica, it is worth considerable time and money to have every possible cause investigated. If the diagnosis has been made, the cure will be facilitated by correcting the underlying trouble. In addition, sedatives and physiotherapy may be required to relieve the pain or disability.

## Shingles (Herpes Zoster)

Herpes zoster, or shingles (the word *herpes* means *blisters,* and *zoster* means *girdle*), is a terribly painful inflammation of the sections of the nerves which have just emerged from the spinal cord. This illness is caused by a virus. Fever and prostration may accompany the pain when the malady first develops. After the illness starts, small blisters or vesicles usually, but not always, appear on the skin along the course of the affected nerves. Frequently, this will be on the chest. But there is a form of shingles which inflames the nerves leading to the face and eyes. This form is specially dangerous because it may cause damage to the vision. The ordinary attack of shingles runs its painful course in a matter of days or weeks, and does not leave any residual difficulties. However, in some instances, most frequently in elderly people, there is a persistence of pain which may be terribly disabling. In this

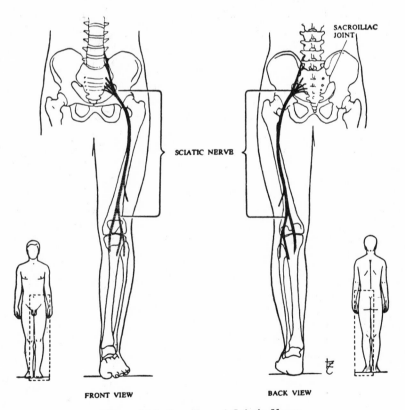

*Figure 34-5. Location of Sciatic Nerve.*

event, special treatments and medicines can be given by your doctor to relieve the pain. Incidentally, there is no truth to the old saying that "the patient will die if the blisters appear on both sides of the body and meet in the center."

Some people think an ordinary attack of "shingles" is too trivial to warrant a doctor's time. Your doctor knows the discomfort and complications this illness can cause, and he is eager to relieve and prevent the symptoms.

### Neuritis of Other Spinal Nerves

Any one of the many nerves traveling out from the spine may be affected by injury or disease. For example, the nerves which lie between the ribs may become inflamed and cause pain in the chest which may resemble pleurisy and even a heart attack. This form of nerve ailment is called *intercostal neuritis* or *neuralgia*. Similarly, the nerves traveling down the neck to the arm may be subject to various injuries and diseases. For example, a chronic pain in the hand or arm is sometimes traced to the irritation caused by the pressure of an extra rib in the neck. Doctors call this the *cervical rib syndrome*. Sometimes, too vigorous pulling on the nerves in the neck, such as might occur in difficult obstetrical deliveries, causes the condition known as *brachial nerve palsy*, which may lead to paralysis of the arm.

### Neuritis of the Cranial Nerves

I have mentioned ailments like sciatica which strike at the spinal cord nerves. However, there are also *twelve pairs* of important nerves leading directly from the brain. These are called *cranial nerves*. I have described Bell's palsy which results from inflammation of the facial or seventh cranial nerve. There is another nerve, the *trigeminal*, or fifth cranial nerve, which also ends in the face and jaws. This nerve may be the source of a neuralgia which causes spasms of pain on one side of the face. This *trigeminal neuralgia* is also called *tic douloureux*. It may be set off by a draft of cold air, by chewing, or by other trigger factors. Both medicines and surgical operations can relieve this terribly painful malady.

The nerves leading to the retina of the eye may be involved in various ailments. This condition is called *optic neuritis* and, because of its potential danger to vision, requires immediate treatment. Any of the other cranial nerves may be damaged by infections, tumors, and toxins. The antibiotic medicine, *streptomycin*, can injure the eighth cranial nerve, which helps control the sense of balance in the internal ear. Any disturbances of vision, hearing, balancing, swallowing, taste, or speech may be signals of trouble in the cranial nerves, and should be mentioned to a physician at once.

### Injuries to Nerves

The peripheral nerves may be cut, bruised, or torn by fractured bones, blows, or gunshot wounds. Nerves have a capacity to heal and regenerate. A torn or cut nerve should be treated by a surgeon who specializes in such work. If necessary, go hundreds of miles for such treatment if your doctor advises it, rather than take a chance on paralysis and other serious consequences of nerve injuries.

Read again my comments in the First Aid chapter (page 337) on how to avoid injury to nerves after a bone has been broken.

## ALCOHOLISM

*Alcoholism is one of the greatest disabling diseases.* I am not referring to moderate drinking, or even to excessive drinking with its hangovers which, although certainly disabling, occur only occasionally. It is hard to draw a fine line between drinking in moderation, drinking to excess, and habitual drinking, or chronic alcoholism. On page 22 I discuss these and also explain the effect which alcohol has on the body. It is not, as it seems to be, a stimulant, but actually a depressant. When I speak of the habitual drinker, I mean anyone who craves and is dependent on alcohol, drinking regularly and excessively, so that it interferes with his or her work, home life, and normal relationships with other people.

Under the effects of alcohol, the drinker may feel he has rid himself of the inhibitions that made him feel shy and inferior. But he also loses those that made him behave in a socially acceptable manner. Under the impression that alcohol makes him feel at ease, he fails to realize, or does not place sufficient emphasis upon, the fact that it slows down his thinking processes and his reflexes. Judgment and coordination are impaired, so that accidents result, especially when driving an automobile. It is impossible even to estimate how much disability has been caused in this way not only to the drinker but to his innocent victims.

## Disabling Illnesses Resulting from Habitual Drinking

In many cases these may be due not only to the effect of alcohol, but also to the fact that habitual drinkers tend not to eat properly. They get their required calories from alcohol itself which is a food, providing fuel for the body. However, although it contains calories, alcohol lacks vitamins, minerals, and other essentials without which the body may suffer from nutritional disorders (see page 37). The appetite usually becomes poor, and general malnutrition results.

1. *Effects on the nervous system.* These include *neuritis,* an inflammation of the nerves, usually associated with pain. In *polyneuritis* or *Korsakoff's disease,* the nerves of the limbs, particularly of the foot and wrist, are affected. It is often accompanied by memory disorders. *Delirium tremens,* or "D.T.'s," is an acute condition which is particularly apt to occur if the habitual drinker is suddenly deprived of alcohol. It is vividly described in the book and the motion picture called *The Lost Weekend.* The patient's fingers, legs, or entire body may shake. He is extremely confused, suffering from hallucinations in which he may see "pink elephants" or feel "ants crawling under his skin." This is a serious disease, and unless he receives proper medical care, the patient may suffer heart failure or get pneumonia. *Mental deterioration* is a real possibility in habitual drinkers.

2. *Cirrhosis of the liver.* I describe this potential killer on page 445. Although it is by no means limited to habitual drinkers, they are more susceptible to it than the average person. It may be caused by nutritional deficiencies that are produced by excessive use of alcohol in place of food.

3. *Involvement of the eyes.* In certain instances, *alcohol amblyopia* or loss of central vision may result. This condition is not to be confused with blindness caused by drinking methyl alcohol (wood alcohol) which is substituted for or mixed with ethyl alcohol (grain alcohol) because it is cheaper or more easily obtained. *Alcohol amblyopia* may result from prolonged use of even the highest quality alcoholic beverages.

4. *Involvement of other organs.* The heart and kidneys may be impaired as an indirect result of chronic alcoholism. Gastric disturbances and circulatory disorders may afflict the habitual drinker. As in the case of cirrhosis of the liver, he is apt to suffer from *acne rosacea* (see page 123), in which the blood vessels of the face, especially of the nose, become enlarged.

5. *Infections.* Habitual drinking usually lowers the resistance to infectious diseases. This is particularly true of *lobar pneumonia* which I describe on page 443 and which has a higher death rate among drinkers than among nondrinkers.

## Why Some People Drink Excessively

There is still no definitive answer to the question of what causes alcoholism. Both physical and psychological factors have been cited. People who become excessive drinkers may or may not be immature or neurotic.

As their addiction takes hold, all alcoholics, whatever their background, tend to become much alike in behavior. The procurement of alcohol becomes their chief concern, superseding other interests, producing a deterioration in their work, social life, and relationships with their families.

There have been studies of intelligent, heavy-drinking people to determine what they consider excessive drinking. Always, it appears, the definition of excessive drinking turns out to be several drinks more than the heavy drinker personally consumes. Some of these people have indicated they see nothing excessive in drinking as much as a fifth of whiskey a day.

Unless they have guidelines, it would appear that even intelligent people who have moved far along the road to alcoholism may not recognize the fact. In an effort to provide such guidelines, the Life Extension Foundation in New York has produced the following for its business executive clients, which I think worth repeating here. Any drinker, the foundation suggests, can consider that alcoholism is approaching

1. If two or three years ago a half hour before dinner was set aside for a drink and now this has stretched to two hours and four drinks

2. If two or three years ago dinner was anticipated with pleasure, and now there is little interest in food and sometimes dinner is completely omitted

3. If two or three years ago cocktails at lunch were for business entertaining only and now one or two are routine

4. If two or three years ago weekend consumption was little more than that of weekdays, but now drinking is started in the morning and continues more or less all day

Dr. Harry J. Johnson of the foundation goes on to urge, very soundly, that every heavy drinker give himself a test to determine whether or not he is becoming an alcoholic.

It's a simple test. It merely requires the heavy drinker to declare a semiannual alcoholic abstention period of not less than one week. If he can get through the week without unpleasant withdrawal symptoms, without a feeling of martyrdom, and with no obsessive desire to return to drinking when the rest period is over, alcoholism is not yet present. If, when time for the test period arrives, the drinker rationalizes and justifies a postponement for any reason whatever, he is entering the twilight zone of alcoholism, and the point of no return may be near.

Alcoholism is preventable. Even the heavy drinker, alert to the danger that he is traveling the road to alcoholism, often may have time to prevent development of the full-blown addiction by limiting alcohol intake.

## Help for the Alcoholic

Once alcoholism has developed, the problem is difficult but not beyond solution. To be solved, it must be approached in no simplistic fashion. Every aspect must receive attention.

An important part of the physician's job is to help the patient recognize, accept, and understand his illness. He must be made to feel, not an outcast, but a worthwhile person who has a definite sickness. Treatment—more properly, re-

habilitation—must be multifaceted: physical, psychological, social, and spiritual. On the physical side, for example, because an alcoholic often is malnourished, his diet must be carefully supervised.

Many forms of treatment have been used. For some well-motivated alcoholics, Antabuse, a drug that causes uncomfortable reactions to drinking, has proved useful. Although hypnosis has been found of limited usefulness in producing aversion to alcohol, it sometimes may help in teaching the anxious person to relax and develop greater self-esteem. Psychoanalysis, as a rule, has produced disappointing results with alcoholics.

In the view of many authorities, Alcoholics Anonymous is of first importance in the rescue and rehabilitation of alcoholics. It has been called by Dr. Ruth Fox, medical director of the National Council on Alcoholism, "a pragmatic, simplified, spiritual approach to life, a prescription for living. For patients who can and will accept it, it may be the only form of therapy needed. There can be an immediate amelioration of symptoms as the isolated alcoholic feels that there is hope for him."

Alcoholics Anonymous is an organization of individuals who have conquered or are trying to conquer their own habitual drinking and to help others with their problems. From their own personal experience, they have learned how to encourage and stimulate others in their desire to stop drinking. Meetings and discussions provide opportunities to air problems, and this is a most useful form of psychotherapy. The organization has branches in many communities across the country, and members are welcomed wherever they may travel. A call to a local branch can bring immediate help. The national headquarters is P.O. Box 459, Grand Central Annex, New York, N.Y. 10017.

## CEREBRAL PALSY

Cerebral palsy is the most common cause of crippling of children in the United States. Almost one quarter of a million persons are afflicted. It is one of the saddest of the disabling diseases because it strikes at infants, many of whom are treated as though they were helpless mental and physical cripples for the rest of their lives. This is particularly tragic because, in the overwhelming majority of cases, a great deal can be done to help the victims of cerebral palsy.

Cerebral palsy is due to damage in one or more areas of the brain. The damage may stem from many possible causes. They include injury to the unborn child during the latter part of pregnancy because of bleeding, toxemia, diabetes, placental problems, or kidney infections; damage to the infant at birth because of lack of oxygen, difficult labor, breech birth, or complications of delivery; and such other possible causes as Rh-incompatibility disease, rubella of the mother in early pregnancy, and brain damage in early infancy from encephalitis, meningitis, or other infection.

We have found that in only a relatively small percentage of cases does the injury cause mental deficiency. It is generally of such a nature that it interferes with the nerves controlling the muscles. As a result, the victim of cerebral palsy may *appear* to be an imbecile, for example, by drooling, grunting instead of speaking, and making strange gestures and grimaces. Of course, many children with cerebral palsy fail to develop normally because they are treated as if they were hopeless idiots.

The injury to the brain may cause (a) *spastic* paralysis, with stiffness and impaired movement of the muscles. Such a patient will walk with a scissorslike gait; (b) *tremors,* and strange movements of the limbs and the head, which may be accompanied by bizarre grimaces; (c) *poor coordination.*

## Treatment

This varies according to the nature and extent of the injury. Certain medicines help to relieve muscular spasms. Some deformities can be corrected by surgical means. But training is the key that has opened the door to a useful, normal life for countless cerebral palsy sufferers. The earlier this treatment begins, the less difficulty there will be in overcoming or avoiding the disabilities.

Usually the parent or physician can observe indications of cerebral palsy when a baby is only a few months old. Such an infant should be examined at a medical center that specializes in this disease. It is extremely important for the parents of children with cerebral palsy to *learn how to help them.* They must understand that it is not kindness to do everything for a child with cerebral palsy instead of encouraging him in the difficult task of doing things himself. Helping such a child learn to talk, walk, and do the many things which are so easy for the average child and so difficult for one whose muscles do not respond in the normal way, requires a great deal of skill and patience. Methods vary according to the type of cerebral palsy from which the child is suffering. For example, *spastic* children are usually timid and shy, while *athetoid* children, whose muscles tend to be relaxed rather than stiff, are apt to be fearless.

The United Cerebral Palsy Association, 66 East 34th Street, New York, N.Y. 10016, which has branches in many cities, can give help and encouragement. It is most heartening to see the miracles which time, patience, and knowledge can work in many cases of cerebral palsy.

Parents whose children are mentally retarded as a result of cerebral palsy should get in touch with the National Association for Retarded Children, 420 Lexington Ave., New York, N. Y. 10017, or one of its local branches. They will find that a great deal can be done to help the retarded child make his maximum contribution to society and to help the family make the necessary adjustments so that the other members will not be unduly affected.

It is never too late for a patient with cerebral palsy to have a complete evaluation of his condition, for good results can be obtained later in life.

## DISABLING DISEASES OF THE MUSCLES

In polio and other diseases that affect nerves or the brain, the muscles are disabled because the nerves leading to them have been injured or destroyed. In other words, in polio, in multiple sclerosis, and in a stroke, there is nothing wrong with the muscles *at first.* However, when the nerves leading to muscles no longer stimulate them, the muscles waste away or atrophy from lack of use.

In contrast to the nerve type of muscle illness, there are several diseases of the muscles themselves which cause severe disabilities. Of these, the two most important are *muscular dystrophy* and *myasthenia gravis*.

## Muscular Dystrophy

This is a particularly sad disabler disease because it strikes chiefly at young children and teenagers. The muscles are weakened and shriveled away gradually by the disease, which, in the childhood type, has usually shown itself by the age of six. It occurs much more frequently in males than in females. The disease affects important muscles, even those of the trunk of the body. As it progresses, it may incapacitate the patient so completely that he cannot even stand or sit. However, there are many forms of the disease, and not all lead to total incapacitation.

There is a less extensive form of muscular dystrophy which usually appears between the ages of ten and twenty. This form is apt to involve the muscles of the face and the shoulders. However, it does not always spare the leg or trunk muscles.

Because of the way this variety of the disease affects muscles, it is referred to as the *fascio-scapulohumeral type*. Usually, patients with this type will live out their years, and the fortunate ones will have rather mild disability.

TREATMENT. At the present time there is no really effective therapy. However, research physicians are studying this illness and hope to be able to improve the condition of these patients. Patients with this illness should be in touch at regular intervals with a doctor or a clinic that treats this illness. The use of the muscles often can be prolonged by exercises, surgery, orthopedic devices, and prescribed activity.

The Muscular Dystrophy Association of America (p. 410) can provide information about rehabilitation centers and the latest developments in treatment.

## Myasthenia Gravis

In myasthenia gravis, there appears to be a chemical defect at the sites where the nerves and muscles interact. As a result, the muscles do not function properly. People with this illness find that certain muscles tire very quickly on exertion.

Also, there is a feeling of weakness in the muscles. Muscles frequently affected are those of the face, eyelids, larynx, and throat. Therefore, the patient may first detect the onset of myasthenia gravis because his eyelids droop, or there is trouble in swallowing a drink of water.

There is no true paralysis of the muscles, and they do not usually shrivel away. However, in severe forms the disease can be terribly disabling or even fatal because it may involve the vital muscles of swallowing or even breathing. Fortunately, there are both medical and surgical treatments which are helpful to a considerable number of these patients. A medicine called *Neostigmine* or one called *Mestinon* will reverse the disordered chemistry at the nerve-muscle junction in a short time. It is one of the most amazing sights in medical practice to see a patient with drooping eyelids, hands that cannot be clenched, arms that cannot be moved because of excessive weakness, suddenly come to life within a few minutes after the administration of Neostigmine.

In addition to this medication, there are several others that are helpful. Removal of the thymus gland has also been found helpful, *even curative*, in some instances.

Patients with *myasthenia gravis* should have a complete evaluation of their illness made by a specialist in this disease. Individuals in smaller communities may have to arrange to go to the large clinics maintained for this disease at Johns Hopkins Medical School, Harvard Medical School, and a number of our other leading schools and medical centers. Your family doctor can make the arrangements.

## Other Disabling Diseases of Muscles

A less common condition of the muscles is *familial periodic paralysis*, in which the muscles undergo temporary, intermittent paralysis. It has been found that this is a functional disease associated with a low content of the vital chemical potassium in the blood serum. Administration of potassium will alleviate or prevent the attacks. Another familial muscle disease is *myatonia dystrophica*, in which there is weakness and wasting of the muscles. Cataracts of the eyes may accompany this illness. Another muscle disabler, which tends to run in families, is *peroneal muscular atrophy*, also called *Charcot-Marie-Tooth disease.* This disease, which can spread to areas other than the leg muscles where it starts, tends to be remarkably slow in its progress. Sometimes there are associated nerve disturbances in the spinal cord.

## LOSS OF EYESIGHT

On page 107, I have discussed everyday care of the eyes, and how to prevent loss of vision, by guarding against glaucoma, infections, and injury.

Unfortunately, despite the best that modern medicine and surgery can do, there are still many people whose vision is severely and irreparably damaged, or who are totally blind.

Let me at this point urge every blind or near-blind person who has not done so to review the situation with his doctor or an eye specialist selected by his doctor. You may not know, for example, that some blind people have had sight restored by the operation in which a cornea, obtained from an eye bank, is grafted in place of the diseased one. Also, many cataracts can now be operated on earlier than was once advised (see page 108). Other newly devised operations are helping people whose condition would have been considered hopeless until a short time ago.

What about those who must accept blindness? Let me first suggest that they take heart by learning about blind people who have lived useful, enjoyable lives. I recommend the inspiring story of famous Helen Keller, blind *and* deaf since early childhood, as well as such books as *Keep Your Head Up, Mr. Putnam,* in which young Peter Putnam tells with humor about his adventures with his Seeing-Eye dog, following the accident that blinded him but also opened many new doors to living, and Dr. Elliott Dobson's story in *When Doctors Are Patients,* which he tells under the title "The Light Within." Although blind, Dr. Dobson continues his large practice of internal medicine and his lectures to medical students. In addition, he has a happy family life and many social engagements. When I had lunch with him recently we talked enthusiastically about medicine, friends, and other things for almost two hours. At no time did the waiter realize that he was serving a blind man, so expert was Dr. Dobson in handling the knives, forks, and hot dishes. I was puzzled when he said, "I got up early and read an exciting novel this morning," for I knew he did not read Braille. He meant that he had enjoyed a "talking book" on his phonograph.

There are many agencies which help blind and partially blind people to find solutions to their problems, including the Braille Institute of America, Inc., 741 Vermont Avenue, Los Angeles, Cal. 90029, The Seeing Eye, Inc., Morristown, New Jersey, and other local as well as national organizations. Federal agencies help provide jobs and other opportunities. When blindness proves too upsetting emotionally, psychiatric assistance should be obtained (see page 183).

Currently, too, many new developments promise to improve the lives and opportunities of many of the blind. Now available, for example, is a laser cane, the result of twenty-five years of Veterans Administration-sponsored development by Bionic Instruments, a Bala-Cynwyd, Pennsylvania, bioengineering firm. It uses thin beams of light that permit a blind person to know when there is an obstacle directly ahead and when he is approaching a dropoff such as a curb or down stairway. A talking calculator for the blind has been produced by Telesensory Systems, Inc., of Palo Alto, California.

Presently under development are several different types of reading machines. One, also produced by Telesensory Systems, is called the Optacon (for optical-to-tactile conversion). In one hand, a user holds a miniature camera about the size of a small pocketknife to read printed material and convert it into impulses. And with the index finger of his other hand, the user can feel the letters and numbers via a 1″ x 1½″ tactile array of 144 miniature vibrating rods contained in a portable, battery-operated electronics section about the size and weight of a portable cassette tape recorder. For example, as the camera moves across an "E," the user feels a vertical line and three horizontal lines moving beneath the finger. A machine that reads aloud to the blind has been developed by Kurzweil Computer Products in Cambridge, Massachusetts.

At this writing, such devices are expensive ($1950 for the laser cane, $395 for the calculator, $2895 for the Optacon, for example). But prices are expected to come down with volume production.

# DISEASES OF THE EAR AND THE LABYRINTH

I discuss care of the ears, detection and prevention of deafness, and hearing aids on page 112. Workers in noisy trades such as riveting should take precautions for the prevention of deafness. Sportsmen often forget that trapshooting and pistol shooting may impair the hearing in the ear nearer to the sound of the shot. It is important to remember that 2 to 3 percent of schoolchildren and 10 percent of adults have some hearing impairment which should be discovered and, if necessary, treated to prevent further disability. Remarkable progress has been made in enabling little children whose hearing is drastically impaired to develop normally, especially if they receive help early.

The hearing nerve is closely connected with the nerve leading from the balancing mechanism located in the innermost portion of the ear. Disturbances of the balancing mechanism, the labyrinth, may cause so much ringing in the ears that hearing is also impaired. One of the principal diseases of the delicate balancing structure is *Ménière's disease,* in which there may be ringing in the ears, *tinnitus,* and some deafness for many years. In acute attacks there may be disabling dizziness, nausea, and vomiting. The individual suffering such an attack may actually keel over from the violent dizziness. There are both medical and surgical treatments for this disease which will require the advice of a specialist in diseases of the ear (an otologist) or examination in the ear diseases clinic of a hospital.

There are a number of agencies, both governmental and voluntary, to help the deaf and hard of hearing. These are listed on page 410.

## LOW BLOOD PRESSURE
(Hypotension)

Low blood pressure seldom causes true illness. Diseases in which chronic low blood pressure occurs are also rare. All these cases combined are so few in number that they would hardly warrant consideration if it were not for the fact that many people *consider themselves disabled*—and arrange their lives accordingly—because their blood pressure is low. *They worry for no adequate reason.*

It would be helpful if these cases were spoken of as "low normal blood pressure" or "lower-than-average blood pressure" rather than as "low blood pressure," which has an ominous sound. Look at it this way: although the average male is about five feet eight inches tall, you surely would not think of saying that a man who measures only five feet has "low height"—*and therefore must be sick!* Similarly, although the average blood pressure of a group of young adult males is about 120, expressed in millimeters mercury systolic pressure, a certain percentage will have blood pressures of 100 or even 90. In most instances, they are perfectly healthy and are just the low normals of the general population. In fact, individuals whose blood pressure tends to be somewhat below the average are apt to live longer than other people.

There are occasional individuals with low blood pressure who have symptoms such as dizziness or faintness, especially during change of position. These cases are very rare. Your doctor can prescribe treatment which will usually relieve these symptoms.

In other rare instances, low blood pressure may be associated with definite diseases such as Addison's disease and inadequate thyroid function. In these cases, the primary disease which causes the low blood pressure usually produces so many other symptoms that the disease is recognized even before the low blood pressure is observed.

Because the occasional case of lower-than-normal blood pressure which causes symptoms may be associated with some other illness, you should have a thorough medical checkup if your blood pressure is 90 to 100 or lower. But if your doctor concludes that your blood pressure is just low normal, consider yourself fortunate. Don't feel you have an abnormal blood pressure at all.

## INFLUENZA

Because influenza, usually called "the flu," often resembles a common cold, many people fail to take it seriously. This is a grave mistake, because pneumonia may go hand in hand with influenza. During the world-wide epidemic of 1918, approximately 20,000,000 people lost their lives from this combination of diseases. This fact may make you feel that the flu is entitled to a place among the killers, but I consider it a disabler because it is seldom the *direct* cause of death. Even though the fever and other symptoms may last only a few days, influenza is apt to leave people as weak and generally disabled as though they had gone through a long siege of illness.

Influenza is caused by a virus (see page 132). Its symptoms include fever, sore throat, cough, a runny nose, and a feeling of misery, chills, sweats, and aches, especially in the head, back, and legs. Like a cold, it is spread from one person to another, most commonly when a person in the early stages coughs or sneezes, spraying the virus into the air which other people breathe (see page 136). It is so contagious that health authorities are seldom able to prevent it from becoming an epidemic, once it appears in a community. Fortunately, these epidemics usually last no longer than a month.

## Prevention

The following precautions will help you avoid catching influenza. Be sure to pay special attention to them when you know that there are flu cases in your community.

Get plenty of rest and avoid getting overtired or chilled.

Avoid crowds and any unnecessary contact with other people. Keep as far away as possible from those who do not smother their coughs and sneezes with a handkerchief or tissue. Be sure to make this a habit in your family.

Be especially careful about contact with anyone who is coming down with "the sniffles." Influenza is highly contagious during its early stages. Regard every cold as potential influenza. This is always a safe rule to follow, as it is often difficult even for a doctor to distinguish between the two.

If someone in your household has the flu, keep him isolated from the other members of the family. His dishes, towels, etc., should be kept and washed separately, and rinsed in scalding water. Don't touch the cloths or tissues he uses as handkerchiefs. He should put them in a paper bag which can be burned or easily disposed of in some other way. Always wash your hands after touching anything with which he has come in contact.

Purchase a gauze mask and wear it over your nose and mouth when you are in his room.

Do not count on being immune because you have recovered from an attack of influenza. It is true that temporary immunity does follow the flu, but there are a number of different strains of the influenza virus, and having had one kind does not keep you from catching another. Similarly, *vaccines* give protection for some months, but only against certain influenza viruses. However, vaccination can be extremely helpful in preventing the flu during some epidemics. Be sure to ask your doctor about this.

## Treatment

The best way to get well quickly and avoid dangerous or disabling complications is to give yourself all the possible odds in your fight against the virus. Go to bed if you have any symptoms of a cold or the flu, or even if you just do not feel well when there is influenza about. If it turns out to be nothing, think of your "wasted" day as insurance against catching the flu. If it's just a cold, be sure to follow very carefully the instructions I give on page 497. Don't overtreat yourself with nose drops, sprays, or antihistamines. If you have any aches and pains or a fever, call the doctor immediately. He will prescribe the medication you need. Although the sulfa drugs and antibiotics such as penicillin will not cure your flu, they are valuable in guarding against pneumonia and some other diseases for which influenza paves the way. Avoid visitors because they may carry in these germs.

Be sure to stay in bed as long as your doctor tells you to, even if your symptoms have disappeared. The fatigue may last several weeks. A great many of the complications of influenza develop because patients insist on deciding for themselves when they are able to be up and about. Influenza is a *serious infectious* disease. If you keep that in mind, you will be going a long way toward preventing it from doing any damage to you and to others.

## THE ANEMIAS

*Anemia* comes from the words "without blood." Actually, it indicates that the red blood cells are below normal. These vital blood cells contain the pigment hemoglobin, which carries oxygen from the lungs to the body tissues. In anemia, the hemoglobin may be reduced, too. If you turn to page 95 you will learn more about the blood.

## How to Recognize Anemia

When the red blood cells and hemoglobin are greatly reduced in amount, the individual becomes pale. However, the skin may appear pale or sallow in normal individuals. Anemia is best recognized by the pallor of (a) the palms of the hands, (b) the fingernails, (c) the inner parts of the eyelids, the conjunctivae. However, mild degrees of anemia are not detectable in this way. Your doctor has instruments for testing the blood for anemia. This is a part of any periodic medical checkup, or of a diagnostic examination.

## Symptoms of Anemia

Mild degrees of anemia may cause only slight and vague symptoms as compared with a severe, disabling anemia. In mild anemia, there may be nothing more than a sensation of lack of pep or of feeling not quite so energetic as one does under normal circumstances. There may be a tendency to greater fatigue. On the other hand, more severe anemia causes actual shortness of breath on exertion. This may be accompanied by pounding of the heart, or palpitation, and a rapid pulse and heart action, or tachycardia. In addition, there may be severe headaches, loss of appetite, dizziness, ringing in the ears, and even fainting spells. In very advanced cases of anemia, swelling of the ankles and other evidences of failure of the heart may appear.

## The Varied Causes of Anemia

There are many causes of anemia. I shall describe the most important ones completely enough for you to recognize them and shall mention briefly most of the others, so that you will know the general methods of prevention.

*Loss of blood.* If there is a massive homorrhage from a wound, the body may lose enough blood to cause severe anemia. This *acute type of anemia* is frequently accompanied by shock (see page 334).

Immediate transfusions are generally required to replace the blood that has been lost.

*Chronic blood loss* also leads to anemia. The slow leakage of blood from an ulcer of the stomach may cause a severe anemia. This may be overlooked because the blood is mixed with the bowel movements. Hemorrhoids may cause loss of blood and lead to anemia. Excessive menstrual flow may act in the same way. A cancer of the stomach or intestines may erode and cause sufficient bleeding to produce anemia.

These anemias will clear up when the cause has been found and corrected. Since iron is necessary to build hemoglobin, medicines containing iron are helpful in these cases, and so are foods with a fairly high iron content, described on page 32. In addition to iron, hemoglobin production requires protein, vitamin $B_{12}$, and other minerals and vitamins; therefore the diet for this type of anemia should be rich in these elements. (See Chapter 2, The Food You Eat.)

A *deficient diet* can cause anemia. If there is not adequate iron, protein, vitamins, and certain minerals such as copper and cobalt, the production of hemoglobin and the formation of red cells will be impaired. That is precisely what happens when people live on inadequate diets because of low incomes. It also occurs in individuals who can afford good diets but who insist on eating "coffee and doughnuts" because of the pressure of work, or who take up some diet fad.

The combination of a poor diet and chronic blood loss makes one particularly susceptible to severe anemia. For example, a child suffering from hookworm disease is likely to live in a low-income area, on an inadequate diet. In addition, the hookworm parasites produce leakage of blood from the intestine where they have attached themselves. The blood loss and the poor diet combine to cause the severe anemia for which the "hookworm belt" has been notorious (see page 300 on hookworm disease).

A periodic medical checkup to detect blood loss is a good precaution against anemia. So are the diets described on page 32 which will give you sufficient iron and other important foodstuffs to keep your blood healthy. There is no need to supplement a good diet with medicines containing iron or other minerals or vitamins, the so-called blood tonics, unless your doctor prescribes them.

## Pernicious Anemia

Pernicious anemia differs from the other types I have been describing. For red blood cell production in the bone marrow, vitamin $B_{12}$ is needed. The vitamin is present in adequate amounts in any balanced diet. But for absorption by the body, $B_{12}$ requires the presence in the stomach of a substance called *intrinsic factor*. In pernicious anemia, intrinsic factor is lacking or operates inadequately. Vitamin $B_{12}$ absorption is then inadequate.

The diagnosis of pernicious anemia is made through the characteristic appearance of the blood cells, examination of a bone marrow sample obtained by simple needle puncture, a finding of acid deficiency in the stomach juice, and other laboratory tests.

Once pernicious anemia was often a fatal disease. That was before the finding that liver extract was helpful because, it was to turn out, it contains vitamin $B_{12}$. Now quite simply pernicious anemia can be overcome with injections of the vitamin. Blood returns to normal. The patient feels well. Once blood values return to normal, a single injection of vitamin $B_{12}$ per month may suffice for good health. When injected, the vitamin, of course, doesn't have to go through the usual absorption process, and so lack of intrinsic factor doesn't matter.

## Anemias Caused by Destruction of the Red Cells

Anemia can also be caused by the *destruction* of red blood cells. These are referred to as *hemolytic anemias*. Some of them are congenital in type. Others are acquired. Some are chronic, others acute. They differ from other anemias, too, in that jaundice may be present because the destroyed red cells release their hemoglobin, and it is converted into the jaundice pigments.

Hemolytic anemias may result from Rh incompatibility (page 241); from mismatched blood transfusions; from industrial poisons such as benzol, TNT, and aniline (see Chapter 8); and from sensitization to many chemicals and medicines, e.g., lead, sulfonamides, quinine, snake venoms, castor bean, or ricin poisoning, fava beans. Sometimes, a hemolytic anemia appears in the course of another disease, such as widespread cancer; leukemia; Hodgkin's disease; liver disease; infections caused by malarial parasites; bacterial septicemias.

Severe hemolytic anemias may lead quickly to a fatal end. Therefore, such patients must immediately be hospitalized so that transfusions can be given and other treatment started. If the cause can be located, and if it can be removed successfully, there is a good chance of recovery.

In some types of hemolytic anemia, surgical removal of the spleen causes great improvement. This is especially true in the congenital form of hemolytic anemia.

## Sickle-Cell Anemia

This is a form of hemolytic anemia that affects blacks. It gets its name from the fact that the ordinarily round red blood cells become sickle-shaped under certain conditions. This is a serious illness. It produces recurrent attacks of fever with pain in the legs, arms, and abdomen. For severe pain attacks, hospitalization may be required to provide relief.

*Sickle-cell anemia* occurs in about 1 of 500 American black people, whereas the *sickle-cell trait* occurs in about 1 in 11. With the trait, there is no anemia and health is usually good unless there is exposure to special stress. People with the trait may suffer when deprived of oxygen at high altitudes or when there is heart disease, shock, or acute alcoholism.

When both partners in a marriage know they carry the sickle-cell trait, they may wish to have genetic counseling to determine the risk in having children.

The treatment of sickle-cell anemia has been largely supportive. It has included administration of oxygen, use of analgesics or pain-killers, and careful monitoring and control of the acid-base balance of the body to help reduce the likelihood of crises at least a little. Drugs such as prednisone have sometimes been of value in arresting painful crises.

Recently, however, there have been increasing efforts to go beyond supportive treatment alone. Various experimental medicines are being tested; some show promise. Compounds under study include urea and cyanate. There is now hope that effective medications may become available before long—medications that can desickle the abnormal cells.

## Anemias Caused by Impairment of the Bone Marrow

The red blood cells are manufactured chiefly in the red marrow of the long bones, the sternum, and the vertebrae. Any disease process that invades, destroys, or depresses the activity of the bone marrow can lead to anemia. For example, a tumor or cancer can invade the marrow spaces and crowd out the blood-producing marrow. The marrow can also be destroyed, or its activity depressed, by the following agents: exposure to radioactivity, for example, excessive x-ray, radium, or the materials and radiation released in the manufacture of, or explosion of, atomic weapons; certain hair dyes; medicines containing gold, arsenicals, or nitrogen mustard; certain types of insecticides; and industrial poisons such as benzene.

This bone-marrow illness is also called *aplastic anemia*. In aplastic anemia, the blood platelets and the white cells are also damaged. Therefore, in aplastic anemia, there will usually be other symptoms besides those of anemia. Bleeding from the nose and mouth and "black and blue" spots on the skin occur frequently. Infections and fever may accompany the debilitation following aplastic anemia. It is a serious condition, and should be treated in a hospital with transfusions and other methods.

## Miscellaneous Anemias

There are many anemias which arise in the course of other diseases. For example, in *chronic kidney disease* there is usually a severe and persistent anemia; in *hypothyroidism,* or myxedema, anemia may be persistent until thyroid medication is given; *sprue* may be accompanied by anemia; *intestinal parasites* cause various kinds of anemia; hookworm has been mentioned; *tapeworms* such as the huge, fish tapeworm may produce a severe form of anemia.

*Mediterranean anemia* is found in people living in the Mediterranean area, or in their descendants who have migrated to other countries. This inherited form of anemia is also called *Cooley's anemia* or *thalassemia major.* This is a severe disease which has often been fatal early in childhood. Recently, with regular, intensive transfusions of packed red blood cells, many children have been living into the teens, some into the early twenties. With such transfusions, however, there eventually builds up a deadly amount of iron in the body. Still more recently, the use of a compound, Desferal, which is capable of removing the excess iron, has been showing promise of further extending life, with some physicians hoping that it may even be possible to attain normal life-spans.

I want to emphasize here that thalassemia takes another form, called *thalassemia minor.* In the minor form, the anemia is mild and the outlook very good. Life-span is normal. Usually no treatment is needed except possibly in pregnancy, when blood transfusion may be used to keep the hemoglobin at a safe level for mother and child.

## ULCERATIVE COLITIS

*Ulcerative colitis* is sometimes confused with a milder, though troublesome, functional disease called *irritable colon* or *functional bowel distress.* This is also known as *"colitis"* or *"mucous colitis."* The words "colitis" and "mucous colitis" are misleading because of their resemblance to *ulcerative colitis.* I shall therefore use the expression *irritable colon* to describe the mild forms of functional illness of the large intestine.

Irritable colon is distinct and different from ulcerative colitis. It is a *functional* disorder; that is, there is nothing wrong with the large bowel or colon itself, but only with the way it acts. No organic disease can be found upon careful examination, including x-rays and other tests. When viewed through a *sigmoidoscope,* a metal tube used to examine the rectum and colon, the lining of the rectum and colon appears normal. X-rays, however, may reveal minor disturbances of *movement,* for example, spasm. People who have irritable colon almost never get ulcerative colitis. Since these diseases are quite different, it is particularly dangerous to follow the advice of some neighbor who has cured his or her "colitis."

*Ulcerative colitis* is a potentially serious disease which can be disabling. Its cause is still unknown.

## Symptoms and Diagnosis

The most common symptom of ulcerative colitis is severe diarrhea. There may be as many as fifteen or twenty watery bowel movements a day. Blood is frequently found in the stools. There is a feeling of weakness, and a loss of weight. In advanced cases, the patient may suffer from arthritis or pains in the joints, or skin disorders.

Careful medical examination and tests are required to diagnose this condition. These include x-rays of the large intestine after it is filled with barium, a metal which is employed as an enema in the form of a milky white liquid. The rectum is also examined with a proctoscope or sigmoidoscope through which the lining of the bowel can be seen. Marked redness and, sometimes, actual ulcers or sores are observed.

## Treatment

Today, prompt medical treatment can prevent the disabling effects of this disease, which may otherwise make the lives of its victims miserable. The diarrhea can be so severe as to be completely incapacitating, and emaciation can reach the degree where the patient's life is threatened. Sometimes, in the most advanced cases of ulcerative colitis, the only recourse is to perform one of several types of operation in which the ulcerated large intestine is placed at rest by making an artificial *anus* leading from the healthy intestine outside through the abdominal wall. Once this operation has been performed, the patient will usually have to continue using the artificial anal opening for the rest of his life. I feel that the decision to operate should be made only if a specialist in ulcerative colitis considers it absolutely necessary. Fortunately, this possibility can usually be avoided by early and proper treatment.

Treatment of acute attacks may include rest, sedation, and good nutrition. Steroids or cortisone-like agents are useful in severe cases.

Helpful in the treatment of severe ulcerative colitis is the use of steroid enemas. Administration of steroids this way, instead of by mouth, helps to prevent occurrence of undesirable side effects of the powerful antiinflammatory agents, such as weight gain, bone brittleness, and diabetes.

# ENLARGED PROSTATE GLAND

The medical names for this condition are *benign hypertrophy of the prostate* and *prostatism*. It is *not* a cancer.

To understand this condition, look at the illustration on page 482 and read the description of this organ, which provides much of the seminal fluid that carries the reproductive sperm. It is situated at the neck of the bladder, surrounding a part of the urethral canal through which the urine is excreted.

In about one of every three men over fifty years of age, the prostate gland becomes enlarged. It can happen earlier, but it is most common in the later years of life.

If the prostate becomes too large, it interferes with the normal passage of urine, by pressing against the urethral canal. The urine, unable to pass through freely, accumulates in the bladder. As the amount of urine in the bladder continues to increase, the pressure increases, forcing it to back up into the kidneys. This is serious, because the kidneys become damaged by the pressure and by the contaminated urine. Furthermore, the accumulation of urine makes it easier for infections such as *acute* or *chronic prostatitis* to occur. Thus, an enlarged prostate can cause disability and even serious illness. No one should disregard its symptoms as being "no more than a nuisance."

## Symptoms

1. The need to get up several times during the night to pass urine, becoming more frequent as time goes by.
2. A decrease in the amount and the force of the stream of urine. Instead of being able to urinate to a distance of a few feet, the person with an enlarged prostate can only manage to dribble urine.
3. Difficulty in starting to pass urine.
4. The need to urinate almost immediately after passing urine. This is due to incomplete emptying of the bladder during urination.

## Diagnosis

In order to determine whether the prostate is enlarged, the doctor will make an examination by

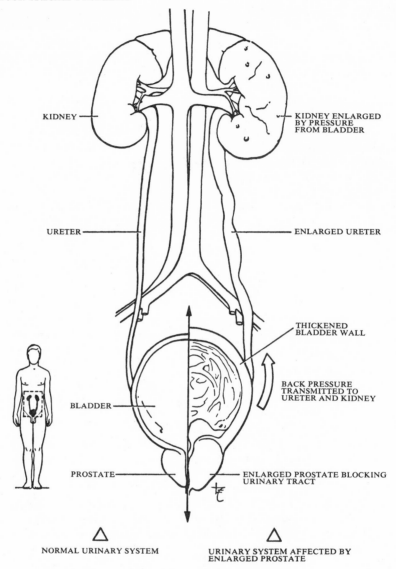

KIDNEY

KIDNEY ENLARGED
BY PRESSURE
FROM BLADDER

URETER

ENLARGED URETER

THICKENED
BLADDER WALL

BACK PRESSURE
TRANSMITTED TO
URETER AND KIDNEY

BLADDER

PROSTATE

ENLARGED PROSTATE BLOCKING
URINARY TRACT

NORMAL URINARY SYSTEM

URINARY SYSTEM AFFECTED BY
ENLARGED PROSTATE

*Figure 34-6. Enlarged Prostate.*

way of the rectum. Through the wall of the rectum he can feel the prostate gland and determine its size, shape, and firmness. He may also want to do a cystoscopic examination. A physician who specializes in diseases of this type is called a *urologist*. It is most important to be examined immediately by a competent private physician or in a hospital clinic, to guard against possible complications due to an enlarged prostate, and to make certain that you do not have a cancer of the prostate. Although prostatism is *not* a cancer, *a cancer can cause the same symptoms.*

## Treatment

The urine which has collected in the bladder may have to be removed by a rubber tube. This is called *catheterization,* and should be performed by a trained person. Existing infections may also require treatment.

If the prostate is sufficiently enlarged, an operation will be necessary. Advertised remedies and "doctors for men" cannot possibly "shrink enlarged prostate glands" and may actually cause the patient additional suffering and injury. Removing a part of the gland so that the bladder is no longer blocked is a *major* operation. But it is safe when performed by expert surgeons. *Even aged men withstand it very well.* They find they are more than repaid for it by increased health and the relief of their disabilities.

## HERNIAS

*Hernia* is the medical term for a rupture. The word rupture is not accurate, since it means tear, and nothing is actually torn. What usually happens is that a weak spot develops in the bands of muscle tissue in the abdominal wall, and the intestines begin to bulge through this, forming a soft lump. When the patient lies down, the intestines slide back to their proper place, and the bulge usually disappears entirely, especially if the hernia is of fairly recent origin.

There are various types of hernias. They occur in men more frequently than in women. They may also occur in children.

The most common type is the *inguinal hernia,* which occurs in the groins of males. The weakest spot in the male's abdominal wall is located in the groin. It is here that the cord leading to the testicles passes. Unfortunately, in some male infants the wall fails to shut tightly around the cord at this spot, leaving it especially weak. In later years, a strain such as that caused by lifting a heavy object may cause the wall to give way suddenly, or constant straining may force it out gradually. The intestines begin to bulge out. At first, this may be hardly noticeable, and there may be little pain. As time passes, the bulge may become as large or larger than a hen's egg. Hernias may extend downward into the scrotum, the bag of skin containing the testicles.

Hernias in women are most frequently located on the upper thigh, just below the groin. This is called a *femoral hernia.*

In *umbilical hernia,* the navel protrudes. This type is unusual in adults. I discuss umbilical hernia in children on page 256.

Among the other types of hernia are those that follow operations in which the scar does not heal properly, permitting bulging to occur.

Hernias may be aggravated by coughing, sneezing, or, especially in constipated individuals, straining to pass bowel movements.

Anyone with a hernia should see a doctor with-

*Figure 34-7. Inguinal Hernias. The left side of this figure shows an indirect hernia which protrudes through the inner abdominal opening and traverses to the scrotum inside the covering of the spermatic cord. The right side shows a direct hernia which comes through the abdominal wall at its external opening. It may pass directly into the scrotum, and thus become complete.*

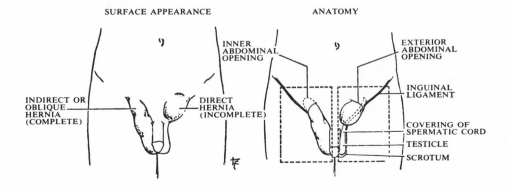

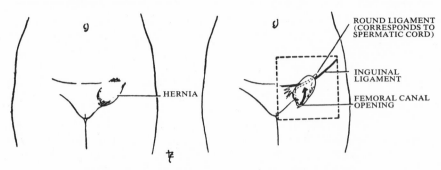

SURFACE APPEARANCE                    ANATOMY

HERNIA

ROUND LIGAMENT
(CORRESPONDS TO
SPERMATIC CORD)

INGUINAL
LIGAMENT

FEMORAL CANAL
OPENING

*Figure 34-8. Femoral Hernia. Insert shows the hernia passing through the canal and sliding up and over the inguinal ligament.*

out delay. One reason for this is that "strangulation" may develop. When this happens, a loop of intestine becomes caught in the bulge, and its blood supply is cut off. This results in gangrene of the strangulated loop of bowel, a condition which is as serious as a ruptured appendix (see page 450). It can cause death. If you have an untreated hernia which suddenly becomes painful, see your doctor *immediately,* or go to the emergency room of a good general hospital. This is an *emergency* calling for quick medical help.

In addition to the constant danger that a hernia may become strangulated, the inconvenience and disability, as well as the unsightliness, of a hernia warrant medical attention.

### Treatment

The best treatment for hernia is an operation to repair the weakness in the muscles responsible for it. This operation is usually minor and quite safe. Even elderly people undergo it without difficulty. No one with a hernia should avoid or delay the operation if it has been recommended. With the modern advances in surgery, almost no reason exists for using a truss or other support. Trusses are inconvenient, frequently uncomfortable, and may add to the injury by enlarging the weak spot. Even a well-fitted truss does not avert the danger of a strangulated hernia. The hernia may continue to grow until the truss can no longer hold it in. Medical opinion today is opposed to the use of

trusses except in unusual circumstances. Furthermore, treatment by injections is not recommended by modern authorities. Apart from small babies, on whom an operation is usually postponed temporarily, the best thing to do is to have the hernia corrected by surgery immediately.

### Prevention of Hernia

1. Get used to doing heavy work gradually, so that your muscles become adjusted to the increased strain.

2. When lifting heavy weights, face the object, keep your feet close to it, and spread them about twelve inches apart. When lifting from the floor, keep your knees bent, and rise slowly, using leg rather than back muscles.

3. As much as possible, carry loads on your shoulder rather than on the hips.

4. Don't reach too high for heavy packages.

5. Always try to have someone help you with unusually heavy lifting.

6. If you work in a factory, use mechanical devices, such as conveyor belts, elevators, and hoists whenever you can.

# INFECTIOUS MONONUCLEOSIS

Infectious mononucleosis, also called *glandular fever,* belongs in this section because it may sometimes cause a degree of disability surprisingly prolonged for what may seem to be a mild illness. A viral disease, it affects mostly young adults, is rare after thirty-five.

Athough it is often called the "kissing disease" because of the age group affected, little is known about how it is transmitted.

The symptoms include fever, sore throat, swelling of the glands of the neck and sometimes those under the arm and in the groin. There is often headache, which may recur daily. Weakness and fatigue are common. In a small proportion of cases, there may be a general rash.

It is now recognized that "mono" may make the spleen vulnerable to rupture and may sometimes affect the liver and be mistaken for hepatitis.

Mononucleosis is infectious for about a week after fever and gland swelling appear. The fever may persist for several weeks, and listlessness may persist for several months.

There is no specific treatment for the illness. But the symptoms may be relieved by appropriate medications. Bed rest during the acute stage is wise. Relapses can occur. Young people tend to think they are cured after the acute symptoms subside and may resume a full schedule too early and perhaps invite relapse.

Diagnosis of mononucleosis is made with the help of blood tests. And medical care is essential because of the possibly serious consequences or complications. Only a physician should indicate when full activity may be resumed. With proper care, total recovery is the rule.

# GONORRHEA

*Gonorrhea* is the most widespread venereal disease in the United States. It is not as dreaded as syphilis because it is not one of the "great killers." However, the old saying that gonorrhea is "no worse than a bad cold" is a dangerous falsehood. *Gonorrhea can become extremely serious.* It causes pain as well as discomfort. Far more important, it is a frequent cause of sterility in men as well as in women and of many disorders of the reproductive system.

If the germs get into the eyes, blindness can result. Most states now require doctors to place a disinfectant in the eyes of newborn babies. This has practically eliminated blindness due to infection during passage through the birth canal of a gonorrheal mother.

The disease can also lead to painful arthritis and destruction of the joints. It can even cause death if the germs enter the blood and lodge in the heart valves.

Gonorrhea is an infection caused by the germ *Neisseria gonorrhoeae*, also called the *gonococcus*, which attacks the sex organs of men and women. It is known by many slang terms including "clap," "dose," "gleet," and "strain." It is almost always contracted by sexual intercourse, *not* by kissing or sitting on toilet seats, except in the case of infections of the eye in children or adults, and vaginal infections in little girls. It is important to realize that little girls can easily be infected with gonorrhea from towels, diapers, and other objects contaminated with the germs of this disease.

## Symptoms and Diagnosis

The first symptoms of gonorrhea usually appear from five to seven days after the sexual exposure. In men there is a whitish discharge from the penis and/or a burning sensation upon urination. Women may develop pain in the lower abdomen with or without a period of burning urination and/or a whitish vaginal discharge. Never disregard any symptoms of gonorrhea.

Because germs other than those causing gonorrhea may cause these symptoms (see page 519), it is necessary that the diagnosis be made on the basis of microscopic examinations performed by a reputable doctor, a hospital clinic, or a venereal disease detection center. Although gonorrhea is a disease entirely separate from syphilis and is caused by a different germ, it is not unusual to contract both gonorrhea and syphilis at the same time. This is another important reason for having the diagnosis made by a competent person. The tests for gonorrhea are easily performed, and no one should feel ashamed to have them made.

## Treatment

Penicillin and other antibiotics are effective in curing gonorrhea. They can be dangerous unless administered by a physician. If, for doctors who advertise, and home remedies. They can be dangerous as well as costly. Many people have been victimized by so-called experts who "treated" them even though they actually never had gonorrhea.

Sulfa drugs, penicillin, and other antibiotics are effective in curing gonorrhea. They can be dangerous unless administered by a physician. If, for example, someone contracts syphilis and gonorrhea at the same time, the symptoms of gonorrhea will appear first. The amount of penicillin required to cure gonorrhea will *suppress* the signs of syphilis without curing that disease. In addition, only a competent doctor will know when the disease is cured and treatment can be discontinued. It is foolhardy to discontinue treatment, even though the symptoms disappear, before tests prove that the disease is cured.

Having an attack of gonorrhea does *not* produce an immunity to the disease. Having been cured once does not protect an individual against later infections.

### Prevention

Although it is now possible to cure gonorrhea, prevention is still the best and safest method of coping with it. Follow the directions for the prevention of syphilis which I give on page 448. In brief, these are (1) avoiding intercourse with an infected person; (2) using a rubber condom and a thorough washing afterward. This is an excellent safeguard, because it is often impossible to tell whether or not a person is infected with gonorrhea or some other venereal disease.

### Other Venereal Diseases

In addition to syphilis (p. 447) and gonorrhea, there are three other less common types of venereal disease: *chancroid, lymphogranuloma venereum,* and *granuloma inguinale.* For these diseases also, we emphasize careful preventive measures. Use a condom and the soap and water wash. Symptoms of these diseases are sores on the genital organs, swellings or lumps in the groin, or sores around the groin and the anal region. If any such symptoms appear, see your doctor quickly.

A relatively new venereal disease which has been increasing very rapidly is *herpes simplex of the genitals.* In just a few years, it has become one of the most common venereal diseases. It is caused by a form, called Type II, of the same virus, herpes simplex, that produces fever blisters on the lips; it is the only important venereal disease caused by a virus.

Transmitted by sexual contact, the disease produces painful blisters on the penis, within the vagina or cervix, in the pubic area, and on the thighs and buttocks. Although the blisters may disappear within a week or so without treatment, recurrences are frequent. The disease, if present during pregnancy, may damage the child. Efforts are being made to develop a vaccine capable of preventing the disease.

## BRUCELLOSIS
(Undulant Fever)

There are several forms of undulant fever, an infectious disease which is known by various names. The word *undulant* indicates that the fever comes in waves, or undulations, instead of being constant. One form was formerly called *Malta fever* because it was prevalent in some of the Mediterranean Islands. More recently, all forms of the disease have been given the name *brucellosis* because they are all due to infections with some member of the germ family called *Brucella* after Dr. David Bruce, who discovered them.

The symptoms of brucellosis usually come on slowly and are rather indefinite, consisting of an irregular fever, chills, sweating, and aches and pains in the joints and muscles. The death rate is not very high. However, it is rare for a patient to recover after only one attack of the illness. As a rule, another attack follows the first and this may be repeated.

Brucellosis is very rarely carried from one person to another. It is, however, constantly carried from animal to animal, and from animal to person. The animals which harbor the germ are chiefly domesticated goats, cattle, and hogs.

The best way to prevent brucellosis is to eradicate the disease in animals. The excellent efforts being made along this line will undoubtedly be successful in the long run. *But in the meantime other preventive measures must be taken,* because it is practically impossible to be sure at any given time that a herd of animals is free from the bacillus. The danger of brucellosis is a powerful argument for universal pasteurization of public milk supplies (see page 137 for "home pasteurization" of milk). Infection by contact with diseased animals or their carcasses is less easy to prevent and is essentially a matter of industrial hygiene (see page 147). Persons who are exposed to brucellosis in their jobs should be fully informed of the dangers and should take precautions against unnecessary exposures.

Treatment is by antibiotics and sulfa drugs, which usually are more effective the earlier in the course of the disease they are used.

# LEPROSY
(Hansen's Disease)

You may be surprised to see leprosy included among the disabling diseases when, for centuries, people have feared leprosy as a horrible killer. The very word "leper" has caused terror to men throughout the ages. During and after World War II and the Korean and Viet Nam wars, there were many anxious inquiries about this disease from the families and friends of servicemen who had been in Asia.

Their anxiety is unnecessary. In the first place, there is no truth whatever in the ancient belief that leprosy can be contracted by touching an infected person or some object he has handled, or simply by passing him on the street. Leprosy is one of the *least* contagious of the infectious diseases. By taking ordinary precautions, doctors and nurses have worked for years among leprosy patients without getting the disease. It is contracted by *prolonged, close* contact with a person who has an *active* case of certain types of leprosy. With modern treatment, most cases of leprosy can be controlled or even arrested.

In the average case, it is not a particularly severe disease. Nevertheless, it is a disabler. Although it is actually quite rare in this country, I include it because the *psychological* disability it causes can be as serious as the physical. In this way, it affects not only the patient and those who

have been in contact with him, but many others who only imagine they have been exposed.

Leprosy is caused by *Hansen's bacillus,* also called *Mycobacterium leprae.* It generally attacks the skin and nerves. It does *not* affect the brain. It is *not* inherited. There are several types of leprosy, one of which often arrests itself even without treatment.

## Symptoms and Treatment

The most common symptoms include the typical leprosy patches on the skin, small nodules on the face and legs, and a loss of feeling in limited areas of the body, such as the fingers. The disease develops slowly and is difficult to recognize. There are specific tests doctors employ to diagnose leprosy.

Treatment with certain medicines effectively halts the progress of the disease and relieves its symptoms. Although certain patients can be treated at home, they usually do best at the U.S. Public Health Service Hospital (National Leprosarium), Carville, Louisiana. Here, specialists in the disease provide expert treatment, restful sanatorium care, and an understanding of the disease, along with freedom from worry about spreading the infection. There is no charge for treatment. Patients can have visitors and, when their condition permits—that is, when they are no longer capable of spreading bacteria—they can visit or return to their families.

# TROPICAL DISEASES

Millions of people, especially in the tropical areas of Asia and Africa, are completely or partly disabled by the so-called tropical diseases. Of these, malaria is the most important, until recently infecting as many as 300,000,000 people throughout the world. I describe malaria fully below, as it is prevalent, to some extent, in this country.

I should like to add a few notes about other tropical diseases because of the many Americans who have been or are at present overseas in the armed services or civilian jobs, and because of the increased airplane travel which brings the tropics, and their diseases, to our door. Men in the armed forces are protected from these diseases by vaccinations, medicines, and the vigilance of their health officers. But civilians are frequently careless or uninformed. If you are going to a tropical or semitropical country for a visit, a vacation, or a job, be sure to ask your doctor about the health hazards you may face, and follow his instructions exactly. I want to emphasize, too, that due to poor sanitation in many tropical countries, there is a great danger from intestinal diseases. Some of these, such as *amebic dysentery,* can be extremely disabling. Other types of intestinal diseases, e.g., *bacillary dysentery, typhoid fever,* and even the dreaded killer, *cholera,* are prevalent in many tropical countries. It seems to me that travelers to distant lands frequently get excited about the exotic diseases such as *schistosomiasis, tsutsugamushi fever, filariasis,* and *leishmaniasis,* and forget that the chief sources of danger are eating and drinking infected foods and water which cause intestinal diseases. Simple precautions which I outline on page 136 will prevent most of the so-called tropical illnesses.

## MALARIA

Malaria is still one of the most prevalent diseases in the world, especially in Asia and Africa. It has been almost eliminated from the United States, but American military personnel and civilians who have lived in tropical regions have been exposed to malaria. Some of them contract the disease, which may recur long after they leave military service. Veterans who have suffered from malaria and later in life have vague, undiagnosed episodes of fever should consult their doctor for diagnosis and treatment.

While malaria is still a health problem in many countries, the intensive efforts of the World Health Organization have succeeded in checking its spread. Malaria does not kill very frequently, but it is disabling because of its high fever and severe chills, and its long duration.

### Cause and Symptoms of Malaria

The disease is caused by a parasite so small that it can live and reproduce in the tiny red blood corpuscles. This parasite is carried from a patient with malaria by the intermediary action of the female Anopheles mosquito. While feeding on such a patient, the mosquito sucks up infected blood. It transmits the infection to healthy human beings on whom it subsequently feeds. About two weeks later the person infected will develop characteristic symptoms. These are chills and shaking, and a high fever which subsides in several hours, leaving the patient drenched in sweat, exhausted, and very sleepy. The types of malaria are named according to the interval between the fevers, e.g., tertian, every third day; quartan, every fourth day.

If the disease is not treated, the chills and fever may continue for months before the body overcomes the acute stages. Even then, malarial symptoms can recur if the patient's resistance is lowered by strenuous activity, alcoholic excesses, or exposure to cold. Patients chronically ill with malaria suffer from anemia, headaches, muscle pains, and general poor health.

*Diagnosis* is made by the doctor when he examines a drop of blood under the microscope. The malarial parasites are generally abundant and easily recognized.

### Treatment

For many years, quinine was the standard treatment. It was not a real cure, but it suppressed the symptoms and kept the parasites out of the blood. Since World War II, when the Japanese cut off the supply of quinine to the U.S.A., there has been intensive research to find new and better compounds for treatment. The search has been rewarded. Doctors now have medicines that can cure this disease. These medicines include chloroquine, pentaquine, primaquine, and quinacrine (Atabrine).

## AMEBIASIS

Amebiasis, caused by a parasite which invades the intestines, was formerly regarded as a purely tropical disease. However, we now know that a considerable number of cases of even the severe form, *amebic dysentery* are found throughout the

United States. It is widespread in its mild form. From 5 to 10 percent of the people in this country may harbor the parasitic ameba in their intestines.

I describe parasites and explain how they are taken into the body in Chapter 7, Keeping the Germs Away (p. 136). I also tell you how to prevent infection from these organisms by taking proper sanitary precautions with respect to food and water.

However, it is not safe to assume you cannot get amebiasis if you follow these precautions, for the disease can be passed to you by someone who handles food and who may not know he or she is harboring the invisible cysts of this parasite. This can happen because individuals with the mild variety may experience only minor symptoms such as headache, occasional nausea, flatulence, fatigue, and bowel irregularity.

It is most important not to neglect any symptoms of amebiasis. You are very apt to give the disease to someone, perhaps a child, who may develop it in its severe form. In addition, mild cases may develop into amebic dysentery, with abdominal pain and diarrhea, often accompanied by blood-streaked stools and, in severe cases, chills and fever. Severe amebic dysentery can cause death. There is also the risk that the parasite may travel to the liver and produce an abscess there. If not treated properly, such an abscess can prove fatal. Finally, even mild amebiasis can make one miserable, run-down, and unable to resist other diseases.

Only a physician can diagnose amebiasis in either its mild or severe form. The patient's stools must be examined under a microscope. Several specimens usually have to be examined because the organism may not always be present. A blood test has also been developed to help in making the diagnosis.

Amebiasis can usually be treated with success. New medicines have been developed for all types of this disease. Even people who have had chronic, resistant cases should not be discouraged, but should again consult their doctors, as they can probably benefit from the new treatments.

## SARCOIDOSIS
(Boeck's Sarcoid)

Sarcoidosis is a long illness which can be considerably disabling at times. Fortunately, despite its chronicity, it usually heals eventually. The disease is more severe in dark-skinned races than in white. In the United States more cases are found in the southeastern rural areas than elsewhere.

In this disease, little fleshy lumps invade the tissues. Most frequently the lungs, skin, and lymph nodes are affected. However, it has been known to occur in almost every part of the body, including the eyes, liver, and bones. Because the disease so frequently affects the lungs, it has been confused with tuberculosis. However, sarcoidosis is not communicable. The patient may live with his family.

In mild forms, there are few if any symptoms. In severer forms, there may be fever, loss of weight, cough, and other distressing symptoms. In some forms of the illness, it is possible to relieve the symptoms by the use of cortisone and ACTH.

# 35
# THE NUISANCE AILMENTS

I wish we had a complete list of all the illnesses that afflict our population. Strange to say, no complete enumeration of diseases is available. It is true that we have a good idea about the *Killer diseases* because they appear on the death statistics. And there has been some approximation of the *Disablers*, based on the extremely valuable information obtained by the United States Public Health Service. But there has never been an accurate account of the minor ailments that do not ordinarily disable or kill, but may cause days and even years of pain, discomfort, worry, or shame. It is my guess that, were we to obtain such a census, we would be amazed to discover how many *person-hours of suffering* are caused by such diseases. For example, the hours of distress caused by *psoriasis* alone must run into millions each year for our population. And besides the actual discomfort, there is the emotional suffering so many of these patients endure.

In this chapter I shall discuss a number of the so-called minor illnesses. Only rarely do they actually disable people. Only very exceptionally do they lead to death. But, in my experience as a doctor, I have found that a tremendous amount of pain and emotional grief are caused by these conditions—most of it unnecessary. That is the saddest part of it! Almost all of these conditions are either completely curable or can be greatly improved by medical or surgical help. All too often people with headaches, sore feet, varicose veins, hemorrhoids (piles), constipation, and so on, suffer stoically for years because they feel that their doctors or the hospital clinics don't

want to "bother about such little things." I've often heard a patient with, for example, varicose veins, say in an apologetic manner, "These veins of mine aren't causing me any great trouble, Doctor, and I really shouldn't take your time simply because I don't like the way they look."

Believe me when I say that any doctor worthy of his M.D. is extremely interested in correcting or relieving these *nuisance ailments*. In the first place, doctors know that appearances affect people's happiness, health, and ability to earn a living. Doctors want them to seek expert advice about anything they consider unsightly—and not try to hide it, when it can be cured, or to experiment with unscientific, often dangerous "cures" or "aids." In the second place, doctors know that the nuisance ailments almost never limit themselves to marring the appearance. They may interfere with sleep, spoil appetites, pave the way for local or general infections; in short, they prevent people from enjoying good health and the positive feeling of well-being that goes with it.

I know that many people suffering from the nuisance ailments have forgotten what it is like to feel *really* well. If you're one of them, this chapter is written especially for you. In it I discuss some of the most common of the minor causes of distress. All of them can be helped, and many can be completely cured.

You will notice that I discuss only a comparatively small number of the "nuisances" in this chapter. That is because I have dealt with many of them in other chapters—for example, in discussing the Care of the Teeth and Gums (Chapter

4), Problems of Women (Chapter 36), The Later Years (Chapter 37) and so on. Here are lists for your convenience in locating the nuisances I discuss elsewhere.

## TEETH, GUMS, MOUTH

Unless you belong to the very lucky and very small minority in this country, you have undoubtedly been bothered by

## SKIN CONDITIONS

These are among the most annoying, both from the point of view of appearance and discomfort, of all nuisances.

## THE HAIR

Actually, disorders of the hair cause less discomfort than they do worry about unsightliness. But they certainly take a lot of our time and energy!

## POSTURE AND WEIGHT

Many of our everyday pains and aches are due to poor posture, which is frequently associated with being overweight. Both these conditions can cause a great deal of distress because of their effect on the general health and appearance.

## EMOTIONAL PROBLEMS

I have written a whole section of this book, entitled You and Your Mind, in order to help you to understand minor, as well as major, emotional difficulties. I have also discussed them in such chapters as Emotional Attitudes Toward Marriage, Our Children's Emotions, and Adolescence. Some of the most frequently encountered "minor emotional nuisances" are

## WOMEN'S PROBLEMS

Doctors no longer assume that a certain amount of pain and discomfort are "the price a woman must pay for being a woman." Nor do they feel that it is foolish for a woman to want to keep up her appearance as well as her health.

## "INDIGESTION"

You notice I put this word in quotation marks. That is because I want to do everything I can to remind you that it is not a disease in itself, but a symptom of many diseases. However, there is such a thing as a *minor digestive disturbance,* which I describe on page 100.

By now you're probably wondering what nuisance ailments are left for me to discuss in this chapter. Unfortunately, there are a great many! Here they are:

Headaches
Insomnia
Colds
Sinusitis, dry throat, cough, etc.
Allergies (including hay fever and eczema)
Constipation
Psoriasis
Disfigurements (including crossed eyes, harelip, unsightly nose and ears)
Rectal troubles (including hemorrhoids [piles], fissures, and pruritus ani)
Varicose veins
Seasickness (motion sickness)
Pilonidal sinus

## HEADACHES

I have given considerable thought to whether or not headaches constitute a nuisance disease or a disabling disease. It is true that migraine headaches—and even tension headaches—may become severe enough temporarily to disable their victims. However, because headaches rarely disable for prolonged periods of time, I am placing them in the nuisance category. I am sure that most of my readers would refer to the two common types, *tension* and *migraine* headaches, as "confounded nuisances," rather than disablers.

You can be helped with headaches. First, a word about their prevalence. It is believed that almost every adult has experienced a headache, and that one in ten has headaches sufficiently frequently or severely to find them a source of genu-

ine discomfort. Another index is the millions of dollars spent each year on aspirin, Bufferin, Empirin, etc., which are used chiefly for relief of headaches.

I am sure I need not describe the symptoms of a headache, since it is exactly what the word implies, although the ache or pain varies considerably in type and intensity. However, I want to stress the point that in *many instances headache is a symptom of some disease.*

### Headaches as a Symptom

Headaches may be due to *sinusitis* (see page 498) in which the membranes of the nose swell and block the sinuses, causing pressure. This makes the head throb painfully, especially on bending forward. *Colds, hay fever,* and *other allergies* can have the same effect.

Headache is an early symptom of many *infectious diseases,* from polio, meningitis, and measles to the flu. In such cases it is usually accompanied by other symptoms such as fever and a general feeling of sickness.

In a serious, though uncommon disease, *brain tumor,* headaches may be repeated and grow increasingly painful, accompanied by blurring of the vision and vomiting.

*High blood pressure* can cause headaches, although this is not nearly so common as most people believe.

Of course, *head injuries* and injuries to other portions of the body such as the neck, cause headaches.

I discuss *menstrual* and *menopausal headaches* on pages 516 and 519.

Anemia, disorders of the intestinal tract—in fact, almost any disease I could name—can be accompanied by headaches. So can hunger, cold, lack of sleep, overexertion, too much drinking, or smoking.

The headaches which some people associate with constipation are actually due to a nervous reaction.

Naturally you don't want to visit the doctor for every headache. However, *I strongly urge you to go* if:

1. The headache does not vanish when the condition you believe has caused it is corrected or relieved—for example, if getting sufficient rest

doesn't stop a headache you thought was due to fatigue.

2. The headache is accompanied by any other symptoms, such as fever, nausea, vomiting, visual difficulties, and so on.

3. The headaches occur often, are severe, or seem to be increasing in intensity, duration, or frequency.

Your headaches may be a symptom of some difficulty that can be corrected, or a disease which should be promptly treated. They may not be, but if they fall into any of the three groups I just mentioned, only a doctor can decide.

If your headache is not of this kind, it will probably be a *migraine headache* or a *tension headache*—the latter being more common.

## Migraine Headache

This is also called a "sick headache." Its cause is unknown. However, it appears to be connected with the psychological makeup of the individual, since it is found most often in certain personality types, and an attack is apt to follow an emotional disturbance. In women, it often coincides with the menses. There is a family tendency toward migraine. Some of the rarer kinds of migraine headaches have been diagnosed when, for example, the doctor learned that close relatives of the patient had headaches following attacks of flickering vision. Therefore, it is important to tell your doctor about relatives who suffer from this disease.

Symptoms of migraine are so varied that diagnosis can often be made only by a skilled and experienced physician, such as a specialist in neurology. A typical attack starts with changes in the field of vision—a flickering before the eyes, flashes of light, or a blacking out of part of the vision. Migraine headaches are almost always one-sided, in either the right or the left part of the head, and scarcely ever involve the entire head. They are frequently accompanied by nausea and vomiting. They are seldom relieved by aspirin. However, the symptoms vary in less typical cases of migraine.

Many migraine sufferers tend to eat foods high in a substance called *tyramine*. It occurs in cheese, especially ripe and aged cheese, yeast, some wines, chicken liver, chocolate, and citrus fruits. Sometimes avoidance of such foods may help in preventing migraine attacks.

Although aspirin is not usually helpful, some victims may obtain relief by applying an ice pack to the head, thus reducing the pain enough so aspirin helps. Resting quietly in a dark room also may help to reduce the pain.

In severe cases, a drug such as ergotamine may be prescribed. Recent studies suggest that propranolol, a drug first employed for some heart conditions, may have value for migraine patients, sometimes significantly reducing the number of attacks.

Recently, too, *biofeedback* has shown promise. Now being used in some hospital clinics, biofeedback involves a procedure such as the following: Temperature sensors are taped to a patient's finger and forehead. A meter shows the difference between head and hand temperature. The patient learns—through such simple methods as repeating a calming phrase such as "I feel quiet"—to relax blood vessels in the hands and thus increase hand temperature. When he or she succeeds, the needle moves. And with the relaxation and warming of the hands comes a redistribution of blood that reduces pressure in blood vessels in the head, ending the migraine headache. Once a patient develops the ability to move the needle, the same technique may be used, without the biofeedback equipment, to cut short a migraine attack.

## Tension Headaches

Tension headaches account for an estimated seven of every ten headaches.

When a job demands a fixed head position (for example, driving against bright headlights), we often set the muscles of our neck, jaw, and scalp in pain-causing postures. We commonly do the same as part of a reaction against psychological pressures. Tension headache victims have been said to "symbolically carry a great weight on their shoulders." Upon feeling harassed or anxious, they may set scalp and neck muscles and develop headache.

What will relieve the pain of tension headaches? In mild cases, aspirin is still the most practical and useful analgesic. An aspirin substitute such as acetaminophen also may be helpful. But for more persistent, severe pain, an analgesic alone often is not enough, nor is a tranquilizer alone. Often what may be needed is a double-pronged approach, using an analgesic to raise the pain threshold and a sedative to reduce tension at least a little. Gentle massage of neck muscles and applications of moist, warm compresses to the back of the neck are helpful, too.

Biofeedback, first studied in migraine, also is showing promise in tension headaches and is being used now in some hospital outpatient clinics. Patients have sensor electrodes applied to the forehead to record muscle tension. If the level is high, the biofeedback machine emits a series of rapid beeps that the patients hear through earphones. As tension is reduced, the beeps slow. And patients learn by simple methods how to reduce tension (see biofeedback discussion under Migraine, page 493).

# INSOMNIA

Most of us who live in noisy cities, work at competitive jobs, worry about our children being in an automobile accident, and don't even relax during our hours of recreation, know what it is to have occasional—or recurrent—sleepless nights.

Talking about insomnia is almost like discussing human nature, because there are as many variations on that theme as there are individuals. Here are some questions to answer in determining the cause or type of your insomnia:

*How much sleep do you need?* Some people suffer from "insomnia" because they think they need more sleep than they actually do. I discuss sleep on page 15 and on page 539. I point out the fact that some elderly people require less sleep than they did when they were younger.

*Are you "too tired" to sleep?* It is hard to relax if you are, and relaxation must precede sleep. Try not to overdo things during the day. Even more important, slow down as evening approaches, so that your "machinery" can coast to a halt.

*Is there a physical cause for your inability to sleep?* Some people are sensitive to things that do not disturb the average person; they are normally light sleepers. Poor sleeping conditions such as noise, light, someone moving around, sharing a

bed with someone they don't want to disturb or who disturbs them, make it impossible for them to sleep well. Would you, if married, sleep better by using twin beds or a separate bedroom? Do you drink too much coffee, tea, or cola drinks? Caffeine in these beverages keeps some people awake. Do you eat heavy meals before bedtime and toss around with gas and "indigestion"; or drink fluids that make your bladder feel distended?

If your insomnia is due to any of the above, try to eliminate the cause.

Some forms of insomnia come from such problems as muscular jerking of the legs, arthritis, ulcers, and hyperthyroidism—and the insomnia may be overcome when these conditions are treated.

One cause, only recently discovered, is sleep apnea, a nocturnal breathing disorder that may affect as many as 50,000 people in the United States and sometimes wakes its victims hundreds of times a night. So brief may the episodes (snore-like gasps for air) be that victims may be completely unaware of them and for years may be unable to account for their daily fatigue. Today it has become possible to diagnose and treat this condition. And if there is some indication that it exists—perhaps your spouse's awareness of your peculiar snoring habits—your physician may suggest consultation with experts at the nearest sleep study clinic.

Insomnia can be the result, too, of psychological disturbances. Anxiety is one. Another common one is mental depression, which may go unrecognized until you take your sleeping problem to a physician. Depression may follow a personal crisis—an injury, loss of job, a marriage problem, for example. But depression may develop gradually without any such crisis, often defying rational explanation. The type of treatment for depression depends upon severity. Antidepressant medication may be used. Sometimes psychotherapy may also be employed.

I must add a special word here about sleeping pills. Under some circumstances, their brief use may be indicated. But there has been excessive resort to their chronic use. Recently investigators at sleep clinics have been finding that as many as forty percent of patients complaining of insomnia can blame the very drugs taken to "treat" it. And when the drugs are eliminated—gradually, to avoid withdrawal reactions of intense dreams and nightmares—they average about twenty percent more sleep, and many become free of insomnia.

METHODS FOR GETTING TO SLEEP—OR RETURNING TO SLEEP IF YOU AWAKEN.

1. Don't be afraid of staying awake. It is not going to hurt you, if you don't worry about it. Many people can simply relax or doze and be perfectly rested the next day. Incidentally, most people suffering from insomnia actually sleep more than they think they do.

2. Make the two hours before you go to bed *peaceful* ones.

3. Go to bed half an hour to an hour sooner than you expect to go to sleep. Read something soothing until you feel drowsy. Then turn off the light.

4. Relax physically. Try to let your muscles "go" and feel yourself sinking down into the mattress.

5. Relax mentally. Try not to think of anything when you start "courting" sleep. Since this usually isn't possible, find something relaxing to think about. The time-honored "counting sheep" is too dull for most people. Personally, I like to imagine I'm sitting in a boat with my fishing rod waiting for a bite as I watch the water. One of my wife's friends sews endless seams. Another friend tries to focus her eyes on the window, knowing they will soon become so heavy she will have to close them.

6. If you don't go to sleep, and lying quietly disturbs rather than relaxes you, begin again by reading for a while or try listening to soothing radio music.

7. Sleep in a cool room.

8. Don't go to bed with a full stomach. Avoid daytime napping. Avoid stimulants, such as coffee and tea, in the evening.

9. Exercise every day if your doctor has approved that, but avoid vigorous activity at or near bedtime.

# NARCOLEPSY (SLEEP ATTACKS)

Narcolepsy is a condition that usually makes its first appearance in the late teens. Its most characteristic symptom is what many victims rightly call sleep attacks because they are so overwhelm-ing. Regardless of how well they have slept the night before, people with narcolepsy may experience many episodes of sleepiness during the day that may last fifteen minutes or so and cause them to fall asleep—even in the midst of a conversation or at the dinner table.

As many as 80 percent of victims have another symptom, called cataplexy. Some or many body muscles may become suddenly and briefly paralyzed when a strong emotion such as fear or anger is experienced.

In addition, some victims may experience visual or auditory hallucinations when falling asleep during the day or at night, and they may experience fleeting paralysis when they wake.

Because the disorder has been unfamiliar to most laymen and even to some physicians, an average of fifteen years elapsed between its first appearance and the diagnosis, and some authorities say that two-thirds of victims, who may number in the hundreds of thousands, are undiagnosed even now.

Narcolepsy often can be diagnosed if the patient gives a full account of symptoms. When there is any doubt, a sleep clinic can help. All-night sleep monitoring is valuable for clear-cut narcolepsy detection. At night, narcoleptics tend to fall directly into the state of sleep called REM (rapid eye movement), while other people usually do not enter REM until more than ninety minutes after falling asleep.

Although the cause of narcolepsy remains unknown and no cure has been found, stimulant drugs can help control the sleep attacks, and other drugs can eliminate the other symptoms or at least render them more tolerable.

Founded by victims of the disorder, The American Narcolepsy Association, Box 5846, Stanford, Calif. 94305, provides valuable information for narcoleptics and their families.

# THE COMMON COLD

The common cold is the most common of the nuisance diseases. Although I have run into people who proudly claim "I never catch a cold!" I have as yet to meet anyone in my own medical experience who has not had at least a few—even though he or she may ignore them, and pass them along to others. All but 10 percent of the people in this country have a cold every year, and over half of us have several.

Colds are a special problem in children, frequently causing ear infections as well as other complications. Also, many childhood diseases start with the symptoms of a cold. For these reasons, I have discussed colds in infants and children elsewhere in this book (see page 289).

I hope I can convince you that colds may also be serious in adults. As you know, they may start with a brief "dry" stage, during which the nose usually feels "prickly," and there is a tickling feeling in the throat. Then the eyes become watery. Sneezing, a "running" nose, a cough and sore throat, headache, and some fever follow. Then the secretions become thick and the cold begins to "dry up." "Three days coming, three days with you, three days going" is an old, and still fairly accurate, description of the course of a cold.

These symptoms are common, and familiarity breeds contempt. Many people feel that there is no need to bother about a cold, and they go their regular way in spite of it. This is dangerous. A cold is potentially serious, because it is frequently accompanied by complications, including diseases such as pneumonia. A cold should be regarded as an illness which must be prevented or treated.

"I'd be glad to, if I knew how!" you are probably saying. "If there were any way to prevent or cure a cold, I'd do it in a minute."

It is true that medical science has not yet discovered any exact method for preventing or curing colds. There is no vaccine, no medicine, certainly no advertised "cure" to do it. The tremendous amount of research devoted to the common cold may bring the answer at any time. However, I want to caution you against putting your faith in any new preventive or cure you may hear about. Even if it is the result of sound scientific work (and most "cures" are not) it will undoubtedly take a long time to determine its exact effectiveness. You can readily see how difficult it is to obtain accurate records of something as universal, variable, and mild as the common cold—compared, for example, to a disease such as smallpox.

Does that mean nothing can be done about colds? By no means. Colds can be prevented in a number of instances. Their duration can frequently be shortened and their complications very frequently prevented.

## The Cause and Prevention of Colds

Colds are caused by a virus to which the body is particularly susceptible when its resistance is lowered. Although this virus itself is not able to do much damage, it may pave the way for more dangerous types of microorganisms.

People who have this virus in its active form—that is, people who have a cold, especially in its early stages—spread it to others. It can be transmitted by close contact, particularly kissing, and by handling contaminated objects such as handkerchiefs. But the *main* method of transmission is a cough or sneeze. Pictures taken of sneezes by high-speed cameras show that a cloud of particles containing the germs is spread around an area extending approximately three feet in front of the person who sneezed (see illustration, page 137). Most of these particles can be caught if the sneeze or cough is smothered by tissues or a handkerchief. *Colds can be avoided if people will take this simple precaution.* It is true you can't persuade everyone to do this, but you can cut down on the number of colds in your own household; and if your friends won't do it, you can avoid them when they have colds. A little tact and the explanation that you are susceptible to colds will often make it possible for you to keep a safe distance or postpone some visit until your sneezing friend has passed the most contagious stage. Naturally you can't stay at home all winter when colds are most prevalent, but you can keep out of crowds as much as possible during a wave of colds, especially if there is much influenza and pneumonia associated with them. Some immunity follows a cold, but it is usually brief, so don't count on it.

Can *vitamin C* in large doses help? Whether it can or not remains controversial. For some, it may be effective; for others, not. Its use to try to head off a cold when one seems to be coming on involves at least two grams a day.

Certainly, it pays to eat a well-balanced diet (see page 35). People in good condition catch colds, but they are better able to resist some of the complications that may follow.

*Chilling lowers the body's resistance to colds.*

This varies a great deal in different people, some of whom become chilled very easily (see page 14). Each of us must learn for himself just how careful to be about sitting in drafts and getting wet feet. Don't let the mistaken notion that it is heroic to go without rubbers or a warm coat increase the number of colds you get and give to others. Be especially careful about working in cold, damp places, and any exposure that leaves you shivering; get into warm, dry clothes as soon as you can after being wet or chilly.

In spite of these precautions, you will probably get an occasional cold. I wish that you would call a doctor when you do. His judgment, based on your condition, will enable him to decide how your cold should be treated—for example, how long you should rest. He will almost certainly be able to prevent complications such as pneumonia.

Unfortunately, most people cannot afford to—or don't want to—call the doctor for an ordinary cold. That is why I'm going to tell you what to do for one. However, *there are certain people who must see a physician.* Even a mild cold can represent a severe threat to their health, possibly to their lives. A doctor should be called promptly when anyone with one of the following diseases catches a cold:

Tuberculosis
Rheumatic fever or rheumatic heart disease
Chronic bronchitis or bronchiectasis
Bronchial asthma
Kidney disease, especially Bright's disease and chronic pyelonephritis
Severe liver disease
Severe diabetes
Heart disease that is severe enough to cause shortness of breath
Asthma
Severe sinusitis

A pregnant woman should also report a cold to her doctor.

## What to Do for an Ordinary Cold

If you possibly can, go to bed as soon as you feel that you are coming down with a cold. You should stay away from others anyway, in order not to spread your cold, so why not go to bed where you, too, will be better off? Stay there, or at least keep warm and avoid changing temperatures, until you are past the "runny" stage. Drink plenty of liquids and eat moderately of anything that appeals to you and doesn't cause indigestion. Be careful about blowing your nose so hard that you force infection into the sinuses and ears. If your nose is badly stopped up, *ask your doctor* to tell you what kind of medication to use. For the general misery of a cold, aspirin or an aspirin substitute such as acetaminophen is valuable. Take one or two tablets every two to three hours if necessary.

*Protect the other members of your family:* Smother all coughs and sneezes in a handkerchief or tissue.

Put all tissues (toilet tissue or paper napkins will do) into a paper bag after using them. Don't handle the outside of the bag. The tissues can then be easily disposed of without contaminating anyone else.

See to it that no one handles objects you have contaminated, or handles them as little as possible, washing his hands immediately. Your eating utensils, dishes, etc., should be washed separately from those of the other members of your family, and rinsed in scalding water.

*Be sure to call a doctor if*

1. You have a fever that lasts for more than two or three days or goes above 101° or 102°.

2. You have a severe headache that does not respond to an aspirin.

3. You have chills, a severe cough, chest pains, blood-stained or rusty-looking sputum.

4. Your back, neck, or any other bones ache. You "ache all over." You have an earache.

5. Your cold symptoms don't clear up. (You may actually have hay fever or some other allergy which I describe on page 498.)

## OTHER TROUBLESOME CONDITIONS OF THE NOSE, SINUSES, AND THROAT

Inflammation of the membranes of the nose, the sinuses, and the throat is a frequent, annoying difficulty. These conditions are called by various names such as catarrh, postnasal drip, sinusitis, irritated throat, and smoker's cough. They can be caused by a number of conditions in addition to colds, e.g., infectious diseases; decayed teeth; enlarged, infected tonsils and adenoids; allergies; irritation by cigarette smoke, and dry or dusty air; vitamin deficiencies.

I discuss sore throat and tonsillitis, which are potentially serious diseases, on page 290. The nose and its care are described on page 112. Here I want to emphasize certain other important points.

Proper treatment of irritations of the nose, sinuses, and throat depends on finding the cause. That is why you should see a doctor promptly. Don't wait until the condition becomes severe or chronic. Incidentally, *chronic* sinusitis is far less common than most people believe; but inflamed sinuses can be extremely painful. People often neglect this condition until they feel they can't stand the pain any longer, and seek relief in an operation. The results of this difficult operation do not always live up to what the sufferers hoped for. Don't decide on one without careful thought and consultation with a doctor who has had a great deal of experience in treating sinuses by other means.

I realize that, unfortunately, many people will not see a doctor for mild cases of these nuisance ailments. If you won't go to a doctor, don't do yourself harm by attempting to cure these conditions yourself. Nose drops, sprays, and inhalers should not be used unless they are prescribed by a doctor. They can do far more harm than good, for example, by irritating the membranes which may be causing the trouble simply because they are unusually sensitive.

For temporary relief, if you cannot see a doctor, do no more than the following:

CATARRH (POSTNASAL DRIP). Avoid cold and dry air and cigarette smoke. Keep one or more pans of water in your room, preferably on or near the radiator. Stay indoors if possible on a cold, raw day; wear warm clothing and don't get chilled. Blow your nose *gently*. Although the accumulation of mucus is unpleasant and irritating, it won't poison you or upset your digestion if swallowed.

SINUSITIS. Avoid cold and dry air, as I have ex-plained above. If the pain is severe, inhaling the steamy vapor rising from a basin of hot water may bring relief, but be careful not to use boiling water as the steam is scalding. An electric heating pad or a hot water bottle, protected by a cloth cover to prevent burns, may be helpful if applied over the painful area on the face or forehead. Ten minutes every two hours would be a good schedule. Take an aspirin or Bufferin tablet every two or three hours to relieve the pain.

IRRITATED THROAT AND SMOKER'S COUGH. Stop smoking, or cut down on it drastically; or try filter-tip cigarettes or a holder with a filter in it. Gargle with a third of a glassful of water in which two aspirin tablets have been dissolved; swallow a small amount of the thick suspension. Aspirin is a mild local anesthetic and helps to soothe the irritated mucous membranes. If this method gags you (as it may, especially in the morning when the symptoms are most in need of relief) try plain warm water as a gargle, or chewing gum, followed by a soothing throat lozenge. Avoid breathing through the mouth.

If these simple methods do not bring relief, *be sure to see a doctor* before these nuisance ailments develop into something *more* than a nuisance. They may be symptoms of more serious illnesses.

## ALLERGIES
(Including Hay Fever and Eczema)

About one person in ten is allergic to something; that is, he is hypersensitive to something which is not in itself poisonous or harmful, e.g., pollen, foodstuffs. The result may be a minor or a major nuisance; it may even be disabling—for example, an allergy that causes asthma (see page 454 for separate discussion of this disabling illness).

There is so much discussion about allergies these days that some people are inclined to think they are new diseases. Actually it is only the word and our knowledge that is new. Centuries ago physicians described this condition, and probably even before records were kept, some people got hives or a rash from eating certain foods, while others suffered from "catarrh" after breathing ragweed pollens.

The impetus for our new scientific knowledge of allergies was provided only about sixty years ago, when doctors discovered that while one injection of horse serum antitoxin would do no harm, a second might cause death. Investigations showed that what we now call allergic reactions are basically similar, although they differ in certain ways.

We still do not know just why allergic reactions occur. Why, for example, should some babies react to an ordinary food substance such as egg yolk? Why should an adult suddenly become sensitive to something that never troubled him before?

But we do know what happens to the person with an allergy. The substance to which he is allergic may be something he eats, breathes in with the air, touches, or is given as an injection. The bronchial tubes, the skin, and the mucous membranes of the nose, eyes, and throat, and the intestinal tract are some of the parts affected. The symptoms vary according to which of these parts becomes congested or irritated; more than one part can be affected by the same *allergen*, as the substance causing an allergy is called. We know, too, that allergies tend to run in families. Also, some allergic ailments may be influenced by emotional factors. People can be allergic to more than one allergen. An attack can, and usually does, make the victim more susceptible to future attacks, although sensitivity may vanish.

## Prevention and Treatment

While air conditioning can neither prevent nor cure allergies, it certainly can bring great relief. Air conditioning is more and more available, and sufferers from various allergies try to spend as much of their time as they can in air-conditioned rooms.

In some cases the victim himself knows what is causing his suffering, but more often it is difficult to track it down. Today we are able to make tests which will show not only the guilty substance but, in many cases, the degree of sensitivity to it. The most common tests are the patch, scratch, and injection methods made by applying the suspected allergens to the skin. A complete screening for allergic sensitivity may require as many as thirty skin tests (see Figures 35-1 and 35-2). These tests must be made by a trained physician. Only an extremely minute quantity of the substances should be used, because severe toxic reactions can occur.

However, it is well worthwhile to find out what is causing an allergic reaction. Treatment and prevention usually depend on this. I advise everyone who suffers from any allergic conditions to do everything possible to find out the cause. This is important not only to comfort but to health itself, as I shall point out below when I discuss various allergic ailments.

Your doctor may require the help of a specialist, an *allergist*. Having discovered the cause of the reaction, the doctor will do some or all of the following:

1.  He will help you to avoid the cause of your allergic reaction.

2.  He may give injections that will desensitize you partly or completely to the allergen or allergens.

3.  He will give you medicines to stop or alleviate the attacks or their sometimes dangerous symptoms. These medicines include adrenaline, usually given by injection, and antihistamines. He may show you how to administer these yourself if necessary. *But they should not be taken except when and as directed by him.* Steroids are valuable in treating allergies. They are not without hazards, and so must be administered only by a doctor with experience in their use.

In addition, the doctor will search for any possible connection between your allergic reactions

*Figure 35-1. Patch Test for Allergy.*

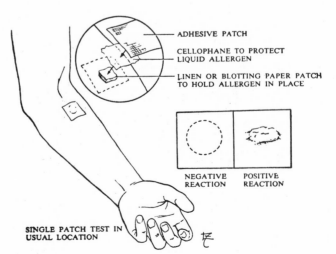

ADHESIVE PATCH

CELLOPHANE TO PROTECT LIQUID ALLERGEN

LINEN OR BLOTTING PAPER PATCH TO HOLD ALLERGEN IN PLACE

NEGATIVE REACTION

POSITIVE REACTION

SINGLE PATCH TEST IN USUAL LOCATION

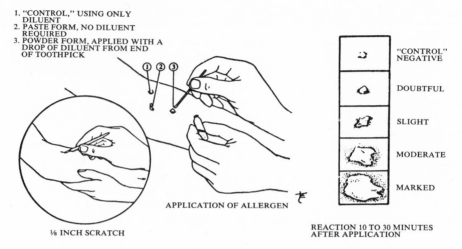

1. "CONTROL," USING ONLY
   DILUENT
2. PASTE FORM, NO DILUENT
   REQUIRED
3. POWDER FORM, APPLIED WITH A
   DROP OF DILUENT FROM END
   OF TOOTHPICK

APPLICATION OF ALLERGEN

⅛ INCH SCRATCH

"CONTROL"
NEGATIVE

DOUBTFUL

SLIGHT

MODERATE

MARKED

REACTION 10 TO 30 MINUTES
AFTER APPLICATION

*Figure 35-2. Scratch Test for Allergy.*

and emotional stresses, and help you to overcome them if they are responsible. He will prevent the secondary illnesses that frequently appear when allergic attacks have prepared the way. And, of course, he will determine whether there are any other illnesses hiding beneath the allergic symptoms.

As I said, allergies frequently involve the bronchial tubes, the nose, the intestines, and the skin. I shall discuss typical examples of each, with the exception of the bronchial tubes, the symptoms of which I describe under asthma, on page 454.

## Hay Fever

This is the term often used to cover most of the allergic reactions in the nose, usually caused by substances which are inhaled. These include pollens, dust, and a number of things such as animal hair and feathers. Foods and medicines can also cause hay fever. Consult your doctor about the common *allergens* and the pollination schedule for different parts of the country. The latter is particularly useful to victims of hay fever when planning a vacation. The different types of hay fever are as follows:

1. *Perennial hay fever.* This occurs at any time of the year. It is due to house dust, animal hair, feathers, and certain other substances, including foods.

2. *Seasonal hay fever.* This is the most common type. If it occurs in the spring, it is due to tree pollens; in the summer, to the pollens of grasses. In the fall, when it is most frequent, it is usually due to ragweed pollen. Of course, there are parts of the country in which pollens are present during almost all of the year.

The symptoms usually center in the nose, eyes, and face. There are tickling, stuffiness, a watery discharge, and itching of the eyes and face. The condition may be mistaken for a cold.

If you have hay fever, *be sure to see a doctor.* It can become far more than "just a nuisance," for it can affect your general health, causing loss of appetite and sleep, and inflammation of the eyes, ears, sinuses, throat, and bronchial tubes.

Treatment varies according to the allergen responsible. In some cases the offending object can be avoided—for example getting rid of a cat or dog will often be sufficient in cases that are due to the "dander" of these animals, or parting with that "sable" coat that is actually made of rabbit fur to which you are sensitive. Or it may be possible to go to the seashore for your vacation if the pollens elsewhere are responsible. If you can't escape from a place abounding in pollens to which you are allergic, an *air conditioner* in your room may mean the difference between misery and comfort. A filter mask or a small filter in the nose may be necessary. In addition, your doctor may be able to give you injections that will prevent attacks. But remember—these injections should be made in advance; it is usually too late if you put them off until the attacks have begun. And it is just a waste of money to start them and then not see them through. Your doctor may also give you medicines to relieve your hay fever, in the form of eye or nose drops, sprays, or pills. As new medicines are constantly being discovered, be sure to see your doctor regularly and do not assume that nothing more can be done for you.

So many medicines are available that you may have to try several before you (and your doctor) find one that works. I know one patient who tried fourteen medicines with never more than very slight relief, and frequent unpleasant side reactions. Finally, number fifteen was the right one for him!

## Allergic Reactions of the Digestive System

Although allergic reactions to certain foods usually cause hay fever and skin reactions (which I shall discuss next), there are some that involve the digestive system, causing nausea, vomiting, and dizziness. Because so many potentially serious conditions can cause the symptoms of "indiges-

tion," I think it is most unwise for anyone to decide they are caused by an allergy. Be sure to read about "indigestion," which I discuss on page 100. Your doctor, or an allergist, can sometimes diagnose intestinal or food allergies by special laboratory tests. Also, he may need your cooperation while he places you on a simple, *nonallergic diet* and then adds each suspected food or beverage systematically.

## Skin Allergies

These can be caused by direct contact or rubbing with sensitizing substances, or in the same way as "nose" allergies—that is, by allergens that are taken in through the nose, eaten, or taken through injections.

It requires a competent doctor, and sometimes a specialist in dermatology and allergy, as well, to distinguish some of these allergic reactions from other skin diseases. It is most important for these conditions to be treated properly, in order to avoid the danger of making them worse. For example, people often think they have athlete's foot when they have a contact allergy or just an irritation, as I explain on page 118. Serious secondary irritations often result from neglect or improper treatment, and potentially dangerous infections can follow.

*Figure 35–3. Dermatitis. Areas and causes of dermatitis due to allergy or irritation.*

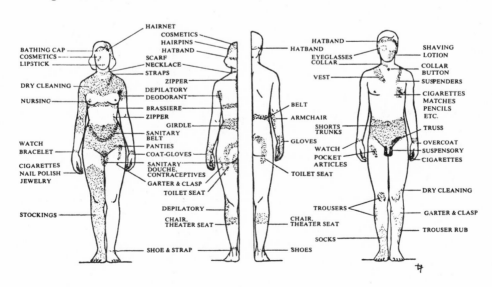

It is usually difficult to desensitize people with skin allergies by means of injections, but the doctor can relieve the condition in other ways, depending on its cause.

SKIN ALLERGIES DUE TO CONTACT (CONTACT DERMATITIS). The most common of these is *poison ivy,* which I discuss fully on page 157. This is so common that we seldom think of it as an allergy, but there are many people who are not sensitive to it. The itching, blisters, and watery discharges with which we are all familiar are quite typical of skin allergies.

A great many other things can cause contact dermatitis, including industrial oils, medicines, cosmetics, perfumes, soaps, mouth washes, clothing made of various materials or treated with certain preservatives, and dyes (see Figure 35-3). One part, or many parts of the body, may break out, as in the case of poison ivy. Sneezing and other nose symptoms may accompany the skin symptoms.

Although, as I have indicated, almost any substance coming in contact with the skin can produce an allergic reaction in some people who happen to be sensitive to it, a recent study by investigators at ten major medical centers has identified what are, by far, the leading troublemakers.

At the head of the list is nickel sulfate, which is often used in the making of inexpensive watches, earrings, rings, and bracelets. As many as 11 percent of those who wear such jewelry eventually suffer allergic reactions.

Another major offender is potassium dichromate, a substance commonly found in tanned leather. Almost 8 percent of the population is allergic to it.

Antiseptics, a common group of household products, are also responsible for many allergy cases. Merthiolate produces reactions in 8 percent.

And an ingredient in many hair dyes, *p*-phenylenediamine, produces allergic symptoms in 8 percent of users.

The purpose of the study was to let physicians know the substances most likely to be responsible for otherwise often mysterious skin problems in patients. But the results can also provide guidance for many of the victims.

## Hives (Urticaria)

Hives are usually caused by foods, but they may also be due to medicines or injections of serum. As a rule, swellings—wheals or welts—suddenly appear on the skin. Usually they disappear again in an hour or two, but they may last a day or even longer. Often the itching or burning is so severe that the sufferer is miserable. For immediate relief, bathe in a tub of tepid water to which two cups of "basic mixture" of Linit starch, made according to the directions on the box, have been added. A cheesecloth sack containing four to six tablespoonfuls of rolled oats can be placed in the tepid tub instead of the starch; the bag can be used to "rinse" the body. If the itching is localized, relief can be obtained by applying a compress dipped in ice-cold milk. It is, of course, important to discover the cause of hives, and to call a doctor in severe cases.

"Giant hives," *angioneurotic edema,* may appear on the skin, lips, tongue, throat, eyes, and other parts of the body. An attack in the throat may interfere with breathing. A person subject to hives should discuss *emergency* treatment with his physician in advance, and not wait until a serious attack occurs.

## Drug Allergies

Any medicine may have more than a primary, desirable effect. For example, an antihistamine may provide some relief for hay fever; that is its primary action. But it may have a secondary effect, drowsiness. In addition, it may have unexpected bizarre actions, producing varied symptoms, sometimes including hives, skin rashes, hay fever, or asthma.

The most feared reaction from administration of a medicine is the allergic condition *anaphylaxis,* or *anaphylactic shock,* in which the patient develops itching, hives, runny nose, and asthmatic breathing, sometimes followed by pallor, cold sweats, low blood pressure, stupor or coma, and sometimes death. In some cases of anaphylaxis, there may be only hives with or without swelling of the throat and larynx.

Another allergic reaction to medicines and serums is the *delayed* or *serum sickness type.* It occurs five to ten days after the sensitizing substance is used and involves itching, hives, and joint pains.

Almost any medication, even aspirin, may produce allergic reactions, either mild or severe, in some people. But certain compounds are noted for allergic potential. Of these, penicillin is one of the most notable offenders. Five to ten percent of patients receiving penicillin have allergic reactions.

The list of medicines that can sometimes cause allergic reactions in the sensitive includes such agents as sulfa compounds, tetracyclines and other antibiotics, insulin, antitoxins, local anesthetics, some of the tranquilizers, mercury, and arsenic. In some cases, a person seemingly allergic to a drug may actually be reacting to milk sugar or other material used as filler for the tablet or a dye used to color the pill.

An important preventive measure for anyone with sensitivity to a medicine is to carry a card or bracelet indicating so, and also to announce the fact to every doctor or nurse who has occasion to take care of him.

A person experiencing a severe allergic or other adverse reaction to a medicine should be promptly treated by his doctor or should go to an emergency room in a hospital. It is not enough to rely on an antihistamine.

## Insect Allergy

The sting or bite of many insects—including wasps, bees, hornets, yellow jackets, and ants—can set off allergic reactions, and in some instances these can even be fatal.

The type of allergic reaction can vary from local swelling to generalized reactions involving the whole body. In a generalized reaction, there may be breathing difficulty, throat swelling, sometimes unconsciousness—and prompt emergency measures may be needed to prevent death.

Fortunately, there are preventive measures. Those who know they are sensitive to insect bites should carry cards indicating so, and should also be trained by their family doctor or an allergist in the use of a special kit available on prescription for emergencies. Also, there is effective desensitization treatment for those allergic to bee, wasp, and other stings.

It makes sense for anyone who is allergic in any way and who receives a bite by a bee, wasp, hornet, or yellow jacket to discuss with his doctor the advisability of carrying an emergency kit, on the assumption that since he is allergic to other things, he might become so to these insects from a second sting.

If you are ever confronted with a person suffering a severe reaction to an insect sting or bite, and if an emergency kit with adrenaline and antihistamine is not available, you can do some good by placing a tourniquet between the bitten or stung area and the heart, applying ice to the inflamed area, and rushing the victim to the nearest doctor or hospital.

## Eczema

*Eczema,* also called *atopic dermatitis,* is manifested by a rash of "weeping" blisters. Later, the area may become dry and scaly. Eczema occurs most frequently in the bends of elbows and knees and on the face and neck. It is common in children, many of whom also have hay fever and asthma. Some children benefit when an allergenic food is found and removed from their diet.

A great deal can be done to help both children and adults suffering from eczema. Don't fail to consult your doctor for suitable treatment. His diagnosis may be required also because many skin disorders resemble eczema.

## If You Have an Allergy

1. *See a doctor, the sooner the better.* Allergies very seldom vanish by themselves. More often, they get worse, which means you'll have to do something eventually. Why not now, before you've suffered too much?

2. *Keep in good health.* Get plenty of rest and fresh air and maintain a balanced diet. This will help you to avoid the infectious diseases which may bring on nose and bronchial allergies, and help prevent the complications that often follow attacks.

3. *Avoid tensions and emotional disturbances.* We do not know the exact connection between allergies and the emotions, but we know that a relationship does exist between them. Certain skin allergies have been shown to be of a psycho-

somatic nature (see page 182). And many people with allergies have clearly recognized the fact that their attacks are more frequent and severe when they are nervous and upset. If this happens in your case, ask your doctor about the advisability of getting psychiatric help (see page 187).

4. *Remember, you can become allergic to practically anything.* Even if the cause of your allergy has been discovered, don't assume you need not look for a *different* allergen if your attacks return. A patient of mine, whose eczema was caused by face powder, later became allergic to *sunlight.*

5. *Take special precautions if you have an allergy, however trivial.* Make sure you are tested before taking any medicines, vaccines, or serums. Your regular doctor who knows about your problem will undoubtedly take it into consideration, but if you see a new doctor, be sure to tell him. You could get a severe reaction to a medicine. *For example, if you need an injection of tetanus antitoxin, your doctor should first try a little of it under the skin or as a drop in the eye* to determine whether or not you are sensitive to it. This is a routine precaution with everyone, but it is especially important with people known to have allergies.

If your attacks are severe, it is wise to carry a card with you stating clearly that you are allergic to, for example, insect stings, followed by instructions from your doctor telling what should be done for you. Tell people about your allergy whenever it is necessary. If you happen to be allergic to oysters, it is foolish to risk an attack by eating some turkey stuffing containing oysters chopped so small you don't realize what they are. The attack could be more severe than usual, disturbing both you and your hostess far more than your questions would. Don't be sensitive about your sensitivity!

Allergies are a nuisance—but your doctor can help you prevent, control, or avoid their highly unpleasant and sometimes serious effects.

## CONSTIPATION

Some years ago, a friend of mine who is a physician told me that he had been telephoned at a dinner party the previous night by a patient who said she couldn't go to sleep because she hadn't had a bowel movement in thirty-six hours. "I was very much tempted to tell her I hadn't either," my friend remarked with a smile. "But, seriously, I sometimes think people would be happier and healthier if they didn't know constipation existed. It's becoming *the* American obsession."

Too many people suffer from constipation that is nonexistent, except in their imaginations, or self-induced, or could be corrected with time, patience, and common sense.

Before I go into this any further, I want to stress the fact that constipation *can* be *organic*—that is, due to actual physical change in some organ. It can be caused by a tumor or cancer which is obstructing the intestines, a stricture which narrows them, or some disease such as a hypothyroid condition. That is why it is important to *consult a doctor if you have constipation*, especially if it has come on fairly suddenly. This is essential for people who are middle-aged or older, in order to make certain that a cancer is discovered while it is in the early, curable stage.

Here is the medical definition of *real* constipation: A person has constipation when the bowel movements are too hard to pass easily or are so infrequent that uncomfortable symptoms result. Constipation does *not* mean failure to pass a stool every day. This may be *imaginary* constipation.

Movements that are too hard to pass easily require straining and can bring about rectal troubles such as hemorrhoids and fissures which I discuss on page 509, or they can aggravate hernias or the tendency to a hernia (see page 483). Constipation can cause a number of uncomfortable symptoms which include nausea, heartburn, headache, or distress in the rectum or intestines, continuing until the stool is passed. You notice I say uncomfortable rather than harmful. That is because these symptoms are due to the nerves which send "distress signals" to various parts of the body when the rectum is distended by the retained fecal matter. *These symptoms are not due to "autointoxication,"* or absorption of poisons from the fecal matter. In experiments, it was found that similar symptoms arose when cotton was inserted into the rectum after all the fecal matter had been removed.

Some people suffer far more than others from these distressing symptoms. This is not due to their imaginations; they are actually more sensitive.

In *imaginary constipation,* the bowel movements are not difficult to pass and cause no unpleasant symptoms, but simply do not occur as often as the individual thinks they should. Very often, it is a fond mother or some other relative who insists the movements should be more frequent. Remember: bowel habits can be perfectly normal without being "average." The "average person" has a movement every day, usually right after breakfast. But countless people are perfectly normal even though they have more than one movement a day, or a movement only every other day —or every third, fourth, fifth, or even eighth day! People vary a great deal in body makeup, type of intestine, eating habits, physical activity, and custom.

By *self-induced constipation* I refer to the kind that is caused by one or more of the following— which I shall discuss when I tell you how to prevent or cure constipation:

Improper diet—eating the wrong things or eating too little.

The use (that is, *abuse*) of laxatives, cathartics, etc.

Irregularity in habits of elimination.

Our modern mode of living, with its strains and stresses and sedentary habits, helps promote these. In some primitive languages, there is no such word as constipation, and no need for it as the condition does not exist.

*Functional constipation* can also be caused by "sluggishness." After food has been digested in the stomach and intestines, the residue is passed along in the form of watery material. The water is absorbed in the colon; that is why the feces become hard and difficult to pass if they remain there too long before being eliminated. The stools are pushed along by a series of wavelike, *peristaltic* movements. These "waves" are irregular; usually they are strongest in the morning, which is why it is easiest to have a bowel movement before or just after breakfast.

In some people, peristalsis is weak. This is apt to happen with increased age; elderly people may have to use some method to help in elimination (see page **537**).

## How to Prevent or Cure Functional Constipation

If you actually have constipation, there are certain things you can safely do to *cure* it. These same methods will also *prevent* you from becoming constipated.

1. *Cultivate regular habits of elimination.* Choose a regular time shortly before or after breakfast every morning for going to the toilet, and attempt to defecate whether or not you have "the urge." Allow ten minutes. Relax and be comfortable. You can read or smoke if you like—the main thing is not to feel hurried or tense. Prop your feet on a footstool so that your knees will be close to your chest. If you go before breakfast, it will help to drink a glass or two of fluid upon getting out of bed; it can be warm or cool water, fruit juice, tea, or coffee.

Teaching your bowels to move regularly is a little like training yourself to wake up at a given hour every morning. It can be done with patience, and once acquired, the habit persists.

2. *Diet.* The residue of the foods you eat is easier to eliminate if it contains what some people have called roughage but is really fiber. In recent years, many investigations have clearly established the validity of what was once considered an old wives' tale: that the diet should contain roughage for health. Certainly it should for overcoming and preventing many cases of constipation. Fiber in food, when it gets into the intestinal tract, swells up and provides "bulk." And it is this bulk that makes for normal passage of intestinal contents.

Fiber is to be found in whole-grain breads and cereals—cereals such as old-fashioned, not "minute" oatmeal, shredded wheat, and those containing the word "bran" in their names. Bran is actually the fiber-containing part of cereal grain which is removed in the process of refining. Fiber is also to be found in many vegetables and fruits, and those that are particularly valuable are the kinds that can be eaten raw or not overly cooked.

It's also useful to drink plenty of fluids—as much as two glasses between meals, or eight or more during the day.

3. *Exercise.* Strong abdominal muscles are helpful in aiding the bowels eliminate gas and stools.

If you do not have a firm, well-toned abdominal wall, be sure to start on the exercises described on page 17. If your job requires much sitting, you should indulge in regular sports or other forms of exercise (page 16). You will feel better, generally, and also have less tendency toward constipation.

4. *Live sensibly.* Try to avoid the strains and stresses of modern living. Get some relaxation. *Don't worry about your constipation.* If your doctor gives you a clean bill of health on your periodical checkups and you follow my suggestions for "home checkups" between visits (see page **388**), your constipation isn't going to harm your health. Usually, these suggestions are enough to prevent or cure constipation. If they are not, and failure to move the bowels causes real discomfort, you may:

5. *Take an enema.* Use a pint of warm water containing a level teaspoonful of table salt. If you use an enema bag, hold it about two feet above the toilet seat; if you use a bulb, don't press it too hard—the water should flow under *gentle* pressure (see page **357**). This should soften the stool so it can be easily passed. You may take one every few days, but remember, this is a "crutch" and the sooner you discard it, the better off you will be. If an enema doesn't help, your doctor can show you how to insert olive oil into the rectum at night through a catheter, which will soften the stool and make it easier to pass in the morning.

6. If you cannot take an enema, *take a mild laxative* such as milk of magnesia.

Do not do this until you have given your bowels a chance to work by themselves. The first step in curing constipation is to stop taking all laxatives and cathartics. Laxatives are frequently the *cause* of your constipation, and seldom necessary in its cure. *Suppositories* can be irritating and cause rectal fissures, or increase their severity (see page **510**). *Mineral oil* may lead to indigestion or interfere with the absorption of vitamins.

A final word of warning: Don't give a laxative to a child—and don't take any cathartic or laxative yourself—if there is any fever, nausea, pain, or general feeling of illness associated with the constipation. It can cause fatal consequences if the condition is caused by appendicitis (see page **450**).

## PSORIASIS

At the beginning of this chapter I said that I had discussed most skin ailments earlier in the book. Although many of them are nuisances, I feel that psoriasis, like eczema, deserves a special place. These two conditions probably cause as much distress as all the others combined.

As far as we know, psoriasis is not an allergic condition. In fact, its cause is not known; none of the research carried out to date has definitely indicated the cause, although it has told us much about the disease. We know that it is not due to an infection, and *it is not catching.* It does not appear to be related to diet. It may run in families. It seems to bear some relationship to lack of sunlight, as it is less common in the tropics, rarely appears on the exposed parts of the body, such as the face, and usually gets worse in winter. There are definite indications that emotional factors play a part in this disease, although it can be found in stolid as well as "nervous" individuals. It is not dangerous to life or health—although it can become so if it is self-treated with some advertised "cures."

Why, then, do I consider it a nuisance worthy of special mention? Mainly because the affected areas are usually so unsightly. Rounded or scalloped reddened patches, with sharp borders, appear on the skin. They are covered by layers of shiny, silvery dry scales resembling the scales of mica rock. They appear most frequently on the elbows, knees, lower back, and scalp. The hair is apt to fall out in the affected scalp areas, but fortunately it usually grows in again. The soles of the feet, folds of the body—in fact, any place can be covered with these patches, and they must often be bandaged to prevent the clothing from sticking.

Young adults are most frequently the victims of this disease. It is rare in children under five, and seldom occurs in aged people—in fact, it sometimes shows marked improvement or even disappears after the age of fifty.

Much can be done for almost every patient with psoriasis, provided the patient will find a doctor skilled in treatment and will cooperate with the doctor.

Some patients benefit, sometimes to the point

of almost complete clearance, by tanning in sunshine. In areas lacking in regular sunshine, treatment may make use of a suitable ointment prescribed by the physician. It may contain a coal tar preparation. In addition to application of the ointment, sunlamp treatment may be used, with the daily dose carefully prescribed.

In some stubborn cases, doctors may prescribe a corticosteroid drug to be taken by mouth to get the lesions progressing toward healing enough for ointment and sunlamp treatment to be effective. Small resistant patches may sometimes be made to disappear by injections of corticosteroid drugs directly into them.

Newer treatments are being developed for psoriasis. None promises to be a panacea—a cure-all for psoriasis in every case. But a newer method of treatment may work for some patients who could not previously be helped adequately.

If you have psoriasis and have not sought treatment before, the chances are increasingly good that you can be helped, with even some likelihood of bringing the problem under complete control. And if you have sought help before, and have given up in despair, it could be wise to seek it again, for a newer treatment may prove valuable now.

## DISFIGUREMENTS OF THE FACE AND BODY

In the past, people used to believe that anyone with a natural disfigurement should, and must, reconcile himself or herself to it. Today, doctors are doing everything possible to change this attitude. We realize that such things as a huge, unsightly nose, protuberant ears, or a badly repaired harelip can cause feelings of inferiority, often resulting in serious emotional disturbances, and that they frequently interfere with the individual's ability to earn a livelihood. We know, too, that there is no need to endure these handicaps, because of the remarkable progress of plastic and reconstructive surgery. Understanding this will also prevent people from putting off operations for fear of becoming disfigured, as I have known people to do, with

tragic consequences, in cases such as an early, curable cancer of the lip.

Of course, we all know of people who *believe* themselves to be disfigured by what is actually only a minor irregularity. That is one of the many reasons why I urge you to discuss all problems involving disfigurement with your family doctor. He will evaluate the situation and if an operation is indicated he will know how to find a good plastic and reconstructive surgeon. Be sure to consult your doctor about wens, fatty tumors, and other growths (see page 126) even if their appearance doesn't particularly trouble you, as it may be necessary to remove them to prevent later difficulty. NEVER consult a self-styled "beauty expert" in these cases. Your doctor will know which ones can be trusted in matters such as the removal of unsightly hair. Countless people have been victimized by quacks who not only take their money for nothing, but often actually disfigure their victims and even endanger their lives.

Remember, too, that while it is certainly advisable to have disfiguring conditions corrected early, remarkable results have been obtained late in life. So there is no need to believe it is too late to do anything for yourself or some member of your family.

## Squints (Crossed Eyes)

I was quite astounded recently to see a potentially very attractive young woman in her twenties whose appearance was marred by a severe squint in one eye. She had not had it corrected in childhood, and just assumed that nothing could be done to help her. Of course, it would have been better to have corrected this disfigurement in early life—but this unsightly crossing of the eye could still be improved by a relatively simple surgical operation. Since the muscles involved are *outside* the eye itself, there is no danger to the vision—provided, of course, that the operation is performed by a competent surgeon.

Although crossed eyes can be corrected late in life, it is most important to consult a doctor early for this condition. It is usually associated with, or gives rise to, some visual difficulty. If it is not attended to in time, the vision may be badly impaired.

Parents often wonder whether or not their babies are cross-eyed. The eyes of little infants tend to waver and turn inward, but this usually corrects itself by the time they are three to six months old. If it does not, or if the eyes are continually crossed in the same way even before the baby is six months old, consult your doctor. He may be able to start correcting the condition quite early. For example, he may put a "patch" over the baby's "good" eye, forcing him to use the weaker one, instead of letting it get worse from lack of use. He may recommend glasses or exercises or both, making it possible to avoid an operation or to keep the condition from doing any damage to the vision until the suitable time for an operation. Incidentally, it is quite unusual for anyone to become cross-eyed after the age of six, but it has been known to happen.

## Artificial Eyes

I also want to call your attention to the fact that people who have lost an eye, or have one which is sightless and disfiguring, can now be fitted with a glass or plastic eye that is indistinguishable from a real one. These *prosthetic* devices have been improved so tremendously that, even though I know about them, I frequently find myself unable to believe they are artificial. Not only is such an eye absolutely identical with the natural one, but it moves in unison with it, being attached to the eye muscles. Even children can be fitted with them, new eyes being provided as they grow so that they are spared the embarrassment of having their handicap noticed.

## Other Prosthetic Devices

Other prosthetic devices such as hands, ears, feet, arms, and legs have been so greatly improved in recent years that they look and function as though they were real. No one, child or adult, need be disfigured today because of an accident or a congenital condition requiring the use of an artificial limb.

## Harelip and Cleft Palate

These two conditions are similar, resulting from the failure of the two sides of the face to unite properly before the baby is born. This disunity may involve only the superficial tissues, or may extend to the uvula or the hard and soft palates. We do not know why this happens, but we do know there is no reason whatsoever to believe the old superstition that it is caused by something the mother did during her pregnancy. I am astonished to discover that there are mothers who feel guilty and blame themselves for the fact that their babies are born with harelips or cleft palates.

The extent of difficulty in sucking and, later, in speaking caused by this condition varies according to its degree. But even if it does not cause much difficulty, it should be corrected by an operation or series of operations as soon as your doctor recommends. These operations are performed · so skillfully today that it is almost impossible to detect any disfigurement. Even if they have been performed imperfectly, excellent results can frequently be obtained by a subsequent operation. It is important to start speech therapy as soon as possible after an operation has united the tissues.

## "Cauliflower" and Other Types of Unsightly Ears

A "cauliflower" ear, which we associate with prize fighters, is caused by bleeding below the skin of the ear, usually as the result of a blow. This blood eventually becomes a hard substance. It should be reassuring, especially to mothers whose sons insist on fighting, to know that this need not happen. The blood can be drawn off with a needle before it hardens and alters the shape of the ear. Of course, this must be done by a competent physician, but it is a simple procedure. Even after the hardening occurs, cauliflower ears can be corrected by surgery.

Large, protruding, or misshapen ears can be operated upon with excellent results. There is no reason for being embarrassed by them, or letting your child run the risk of becoming shy and anxious because of constant teasing about his or her ears.

## Misshapen Nose

Most people have heard about the truly remarkable results that are obtained by plastic operations to correct the size and shape of the nose. It is even possible to rebuild crushed and destroyed noses by means of implants of tissue from other parts of the body, or replace them with substances such as silver and latex. I have seen some of these which are impossible to distinguish from a natural nose. However, I do want to caution you against having your nose, or that of your child, operated upon by anyone but a *really competent plastic surgeon,* as some people are tempted to do when a friend who has had such an operation says "there's nothing to it!" ANY operation can be dangerous if performed by an unskilled quack.

## Other Conditions

I have mentioned the body disfigurements caused by clubfoot on page 462, congenital dislocation of the hip on page 462; pendulous breasts, page 523; severe freckles, page 121; scarring from acne, page 123; and excess facial and body hair, page 120.

## HEMORRHOIDS AND OTHER RECTAL TROUBLES

Hemorrhoids, or piles, are enlarged, dilated veins situated inside or just outside the rectum. They are somewhat like varicose veins in the legs, which I describe on page 510. They cause itching, discomfort, and pain, and are frequently accompanied by bleeding.

Aside from the fact that they are a nuisance, there are two important reasons for seeing a doctor promptly if you think you have hemorrhoids. The first is that they may be caused by something potentially serious. Usually, the cause is a local one, such as the hard, dry stools and straining which accompany constipation; this irritates the veins and slows the flow of blood (see page 505 for treatment of constipation). In pregnancy, the enlarged womb sometimes presses on the veins. However, the pressure can be caused by a disease in the liver or even the heart, or by a locally situated tumor or cancer. Rectal symptoms which you casually attribute to hemorrhoids may actually be caused by a curable cancer. This is one reason why it is important to see a doctor promptly if (a) the enlarged vein inside the rectum pushes out and can be felt, (b) there is persistent aching, discomfort, pain, or itching in the rectal region, (c) you notice any bleeding from the rectum, either in the toilet bowl or on the toilet tissue after bowel movements.

The other reason for seeing a doctor promptly is that hemorrhoids should be treated before they cause complications that can be more than a nuisance. For example, the bleeding which appears to be slight can be so continuous that it causes anemia (see page 477). If a blood clot should form in the vein, it can be extremely painful until a surgeon opens the vein and removes the clot. This is usually an office procedure. The veins can also become inflamed or infected and even rupture, causing a hemorrhage.

*Don't* use any advertised hemorrhoid "cure" that promises "instant relief from piles." These do not get at the cause of the difficulty, and often only make the symptoms worse. Cathartics and laxatives encourage constipation which is one of the main causes of hemorrhoids.

For *emergency* treatment of painful hemorrhoids, apply very cold water on tissues or a cloth directly to the anal area. Continue for five to ten minutes until the pain is allayed. Witch hazel can be employed instead of cold water.

A hot tub bath morning and night may also help bring relief. A soothing rectal suppository is worth trying, but regular use of suppositories or ointments may prove irritating after a few days. These are emergency measures to be used only until you can see your doctor, who will determine the exact cause of the hemorrhoids and suggest therapy.

Don't delay. Medical care is necessary not only for relief but also for safety. Many cases of hemorrhoids can be cured by nonsurgical methods. Others need an operation. It is not a serious one, although, of course, it must be performed by a competent surgeon.

New surgical techniques for hemorrhoid removal are now in increasing use. No longer is the standard hemorrhoidectomy operation—simple and effective but followed by discomfort for some days afterward—the only resort. One technique, cryosurgery, involves touching the hemorrhoid with a special extremely cold probe that quickly freezes it. Later, it disappears. This procedure can be carried out in the doctor's office with only moderate discomfort. There may be only a slight discharge for a few days and healing is good.

Another technique, called rubber-band ligation, is often used now for internal hemorrhoids. The procedure is essentially painless and can be done in a doctor's office. With a special instrument, the doctor places a special latex band over the neck of a hemorrhoid. The band ties off the hemorrhoid so it receives no blood, dies, and sloughs off, usually within three to nine days. The ligated hemorrhoid may produce a sensation of fullness for a time. When the hemorrhoid drops off, there may be some brief spotting of blood. And itching may be aggravated for a time when the hemorrhoid drops off.

## Pruritus Ani (Anal Itching)

This is a frequent and terribly annoying condition. Don't let false modesty stand in the way of having it cured. Doctors know how much distress it causes, and serious medical journals contain many articles discussing the best methods of relieving it.

It can be caused by worms, allergies, contact with irritating chemicals, and in many other ways. Sometimes emotional factors are responsible for the "nervous itching" that makes the patient scratch and irritate this sensitive area. Often the cause is not clear, and it takes some time for the doctor to find it, although he frequently can relieve the condition while he is seeking the cause. Be sure to give your doctor a chance to help you, because pruritus ani can result in infections or even interfere markedly with your general health by disturbing your sleep or by making you tense and inefficient at work.

I discuss *pruritus vulvae*, or itching of the external female genitalia, on page 521.

## Anal Fissure (Fissure-in-Ano)

An anal fissure is an ulcerated crack in the anal canal. It may start as a superficial crack caused by passage of large, hard stools. When the crack fails to heal because of distension and contraction of the canal with passage of stools, it may deepen and become inflamed. It then leads to spasm, or involuntary contraction, of the anal sphincter muscle and can be very painful. Distress can be particularly severe when the anus is stretched during bowel movement.

A cure for a fissure often can be obtained in a few weeks with medical measures, which may include use of stool softeners, anesthetic ointments, and sitting in a warm tub of water (sitz bath) after a bowel movement to help relax spasm.

When a fissure becomes chronic, it can be eliminated surgically. The operation is relatively minor, takes half an hour or less, and is almost invariably successful.

## Anal Fistula (Fistula-in-Ano)

An anal fistula is an abnormal tunnel from inside the rectum to the skin outside. Usually it stems from infection that may start in the wall of the rectum or anus and form a painful "boil" that breaks through the skin near the anal opening and discharges pus. The boil, or abscess, may seem to heal only to open and discharge repeatedly over a period of weeks and months, leading to the establishment of a tunnel.

An anal fistula never heals spontaneously but must be surgically removed. Symptoms consist of a pus-containing discharge near the anus, often with skin irritation, itching, and repeated abscess formation.

In the vast majority of cases, surgery is curative. The hospital stay may be a week or less.

## VARICOSE VEINS

Varicose veins are knotlike, twisting enlargements of the veins, usually just below the skin of the legs. They are the result of a breakdown of the valves which are found at regular intervals in the veins. It is through these valves that the blood flows back to the heart, after having been pumped to the extremities through the arteries. These valves divide the veins into sections, each valve forming a floor to support the blood above it. When a valve is faulty or degenerates, it cannot support the blood; when a number of valves in a surface vein break down, the weight of the column of blood becomes sufficient to distend it.

Varicose veins are seen most frequently in people whose work requires them to stand or to sit upright for long periods. A tendency toward valves that break down easily has been found to run in families. Increase in the internal or back pressure of the blood in the veins is also a strain on the valves. This can be caused by constipation and straining at stool, heavy lifting, abdominal tumors, and pregnancy. There may also be a connection between the endocrine glands and the valves, which tend to degenerate with age.

In addition to being unsightly, varicose veins usually cause some trouble eventually, generally in the form of dull, nagging aches and pains. The ankles may swell. The enlarged veins can become the site of an infection and, since the resistance of the surrounding tissue has decreased, a bruise or injury can become serious. The resulting varicose ulcers are not easy to clear up, especially in elderly people or diabetics; they may refuse to yield to medication, and require surgery, including skin grafting.

In mild cases, varicose veins can be handled adequately by such measures as eliminating tight shoes and tight garters that restrict the circulation; elevating the feet at intervals, and walking about occasionally instead of standing still for long periods. Sometimes wearing an elastic stocking or bandage for even part of the day will support a varicose vein and prevent it from becoming more distended. In severe cases, or with individuals to whom appearance is especially important, varicose veins can and should be eliminated. There are two ways in which this can be done. One method is *surgical;* the distended veins can be cut out, or else ligated (tied off). Afterward the blood will flow through other veins. The other method is *medical;* a fluid is injected into the varicose vein, causing it to harden, after which the blood can no longer flow through it

and seeks a new course. The technique for injecting veins has been steadily improved during the hundred years since it was first attempted, and it is now perfectly safe in experienced hands.

Surgical treatment of varicose veins has usually required three to six days of hospitalization. But recently excellent results have been reported with surgery on an ambulatory basis. Typically, the patient arrives at the hospital early in the morning, undergoes surgery, three hours later walks with assistance, by midafternoon walks without aid, and an hour or two later goes home. The next day the patient performs all normal activities and returns for a checkup, and then a week later returns again for suture removal. Not only has the one-day surgery meant convenience and financial benefit to patients, but the reports also indicate that early return to activity has greatly decreased postoperative discomfort.

## MOTION SICKNESS
(Seasickness: Car Sickness)

Why seasickness (the term given to all forms of motion or travel sickness) should be considered funny is a mystery to anyone who has ever suffered from it. There is probably nothing to compare with the misery its victims endure. Nausea, dizziness, headache, and vomiting can be so severe that prostration results; it has even been known to cause death. Fortunately, however, it usually vanishes quickly, leaving no ill effects.

The exact cause of seasickness is not fully understood. We do know that it is related to stimulation of the eye and the labyrinth of the ear (which is an organ of balance as well as of hearing, as I explain on page 476). Psychological factors can also be important. You have probably suspected this from knowing someone who becomes violently seasick even before the ship sails.

There are countless ways to help ward off seasickness. Here are some useful suggestions; of course, it is not always possible to follow them all:

Be sure you are rested and in good condition; you should not have constipation.

Get plenty of fresh air; avoid stuffy rooms and unpleasant smells. Sit on deck with your eyes facing the ship, not the ocean.

Keep warm.

Get some exercise unless you become actively ill, in which case lying down with the head low often helps.

Don't overload your stomach. Small amounts of food, taken frequently, are usually better than a large meal.

Avoid rich, indigestible food.

Alcoholic beverages make some people feel less nervous, and in that way help to ward off seasickness. Also, iced creme de menthe and other pleasant-tasting drinks may help "settle the stomach." But, of course, alcoholic drinks in excess can also upset the digestion.

Don't take advertised remedies. They are usually useless, and in some cases even dangerous.

There are other things your doctor can do to help. Be sure to consult a doctor if you know from experience (or if you fear) that you are going to have motion sickness on a boat, car, train, or plane. He may give you a sedative such as phenobarbital for a few days before the journey.

He may prescribe medicines such as Dramamine or Marezine, which have worked wonders in preventing or curing seasickness, and other types of motion sickness. These must not be taken except on a doctor's orders.

## PILONIDAL SINUS

A pilonidal sinus or cyst is a congenital defect in the skin at the base of the spinal column, the "tailbone." It varies from a small dimple in the skin to a series of small tunnel-like openings. A pilonidal sinus rarely causes trouble until adolescence or later when it may become acutely or chronically inflamed. If trouble persists, it must be excised. The operation is a fairly extensive one because surgeons have learned that unless every bit of abnormal tissue is cut away, the condition recurs. Nevertheless, the operation is considered minor and without danger.

# 36
# PROBLEMS OF WOMEN

You may wonder why I should write a chapter dealing specifically with women's problems. "Haven't you covered the subject in your chapters on pregnancy, childbirth, and the period that follows it, and in discussing the glands, the skin, adolescence, marriage, and so on?" you may ask.

I have two main reasons for writing this chapter. In the first place, the childbearing organs, the remarkable functions which enable them to play the major role in bringing new life into the world, are an integral part of women—when they are not bearing children as well as when they are. Discussing them solely in relation to maternity is not enough. In the second place, certain physical and emotional problems persist in women because of their status in the past, and because of the fact that many women are housewives. The very nature of this work has, for example, made it extremely difficult to compile statistics and conduct research into its "occupational disorders," which afflict many women.

## ARE WOMEN PEOPLE?

Undoubtedly you will laugh at such a question. Yet less than a hundred years ago it was being hotly debated by a small group of the most advanced thinkers in the most enlightened countries. Everyone else took it for granted that women, although extremely spiritual, were mentally and physically quite inferior to men. In addition, they were almost universally regarded as being so fragile morally that one unfortunate sex experi-ence might shatter a woman's life permanently. When my grandmother was a girl, American wives were not permitted to own or inherit prop-erty, sign contracts, keep their own wages if they worked, or have any rights to their own children. A father could give his children away for adop-tion without even consulting the mother who bore them. In short, a woman's legal position was simi-lar to that of a minor child, an imbecile, or a slave—although the law did provide that a hus-band could not beat his wife with a stick larger around than a thumb, without, however, specify-ing exactly how large a thumb might be!

The church regarded women as morally in-ferior, on the grounds that Eve was responsible for the fall of man. Society and the law generally assumed that woman had been endowed with less strength and intelligence than man, so that all her energies could be devoted to childbearing. Since the earliest times, this tendency to regard women as little more than instruments of reproduction helped make the sex "inferior." Primitive people, feeling that supernatural elements must be ac-tively involved in the process of childbirth, sur-rounded the childbearing sex with superstition and taboos.

The fact that women menstruate seemed to in-dicate their close connection with supernatural forces. Menstruation involved a discharge of blood, which itself was surrounded by supersti-tion, fear, and horror. Traces of these emotions still persist today. But more important was the fact that menstruation is of a cyclical nature, similar to the period of time involved in the waxing and waning of the moon. It was called the

513

lunar sickness, and seemed to prove conclusively that women, unlike men, were acted upon regularly by forces outside the world.

Among civilized as well as uncivilized peoples, menstruation was regarded as, at the least, dangerous and unclean. Many laws made outcasts or pariahs of menstruating women, and they were required to go through rituals of purification before being considered fit to resume their place in society. They not only were taboo as far as sex was concerned, but had to refrain from ordinary activities because it was feared that their touch would bring disaster. As the great naturalist Pliny, who lived in the first century after Christ, put it, menstruating women "blighted crops, blasted gardens, killed seedlings, brought down fruit from the trees, killed bees, caused mares to miscarry. If they touched wine, it turned to vinegar; milk became sour." Is is any wonder that such "creatures" were put in an inferior position!

The advent of manhood was almost invariably welcomed with ceremonial rites which, though strenuous or unpleasant to the boy in some societies, were nevertheless great events accompanied by honors and privileges. The coming of womanhood, however, was not a cause for rejoicing. Certain groups had a grim method of "welcoming" a girl into maturity. At the time of her first menstruation, the girl's mother would slap her face and say, "Remember, now you are a woman."

As late as the 1870's and 1880's, doctors almost universally agreed that menstruation was an illness. Because of it, women were incapable of sustained physical or mental efforts—especially mental efforts, since menstruation was regarded as a "temporary insanity."

Some of these attitudes persist today, although often in an unconscious manner. My wife tells me that there are still many women who avoid touching a flower when they are menstruating because they are sure it will promptly fade. I am constantly astonished by the lengths to which even well-educated women will go in order to avoid saying the word menstruation. They call it "the curse," "the cramps," "falling off the roof," or "my periods." Even today, few women are entirely free from completely illogical attitudes toward menstruation. Many of these arose before

or during adolescence, as I explain on page 313. There is no doubt that these attitudes account for many of the menstrual difficulties which are the most common and the most important of the genital disorders of women.

## MENSTRUAL DISORDERS

Menstruation is a normal physiological function, which I describe fully on page 84. From the time a girl reaches the childbearing age, the lining of the womb disintegrates at regular intervals, unless she is pregnant, and is discharged in a flow of blood. Girls begin to menstruate at the age of puberty, usually when they are from twelve to fourteen years old. They continue until they reach the end of their childbearing years, usually when they are in their late forties or early fifties. The period when menstruation ceases is called the menopause, the climacteric, or "change of life."

At first the periods may be irregular, but once established they continue at regular intervals until the menopause, when they may again become irregular. Many women menstruate every 28 days. However, it is entirely normal to have periods at intervals of from 21 to 35 days. Every woman usually has a fairly definite rhythm.

Menstruation generally lasts from three to seven days. The average amount of blood lost is about three ounces. However, it is difficult for a woman to estimate this. The number of pads or tampons which she uses may depend less on actual need than upon considerations of personal daintiness. However, the amount tends to remain about the same during each menstrual period, usually diminishing after the first day or two. Its quantity is no indication of "womanliness." A woman may not menstruate at all, even though she is a completely feminine person.

As I explain in the chapter on adolescence (p. 308), the normal, healthy woman experiences no difficulties, aside from the inconvenience, during her menstrual periods.

Menstrual disorders such as pain, irregularity, excessive flow, and the absence of menstruation are not diseases in themselves, but are symptoms that something is wrong.

## Absence of Menstruation (Amenorrhea)

The term *primary* amenorrhea is used if menstruation has not occurred, although the age of puberty has been reached. If it begins and then ceases, it is called *secondary* amenorrhea. Secondary amenorrhea is, of course, normal during pregnancy and often while the mother is nursing. It is quite apt to occur sporadically in the first and last months of a woman's childbearing years.

In rare cases, *primary amenorrhea* is caused by malformed or underdeveloped female organs. For example, the hymen (see Figure 14-1, page 213) may completely block the vagina, causing retention of the menstrual blood. It may be due to glandular disorders, in which case it can often be cured or at least partially corrected by taking the proper hormones—but *never without a doctor's prescription*. Primary and secondary amenorrhea can be caused by general poor health, a change in climate or living conditions, and by emotional factors such as a shock or the fear or hope of being pregnant.

*Scanty menstruation,* menstrual flow which may be so slight as to amount to little more than "staining," sometimes results from the same causes. It is frequently due to anemia (see page 477).

## Excessive Menstruation (Menorrhagia)

This means an exceptional amount of menstrual flow at the regular periods. The term *irregular endometrial shedding* is used for "extra" menstrual periods. It is not easy to describe the amount of menstrual flow that constitutes menorrhagia. However, if ordinary pads do not afford protection or *if the menstrual blood forms into large clots,* be sure to consult a doctor.

Tumors, polyps, cancers, inflammations, and certain diseases such as rheumatic fever can cause excessive bleeding. It can also be due to disorders of the glands whose hormones set off the process of shedding. Abnormalities of the organs may be responsible. Emotional factors frequently cause excessive menstruation.

A pelvic examination so thorough that it sometimes requires an anesthetic may be necessary to discover the cause of this disorder. The uterus is scraped and the scrapings examined. This latter procedure is called curettage, and will sometimes correct excessive bleeding.

## Irregular Menstruation

During her childbearing years, menstruation usually occurs at definite intervals in each woman, starting almost exactly the same number of days apart. Irregularity may be due to a harmless change in nature's timing, which will correct itself spontaneously, or to changes in climate or living conditions, or to emotional factors. On the other hand, it may result from a disease in some other part of the body, such as a thyroid gland problem, which should be diagnosed and treated as soon as possible. It may be caused by a tumor of the womb or the ovaries. Most important of all, bleeding between periods can be a warning of cancer (see page 432). *It should always be reported immediately to a doctor.*

I am surprised by the number of women patients who do not know the dates of their periods or the number of days in their menstrual cycles. If you have not passed the menopause, make a habit of marking on your calendar the start and end of your current period and the expected date for the arrival of the next one. This will be extremely useful in determining your fertile period (see page 227) in case you wish either to facilitate conception or to avoid becoming pregnant. A menstrual calendar will be a convenience in planning your social life in such a way that you will not arrange a beach picnic or have to prepare a big dinner party on the day or days when excessive flow or discomfort might be anticipated. And it will enable you to become aware immediately of any irregularity or bleeding between periods.

## Painful Menstruation (Dysmenorrhea)

Many, if not most, women experience some discomfort at the onset of their menstrual periods. It is very difficult to draw a boundary between this and pain, since individual reactions vary tremendously. For practical purposes, I would say that a woman has dysmenorrhea if her menstrual cramps do not yield to aspirin or other mild pain-relievers, and if they prevent her from engaging in her work or social life.

Painful menstruation can be due to physical causes, such as an inflammation or *endometriosis* (see page 523), which require treatment. In many instances it is associated with constipation, and vanishes when this condition is corrected. In the past, there was a tendency to believe that "cramps" were always due to some organic cause, usually the fact that the cervix, the mouth of the womb, was narrow and needed to be stretched, or dilated, or that the uterus itself was not in the proper position. Operations were frequently performed to correct this. In many cases, the pain was not relieved.

Today we believe that dysmenorrhea is often of the *primary* type; that is, it cannot be accounted for by any organic condition. Such illnesses are called *functional*. We do not fully understand this, any more than we fully understand *colic* (see page 272), which causes a similar spasmodic kind of pain. But we do know that this kind of painful menstruation is almost never found in women who have had a number of children, is found only occasionally in married women, and occurs most often in virgins, especially young girls or women in certain types of occupations. In many cases there is conclusive evidence that it is caused by emotional factors.

I do *not* mean that this pain is imaginary. It is quite real, and can be relieved by medicines known as antispasmodics, analgesics, and sedatives.

## Intermenstrual Pain

Some women experience pain approximately midway between their periods, at the time of *ovulation* (see page 227). It may be accompanied by leukorrhea or a slight show of blood. As a rule, the pain is brief and moderate. Sometimes, however, when the ovum breaks through the wall of the ovary to start its journey toward the uterus, it may cause quite severe pain. When it is located in the right ovary, which lies near the appendix, there may be concern that appendicitis is developing. If the doctor knows the exact dates of the menstrual period, he can estimate the day of ovulation. On the basis of this information and a careful examination, together with certain laboratory tests, he can make the correct decision. This is very important because acute appendicitis (see page 449) requires an operation, whereas a ruptured egg sac is perfectly normal except in very rare instances. (The medical name for the ruptured egg container is *corpus hemorrhagicum*.)

## Premenstrual Difficulties

Headache, depression, irritability, slight nausea, and puffiness of the abdomen, skin, and other parts of the body may precede menstruation. The reasons for premenstrual tension are not fully understood, but we know that they are associated with a disturbance of the salt balance, resulting in the accumulation of water in the tissues. Often these symptoms vanish with medication or a salt-free diet.

Menstrual disorders may not mean anything and, in fact, usually correct themselves. However, it is always important to consult a doctor about them. They may be warnings of some potentially dangerous condition. *I cannot remind you too often to be sure to consult a doctor if there is bleeding between periods or if it occurs after the menopause.* In addition, many menstrual difficulties can be easily corrected, and it is unnecessary to be troubled by them.

It is usually possible for a doctor to rule out the possibility of potentially serious conditions fairly rapidly. To discover the exact cause of the symptoms, your doctor may refer you to a *gynecologist* who specializes in the diseases of the female organs. If he cannot find the cause of the disorder, it may be necessary to consult an *endocrinologist*, a doctor who specializes in conditions of the endocrine glands. If this specialist, too, cannot find what is wrong, a *psychiatrist* (see page 188) may discover that tensions and emotional problems are responsible.

Never attempt to treat menstrual disorders yourself. *Never take any medicine containing hormones.* Only a doctor can determine, after a thorough examination, whether you need additional hormones, what kind, and how much you require. The wrong kind or quantity can be very dangerous, as I explain on page 74.

Be sure to mention even mild menstrual disorders to your doctor at your regular checkup. He may be able to help you. In addition, it will give him information that will be valuable in case the condition should become aggravated.

## THE MENOPAUSE

The childbearing period of a woman's life is limited to the years of ovulation and menstruation, that is, to her regular monthly cycles. At the end of this period, ovarian function declines and ceases, and menstruation ends.

The *average* American woman is from forty-seven to forty-nine years old at the menopause. Almost 75 percent of all women reach the menopause while they are in their forties, and about 99 percent between the ages of thirty-five and fifty-five. In general, the younger a woman is at the onset of her periods, the *menarche*, the older she will be when they cease. However, certain diseases and surgical operations can cause a premature menopause.

Several women have told me that they know of "change of life" babies. Strictly speaking, this is not possible. Once the follicles cease expelling eggs into the tubes, no pregnancy can take place. What might have happened was that the woman was undergoing the menopause, but the process was not completed; and although she was no longer menstruating regularly, she was still ovulating, or producing eggs. The length of time for the completion of the menopause varies in different women. As a rule, it takes from six months to three years. The menstrual flow may become smaller in amount, then irregular, and finally cease. The time between periods may lengthen, until there may be a lapse of several months between them.

Some women complain because their childbearing years are more definitely limited than are those during which a man can become a father. In some cases, this extends well into the period of old age. But nature is indeed being very wise. Think for a moment how difficult it would be, for both the mother and the child who requires her care, if women could continue to have babies until extremely late in life!

Some women recognize this fact with gratitude. I was quite surprised when an extremely youthful-looking woman of thirty-nine told me with perfect sincerity that she was glad she was having the menopause. When I questioned her a little about her attitude, she said, "I've had my family, so why on earth should I want to keep on having menstrual periods? They're just a nuisance, and they won't stop me from being a year older each year. Menopause or no menopause, I'm going to be forty on my next birthday." I couldn't help thinking what a priceless gift this woman's attitude would prove to be to her three daughters.

I remember, too, a woman of fifty who burst into tears when she told me she was having the menopause, crying, "Now I can't ever have a baby!" This was a tragedy to her—but it had nothing to do with the menopause. The tragedy resulted from her thirty years of sterility.

### Emotional Problems of the Menopause

Unfortunately, many women have a tendency to attribute to the menopause every sign of the fact that they are no longer young. For them, it is a time to mourn over what might have been.

Making an unpleasant milestone of the menopause is responsible for many of the emotional disturbances associated with it. It is a good thing to look back in order to determine one's best path for the future. But it is devastating to look back for the sole purpose of brooding over failures and omissions! The desperate desire to make hay while the sun is still shining has driven many a woman into sexual adventures, real or imaginary, of a most immature kind. No matter how much we may want to go back, we cannot lead our lives over again.

It is *not* true that the childless woman or the woman who has never had sexual intercourse will wither or dry up or suffer unduly in some other way when she reaches the menopause. Being childless or abstinent can cause problems, but these can and have been solved by countless women who have led rich and happy lives. *Untold suffering has been caused by the many superstitions associated with this period of life:* that women are apt to lose their minds, or have nervous breakdowns, or become unattractive, or lose the ability to enjoy and give enjoyment in sexual relations.

These superstitions have no foundation in fact. Some of the most famous women of our time, whose careers depend on their looks, personality, brains, and glamor, are well along in their forties and fifties. Many of them are proud to be grandmothers. A number of women find, to their surprise, that sexual intercourse is even more enjoyable than it was before the menopause. Since they can no longer become pregnant, their attitude toward sex is more relaxed, free of anxiety over its possible consequences. Premenstrual tensions and the discomforts of menstruation being over, they may feel better than they ever did. The expression "change of life" doesn't seem appropriate, when so few changes in living actually take place.

## Adjusting to the Menopause

It is true that most women in their forties must make adjustments. A mother may find that her children are freeing themselves from dependence on her, just as she once had to cut the knot tying her to her own mother. This can be a painful process, as I point out on page 310. An unmarried woman must relinquish her dream that she can become a mother if she should yet marry.

But, fortunately, the maternal urge to create can be fulfilled in other ways than bearing children. Intellectual and artistic creation, and the "mothering" of ideas, causes, and individuals or groups, give it constructive and satisfying outlets. Maternal instincts often find new and rich forms of expression in a relationship with a son-in-law or daughter-in-law and in the great joy of being a grandmother. Thus, a woman who has had her menopause can consider herself as entering a new and very important phase of life. Having put her childbearing years behind her, she can develop latent talents and new interests that will make her life fuller and more meaningful. If the rich years still ahead of her are used wisely, she can develop into an even more interesting and charming person.

"You're not a woman, so it's easy for you to talk that way!" you may be thinking when you read these lines. "It's not so easy for us to get over a lot of ideas that were put into our minds when we were very young, even though we realize they aren't true."

You are quite right. No matter how intelligent a woman may be in understanding the menopause, she can be influenced by the things she has heard, or half-heard, in the past. Whispers about "poor Aunt Ida, she had to be put away when she had the change." "Isn't it awful, the way Martha Brown's making a fool of herself with that scoundrel when she has a lovely husband and family! She was such a nice woman, too, until she reached the dangerous age." "Mother can't help being cross and crying so much—it's her time of life." "They say that Mrs. Jones——"

Don't be ashamed of any fears, however absurd or vague, that may remain after you have read the facts about the menopause. The best way to dispel your fears and solve your problems is to discuss them with your doctor or some qualified person he recommends (see page 188). Above all, do not depend on your friends to solve the problems which a doctor is far better qualified to handle.

## Physical Symptoms of the Menopause

I certainly do not mean to imply that all the disturbances associated with the menopause are caused by emotional attitudes. When ovulation ceases, certain hormones are no longer produced, and the whole "switchboard" of the endocrine gland system is temporarily "jangled." The endocrine glands affect the emotions, and the emotions affect the endocrine glands. Therefore we cannot say which comes first or is more directly responsible for the physical and emotional symptoms of the menopause.

Fortunately, however, these symptoms will usually vanish when the missing hormones are supplied artificially—that is, in tablets or injections. I repeat what I have said before: *These must be taken only with a doctor's prescription.* After the balance has once more been established by nature, the medication is no longer required.

I see no reason for prescribing hormones as a routine matter. In about 85 percent of all women, menopausal symptoms cause no more than mild, occasional discomfort. This is a nuisance, like menstruation, but one which the average woman can put up with if she has some help from her sense of humor! On the other hand, there is no reason why a woman should suffer if she belongs to the 15 percent that is really troubled by these symptoms.

I think there is a slight, but real, danger that the sane, modern attitudes toward the menopause may prevent some women from seeking help because they feel their symptoms are purely psychological or silly. One very sensible woman I know was secretly ashamed of herself for being disturbed. Always a light sleeper, she would awaken at night feeling hot, throw off her covers, and barely manage to get to sleep again before she awakened, chilled, to repeat the entire process. Her doctor could have given her some medicine to help her enjoy the good night's rest her busy days required.

These *vasomotor disturbances,* known as hot flashes or flushes, are the most common symptoms during the menopause. They are frequently its first sign, and disappear gradually after the menstrual periods have ceased. They may be limited to the face and neck or extend to the entire body. They may be accompanied by an embarrassingly telltale flushing, or perspiration, or a sensation of "closeness of air" that makes a woman throw open the window on the coldest day. There may be headaches. The hands and feet may, surprisingly, be cold. Their frequency varies a great deal, some women experiencing only a few hot flashes during the entire period of the menopause, while others have many, every day and night.

Some women have other unpleasant physical symptoms, including fatigue, a nervous irritability of the bladder with a consequent need to urinate, and a kind of dizziness or giddiness, *vertigo,* occasionally associated with nausea or loss of appetite. The blood pressure may rise considerably.

It is important to consult your doctor during this period in your life. Don't tell yourself to "grin and bear it." Let your doctor make this decision—*after* he has determined whether or not something should be done to relieve some symptom. He must also eliminate the possibility that a symptom is not due to the menopause at all, but to a potentially dangerous disease.

*Estrogen therapy* can be safely used on a short-term basis, under your doctor's supervision, to control such disturbances as hot flashes.

There has been a recent vogue of using estrogen in all postmenopausal women as a possible means of preserving youth and of preventing osteoporosis, a thinning of bone structure which may afflict some women after menopause. But some evidence has begun to suggest that the risk of endometrial cancer may be increased by long-term estrogen therapy in postmenopausal women. Important in preventing osteoporosis are diet and exercise.

I believe that after a woman has experienced menopause, she should consider very carefully with her doctor the advisability of long-term use of estrogen rather than insist upon it because it may be in vogue.

Always see your doctor immediately for excessive bleeding. It is true that this may be due to the menopause, but it *can* indicate cancer. There is no actual connection between cancer and the menopause, but women in this period of their lives have reached the age when cancer is apt to strike. For that reason, they must be particularly alert to its danger signals (see page 432). Always see a doctor immediately for bleeding that occurs after your monthly periods have ended. Don't decide it's "just an extra period." If it is, your doctor will tell you so; but if it isn't, you don't want to delay finding its cause.

## LEUKORRHEA

Nonbloody vaginal discharges, usually called *leukorrhea* or "the whites," are almost as troublesome as menstrual disorders. They, too, are symptoms rather than diseases, and may be due to something relatively minor or potentially serious.

A certain amount of fluid is necessary to moisten the genitals. Sexual excitement, whether or not intercourse takes place, increases the lubricating fluid, as I explain on page 213. Many women have a mucuslike discharge at the time of ovulation (see page 227).

Some women are disturbed by even the slightest discharge, and make every effort to get rid of it by using antiseptic and astringent douches. I have issued several warnings against this practice in the course of this book (see page 107). Douches administered under pressure, or consisting of anything except a little salt or vinegar, often increase the discharges they are intended to eliminate. This is because such douches may be irritating, or may alter the normally acid nature of the secretions, which inhibit the growth of troublesome bacteria.

The genitals need only to be kept clean by bathing and washing. However, the proper kind of douche will do no harm and may contribute to the feeling of personal daintiness. Always use a douche bag, rather than a bulb, and do not hang the bag so high that the douche is administered under pressure. Hold or hang it at arm's length. Use two quarts of warm water with four level teaspoonfuls of table salt, or two to three tablespoons of a good quality of ordinary vinegar. Wash the nozzle before douching, and *never* use one that anyone else has used, because germs can be spread in this way.

An *excessive* discharge can be due to any condition that causes inflammation or disturbs the circulation in the vagina or uterus. In other words, it can be due to practically any disease of the genital tract, including gonorrhea and syphilis, other infections, cancer, polyps, lacerations of the cervix which sometimes occur during childbirth, or the irritation caused by an ill-fitting pessary. Occasionally, it is due to some condition outside the genital tract—for example, malnutrition or even pelvic congestion associated with heart disease. Surely you can see how important it is to discover and treat the *cause* of a vaginal discharge, and not merely to try to relieve the symptoms with home remedies. Always consult a doctor for persistent leukorrhea, or any discharge that is not colorless or that is accompanied by itching or irritation.

Some women are reluctant to consult a doctor about leukorrhea. As one woman expressed it, "I was afraid he'd think I had a *reason* to be worried about a veneral disease." Let me reassure you. In the first place, doctors know that venereal diseases are only one of the many possible causes of a vaginal discharge. In the second place, we know that women (and men) can worry about venereal diseases without having a "reason" to do so. And finally, it is our duty to treat diseases of all kinds and not to pass moral judgment. To us, the terrible thing about syphilis and gonorrhea is the fact that they cause untold suffering—which is needless because these diseases can be cured. *Be sure* to read pages **485** and **447** in which I discuss venereal diseases.

Leukorrhea is frequently caused by a one-celled microorganism known as *Trichomonas vaginalis*. This organism causes a yellowish discharge with an unpleasant odor, often accompanied by itching of the external genitals, and sometimes leads to a chronic inflammation of the cervix. By examining a drop of the vaginal discharge under the microscope, the doctor can identify the infecting organism.

We do not know where this protozoan comes from, although there are indications that it exists in the rectum, where it does no damage. If only for this reason, women should be careful to avoid contaminating the vagina with fecal material after a bowel movement.

Treatment may be with a drug, metronidazole, taken by both husband and wife simultaneously for ten days, but this drug should not be used during pregnancy. Or your physician may use alternatives such as vaginal tablets of diiodohydroxyquin or vaginal suppositories of furazolidone, perhaps with a vinegar douche prior to application of the tablets or suppositories.

Another, though not quite so common, cause of leukorrhea is the yeast known as *Monilia albicans*. It produces similar symptoms, and usually yields readily to medical treatment.

*Nonspecific infections:* these may be caused by some very ordinary kinds of germs, which sometimes produce leukorrhea. This type yields most readily to treatment, although occasionally it is necessary for the doctor to prescribe various medicines in tablets and douches.

The *cervix* may become inflamed by the same condition that causes leukorrhea, and also by injuries during childbirth and irritation of various kinds. *Chronic cervicitis* is usually cured by cauterization, which removes or destroys the inflamed area. It is not a painful procedure. An inflamed cervix should be treated promptly, because it is a fertile area for cancer.

*Cervical polyps,* a type of small tumor, should always be removed. They should then be examined under the microscope because they may be malignant, that is, cancerous. Although this is seldom the case, it is most important to discover it immediately so that the area around the polyps can be removed, to prevent future danger.

*Atrophis vaginalis.* Elderly women are very prone to have vaginal infections. This is due to

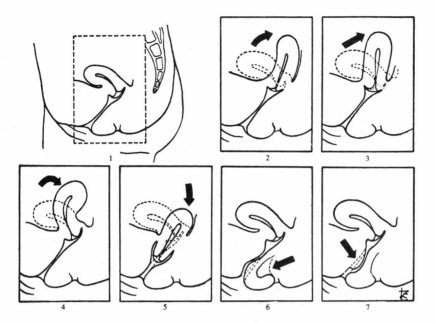

*Figure 36-1. Positions of the Uterus and Vagina.
1. Usual position of the uterus. (Dotted outline indicates the area shown in the following pictures.) 2. Retrocession. The uterus sags backward. This seldom causes any difficulty. 3. Retroversion. The uterus tips backward. This seldom causes any difficulty. 4. Retroflexion. (More pronounced retroversion.) The top of* the uterus bends back. This seldom causes any difficulty. *5. Prolapse. The uterus sinks into the vagina. 6. Rectocele. The rectum pushes into the wall of the vagina. (Normal position of vagina shown by dotted lines.) 7. Cystocele. Part of the bladder pushes into the wall of the vagina.*

the aging of the tissues. After the doctor has eliminated the possibility of cancer and other diseases which might cause the vaginal discharge, he can usually relieve the condition by treatment with vaginal suppositories containing the ovarian hormone estrogen.

*Pruritus vulvae,* or itching of the genitals, is frequently caused by leukorrhea, and vanishes when it is corrected. However, it may also be due to irritation from the urine, especially that of diabetics, to skin diseases (see page 125), and to mechanical irritations such as chafing or nervous scratching of a very minor inflammation. The possibility of an *allergic reaction* (see page 498) should not be overlooked. Pruritus vulvae is most frequently found in women who are in their later years, because of changes which take place in the genital tissues during aging.

It is obviously important to discover and eliminate the cause of this symptom. It is also important to relieve it as quickly as possible, for itching can make life miserable. The external genitals should be kept clean and dry, and harsh soaps, rough materials, scratching, and rubbing must be avoided. Medicines like phenobarbital or other sedatives often greatly relieve the nervous tension which is caused by the itching and which, in turn, aggravates it. This will enable the patient to sleep soundly without unconsciously scratching herself during the night.

## OTHER DISORDERS OF THE REPRODUCTIVE ORGANS

Infections of the ovaries, fallopian tubes, and uterus were extremely common in the past. The overwhelming majority of them were caused by gonorrhea, puerperal, or childbed, fever, or tuberculosis. Today, these diseases no longer cause untold misery to women. However, the fact that any woman still suffers from them is a needless tragedy. Other types of infectious diseases which may attack these organs are also yielding to modern medicines.

Injuries usually resulting from pregnancy and childbirth, such as the following, have also been tremendously reduced by modern obstetrical methods. (See Chapter 17.)

*Lacerations* (or tears) of the perineum, vagina, and cervix may cause trouble if they do not heal properly. As a general rule, no treatment for laceration of the cervix is necessary unless there is inflammation or some other symptom. However, it is *most important* to have your doctor check this condition at your regular medical examinations, because early cancer of the cervix may present a similar appearance. *Vesicovaginal fistula*, an opening between the bladder and the vagina, or *rectovaginal fistula*, an opening leading from the rectum into the vagina, may be caused by lacerations. These should always be repaired by surgery.

*Relaxed tissues* or *muscular injuries* can cause *hernias* (see page 483). They can also cause a *cystocele*, a bulging of the bladder, due to the weakness of the vaginal wall, or a *prolapse of the uterus*, in which the cervix is pushed far down into the vagina, or a *displacement of the uterus*. If any of these conditions is severe, surgery may be necessary. Often, however, they can be treated by other means.

Operations for displacement of the uterus are performed far less frequently today than they were in the past. Because many women who had a misplaced uterus often suffered from dysmenorrhea, backache, and some complications of pregnancy, doctors hoped that correcting the position of the womb would cure their symptoms. Often the desired results were not obtained. In many cases, it became perfectly clear that the misplaced uterus was not the cause of the painful symptoms. Backaches, for example, may be due to many causes, as I explain on page 458. I feel quite strongly that a woman should consult a specialist in gynecology before having an operation to restore her womb to its proper position.

## Hysterectomy

Hysterectomy means removal of the womb. Once removed, this organ cannot be replaced, and

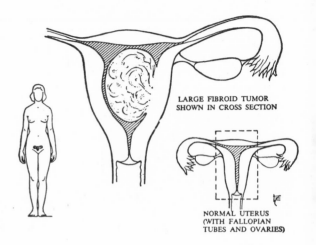

LARGE FIBROID TUMOR SHOWN IN CROSS SECTION

NORMAL UTERUS (WITH FALLOPIAN TUBES AND OVARIES)

*Figure 36-2. Fibroid Tumor.*

a woman without a uterus is not able to bear a child. The *unnecessary* removal of the womb is particularly tragic to women who want to have children, or may want to have them in the future.

Do I imply that hysterectomy is sometimes performed without sufficient cause? I do. We must face the facts squarely. They are proved by hospital records. Examinations of the organs *after* operations have clearly indicated that, in a number of cases, their condition did not justify their removal.

"This is deplorable!" you will say. "Why is it permitted?" There are several reasons.

1. Doctors differ in their opinions about the need for operating upon benign, or noncancerous, tumors in the wall of the uterus.

2. Unfortunately, some doctors are unduly hopeful that removing the womb will cure symptoms such as backache and pelvic pain.

3. It is very difficult to determine whether or not the uterus should be removed when there is a large tumor. These growths cannot be visualized by x-ray. There are no simple laboratory tests to indicate whether or not a fibroid tumor is large enough to necessitate removal of the womb. The diagnosis depends almost entirely upon the doctor's impression as he examines the womb during his pelvic examination. In some cases, it depends on his ability to decide, during an operation, whether or not the growth can be removed with-

out removing the uterus as well. A small fibroid tumor, polyp, or cyst, which is a hollow growth containing fluid, can be removed without taking out the entire womb.

It should be obvious that some doctors have more skill and experience than others in making a diagnosis of this kind. A specialist who has devoted the major portion of his time to this type of complaint may be able to determine with accuracy that a hysterectomy is not essential, whereas a doctor without a corresponding amount of experience may feel that he must suggest one.

Therefore, I recommend, even more strongly than I would for an operation on a displaced uterus, *that a hysterectomy never be performed unless two physicians agree on the need for it.* One should be your family doctor, the other a certified specialist in gynecology. If such a specialist is not available in your community, there will be one in the nearest large city, medical center, or medical school. Your family doctor can make arrangements for an examination and an opinion by a specialist in gynecology.

When I stress this matter, it is *not* because I consider a hysterectomy "a terrible operation," from which a woman will emerge prematurely aged or a semi-invalid. Quite the contrary! In almost all cases, the fallopian tubes and the ovaries, or at least a part of the ovaries, are not removed, and the glandular function will continue even though the woman ceases to have her menstrual periods. If the ovaries do have to be entirely removed, the patient can be given hormones to help her through this artificial menopause. In women who no longer wish to have children, removal of the uterus should not inflict any severe emotional injury. But, *hysterectomy is a major operation.* Because all major operations involve some risk—in addition to time, money, and discomfort—they should never be undertaken unless they are absolutely necessary.

ENDOMETRIOSIS. Many unnecessary hysterectomies have been performed for cases of endometriosis. In this condition, the cells lining the inside of the uterus "run wild." Instead of being *on* the walls of the womb, they may also appear *in* or outside these walls, and even in other tissues as well. Endometriosis may cause sterility, pain, and excessive menstruation. Surgical treatment, but not necessarily a hysterectomy, may be required in some cases, while others are treated successfully with various hormones.

## THE BREASTS

The breasts, or mammary glands, are made up of glandular tissue which is arranged in a complicated pattern of lobes, somewhat in the form of a wagon wheel. The milk ducts lead into the nipple, which is at the center or hub of this wheel. When the muscles of the nipple contract, it becomes hard and smaller. In some women, it is only slightly erectile or may be actually *depressed.* Fatty tissue fills out the breast, making it round and smooth. The amount of this tissue varies considerably in different women.

Many women are unhappy because their breasts are too large or small for the prevailing fashion. Certain exercises (see Figure 36-3) will develop the muscles in the vicinity of the breasts, making them seem larger and firmer. Losing weight will often get rid of some of the fat and make the breasts smaller. Extremely large breasts or too early development of the breasts can be the sign of a glandular or other disorder, which requires the help of a doctor. If the breasts are tremendous, an operation can be performed to remove the excess tissue. Enlargement of small breasts is possible through surgery (augmentation mammoplasty) in which plastic implants may be used.

Breasts may be firm and high or flabby and pendulous. The latter condition is not always due to having worn constricting brassieres. In fact, the shape of the breasts appears in many cases to be inherited.

For flabby breasts, as for breasts that are "too" large or "too" small, a well-fitted brassiere can do wonders. It can be slightly padded to make small breasts seem larger. However, never wear a brassiere that actually constricts the breasts. It should give support and protection without pressure, and there should be no irritating folds or seams.

The breasts should be kept clean and dry, especially if they are large and flabby, in order to prevent chafing, itching, and other skin complaints.

See page 260 for care of the breasts in nursing mothers.

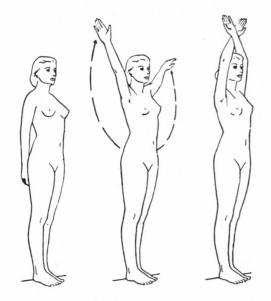

*Figure 36-3. Exercise to Improve the Bust. 1. Stand with arms at side and with heels, calves, buttocks, shoulders, and back of head touching the wall. 2. While inhaling slowly, raise arms slowly and steadily against your own resistance, until they cross above the head as much as possible without substantially bending the elbows. 3. Still touching the wall, keep arms stiff and exhale as you slowly bring them back to your sides.*

The most serious disorder of the breasts is cancer, which I discuss fully on page 433.

Various forms of *mastitis* (inflammation of the breast) are quite common. They may follow childbirth or an injury. Mastitis may become chronic. Chronic interstitial mastitis and chronic cystic mastitis, which are the chief types of breast inflammation, are often confused with cancer. They are usually not serious, although they can be quite painful, especially before the menstrual periods. Never attempt any home treatment of mastitis except to give the breasts proper support and protection.

*Cysts* and *tumors* occur fairly frequently in the breasts, and *abscesses* may result from infections, for example, from germs entering through a cracked nipple after childbirth. A rather rare type of cancer of the breasts, known as *Paget's carcinoma*, frequently involves the nipple, causing itching and burning until the nipple becomes ulcerated.

Always consult a doctor for any lump, pain, injury, or change in the breast, or for any discharge from the nipple.

## SKIN AND HAIR

I describe the care of the skin and hair and the various diseases which affect them, such as acne, growths, and dandruff, as well as cosmetics, beauty aids, dyeing, excess body hair, and permanent waving, on pages 118 to 129.

## "WOMAN'S WORK"

Housework has always been the Cinderella in the family of useful occupations, taken for granted, ignored, or looked down upon. In the past, the average woman in her thirties looked and felt old. But nobody considered it worthwhile to determine whether or not her daily tasks had anything to do with this and, if so, whether it could be prevented.

Modern laborsaving devices have brought about a revolution in housework but, unfortunately, in a hit-or-miss manner. Not until very recently has a beginning been made in studying housework in relation to health, including, for example, the designing of homes, furniture, and equipment.

The hazards of housework do not, naturally, compare with those of certain other occupations such as coal mining. However, even today housework is the cause of injuries and ill health which could often be avoided. Because of the difficulty of collecting statistics, research in this field is necessarily slow.

The form of bursitis (see page 461) known as "housemaid's knee" is probably the only occupational disease of housework that comes to your mind. It occurs less frequently today than it did when it was customary to have wooden floors and to scrub them by getting down on one's knees. In England, during and following World War II, when women had to carry heavy market bags and wait for hours in line to buy provisions, the house-wife's carrying shoulder was afflicted with fibrositis, a form of rheumatism due to inflammation of the fibrous tissue around the joints.

The many new soaps, detergents, and other products so excellent for cleaning have caused a condition of the hands which some doctors speak of as "housewives' dermatitis." But, in the main, housework is not responsible in so *direct* a manner for physical disorders.

Through the cooperation of women physicians in many countries, the American Medical Women's Association has conducted investigations into the diseases and ailments which afflict women who do housework. A British study of a group of house-wives revealed a tremendous number of women who had foot trouble, colds, headaches, varicose veins, depressions, and many other "nuisance ailments" (see Chapter 35). Those who had to do housework in addition to an outside job were found to have the poorest health. Since no similar studies are available for women who do not do housework, or even for women as a whole, the figures compiled do not prove that housework is to blame; but they do indicate that most house-wives are plagued by one or more ailments.

Many housewives have trouble with their reproductive organs, often because they had to work too soon and too hard after giving birth to a baby. Others injure themselves lifting and carrying things that are too heavy for them. Women suffering from a chronic illness or a disabling condition frequently make themselves worse by doing housework. In this connection, I want to urge all such women with chronic illnesses to learn about organizations such as the American Heart Association (see page 409), which can provide useful help and advice to supplement your doctor's care.

A great many things which housewives can do to protect their health have been discussed throughout this book, especially in the chapters dealing with general care of the body, care of the individual parts of the body, diet, pregnancy and childbirth, housing and health, home nursing, and so on. Here I shall present some suggestions relating specifically to housework. I hope they will help you to solve your own problems, but I would be even more pleased if they stimulate women,

as a sex, to work out solutions through clubs and other organizations.

1. *Make a "job study" of your work.* Most women are taught to do housework by their mothers, with the result that old-fashioned methods tend to linger on longer than they do, for example, in modern factories. Think over what you do, and why and how you do it. Do you really need to dry dishes in these days of new soaps and detergents and plenty of hot water? Perhaps if you had two dish-racks and a spray attachment on your tap you could rinse all your dishes and let them drain dry, a very sanitary method, by the way. Do you have to iron ruffled curtains or to stretch lace ones on frames? Nylon or paper curtains can save a great deal of time and energy. Do you exhaust yourself twice a year doing a big spring and fall cleaning because your mother used to, when you, personally, would rather do a part of it each week?

Give special thought to the routines you find distasteful or tiring, and see how many of them you can eliminate or modify. Do this with everything your husband and children consider unnecessary. Consider your efficiency at specific tasks. Do

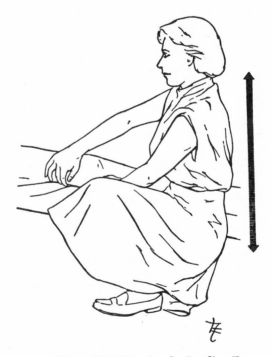

*Figure 36-4. Stooping by Bending Knees.*

you walk more than you need? How many unnecessary motions do you make? If you can manage to cut down strain and fatigue by only infinitesimal amounts here and there, it will make an appreciable difference as the days and weeks go by.

2. *Consider yourself in relation to your work.* Are you taller or shorter, weaker or stronger, than the *average woman?* It was such a mathematically averaged "she" that designers had in mind when they decided on the height and weight of household objects. Reaching and stooping are often unnecessary evils. Even so simple an object as a broom should be light enough not to tire a woman who is not muscular, and large and heavy enough to enable an unusually strong one to get through the job rapidly. Whenever you buy something new,

*Figure 36-5. Working at a Table. Whenever possible, avoid strain and fatigue by working at a table of the proper height. Bend forward from the hips rather than from the shoulders.*

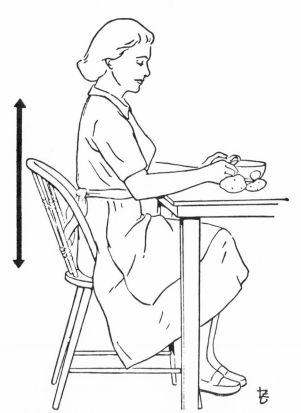

from a stove or sink to an ironing board, find out what can be done to make it the proper height for you. If you have to make do with what you have, perhaps you can put something under the dishpan in the sink to raise it to the proper height, or sit on a high stool if you are so short you have to stretch. Perhaps you can cut a piece off the legs of your ironing board, or raise them in some way. Is there a chair so heavy you strain yourself each time you clean the rug under it? Perhaps casters will solve the problem. The man in your household can probably help you.

There are some household tasks you may not be large or strong enough to tackle by yourself. I know one frail little lady who tortured herself every week turning a huge mattress. Her husband, who had a weak heart, had hired someone to empty the trash barrels, but it never occurred to her to get the hired man to turn the mattress. And I will never forget a young mother who weighed only 95 pounds and who told me she couldn't imagine what was wrong with her back—until I informed her that nature had not intended her to carry around her 30-pound baby for many hours each day! Fortunately her back improved rapidly after she adopted the habit of moving him around in a baby carriage, and lifted him, when it was absolutely necessary, by bending her knees rather than her back (see Figure 36–6). Always keep your feet flat on the floor and bend your knees rather than your back, to lift.

Once the tasks with which one needs help are recognized and listed, it is usually possible to get assistance. The male of the household probably would not object to doing some of them if they could be organized at convenient times for him. Or two housewives who are neighbors can sometimes pool their efforts.

3. *Become posture-wise.* Poor posture is responsible for many of the strains and injuries, to say nothing of the aches and pains, from which housewives suffer. Figures 36-5 and 36-6 show how to hold your back while working at a table and lifting. Be sure to study the illustrations in Chapter 1 (pages 20 and 21), which show the correct and the incorrect way to stand and to sit. When you do the dishes, keep your weight evenly distributed on both feet and your toes slightly turned in. If you do not sit down while ironing,

keep your back straight and your abdomen in; do not hunch up your shoulders. When sweeping, put one foot forward if you reach out in order to get under a table or into a corner. Avoid sudden twisting or movements while you are off balance.

Exercises to strengthen your back are shown on page 17.

*Posture begins with the feet.* The average housewife spends from 80 to 90 percent of her working day, which lasts from nine to twelve hours, on her feet. Be sure to read what I have to say on the care of the feet (p. 115). Nothing could be less economical than saving old shoes with run-over heels to wear in the house.

4. *Take care of your hands.* The new cleansing products are much better than the old-fashioned ones our mothers had to use. They save time and trouble, mainly because of the speed with which they dissolve grease. Unfortunately, they also dissolve the natural oil or fat needed to lubricate the skin. Dry-cleaning fluids, turpentine, gasoline, and other paint removers also have this disadvantage. Fruit and vegetable juices can cause irritation. As a result, many women suffer from skin diseases and infections resulting from minor inflammations.

If you don't like to wear rubber gloves, observe the following suggestions: Discover how much soap or detergent is necessary for efficiency, and save money as well as possible skin trouble by not using too much in your dish water. Don't have the water too hot, as this, too, removes the natural oils and causes irritation. Dry your hands thoroughly, and use a lotion, especially in cold or dry weather. Use an oily lotion before going to bed (see page 122). During winter months, and in desert areas throughout the year, an air humidifier in the home (see page 15) will help keep your skin from getting too dry. Be careful of the skin under your rings, always drying it thoroughly and being on the alert for sores or inflammations that start there. Never neglect cuts or sores of any kind (see page 338). A rubber "finger" or glove, obtained from your druggist, should be worn to protect any injuries.

## The Housework Blues

No matter how efficiently it is organized, housework retains some unattractive features. I feel certain that this fact accounts, at least in part, for the

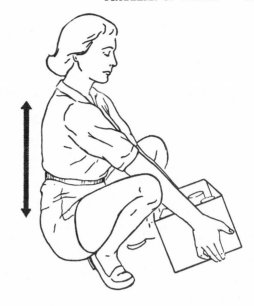

*Figure 36-6. Lifting. Bend the knees and use the leg muscles when lifting, to avoid straining the back.*

headaches from which housewives frequently suffer.

"No matter how thin you slice it, it's still housework!" "It's never done—and when it is, it doesn't *stay* done." "No matter how dull a man's job is, he at least has the satisfaction of earning money for the family."

In my opinion, these complaints are justified. Although housework is essential, it is not productive in a certain sense of the word. And it is seldom possible, especially if there are children, to limit its hours.

The wife and mother who has an outside job carries a heavy burden. Even with the most co-operative husband, she usually assumes the responsibility for the home and children, if only because of her training and experience.

A young girl once told me that she thought Freud was on the wrong track when he said women were envious of men for sexual reasons. "If it weren't for all the chores I have to do, I wouldn't envy my brother the least little bit," she said, only half-jokingly. "We both go to work and come home at the same time, but I have to help with supper and the dishes, I have to wash and press and mend my clothes, shampoo and set my hair, manicure my nails, and do a little shopping for the family during my lunch hour. The only thing *he* has to do is shave, and he makes such a production out of it that I feel I ought to do it for him!"

Of course, the girl's brother countered with an excellent set of arguments, which do not belong in this chapter. The fact that men, too, have difficulties may help women to be philosophical, but it won't make housework attractive.

Here are some suggestions for minimizing its worst features:

*Try to get a day off*, or part of a day off, every week. As you recall, I spoke about the importance of having time off from one's job (see page 15). The five-day week or even the six-day week is impossible for most housewives, but women can usually

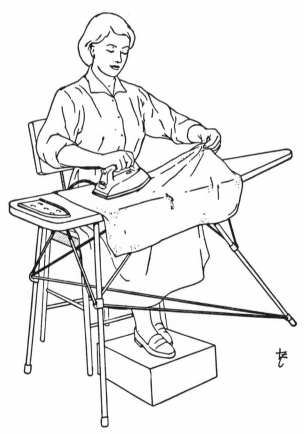

*Figure 36-7. Ironing While Seated.*

arrange for a free morning or afternoon. Ideally, this should come at the same time every week, preferably not over the weekend, when the family should be together.

I realize it is not easy to do this. Sometimes it may seem to be more trouble than it is worth, but if it is at all possible, it will be very good for you. Do something that is a complete change—go to a movie, or window shopping, or to a church or club meeting, or for a visit. Perhaps you and a neighbor can alternate in caring for the children, or pool your resources to engage a sitter. Plan an easy-to-prepare supper and see whether some other member of the family can fix and serve it. Most families will cooperate in giving mother her day off if she shows her appreciation.

*Arrange to get some rest during each day.* Again, this will take some planning and may seem scarcely worth the trouble, but it will repay your efforts. You will feel better physically and emotionally, and be able to accomplish more in less time, if you take a complete break both morning and afternoon, preferably one fairly long one if possible, but at least two fifteen-minute periods to rest and relax, with your feet up and an imaginary "Do Not Disturb" sign out.

*Organize your housework in such a way as to break its monotony.* Many chores must be attended to every day, but it is usually possible to put some of them on a biweekly or even a weekly basis. An athletic young wife in our neighborhood worked out the following system: Three mornings a week she got into a sweat shirt and dungarees and did all the work that, as she put it, could come under the heading of exercise. "I don't kid myself it's tennis," she said. "But by going at things hard and fast, and then taking a rest and a shower, I at least feel as though I've had a good workout." Of course, this method is not suitable for everybody, but the idea underlying it is sound.

Here are some ways of getting over the *"being-a-woman blues"*:

*Talk to a good and trustworthy friend*, that is, anyone who serves in that capacity, including a relative, your clergyman, or a neighbor. Talk about your problems, or just talk. *But establish communication with someone.* That is one of the great advantages of having a telephone, especially in the suburbs or in rural areas. Some women find they can work off the blues by *doing something active*, anything from taking a walk or playing golf to cleaning out the closet. If a feeling of inadequacy accompanies your blues or, perhaps unconsciously, is the cause of them, it will help to do *something useful or creative*. Having done something for someone else is a wonderful restorative for the faith in yourself that has temporarily deserted you. So is the satisfaction of creating something, which may be a drawing, a good letter, a new dress for your daughter's favorite doll, or a cake with fancy icing. On the other hand, perhaps you should pamper yourself, as you would anyone else who was unhappy. In that case, *do something frivolous*. Buy yourself those gloves you don't absolutely need, or read a light novel instead of the good book you "ought" to read, or indulge yourself, just this once, in a fattening ice cream soda in an attractive place.

*Maybe a medicine will help you.* Perhaps a mild stimulant is what you need—a good cup of tea or coffee, a cola drink. An aspirin, Bufferin, or Empirin tablet may do away with that nagging little headache you have been too blue to notice. There are also new *medicines which your doctor may recommend*.

*Consider part-time work.* Once your children start going to school, you will have several daytime hours free of responsibility for them. Many jobs are open to women, and most cities have placement offices that specialize in filling office or other types of positions where a clerk, typist, bookkeeper, secretary, or other worker is needed to handle peak work loads. No woman should feel guilty because she wants to do something besides housework!

Don't say to yourself that you ought not to get the blues. Every normal person is susceptible to the stresses and strains of living. Try to find out what is causing your blue mood. It often helps simply to know that it is the weather, or the fact that your menstrual period is due, or that you are tired. Then do something about it if you can. If you can't do it alone, enlist the aid of your doctor or someone he recommends.

Most important of all, accept the fact that you are human, which means that you are remarkably sensitive and reactive. In other words, you are apt to become depressed—but fortunately, it won't last. In the beautiful words of the Thirteenth Psalm, "Weeping may endure for a night, but joy cometh in the morning."

# 37

# THE LATER YEARS

This chapter is written for readers of all ages. Naturally, the problems of aging are of little or no immediate concern to young people. But almost everyone has parents, grandparents, uncles, and aunts who are beginning to get along in years. If you are one of my younger readers, you can learn how to make the later years good ones for the old people you love—and they will be grateful for your knowledge of their special problems. It is a source of abiding satisfaction to me that my mother used to say, when she was seventy-five, that she felt better than at any time during the previous forty years. Then, too, by understanding the needs of the aged, we can unconsciously and gracefully prepare for the fullest enjoyment of our own geriatric period. The best way to rob old age of its terrors is by seeing elderly people who are well and happy!

Most prudent folks start making plans for their future financial security at an early age. I hope that you will also give some thought to the kind of investments that will pay off in physical and emotional health. No matter how old you are, you'll want to continue this. Even if you have passed the mark of the Biblical three-score years and ten, you won't have to fold your hands and say, "I have reached my goal." As a scientific article I read recently pointed out, it is not enough to add years to life; we also want to add life to years.

Remarkable progress has been made in adding years to life. The average American of today lives twice as long as he might have had he been alive when this country was founded, and practically twice as long as does the average of the world's population.

This tremendous increase in life expectancy is due in great part to the fact that such diseases as cholera, typhoid fever, smallpox, diphtheria, and yellow fever have been practically eliminated. The greatest reduction in mortality has been in infants. However, the mortality of people *over seventy-five* has been reduced by one-fifth during the first half of this century. According to present figures, the average white, male American who has today reached the age of sixty-five will live for another dozen years, and the average woman will live another fourteen. These estimates are constantly being revised upward, so that before those years actually pass, life expectancy will be longer than it is at present.

## HOW OLD IS OLD?

Everyone has an answer to this question. "An old person is anybody who is ten to twenty years older than you are." "The process of aging begins at birth." "It all depends on what you're doing; a combat pilot, a baseball player and a prize fighter are old at thirty, while a scientist is young at fifty." "You're as old as you feel, or as old as you look."

Like most doctors, I am frequently impressed by the great mental and physical differences between patients of the same age. However, since it is convenient to set some sort of boundary, the age of sixty-five is usually chosen. Personally, I rather like Victor Hugo's remark that fifty is the youth of old age, because it shows an awareness of the fact that old age does not arrive suddenly. Like other periods, it depends on what went before. For this reason *gerontology*, which is the science of the process of aging, does not actually limit its studies to a single group. This science has shown us that, in the later years, as in the others, a great deal can be done to correct the errors and omissions of the past. The medical specialty concerned with diseases of the aged is called *geriatrics.*

Medical science can help to add years to life and life to years. But—perhaps more than at any other time—the part played by the individual is a vital one. That is why I am so eager to impress on you the fact that it's never too early or too late to plan for the later years.

## ASSETS AND LIABILITIES

Many of us are accustomed to think only of the limitations and liabilities of old age; we tend to overlook the physical, mental, and emotional assets of this period.

### Mental Assets

I will start with these because here the ledger shows many assets and very few liabilities. It is encouraging to know that the mind, at least, does not wear out from use or even "overuse." We heard a great deal about "brain fatigue" and "brain exhaustion" in the past. Now we know that these symptoms and illnesses are actually due to tensions or emotional problems and conflicts which drive people to push themselves beyond the limits of their physical endurance. One cannot conserve "brain power" by not using one's brains. On the contrary, the more a physically and emotionally healthy person uses his brain, the better it will be in the later years.

We have all seen examples of this in people like the scientist Einstein and Toscanini, the orchestra conductor, whose abilities certainly did not wane when they reached old age. The doctor-author Oliver Wendell Holmes began writing *Over the Teacups,* and at the same time continued his important medical work, when he was seventy-nine. Darwin wrote one of his major scientific books when he was over eighty. Benjamin Franklin was chief executive officer of the state of Pennsylvania from the time he was seventy-nine until he was eighty-two. Tennyson wrote the beautiful poem, *Crossing the Bar,* at eighty-three. Verdi composed *Ave Maria* and *Te Deum* at eighty-five. Galileo's scientific discoveries continued when he was in his nineties. Florence Nightingale engaged in effective health crusades until she died at ninety. Titian, who was born in 1477, painted *The Last Judgment* when he was over eighty, and was still producing masterpieces when, at the age of ninety-nine, he died of the plague, in 1576.

These are only a very few of the many great things that have been accomplished by old people. Isn't it encouraging to realize that the work they did in their later years equals or excels their remarkable accomplishments when they were in the so-called prime of life? In other words, their brains certainly did not wear out from being "overworked"!

I also want to call your attention to a few of the many people who embarked on new ventures late in life. "Grandma" Moses began to paint when she was seventy-nine, and was almost immediately successful. Clara Barton, having founded the American Red Cross, became its president at the age of sixty-one; when she resigned twenty years later, it was to establish the American National Association for First Aid, and at eighty-nine she learned how to type in order to help her work. The Roman statesman Cato began to study Greek when he was over eighty, and Supreme Court Justice Oliver Wendell Holmes, the son of the doctor-author, decided even later in life that he wanted to learn this language.

From the scientific point of view, there is nothing astonishing about the fact that these people could learn so late in life. Tests have been made which prove conclusively that there is no truth to the saying "You can't teach an old dog new tricks." It all depends on whether the old person wants to learn. These tests show that older people tend to learn a trifle more slowly, but they also learn more thoroughly, so that they actually *master* a new subject in the same length of time as do younger students.

We used to believe that memory faded with age. It is true that many old people forget names and recent events, while recalling the past in great detail—and often bore their young friends by recounting it. Now we know that memory is directly related to interest. Many of us suspect this when we hear a boy, who cannot remember when Columbus discovered America, rattling off the batting averages of his favorite ballplayers. Older people do, indeed, forget recent events, because many of them are interested only in the past. Then, too, remembering is an art or skill that can be developed, and it is possible to do so late in life. It is not at all unusual, in the theatrical profession, to find elderly actors and actresses who learn long and difficult parts in record time.

Older people have a natural advantage when it comes to judgment, which depends not only on the ability to reason, but on experience.

## Emotional Assets

I am sure that emotional assets and liabilities compare pretty well in the later years with those we find on the ledger at any period of life. The mental, or emotional, diseases that result from physical causes, such as the *psychoses* due to *cerebral arteriosclerosis,* are far more common in the aged than in the young, but most *manic-depressive psychoses* appear between the ages of twenty and sixty, while *schizophrenia,* which accounts for over half the inmates of mental institutions in this country, is most likely to afflict people in early maturity. The large number of elderly people in institutions is due, at least in part, to family situations which make it impossible to care for them at home. No less important is the indifference found in the overworked personnel of mental institutions and in the general public.

*Fear, anxiety, and insecurity are extremely damaging to the emotional health of old people—as, indeed, they are at any time.* The irritability of the aged is frequently due simply to fatigue, and responds readily to rest. The dislike of change, and a suspicious attitude toward anything or anyone new, often stem from a lack of self-confidence or a loss of self-confidence. It is not characteristic of old people who are emotionally secure, although elderly people may tend to be conservative.

It is true that there are special emotional difficulties in this, as in other, periods. It is not surprising that many of them occur in the "youth of old age," for as I pointed out in Chapter 21, which deals. with adolescence, it is not easy even for young people to make a transition. I discuss some of these problems in dealing with the "change of life" in women, on page 517.

It is after we pass the midway mark that many of us face the fact that we are mortal and must die. We face it as a personal, emotional matter and not merely as an intellectual one. Some people accept it with equanimity. But to a great many others, this "shock of recognition," as it has been called, is profoundly disturbing. If you experience it, don't feel that there is anything wrong or weak —and certainly, nothing "insane"—about you.

*Can the fear of death be overcome or at least minimized?*

I have discussed this problem with philosophers and psychiatrists, and with clergymen and doctors who, like myself, have often been in the presence of death. Here are some ideas I have found helpful, both personally and for others. Each of us has noted that people will go to great lengths to escape from this universally feared and dreaded enemy; and we have expected the terror to increase when escape is no longer possible. But this is not the case. Quite the contrary. We physicians have seen patient after patient accept death with equanimity when the time has come. We have even heard them express the sentiments of William Hunter, the distinguished anatomist, who said on his deathbed, in 1783, "If I could hold a pen, I would write how easy and pleasant a thing it is to die." The great physician, William Osler, made a careful study of a large number of deaths. "The great majority," he wrote, "gave no sign one way or the other; . . . their death was a sleep and a forgetting." To the dying, then, the face of death is not that of a terrible monster. I cannot tell you how or why God, or nature, has made it so. But surely this fact should help us overcome our fears.

I will never forget the remark made by a young patient who was facing a dangerous operation. "I'm not worried about dying any more," he said. "I got to thinking about all the wonderful people who have died, and it seems to me, it can't be too bad if they've all done it."

This boy had established an identified emotional unity with the dead. It is one excellent way to minimize the fear of dying. Try to identify with people who stood for the finest things you live by —your own grandparents or parents, or some great men and women who have inspired you.

Be proud of your own life. Realize that each of us has contributed in an important manner, even if we have led the simplest kind of life. There could be no human, social living if it were not for the joint cooperative efforts of ordinary individuals. Each thread is an essential part of the pattern of life, touching and supporting the lives of others.

Talk about the meaning of life and death with members of your family or your closest friends. It will help you to work out your own adjustment. If there are things in the past that weigh heavily on your conscience, or if you fear death excessively, discuss the matter with your clergyman or doctor or a psychiatrist. Shakespeare said,

> Cowards die many times before their deaths;
> The valiant never taste of death but once.

In my opinion, he should have said, "The badly adjusted die many times before their deaths." One must be able to adjust to life in order to accept the fact that it will end.

Once the adjustment has been made, there are real rewards that come with aging. Many intellectual powers increase. Experience and wisdom are rewards of later life. The well-adjusted older person approaches true freedom because he has overcome the self-consciousness that causes so much pain and frustration in the early years. He gains in poise and self-control, becoming more tolerant of himself and others. Although emotional experiences are less acute and intense, they are richer, deeper, and more subtle. Past efforts are rewarded and promises fulfilled in the harvest season, and Indian summer is the most beautiful time of all.

## Physical Assets

People usually assume that all the items in this category will be entered in red ink. This is not so. Many of the physical liabilities of old age are relatively minor; and there are even some assets.

It is true that certain changes occur in the body with the passing of years, but the organs and tissues of an aged person often compare very favorably with those of his juniors. We all know people of advanced years who have no infirmities and whose health any young person could envy.

The process of aging is usually an uneven one. For example, the *thymus gland* atrophies and disappears after puberty, and the *tonsils* are senile when we are fifty. In most individuals, certain organs will show signs of impairment while others remain "young." I can't recall finding an elderly person suffering from a condition which I have not seen in individuals one or even two generations younger.

The *eyes, ears, and teeth* are a good example. Few people reach the age of sixty-five with a full set of natural teeth, even with the best of dentists, care, and luck. But how many of your acquaintances haven't had a tooth pulled by the time they reach forty-five or thirty-five—or even twenty-five? As a rule, cavities occur less often with advancing age, and this tends to compensate for the toll exacted by constant wear and tear.

By the time we reach fifty, most of us need glasses for reading. But how many of us have had to wear glasses since childhood? Occasionally we even hear of an older person who can actually see better than when he or she was young.

While it is true that our hearing ability decreases from the time we are in our twenties, the rate of decline appears to be more closely related to inheritance than it does to age. An operation may correct the form of deafness due to *otosclerosis*, the hardening of the tiny bones of the ear. More important, however, is the fact that the types of deafness attributed to "catarrh," actually due to infections or allergies, are being prevented by early treatment. And the older person is far less susceptible to the middle-ear infections from which so many children suffer.

In our society, which places such a high premium on sex, many people worry about the effect of aging on their sexual powers. This troubles men more than it does women. It therefore comes as a welcome surprise to them to learn that sexual potency persists surprisingly late in life. Many experts state that the period of *full potency* in the male extends into the fifties and even well past the sixtieth year.

It seems to me that nature usually permits sexual activity in normal people as long as they need it. When the need vanishes, the desire also fades.

Of course, a kind of wistful nostalgia may remain. Supreme Court Justice Oliver Wendell Holmes jokingly expressed this when, at the age of ninety-four, he looked at a pretty ankle, and sighed, "Ah what wouldn't I give to be seventy again!"

There is no physical limitation to the sexual potency of women, such as the problem of erection in the elderly male. The matter is almost entirely an emotional one—of the sexual needs of the particular individual. As in men, when this need vanishes, the equivalent of sexual tenderness can be found in nonsexual affection or love.

There are, occasionally, elderly people who cannot restrain their sexual impulses. This may cause distressing or dangerous situations. Be sure to bring such instances to the attention of a doctor immediately; they are emotional problems, probably associated with true senility.

## DISEASES IN THE ELDERLY

Scientific studies of the *causes of death* in aged individuals indicate clearly that, in the majority of cases, the disease originated when they were in ,eir middle years. This is one more of the many arguments for regular medical examinations and health education.

We cannot say that *any* disease is actually *caused* by old age, in the same way that, for example, we can say certain diseases are caused by childbirth. However, there are illnesses which are most likely to occur in the later years. In addition, diseases often run a somewhat different course in the aged, whose health and hygiene requirements change with the passing years.

As people age, they are less apt to suffer from infectious diseases. This is true not only because they cannot catch certain diseases which they had in the past, but also because they have acquired a partial immunity to other infections without ever being ill—and even some immunity to colds.

When older people do develop one of these illnesses, it usually is less severe than it would be in a young adult. For example, tuberculosis is less dangerous to an elderly person than to an adolescent. Incidentally, this is also true of some noncontagious diseases such as diabetes.

The fact that the symptoms are less acute and severe is not an unmixed blessing. An elderly person with tuberculosis may think he or she has "just a bronchial cough," and may infect a young member of the family—with serious consequences. On one occasion I visited a family and, inquiring about the grandmother, was told that she had taken to her bed because she was feeling tired. I went to her room mostly as a matter of courtesy. "I guess it's my age; or maybe I'm getting to be a hypochondriac," she said apologetically. "I'm sure there's nothing the matter with me because I took my temperature and it was practically normal. But I feel very poorly." Examination revealed that she had pneumonia, which could have been fatal if it had remained untreated.

Another good example of this is the vigorous old lady who had organized some of her contemporaries into a group called "Never Too Late." One afternoon she telephoned her doctor to say she had caught the "intestinal flu" that was making the rounds, and to ask for some medicine that would enable her to address her club. Although her doctor told her to stay home until he could examine her, she went to the meeting. By the time she had delivered her speech she felt so ill that she took a cab to the doctor's office, where she collapsed—with a ruptured appendix. Fortunately she survived the peritonitis which set in, and learned the lesson, as she ruefully puts it, that "it's never too late" for appendicitis.

### Surgery in the Aged

The fact that older people are able to withstand operations extremely well in these days of *improved surgical techniques* has, in my opinion, done more than anything to rob old age of its greatest tribulations. It is now possible to carry out a four-hour operation on an eighty-year-old patient with practically no danger. I marvel every time I see one of these patients suffering only a minimum of shock, recalling how severe the symptoms used to be only a few decades ago. In those days, many elderly people were forced to endure painful, disabling, and even dangerous conditions which can safely be corrected by surgery today.

Among these diseases are *enlargement of the prostate, hernia, cataracts,* and a *prolapsed* or *fallen bladder, rectum,* or *uterus.* To break a bone once spelled disaster. It could mean the end of an active life for an old person—especially if the bone was in the hip or thigh—for bones knit slowly in the aged. Today, operations have been perfected for nailing the bones together, so that they heal adequately. This type of surgery requires the expert work of a specialist in *orthopedics*. If such a surgeon is not available in the patient's community, a trip to the nearest medical center is a most worthwhile investment. It may save an old person—and his or her family—from the problems of a crippled existence.

Can an elderly person benefit from surgery for cancer? A recent review of 226 colon cancer patients at least 80 years old shows gratifying results—strikingly, a five-year survival rate, even better than the survival rate overall for patients with the disease regardless of age. Apparently, the outlook in surgically treatable colon cancer is more favorable for the aged than for younger persons. There have been recent similarly encouraging reports on results in elderly patients treated surgically for lung and prostate cancer.

Remarkable strides have been made in open-heart surgery. Recent reports indicate success rates of 80 percent and even higher in the elderly needing heart surgery for valve and other problems.

*Unfortunately, many old people and their families do not realize the tremendous advances that have been made in surgery.* They suffer needlessly because they are afraid of an operation. My own mother was no exception. At sixty-five, she began to lose her eyesight, due to *cataracts* (see page 108). We, her three sons and three daughters, explained that her sight could be restored by an operation. She seemed strangely hesitant. One excuse after another was advanced to delay the operation. Yet she appeared to have the fullest confidence in her ophthalmologist and her own family doctor; and she knew that I, too, approved the operation.

After nearly six months, the cause of her hesitation became clear. She had never been a patient in a hospital. All her babies had been delivered at home. To her, as to many old people, a hospital had always represented a place for patients suffering from fatal diseases.

To further complicate the problem, the eye specialist operated at a medical center fifty miles away from Mother's home. She knew she would be temporarily blind for several days after the operation because both eyes would have to be completely bandaged. It was too terrifying a prospect for her to face even with the assurance that the reward would be renewed eyesight.

The solution was easy when the problem was understood. Mother had developed a great fondness for a nurse who spent five years with her during my father's last illness. We arranged to have the eye surgeon engage this nurse for my mother's hospitalization, and to have her live in the hospital. The moment the arrangement was mentioned to Mother, she started to pack for the trip. She really had been extremely eager to have that operation.

From that experience, I learned a good deal about how old people react to hospitals. The average young or middle-aged person requiring an operation asks, first of all, "Who is the best doctor for the job?" Then, later, "Which hospital does the doctor consider best for this type of surgery?" He wants to get it over with in the shortest possible time. Not so with elderly patients. They are confident that a capable doctor has been engaged for them and that all the technical arrangements will be satisfactory. What really troubles them is the terrifying prospect of undergoing a new and potentially dangerous experience.

Old people need to be thoroughly reassured about impending surgical operations. All possible details should be explained to them, even those that seem to be quite insignificant. If it is feasible, the patient should visit the hospital to see the room he or she will occupy and to meet the nurses. It is important for them to know the people involved. If the family doctor is calling in a surgeon, elderly patients should become acquainted with him well in advance of the scheduled operation.

## Partial Restoration of Function

*I want particularly to emphasize the importance of partial restoration of function as far as old people are concerned.* Physicians understandably hesitate to take money from elderly people for prolonged therapy that may produce a return so small as to be barely measurable. Make it clear to your doctor that you do not expect him to present you—or your parent—with the fountain of youth, and that you will be grateful for a small improvement. It can make a tremendous difference. For example, an elderly person may be quite miserable when confined to bed, whereas being able to get up for meals and go for an occasional drive or short walk will make life happy and normal. Again, I'd like to illustrate my point by referring to my mother's experiences.

The grim hand of old age really seemed to be gripping Mother when she was seventy-three. She was often seized by a painful cramp in the calf of the leg. On some nights it was so severe that she was awakened by it. Poor Mother! She consulted her friends and neighbors instead of the doctor, and they told her, "It's hardening of the arteries. Nothing can be done."

Finally Mother called me in distress to tell me that an ulcer had formed on her foot. It just wouldn't heal, she said.

Careful continuous medical attention was necessary. Slowly the circulation in the hardened arteries improved enough so that she could again attend to her daily chores and enjoy short walks. Her sleep was no longer interrupted by pain. When the improved circulation brought more blood to the leg, the ulcer eventually healed. Mother was lucky. She was treated early, and her arteries were still flexible enough so that this helped her circulation. I'm certain she was not *cured*, but the *partial improvement* made it possible for her to visit her many friends and her twenty-one children and grandchildren.

Similarly, her deafness was not "cured." But with the help of a hearing aid she was again able to enjoy the movies, the radio, and "visiting" —instead of feeling alone and isolated. It was during this experience that I learned something else about the reactions of elderly people to health problems. Although partial restoration of function is extremely important, the doctor's approach must not be negative. He must avoid warning the patient not to expect too much. Most old people don't expect to attain perfect health again, but unless the doctor makes his recommendations with force and enthusiasm, they may take the path of least resistance.

It was not easy to persuade my mother to go to an *otologist* (ear specialist). Being quite sensitive and dreading the idea of a hearing aid, she tried to conceal her deafness. Finally she went to an excellent doctor, but he failed to offer her sufficient encouragement, and it took time and patience—and a second and stronger recommendation on his part—before she was willing to try a hearing aid. Failing to plan carefully enough, we turned Mother over to a competent instrument company where, unfortunately, the technician was rather inept, and tuned the instrument so loud that the strange blares, scratchings, and static startled Mother, and she immediately decided the whole procedure was senseless.

After another six months, we tried again, this time more thoughtfully. We found an agency which, on a nonprofit basis, demonstrates various hearing devices for the sole purpose of helping people select the most suitable instrument. We described Mother's unfortunate experience to one of the technicians in advance. Her tact and patience were rewarded, for she convinced Mother that an apparatus would be very valuable.

One reason I have told these stories is to admit frankly that it isn't always easy to guide older people in matters of health—even when one happens to be a doctor as well as a devoted son! But it is worth everything you put into it.

Naturally, choosing the right doctor is especially important as far as older people are concerned. If they do not have confidence in a "youngster," they should have an older physician. On the other hand, elderly patients may find that a younger physician transmits some of his vitality to them. There are advantages in having the same doctor attend both the older and younger members of a family. This keeps children in close touch with the medical status of their elderly parents, and also promotes the "teamwork" so valuable in solving medical problems.

People who do not have the blessings of children and grandchildren will find a trusted doctor one of the greatest comforts of their old age. Like their clergyman, he can always be depended upon. That is why I urge older people, especially, to stick to one doctor, and get to know him well —and let him know them, too, not only as patients but as individuals.

# DISCOMFORTS AND MINOR IMPAIRMENTS OF OLD AGE

It is true that old age brings inevitable changes in the body, and many of these may be reflected in discomfort and minor impairments. The joints and *bursae* (see page 461) aren't so well lubricated as they are in younger people. For this reason, certain forms of rheumatism and arthritis frequently occur. Usually, these are not the crippling types, but they do cause discomfort. These symptoms, as well as many others such as buzzing in the ears, insomnia, dry skin, and so on, can be greatly relieved by your doctor. Give him a chance! I've heard of more than one person who, without saying a word to his doctor, failed to take the aspirin he prescribed, because it was thought to be "habit-forming" or "a heart poison." This old superstition has been completely disproved by medical research. Aspirin, or a similar preparation, can be very helpful to elderly people suffering from headaches, rheumatism, and a number of other complaints. Your doctor may also advise the use of a heating pad, or some other form of physiotherapy such as warm baths or Swedish massage, to relieve aches and pains.

*Constipation,* and the consequent use of laxatives, has often become a fixed habit by the later years of life. (See page 504 for my discussion of constipation.) Although mineral oil is the best remedy, I consider it wise to accept the one which an elderly person is accustomed to, unless I feel that some real harm is being done—whether it's hot lemon water at 6:45 A.M. or the enema which some old people insist has magical virtues. The important thing is to watch for a sudden change in established bowel habits. For example, the onset of constipation in someone who has always been regular warrants an immediate examination because it might indicate an obstruction due to a tumor.

*Skin and facial changes* occur as old age approaches. The skin becomes drier and less elastic. It may sag or wrinkle. If a number of teeth are missing and have not been replaced by dentures, the face is frequently disfigured.

Facial massage, lubricating cream or oil, care-

ful tanning in the sun, and exposure to fresh outdoor air will help keep the skin in a more youthful condition. As a rule, I prefer to advise people to accept the changes of old age, let nature take its course, and invest any spare money in good meals, vitamins, and a full set of false teeth, if these become necessary. However, if wrinkles and sagging cause serious concern and worry, they can be helped by a skin specialist. He can be extremely helpful to actresses, actors, and others to whom a youthful appearance is extremely important. It is even possible to remove or to stretch badly sagging or wrinkled areas of the skin on the face and neck. *This must be done only by a qualified expert in plastic surgery.* AVOID QUACKS. Always consult your own doctor. He has a list of accredited specialists in cosmetic surgery.

Despite the complaints we make about it, our *digestive systems* usually hold out pretty well. Death is very seldom caused by the "wearing out" of our digestive organs.

Some old people do develop finicky appetites, partly because they actually need less food, but often because of trouble with their teeth. They may avoid meat if chewing is difficult. It is important for older people to maintain an adequate diet, especially one containing plenty of proteins and minerals, rather than one high in starches and sugars. Meat, fish, eggs, and cheese are good sources of protein. Milk, which is high in protein, is the best source of minerals such as calcium and phosphorus. A pint of milk a day is essential for old people. Those who do not like to drink milk can take it in soups, desserts, and various other milk dishes. Fat-free (skimmed) milk is very good for elderly people because it provides the necessary minerals and protein, without the extra calories from the butterfat in whole milk. Consult my discussion of diet on page 30. Elderly people who must live on limited incomes can purchase the more economical types of protein and mineral foods.

I like to prescribe extra vitamins for people who are over sixty. Usually a capsule or two a day of multivitamins is sufficient. If the supplementary vitamins cause troublesome intestinal gas, natural foods can be substituted for them: cereals, liver, and pork chops for the B vitamins, orange and tomato juice for vitamin C, and cod-liver or halibut oil for vitamins A and D.

## Diseases of Overweight

Most of the problems connected with digestion do not arise from eating too little, but from eating too much. This is particularly true in elderly people. In fact, many of the illnesses which are spoken of as diseases of old age could more properly be called diseases of overweight.

Be sure to read my discussion of overweight on page 44. Life-insurance figures show that obese people are more apt to suffer from diseases of the circulatory system (the heart and blood vessels) which cause half of all the deaths in the elderly. People who are overweight are also more apt to suffer from cancer, which causes one eighth of all the deaths in people of advanced years. Being obese in later life increases the incidence of diabetes, heart disease, diseases of the gallbladder, backache, and footstrain.

A chart showing the death rate of men whose weight is normal and of men who are overweight reveals the startling fact that, between the ages of forty-five and fifty, men who weigh 60 pounds more than they should have a death rate that is 67 percent higher than that of men whose weight is normal. In other words, each extra pound increases their chances of dying by a bit more than one percent. However, before you start worrying about that extra pound, be sure to read page 543 of my chapter on The Calculated Risk in Health. In this chapter I also discuss the shortsightedness of attempting to lead the existence of a vegetable in the hope of adding a few years to life.

# HOW TO LIVE TO A RIPE OLD AGE

In ancient Rome the average person lived to be twenty-three, while during the plague-ridden sixteenth century, life expectancy was under twenty-one. Yet even in those days some people managed to live well into the eighties and the nineties. In fact, although far more people reach old age today than in the past, *the actual life-span has not been increased.* We hear of people who live for a decade or even two past the century mark, but very few of these cases have been verified. Today, as in the past, a hundred years or so appears to be the limit of man's stay on earth.

Scientists are studying the question of the life-span. Why, they want to know, should a three-year-old rat be as aged as a five-hundred-year-old Galápagos turtle? Why should certain cells be practically immortal, while others live for only a short time? Facts are being assembled, and these fascinating questions will, I am confident, eventually be answered. Perhaps an increase in the life-span of human beings will then be possible.

In the meantime, let us consider how some people—even in the days of a low life expectancy—managed to reach a vigorous old age.

There is a lot of truth in the joking remark that one way to live a long time is to choose the right ancestors. Careful statistical studies have shown that almost 87 percent of the people who live to be ninety had at least one parent who passed the seventy-year mark, and about the same number had two grandparents who reached a ripe old age. These figures are particularly significant when we realize that some of the parents of the remaining 13 percent of these long-lived people undoubtedly died as a result of accidents, wars, and other causes not connected with longevity.

Many other reasons have been advanced by aged people who felt they knew the secret of long life. Some, like Cornaro, a famous Venetian who lived for almost a hundred years, recommended leading a sober and unemotional life, never experiencing anguish or joy. On the other hand, Titian was an intensely emotional man, and he lived to be ninety-nine. Some say that the elderly should, above all, avoid sexual excitement—while others point to Doctor Hahnemann (the founder of homeopathy) who married a young woman when he was eighty and, having been almost decrepit, became vigorous again. George Bernard Shaw adhered to a vegetarian diet. Connie Mack, one of baseball's great names, who was managing a major league team when he was in his mid-eighties, urged people to eat small meals and to get nine hours of sleep each night. For every old man or woman who insists that the way to live long is to avoid tobacco and alcohol, there is another who gives credit to a corncob pipe or a daily tot of rum.

Despite all their contradictory secrets of success, we notice that most of these people have one thing in common—*an interest in, and an enthusiasm for, life.*

I put this at the head of the list. Close to it, in importance, I put: *avoid preventable death,* due to accidents and illnesses which, if detected in time, would not be fatal; and *observe the rules of health and hygiene.*

Although I have covered these two points in other parts of this book, there are some specific rules of health and hygiene for elderly people.

## Exercise

Most doctors feel that the benefits of strenuous exercise have been overrated for older people, and that recreation and regular, mild activity are far more valuable. Some older people enjoy vigorous exercise and are able to engage in it all their lives. However, older people should *always avoid strain and exhaustion.* By the time you are forty, you should have established the custom of consulting your doctor before you undertake any new form of exercise. After that, always speak to him at your regular medical checkups about how much and what kind of exercise you may take. A busy doctor may forget that you are a tennis addict, and will fail to tell you when the time comes for you to give up singles in favor of doubles, or doubles in favor of golf.

Always stop exercising as soon as you feel tired, long before you feel exhausted. Try to be a philosopher, not a sprinter, when you're tempted to chase after that streetcar—or anything else. Stairs have a way of becoming a menace as we grow older. Avoid running up or falling down them.

## Rest

This becomes increasingly important in the later years. Try to rest for half an hour after meals and at intervals during the day. Older people whose work does not permit them to lie down should take advantage of "breaks" or rest periods to relax as completely as possible, with their feet elevated, perhaps on a chair, if it is at all feasible. However, *avoid inactivity.* If you happen to be ill and the doctor says you should get up, by all means make the effort to do so. A prolonged, unnecessary stay in bed is harmful, rather than helpful, to the aged.

## Sleep

People tend to need less sleep as they grow older. If you required eight hours when you were forty, the chances are that six hours will do when you are seventy. Stay in bed longer than that if it rests you, but don't lie there worrying about your insomnia. (There are suggestions for older people in my section on *insomnia,* page 494.)

## Watch Your Weight

As I said earlier in this chapter, people tend to require less food as they grow older. I can't tell you just how much this is in your case—but *your scales will.* If you put on weight, talk it over with your doctor. *Older people should always diet under a doctor's supervision.* If you are overweight, the only thing safe for you to do on your own is to cut out candy and other sweets, and starches between meals, making certain you are eating the well-balanced meals which I describe in my chapter The Food You Eat (p. 30) and on page 537 of this chapter.

## Alcohol and Tobacco

People who smoke and drink in moderation usually do not have to stop in later years, provided they are healthy. However, moderation is essential. It is usually easier for an elderly person to cut down gradually than to make a sudden change. Tobacco is more apt to cause distress than alcohol—for example, dizziness and indigestion. It is frequently forbidden in cases of even relatively minor illnesses such as a tendency to bronchitis, to which elderly people are very susceptible, or high blood pressure. Be sure to abide by your doctor's decision if he tells you to cut out smoking or drinking. On the other hand, he may prescribe small amounts of an alcoholic beverage for medicinal purposes.

## Worry

If you have not learned how to keep from worrying unnecessarily, start right now. This is a luxury you cannot afford. By now you should know yourself well enough to find ways of eliminating or cutting down on those needless worries. Of course, some worries are unavoidable. I remember my mother's "heart trouble" which, her doctor told us, was caused by her sleepless nights during the long months when two of her sons were facing the unpredictable dangers of World War II. When they were safe again, her "heart trouble" vanished. But she could have been spared at least some of it if she had mentioned it sooner. Even when there is real cause for worry, the doctor can help—for example, by giving you a sedative at night—if you will only tell him about it.

## Climate

Older people should be particularly careful not to exert themselves when the cold or, even more important, the heat and humidity lower their vitality. However, as far as pulling up stakes to find a more moderate climate is concerned, remember that older people find it particularly difficult to adjust to new surroundings. Their old friends, the church they attend, even the sight of their own street, are often better medicine for them than anything Florida or California can offer in the way of climate. All the warnings I issue in my chapter Climate and Illness (p. 163) are particularly applicable to older people.

## Medical Insurance

New insurance programs, private and public, have taken much of the worry about illness out of old age. (See Chapter 32, Health Insurance and Community Services.) The federal government's Medicare program offers financial assistance with hospital, nursing home, and private medical care. Other insurance plans, like Blue Cross and Blue Shield, have special provisions for the elderly. Investigate these carefully, so that you know you will be able to afford the special medical attention often required in the later years.

## RETIREMENT

Many of us look forward to retiring someday. But how often we hear of someone who, having worked hard all his life with that goal in mind, begins to fail mentally and physically the moment he actually reaches it!

In order to retire successfully, one must have far more than money in the bank. *One must have a reserve of interests that make life worth living.* That is why I urge young people to cultivate hobbies and recreational activities they can continue in their later years. As Dr. George Lawton, the authority on gerontology, puts it, "To grow old successfully, a man must learn to push around, not his body, but his mind. If his speed, strength, and endurance decline with the years, then he must train in advance skills which will hold up with age and even improve." People who can slip from a business into a hobby or avocation, who can gradually devote less time to work and more time to their outside interests, usually make the transition quite successfully.

This is seldom possible when retirement is involuntary. The dangers of sudden, enforced retirement are clearly revealed by statistics. For example, in railroad men the incidence of mortality reaches a peak in the first year after they stop working. We can only guess at the tremendous increase in emotional disturbances and physical ailments, as these are seldom reported by elderly people or their families.

Many people are forced to retire when they not only are capable of working and want to work, but actually need the full income they were receiving. The older person whom no one will employ is often a tragic figure. This problem is far larger than any individual. I think it can be solved, but only when all of us who expect someday to be old work together to solve it through our communities and our government.

National Conferences on Aging, held in Washington, D.C., are a step in this direction. They have stimulated research into measures for employment, as well as health, recreation, education, and rehabilitation, to benefit our older citizens and, through them, the country as a whole.

A number of organizations provide opportunities along these lines. Clubs of all kinds for elderly people are springing up throughout this country and in other countries. Your town hall, church, community center, or library can tell you about those in your community. If your community does not have a Day Center, McGuffy, Darby and

Joan, Golden Age, Old Guard, or Old Timers group, why not organize one? Your state legislature may be persuaded to give financial assistance. Your local department of welfare should help you, or at least tell you where to go for assistance and advice. The federal government can give you additional information. Write to the U.S. Public Health Service, Bethesda, Maryland 20014.

## INDEPENDENCE, USEFULNESS, AND INTEREST

The basic needs of older people will be satisfied if they are independent, useful, and interested. Please don't be hasty about saying "That lets me (or my parents) out!" It may be true that you have no income and must depend on a son or daughter for support; or that a parent is living with you who just doesn't seem to be interested in anything. Even so, *some degree* of usefulness, independence, and interest may be possible. It will make a tremendous difference.

I know how difficult family situations can become when old people must live under the same roof with their children. That is one reason why it is usually best for the elderly to maintain their own homes as long as possible. Often a room in a light-housekeeping hotel or boarding house proves satisfactory if a house or apartment cannot be maintained. Some boarding houses are run for older people, or can be set up for that purpose. They provide whatever is necessary, which may be simply doing the heavy housecleaning or may be the kind of complete care offered by nursing homes or by individual families which provide "foster homes for the aged." Some "old people's homes" are excellent, although the majority are inadequate and depressing, because of the indifference of the community.

As older people become a proportionately larger part of our population, and as the public becomes more aware of their needs, apartment houses and entire communities have been organized to appeal to the special needs of the elderly. Some of these are operated entirely by private owners; some are built by church, synagogue, or charitable organizations.

I urge older people to investigate these places, because many of them offer excellent facilities—physical, social, and medical. But be sure to consult both your doctor *and* your lawyer before you agree to anything in writing. See your doctor because you want to be sure that you are in sufficiently good health to settle in a new apartment or community, and because you want to ascertain that the medical facilities and staff will be adequate for your special needs. See your lawyer because you should not sign away your property or income or commit yourself to a heavy financial obligation without being absolutely sure of what you are doing.

When elderly people must live with their children, it is usually best not to separate a husband and wife. If they are inclined to quarrel with one another, you will certainly often wish they would at least visit you and your brothers and sisters alternately. But they undoubtedly enjoy each other much more than you realize, so try to remember that they had to put up with many quarrels when you were children!

It isn't easy for elderly people to divide their time between their various children, although this is usually the only fair arrangement. The difficulties can be minimized by establishing definite dates. Any uncertainty is very trying for old people. If possible, make the changes seasonal, as it seems natural to spend the winter months in one place and the summer ones in another. Having a room of their own awaiting them, with some of their cherished possessions in it, adds immeasurably to their feeling of security and independence.

Every effort should be made, on the part of both generations, to find means of achieving a degree of independence. Often, it is easier for a woman to feel she's "paying her way" than it is for a man, since she can help with the housework and the care of young children. But elderly men can be extremely useful, too, if enough time and thought are put into it. Hobbies, crafts, and "handyman" skills often make it possible for them, too, to "earn their keep." I know of a "Rainy-day Stamp Collectors' Club" which, under the guidance of a grandfather, was a boon to the mothers of the neighborhood and a source of cigar money to him. Another old man became the favorite model in a local art class. The important thing is to find something for each individual to do—which should, of course, be appreciated by the younger members of the family.

Projects outside, as well as within, the home help to bring a feeling of independence and prevent the irritations of too much personal contact. Those who can go out benefit tremendously from this. Some older people go to a day center to work, or for study and recreation, as regularly as they once attended business. Clubs, church, or charitable affairs and visiting, if possible on a regular weekly basis, are interesting and stimulating breaks in otherwise monotonous routines. I know one elderly lady whose "job" consists in escorting an infirm friend, a retired teacher, to a local institution so she can read to those whose eyes have failed them. She always complains that her friend is quite capable of going without her, but the truth of the matter is that she enjoys the excursion because she feels useful. Doctors, clergymen, and social service workers can often find a need for the older person to fill. This is particularly important for those who do not have families or friends whom they can serve. And when I say "serve" I want to remind you that one can be a useful member of society even if one can do no more than be a pleasant part of a family or other group.

In this chapter I have spoken very little of true senility or "morbid senility" as contrasted with normal aging. That is because it is a mental illness which I discuss at various places in Chapter 13. Even when this condition manifests itself in mental decadence, the patient's family must not conceal it out of shame or misplaced feelings of duty. Like any other illness, it requires a doctor who may or may not be able to alleviate its symptoms. As in the case of other illnesses, his advice must be followed.

Attitudes toward the aged vary tremendously in different forms of society. Among the Eskimos, it was customary to set them adrift on an ice floe to die. Among the Chinese, they were venerated.

Surely the most civilized attitude to take is to regard old people simply as *people*—who have lived a long time and who have special problems, as we all do at every stage of our existence. The better we can solve these problems, the more valuable these years will be to the individual and to society.

# 38

# THE CALCULATED RISK IN HEALTH

## OR HOW TO AVOID BEING A HYPOCHONDRIAC

---

When one of my nonmedical friends learned that I was writing this book, he said it was a wonderful idea and he'd like to order a copy immediately. Then he added somewhat doubtfully, "But don't you think there's a danger that it will make some people worry about themselves—that they'll get to be hypochondriacs who think they have every disease they read about?"

Other friends expressed the same concern, quoting "Where ignorance is bliss, 'tis folly to be wise," or "A little learning is a dangerous thing." One of them called my attention to a story by a British humorist about a man who went happily into the library to look up some illness he thought he might have. He went right on reading his way through the medical book, and feeling certain he had all the diseases in it (except, possibly, housemaid's knee), he "crawled out a decrepit wreck." Fortunately he went to his doctor who gave him a prescription which turned out to be as follows:

1 lb. beefsteak with 1 pt. bitter beer every six hours.
1 ten mile walk every morning.
1 bed at 11 sharp every night.
And don't stuff up your head with things you don't understand.

Stories of this kind are always making the rounds of medical schools. There's usually one about a student who suffered from every symptom he studied, and who refused to take the course in obstetrics because he dreaded the labor pains. Others concern patients who managed to catch a glimpse of their medical histories or charts, and fainted at the sight of a word like *prognosis* or *alopecia*, thinking it meant they had a fatal illness. (*Prognosis* means a prediction about the course of a disease, and *alopecia* means baldness!)

However, doctors know that patients don't need to read about actual diseases in order to suffer from imaginary ones. We have all had patients who could invent more and better ailments than medical science ever dreamed of. Still, medical books can be alarming, especially old-fashioned ones. I glanced through one of them recently, and was struck by the number of diseases about which the author was extremely pessimistic—from *Anemia, Pernicious,* which was formerly always fatal, to *Zymotic Diseases,* the name given to diphtheria, scarlet fever, and similar contagious illnesses which no longer constitute a serious problem today.

Doctors know that ignorance is *not* bliss in the case of countless people who suffer and even die from preventable diseases or permit a beloved child to die simply because they lack the knowledge to heed nature's danger signals. And no one would say that "a little learning is a dangerous thing" when a person who has no intention of studying electricity or mechanics acquaints himself with the fact that he'll get a shock if he touches a live wire or a blowout if his tires get too thin.

However, it is true that after each health campaign or drive to raise funds for a health organization, doctors are besieged by people who are afraid they have the disease that has been publicized. Campaigns concerned with cancer, tuberculosis, heart disease and high blood pressure, diabetes, obesity, rheumatism and arthritis, multiple sclerosis, cerebral palsy, muscular dystrophy, and venereal disease, give suggestible people something to worry about all year long.

Here are a few examples from some of my own recent experiences.

A middle-aged businessman confronted me with, "Doctor, I want a *yes* or *no* answer. Will my being twenty-five pounds overweight shorten my life?"

A college student asked me whether he would get cancer of the lungs if he continued smoking. "I tried to cut it out," he said. "But I got so jittery I couldn't study for exams."

For years a woman had taken for granted a number of knotty little lumps in her breasts. Her doctor had diagnosed the condition as a mild chronic mastitis, which is merely an inflammation of the mammary glands. This patient carefully followed the directions she had read in an excellent article about self-examination of the breasts for cancer. Her breasts were quite large, and she found herself worrying about each little nodule she encountered: had it been there before? Was it like the others? Or was it a cancer? She would tell herself it was nothing and there was no need to see her doctor again—but she couldn't keep from feeling her breasts from time to time all day long. Eventually they became quite sore.

Later in this chapter I will tell you what I said to these people. At this point, I want only to mention them as typical examples of the anxieties caused by certain campaigns. Most doctors are familiar with this. An outstanding physician recently told me, only half-jokingly, "The blood pressure instrument is the most dangerous medical invention of modern times! I can't tell you how many patients ask me how high their blood pressure is, as though I were about to pronounce their death sentence. Unless I can show them that the reading is exactly right, they worry terribly—usually without any reason."

In speaking of a campaign against venereal disease, the psychiatrist Dr. Alfred Blazer called it "a war of nerves on our youth." He said that syphilophobia, which is a morbid fear of syphilis, "even afflicts young people who are virgins. For them every doorknob is covered with germs." Many other campaigns have waged a similar "war of nerves" on the public who must go to and from work every day in the subway, looking at posters on which a finger points directly at them as potential victims of some fatal disease.

## THE VALUE OF HEALTH CAMPAIGNS

I do not want to give the impression that I am opposed to health campaigns. On the contrary, I feel that they, and the voluntary or governmental agencies sponsoring them, do wonderful work. They alert and educate the public. They raise money to carry out vital research and to assist the victims of various diseases, and they deserve great credit for helping to eliminate or control many illnesses that formerly took a terrible toll from our population.

The hush-hush attitude toward venereal disease in the past was broken down by the excellent campaign instituted by the U.S. Public Health Service. The sale of Christmas seals has indeed helped to "stamp out tuberculosis," which only a short time ago was as dreaded a disease as cancer. It is impossible even to estimate the number of lives that have been saved and the amount of suffering that has been prevented by the efforts of the Heart Association, the Diabetic Association, the National Foundation (formerly National Foundation for Infantile Paralysis), and similar organizations. The endless, tireless—and little known—work of our local public health departments protects us against typhoid fever, dysentery, undulant fever, and other milk-, water-, and food-borne diseases. It has all but eliminated malaria, smallpox, and yellow fever.

Today we are no longer a prey to the panic our grandparents experienced when epidemics threatened: "acute community hypochondriasis," it could be called. For example: before 1900 martial law was frequently proclaimed if yellow fever struck a community, and anyone who attempted to flee was shot down. This was considered essential if the disease was to be kept from spreading. Not so very long ago, a man who was even suspected of having leprosy might be stoned to death, and people who had so much as touched him were apt to commit suicide. These were panics of ignorance for, as we now know, yellow fever is transmitted by mosquitoes, *not* human beings, and the danger of catching leprosy by touching a leper is, practically speaking, non-existent.

Now that we have eliminated the ignorance responsible for these panics, must we pay for our knowledge by becoming a nation of chronic hypochondriacs?

My answer is NO. We can have the tremendous advantages that come with enlightenment, and at the same time avoid the danger of being frightened into hypochondriasis, by (1) *continuous health education,* (2) *routine, periodic medical examinations,* and (3) *a sensible attitude toward the calculated risk in health.*

## CONTINUOUS HEALTH EDUCATION

Most of the harm done by campaigns against the killing and disabling diseases stems from the fact that these campaigns are conducted in a relatively short period of time. Organizations that do excellent work every day of the year are limited to a week or so in which to educate the public and publicize their work in order to raise the major portion of their funds. Whether they want to or not, they must in a sense compete with other valuable organizations. If they want to put across their message, they must use advertising methods and publicity techniques similar to those intended to sell a commercial product. Health organizations cannot depend solely on serious scientific articles to catch the attention of a public which has grown accustomed to clever high-pressure radio, television, newspaper, and other advertising. The public must be reached directly. People must be awakened to a sense of personal danger. Unless they participate personally, the warning signals of cancer, tuberculosis, diabetes, heart disease, and other diseases will go undetected until the time comes for a regular medical examination or the symptoms become severe enough to cause distress. By then the disease may have progressed beyond its curable stage.

This situation would be greatly improved if these organizations could obtain the money they need without having to engage in intensive fund-raising campaigns; for example, by increased donations from individuals and foundations and by aid from the government. It would also help if the campaigns placed even more emphasis on the fact that the diseases they are publicizing can be cured or controlled if they are detected early enough. As an example, this positive approach to the dangers of childbirth has done a great deal to eliminate fear and anxiety in prospective mothers.

But, most important of all, health education should be a *continuous* process, so that organizations would not have to crowd their warnings and recommendations into a single intensive week.

*Health education should begin in childhood.* Some primary and grammar schools train small children in many of the essentials of health and hygiene. Some high schools continue this excellent work, teaching first aid, human biology, and the prevention of disease. How about *your* school? Parents can see to it that their children's health education is not neglected, by working through parent-teacher associations or by organizing interesting after-school programs.

This education should not end when young people leave school. Our knowledge must keep pace with the rapid advances of medical science. Churches, adult education centers, clubs, trade unions, and other organizations should keep health on their agenda, working out ways of interesting their members by means of lectures, demonstrations, exhibits, and so on, and of bringing these projects to the entire community.

The public health department can be of great assistance. Many of us tend to overlook this valuable agency. Dr. Logan Clendening, a noted authority in medicine, put the rise of public health at the top of his list of the most important advances in medical science occurring in the first half of the twentieth century.

The effectiveness of your local health department depends to a great extent on the interest of the citizens of your community. Public health departments and county health officers have learned how to get excellent results without resorting to scare techniques. These methods need not be limited to the communicable diseases.

Mental illness, for example, is not "catching" in the strict meaning of the word, but we all know that the effects of mental illness in any individual are, in the broad sense, communicated to others in the family or even throughout the community.

## ROUTINE PERIODIC MEDICAL EXAMINATIONS

I have devoted an entire chapter (see page 378) to the importance of periodic medical examinations, and I have emphasized this point at various places throughout this book. But I have limited myself to convincing you, as an individual, that you should have checkups at regular intervals. Here I am going to go further; I am going to advocate *compulsory periodic medical examinations for everyone.*

At the beginning, these compulsory examinations could be restricted to searching for *communicable diseases* such as tuberculosis, dysentery, and syphilis. The principle behind this is entirely consistent with the ideals of our democracy. We accept the fact that our community water and milk supply and the food we eat should be subject to inspection. We take it for granted that our children should be vaccinated against smallpox. We agree that individuals have a social obligation not to transmit illnesses to others. This is the principle behind the laws requiring that individuals who handle food must be examined to make certain they do not harbor the germs of typhoid fever or dysentery. A small, but significant, number of people are carriers; that is, they carry certain germs without being made ill by them. Such individuals are not permitted to work in places where they could transmit the germs to others, with sometimes fatal results. Some states require a premarital blood test to detect syphilis so that neither partner will infect the other, perhaps unknowingly, or be responsible for bringing syphilitic children into the world. Nurses and individuals in certain other professions and jobs are examined regularly.

It seems obvious to me that this practice should be extended. Teachers, houseworkers, and babysitters, who are in close contact with our children, should certainly be examined periodically to make sure they are free from such diseases as tuberculosis. Why not include *everybody*, in these days when we come into close contact with total strangers every day in subways, stores, movies, swimming pools, and so on? Compulsory medical examinations are merely an extension—and a most important one—of existing health programs to protect ourselves.

The cost of these examinations could be borne by either the individual, the government, or both. Those who could afford to, and wanted to, could be examined by their own doctors and pay the entire fee. Others could visit clinics at which the local, state, and federal government could share the cost or assume it entirely. Again, this is merely an extension of existing programs which cover vaccination against smallpox and inoculations against other diseases. The expense to the community would be more than compensated for by the number of lives that would be saved and the disabilities that would be prevented or curtailed —if the prevention of suffering alone does not seem sufficient justification.

In addition to the *compulsory* examinations and tests for communicable diseases, *optional* examinations for other potential "killers" and "disablers" could be provided, again on a free, partially paid, or privately compensated basis. These would include tests for diabetes, cancer, heart and kidney diseases, and other illnesses, according to the age or condition of the individual being examined.

I feel that this is necessary because many people, especially if they have not received the proper health education, are not sufficiently aware of the need for checkups to be willing to overcome their inertia and pay the cost of such examinations.

Naturally, I realize that this program will not be introduced today or even tomorrow. I hope some of you will help to speed its realization. But there are only a few people whose inclinations and abilities lie in that direction.

### What You Can Do

*Everyone* can help in some way. There is bound to be something you can do to encourage regular, periodic health examinations—for expectant mothers, infants, preschool and school children, industrial and other workers, people in rural areas—for anyone and everyone. As an individual or through your church, clubs, trade union, parent-teacher association, or other organizations, you can help make the examinations that already exist better and more easily available, and you can encourage people to take advantage of them.

Perhaps you can extend or add to these examinations. How would your lodge or club, business or industry, feel about providing its members and their families with medical examinations on a free or low-cost basis? How would your community respond to the idea of medical tests for those who use the swimming pool? Shouldn't you insist on having the personnel of your children's camp and the campers themselves examined? I have been astonished by the fact that some parents wants to know whether a camp has checked the social background of the youngsters with whom their children will come in contact—and fail to find out whether the camp has checked their physical condition.

Why shouldn't *your* town or the factory in which you work have the advantages of the *partial* physical examinations which may be readily available? Countless people have had chest films made in mobile x-ray units that come practically to their doors. Tests for diabetes have been provided in a number of communities.

As people come to accept such examinations and tests as a part of their regular lives, diseases can be prevented or cured without arousing alarm. Some years ago, anybody who was going to have a chest x-ray taken would probably lie awake worrying all through the previous night. Today, people sail in and out of such x-ray examinations without even asking when they will learn the results. It is mere routine to them. Similarly, young people take their "physicals" in school and college as a matter of course.

When procedures become routine, the fears connected with them become minimal. Soldiers know that. So do civilians. Their terror of bombs during the war was greatly reduced when there was a regular routine procedure for them to follow.

Why, for example, should any woman have to decide "Should I, or shouldn't I, have a test made for cancer of the womb?" (see page 435) or a man have to make up his mind when and how often his blood pressure should be taken? These and similar tests should become routine affairs. In this way, we could all have the benefits that come with knowledge, and yet avoid the anxiety of having to make repeated decisions.

# THE CALCULATED RISK IN HEALTH

A long-range program of health education and routine medical examinations will be extremely important in preventing us from becoming hypochondriacs. In addition, each of us must realize that, no matter how well we guard against it, we cannot entirely eliminate the possibility of disease or accidental injury. At present, and in the foreseeable future, there will always be a chance that sickness may strike. If we are realistic, we will accept the *concept of calculated risk in health.*

I can best explain this by discussing the individuals I mentioned on page 544 who worried about smoking, being overweight, or having cancer of the breast. What could I, or any doctor, tell them?

On the basis of the knowledge we have now, the college student's smoking clearly increases his chances of someday getting a cancer of the lungs and could contribute, too, to increasing his risk of coronary heart disease. The middle-aged businessman would, statistically speaking, live longer if he lost twenty-five pounds. About the woman patient: there is no doubt that the danger from cancer of the breast is tremendously reduced if it is detected early.

These problems varied, and I discussed each of them individually. "We all run some risks every day of our lives," I pointed out. "If we walk across the street we may be hit by an automobile and killed or maimed. Riding in a train, subway, or car may mean an accident. How do you react to this?"

Normal, sensible people do not react by staying at home and trying to protect themselves by withdrawing from life in some neurotic manner. They are not continually tense and frightened because of the potential dangers they face. On the other hand, they do not ignore the existence of these dangers. They don't cross the street without looking where they're going, or drive seventy miles per hour on an icy road, or dive into the water without knowing how deep it is. In other words, the sensible, normal person is neither an *ostrich* nor an *alarmist*. He is what I call an *alertist*.

Suppose you want to go on an automobile trip over a holiday weekend. You know that you run a greater danger of having an accident than you would on an ordinary weekend or during the week. You weigh these risks. If you think they are going to worry you too much, you may decide to take the train. If you make up your mind to drive, you may decide to reduce the hazards you face by leaving early in order to escape the heaviest traffic. Undoubtedly you will take the precaution of having your brakes, tires, and lights checked before you leave. In other words, you calculate the risk as well as you can, you decide whether or not you want to face it, and you take steps to minimize it. After that, you tell yourself it is "in the lap of the gods," and don't let worry spoil your weekend.

That is the attitude I hope you will take toward your health. Be an *alertist,* not an *ostrich* or an *alarmist.* Here are some specific suggestions:

1. Try to estimate the risks. To do this in regard to your health, you must have a certain amount of information, just as you must know certain facts in order to avoid unnecessary dangers when you drive a car. You can, and should, have yourself and your car regularly checked by an expert. Unfortunately, most people can't take a doctor or a garage mechanic along with them wherever they go. They have to be able to evaluate certain risks themselves.

I do not mean to imply that you (or, in most cases, even a scientist) can determine *exact* percentages regarding various risks to your health. But we can arrive at an approximate estimate of them.

For example, although a rise in blood pressure must be regarded as a danger signal, it does not necessarily mean trouble if it is a small rise and a fleeting one. A few points of elevation showing up with one measurement but not again with succeeding measurements need cause no concern.

At the other extreme: anyone who takes a narcotic (morphine, cocaine, or heroin) regularly without medical supervision will become addicted to it. In such cases the risk is almost a certainty. The only time a doctor is justified in ignoring it is when a patient is suffering from a painful, fatal disease.

Most risks lie between these extremes. Kissing anyone who has active tuberculosis of the lungs is extremely dangerous. People have been known to do so without catching the disease. But no sensible person will deliberately take chances by kissing a tubercular person on the mouth.

How about smoking and cancer? We now know that there is a definite connection between smoking, particularly heavy smoking of cigarettes, and cancer, especially cancer of the lungs. Smoking also adversely affects the circulatory system and the heart. In my opinion, *everyone* who smokes ought to do so as lightly as possible. I don't state flatly that no one should smoke at all because I know how difficult it is to stop. But we should all realize the risks involved and balance the pleasure against the possible damage to our health. Anyone with a definite family history of cancer, especially of the lungs, larynx, lips, and tongue, not only should stop smoking but should be especially alert in watching for signs of cancer, such as coughing, hoarseness, and sores on the mouth, lips, and tongue. Anyone who persists in smoking heavily should have his mouth, tongue, and larynx checked by physical examination and his lungs x-rayed at least once a year (really as often as your doctor advises).

2. Don't try to eliminate all health risks. In the first place, as I said before, it isn't possible to do this and still lead a normal life. In the second place, it defeats its own purpose. I have often had people ask me to tell their beloved parents not to do this, that, and the other in the hope of prolonging their lives. Many of these suggestions are good, but occasionally they reach the point where I have to say, "What use will a few more years of existence be to your parents if they can't do anything they enjoy? Do you want them to live like *vegetables* instead of *humans?* Besides, there is no guarantee it will actually prolong their lives."

I was struck by this fact in the case of a mother who lived alternately with her two daughters. One of them was quite well to do, and the old lady was waited on hand and foot while in her home. The other daughter, who had a large family and a modest income, came to me saying that her sister had offered to keep their mother permanently. "Do you think I ought to let her, for mother's sake?" she asked. "She insists on washing the dishes and helping out in other ways while she's with me, and she's so feeble I know it can't be good for her."

I surprised her by answering, "Theoretically, your mother is better off when she doesn't have to exert herself. Actually, however, she's in better condition during the time she stays with you. Knowing that she's being useful more than makes up for the added strain."

This brings me to my third suggestion:

3. Remember that you are a person, not a statistic. Statistics are of great help in calculating the risks we run. But they do not tell the entire story. Each of us is an individual, not a number on a piece of paper. That is why doctors feel they must see and examine their patients, and not depend on laboratory tests alone for their diagnoses. As the medical saying goes, "It's just as important to know what kind of patient the disease has, as to find out what kind of disease the patient has."

It is much safer, statistically speaking, not to be obese in later life. Yet we all know people who are somewhat overweight and still lead long, happy, and healthy lives. I am inclined to doubt that Winston Churchill, Queen Wilhelmina, and Sophie Tucker (to give just a few examples) would have been any better off had they dieted. In fact, I've known some really fat people who were in excellent health until they tried to lose weight. Then they became tense and irritable and suffered as a result.

The woman who could not make up her mind about the lumps in her breast should, as I told her, admit frankly, "Self-examination of the breasts is not for me." Her doctor was quite willing to make an arrangement for a brief examination of her breasts at intervals between her regular checkups. She told me she felt she was being silly, but I convinced her that no one need be ashamed of being human.

If some disease happens to alarm you unduly, because someone you know suffered from it, or for any other conscious or unconscious reason, do not feel ashamed of your fears because they seem exaggerated. Try to understand yourself and accept yourself. *You* are important.

As our rapidly growing understanding of psychosomatic illnesses has shown us, tension and worry can cause or aggravate a number of diseases. Thus, to a certain extent at least, each individual tends to make his own luck.

Today, when medicine has taken such tremendous strides toward eliminating, curing, and controlling disease, there is little need for anyone to avoid the facts. By learning to understand the marvelous bodies and minds with which we have been endowed, we can enjoy the extra years and the additional good health medical science has made possible.

Some of these benefits will come our way regardless of what we do. However, to reap the *full* benefit, without becoming hypochondriacs and worrying unduly, we must each play our part. We must be informed and alert, rather than ignorant and alarmed.

Because of my complete confidence that this will be your attitude, I have written this book.

# DICTIONARY AND GLOSSARY OF MEDICAL TERMS

This is a comprehensive set of definitions of medical terms intended to be used as a *supplement* to the text of the book itself. Terms discussed at some length in the text may not be found here, but the page references for the more complete discussions will be readily located in the Index.

*Most medical terms can be broken down into parts. By understanding the meaning of these parts you can figure out the meanings of many terms you may never have seen before. Some of them refer to sections of the body, such as the following:*

| Term | Meaning | Example |
|------|---------|---------|
| aden- | gland | adenoma |
| cardi- | heart | cardiogram |
| -cyte | cell | erythrocyte |
| derm- | skin | dermatitis |
| gastr- | stomach | gastric juice |
| hem- *or* | blood | hematuria |
| -em- | | anemia |
| lingu- | tongue | lingual |
| myel- | spinal cord *or* marrow | poliomyelitis |
| myo- | muscle | myoma |
| nephr- | kidney | nephrectomy |
| *or* ren- | | adrenal |
| neur- | nerve | neuritis |
| os- *or* ost- | bone | ossification |
| | | osteitis |
| psych- | mind | psychiatry |
| pulmo- | lung | pulmonary |

Others describe position, shape, or amount:

| | | |
|------|---------|---------|
| a- | lack of | apnea |
| dys- | bad, abnormal | dysphagia |
| endo- | inside | endothelium |
| epi- | upon, in addition | epiglottis |
| hyper- | above, extreme | hyperthyroid |
| hypo- | under, below | hypodermic |
| macro- | long, large | macrophage |
| mal- | bad, abnormal | malnutrition |
| micro- | small | microcardia |

Some refer to substances of the body:

| | | |
|------|---------|---------|
| pneum- | gas | pneumonia |
| py- | pus | empyema |
| -rrhag- *or* | flow | hemorrhage |
| -rrhea | | dysmenorrhea |

Suffixes may mean condition, operation, or study:

| | | |
|------|---------|---------|
| -algia | pain in | neuralgia |
| -ectomy | cutting out | tonsillectomy |
| -ia *or* -osis | disease | anemia |
| | | neurosis |
| -itis | inflammation | appendicitis |
| -lysis | dissolving or loosening | hemolysis |
| -mania | excessive preoccupation | nymphomania |
| -oid | similar to | adenoid |
| -ology | study of | neurology |
| -oma | tumor | carcinoma |
| -ostomy | making an opening | colostomy |
| -otomy | cutting into | lobotomy |
| -phobia | fear | claustrophobia |

A

**abasia** (ah-bay′zhe-ah). Inability to walk because of an injury to the nerves or brain affecting muscle coordination.

**abdomen** (ab-do′men). The portion of the body between the chest and pelvis. It is a cavity separated from the chest area by the diaphragm. It contains the stomach, large and small intestines, liver, spleen, pancreas, kidneys, and other structures.

**aberration** (ab-er-ay′shun). A deviation from the normal.

**abort** (ah-bort′). 1. To miscarry or induce the expulsion of a fetus before it is able to live, usually within the first four months of pregnancy. 2. To stop the development of a disease.

**abrasion** (uh-bray′zhun). 1. Wound caused by skin being scraped off. 2. In dentistry, the wearing away of the surface of a tooth as a result of chewing.

**abscess** (ab′ses). A collection of pus in an area where the tissues have broken down.

**absolute alcohol** (al′ko-hol). Alcohol with less than 1% water.

**accommodation** (uh-kom-o-day′shun). In the eye it refers to the change in the curve of the lens to bring objects to a focus, the curve becoming more convex the closer the object.

**acetanilid** (ass-eh-tan′il-id). A medicine which relieves pain and reduces fever.

**acetone** (ass′eh-tone). A substance found in small amounts in normal urine and in larger amounts in the urine and blood in cases of diabetes.

**acetophenetidin** (ass-et-o-feh-net′id-in). A medicine used in treating fevers and neuralgias. It relieves pain and reduces fever.

**acetylcholine** (ass-et-il-ko′leen). The substance believed to carry the nerve impulse at the nerve ending.

**Achilles′** (ah-kil′eez) **tendon.** The tendon at the back of the ankle that connects muscles of the leg to the bone.

**Achromycin** (ak′ro-my′sin). See **tetracycline.**

**acidosis** (ass ad-o′sis). A condition in which the amount of sodium bicarbonate (alkali) in the blood is reduced. It is associated with several disorders including advanced diabetes.

**acne** (ak′nee). Pustules caused by inflammation of the oil glands of the skin, usually on the face, back, and chest; pimples.

**acromegaly** (ak-ro-meg′uh-li). A chronic condition caused by an overactive pituitary gland. The facial features, hands, and feet become enlarged.

**acrophobia** (ak-ro-fo′bi-uh). Fear of high places.

**ACTH.** Abbreviation for adrenocorticotropic hormone, a substance produced by the pituitary gland and capable of releasing cortisone and other hormones from the adrenal gland.

**actinomycin** (ak-tin-o-my′sin). Antibiotic substance isolated from a fungus and active against many bacteria and fungi.

**actinomycosis** (ak-tin-o-my-ko′sis). Infection with a type of fungus. It may affect lungs, skin, intestines, or jaw.

**acupuncture** (ak′u-pungk″tur). A Chinese system of medicine which employs insertion of needles into the body at several hundred points for therapy and anesthesia.

**acute** (uh-kyoot′). When referring to disease it means one having a short course; not chronic.

**Adam′s apple.** The projecting portion of the larynx.

**addict** (ad′ikt). **One who** habitually follows some practice, especially the use of drugs or alcohol.

**Addison, Thomas** (1793–1860). English physician who gave the classic description of pernicious anemia and contributed to knowledge of the ductless glands.

**adenitis** (ad-eh-nigh′tis). Inflammation of the glands.

**adenoid** (ad′uh-noyd). Means glandlike; in the plural it refers to a tonsil-like growth in the small lymph nodes in the back of the nasal passage where it joins the throat.

**adenoma** (ad-eh-no′mah). A glandlike growth, usually a benign neoplasm. If malignant, is is called *adenocarcinoma.*

**adhesion** (ad-hee′zhun). 1. Union of two surfaces abnormally; any fibrous band which connects them. 2. In dentistry, the force which holds upper dentures in place without vacuum chambers.

**adipose** (ad′eh-pose). Fatty.

**adolescence** (ad-uh-less′ns). The period between puberty and adulthood.

**adrenal** (ad-ree′nl) **gland.** A small gland located just above the kidney. Its secretions affect the function of glands and organs in many important ways. See **cortisone, ACTH.**

**adrenaline** (uhd-ren′uh-lin). See **epinephrine.**

**adulterate** (uh-duhlt′er-ate). To add one substance to another for the purpose of cheapening or weakening it.

**aerobe** (air′obe). A germ which needs air or oxygen to live.

**aerosol** (air′o-sol). A spray for the purpose of sterilizing the air of a room, or an atomized solution to be inhaled.

**Aesculapius** (es-kuh-lay′pi-uhs). The god of medicine of Greek mythology, son of Apollo, known for his powers of healing.

**afferent** (af′er-ent) **nerves.** Those which carry impulses to the brain or spinal cord from other parts of the body.

**afterbirth** (af′ter-berth). The special tissues associated with the development of a baby, such as the placenta, which are expelled after the birth of the baby.

**agalactia** (ah-gah-lak′she-ah). Failure to produce milk after the birth of a child.

**agar** (ag′ar). A gelatinous substance extracted from seaweed and used to treat constipation. It is also used for growing bacteria and other microorganisms.

**agglutination** (ah-gloo-tin-ay′shun). Clumping; the drawing together of bacteria suspended in fluid when a serum is used against them.

**agranulocytosis** (ah-gran-yoo-lo-sigh-to′sis). Decrease in the number of granular white cells in the blood. It is often accompanied by ulcerlike sores in the throat and other mucous membranes and sometimes follows use of sulfonamides or other drugs, such as Pyramidon.

**ague** (ay′gyoo). Malarial fever; any chill.

**albino** (al-bigh′no). A person with little or no pigment in skin, hair, and eyes.

**albumin** (al-byoo′min). A protein commonly found in plants and animals and in the white of eggs. Its presence in urine (albuminuria) may be associated with disease.

**alcoholism** (al′ko-hol-izm). Poisoning with alcohol.
  **chronic alcoholism.** Unhealthy conditions chiefly in the nervous and digestive systems caused by habitual use of alcohol in poisonous amounts.

**alimentary** (al-uh-men′tuh-ri). Relating to food.

**alkali** (al′kuh-ligh). Opposite of acid; capable of neutralizing acids. The chief one in the body is sodium bicarbonate.

**allergy** (al′er-ji). Hypersensitivity to one or more specific substances, usually protein. Hives, rash, or cold-like symptoms may result from exposure to the substance. Hay fever is one example of allergic diseases.

**ambivalence** (am-biv′uh-lens). Having opposing feelings, such as love and hate, toward the same object.

**ameba** (uh-mee′buh). A one-celled animal, such as a protozoan, that moves by changing shape and flowing along. Amebic dysentery is caused by organisms of this type.

**ameboid** (uh-mee′boyd). Like an ameba in form or movement.

**amino** (uh-meen′o) **acid.** An organic acid containing nitrogen. Amino acids are used by the body in building muscle and other tissues. The essential amino acids which must be provided by eating protein foods are as follows:

| | |
|---|---|
| arginine | methionine |
| histidine | phenylalanine |
| isoleucine | threonine |
| leucine | tryptophane |
| lysine | valine |

Other important amino acids are alanine, cystine, glycine, serine, and tyrosine.

**ammonia** (uh-mohn′yuh), **aromatic spirits of.** An ammonia solution which is a stimulant when inhaled; used for reviving after fainting spells.

**amnesia** (am-nee′zhuh). Loss of memory.

**amniotic** (am-nee-ot′ik) **fluid.** The watery fluid surrounding the developing fetus.

**amputation** (am-pyoo-tay′shun). Cutting off.

**amylase** (am′il-ays). An enzyme which breaks down starch; found in saliva, pancreatic juice, etc.

**Amytal** (am′-i-tal). A proprietary name for a sedative similar in its action to phenobarbital.

**anaerobe** (an-air′obe). A germ that lives without air or free oxygen.

**analgesic** (an-al-jee′zik). Pain reliever.

**anaphylactic** (an-uh-figh-lak′tik) **shock.** A violent, possibly fatal attack caused by the injection of a substance to which the body has become sensitive from previous injection. Horse serum, which is used for tetanus antitoxin, sometimes causes this reaction.

**anatomy** (uh-nat′uh-mi). Body structure.

**ancylostomiasis** (an-sil-os-to-my′uh-sis). Hookworm disease.

**androgen** (an′dro-jen). A substance, usually a hormone, that produces male characteristics (see **testosterone**).

**androsterone** (an-dros′ter-ohn). A specific hormone that produces male characteristics. It is excreted in the urine.

**anemia** (uh-nee′mi-uh). Deficiency in the blood

brought about by a decrease in the number of red blood cells or in the hemoglobin of the blood.

**anesthesia** (an-uhs-thee′zhi-uh). Loss of feeling.

> **general anesthesia.** Loss of feeling in the entire body.

> **local anesthesia.** Loss of feeling limited to a particular area.

**anesthetic** (an-uhs-thet′ik). A substance used to produce anesthesia.

**aneurysm** (an′yoo-rizm). A blood-filled sac formed by an abnormal widening in a blood vessel.

**angina** (an-jigh′nuh). Any disease in which one gets a suffocating feeling.

> **angina pectoris** (pek′tuh-ris). Heart disease in which the patient suffers from suffocating contractions in the chest and pains radiating from the heart down the left arm.

> **Vincent's angina.** Trench mouth; a very contagious infection of the mouth.

**ankylosis** (ang-kil-o′sis). Stiffness of a joint.

**anomaly** (uh-nahm′uh-li). Any deviation from the usual, such as in location or shape.

**Anopheles** (uh-nof′el-eez) **mosquito.** The mosquito that carries the parasites that cause malaria.

**anorexia** (an-o-rek′si-uh). Loss of appetite.

**anoxia** (an-ahk′si-uh). Lack of oxygen in the body.

**Antabuse** (an′tuh-byoos). A substance used in treating alcoholism. It makes drinking unpleasant.

**antacid** (ant-ass′id). A substance that neutralizes acid.

**antepartum** (an-ti-par′tum). Before childbirth.

**anthrax** (an′thraks). A disease of cattle which can also occur in man either as a hard swelling of the skin or internally as infections of lungs, intestines, etc.

**antibiotic** (an-tigh-bigh-aht′ik). A substance produced by an organism that tends to inhibit the growth of other organisms. Usually refers to extracts of molds or bacteria, such as penicillin, streptomycin, Aureomycin, Terramycin.

**antibody** (an′teh-bod-ee). A type of substance formed in the body in immune or allergic persons. The antibody produced by each disease or antigen is different.

**anticoagulant** (an′tee-koh-ag′you-lant). A drug capable of slowing the clotting of blood.

**antidote** (an′ti-doht). A substance that can counteract the effects of poison.

**antigen** (an′ti-jen). A substance that induces the production of antibodies in the blood. It is usually a protein such as is found in germs or serum.

**antihistamine** (an-ti-his′tuh-min). A compound that counteracts the effects of histamine; used in various allergic conditions, such as hay fever, serum sickness, etc.

**antihypertensive** (an′tee-hy-per-ten′siv). A drug used to lower blood pressure.

**antipyretic** (an-ti-pigh-ret′ik). Relieving fever.

**antiscorbutic** (an-ti-skor-byoo′tik). Correcting or curing scurvy.

**antiseptic** (an-ti-sep′tik). A substance that prevents the growth of germs.

**antiserum** (an-ti-seer′um). Blood serum that contains antibodies; sometimes given to patients to help them fight disease; also used in diagnosis to identify bacteria from a patient by the anti-body-antigen reaction.

**antitoxin** (an-ti-tahk′sin). A substance produced in the body to act against a poison.

**anuria** (ah-nyoo′ri-uh). Scanty urine.

**anus** (ay′nuhs). Outer opening of the rectum through which feces are expelled.

**anvil** (an′vil). Also called "incus"; one of the small bones of the middle ear, important in transmitting sounds.

**anxiety** (ang-zy′i-tee). A feeling of apprehension, the source of which is not recognized.

**aorta** (ay-or′tuh). Largest artery of the body. It arises from the left ventricle of the heart, and branches from it carrying blood to all parts of the body.

**aphasia** (uh-fay′zhi-uh). Inability to speak due to brain damage. The voice box and other organs of speech may be uninjured.

**apnea** (ap-nee′uh). State of not breathing.

**apoplexy** (ap′uh-plek-si). A stroke producing paralysis and coma.

**appendicitis** (uh-pen-di-sigh′tis). Inflammation of the vermiform appendix, which is a worm-shaped projection from the large intestine on the right side of the body.

**aqueous** (ay′kwi-uhs) **humor.** The liquid which fills the anterior part of the eyeball.

**areola** (uh-ree′o-lah). 1. One of the spaces in tissue, such as those in the lung. 2. A pigmented ring around a central point, such as the nipple of the breast.

**Argyrol** (ahr′ji-rohl). A proprietary antiseptic for gonorrhea and eye inflammations; it is a compound of silver and protein.

**arrhythmia** (ah-rith'mi-uh). Variation from the normal rhythm of the heart beat.

**arsenical** (ar-sen'ik-uhl). Compounds which contain arsenic. Before the discovery of antibiotics they were the best treatment for syphilis. Arsphenamine (Salvarsan) is one.

**arteriole** (ar-tee'ree-ohl). A minute artery leading into the capillaries.

**arteriosclerosis** (ahr-tee-ri-o-skle-ro'sis). Hardening of the arteries; a condition in which the walls of the arteries thicken and lose elasticity. See also *atherosclerosis*.

**artery** (ahr'ter-i). Blood vessel that carries blood away from the heart to other parts of the body.

**arthritis** (ahr-thrigh'tis). Inflammation or pain in the joints.

**articulate** (ahr-tik'yoo-lit). Jointed.

**ascites** (ah-sigh'teez). Accumulation of fluid in the abdomen.

**ascorbic** (as-kawrb'ik) **acid.** Vitamin C; a substance found in fruit, such as oranges and lemons. It is needed by the body to prevent scurvy.

**aseptic** (uh-sep'tik). Free from poisonous material or germs.

**asphyxia** (as-fik'si-uh). Suffocation from lack of air or from breathing carbon monoxide.

**aspirator** (as'pi-ray-tor). Device for removing liquids from the lungs or other body cavities.

**aspirin** (as'pi-rin). Acetylsalicylic acid; a relatively harmless drug used to relieve pain and reduce fever.

**assimilation** (uh-sim-il-ay'shun). Process in which the body transforms digested food into tissues.

**astigmatism** (uh-stig'muh-tizm). Inability to focus the eye properly because of an irregularity in one of the surfaces of the eye.

**astringent** (uhs-trin'jent). Causing contraction. Such substances are used to lessen secretions or to stop bleeding.

**Atabrine** (at'uh-breen). A proprietary name for a medicine used to treat malaria; developed when quinine was scarce.

**atherosclerosis** (ath-er-o-scle-ro'sis). The most common and serious form of arteriosclerosis, in which fatty and other substances collect in the inner lining of arteries, forming plaques that encroach upon the passageway and gradually obstruct the flow of blood.

**athlete's** (ath'leets) **foot.** Fungal infection of the foot in which small sores and cracks appear on the skin, particularly between the toes.

**atrophy** (at'ruh-fi). Reduction in size; wasting.

**atropine** (at'ro-peen). A medicine used to relax muscles of the intestines, lungs, and other internal organs. Also used for dilating the pupil of the eye.

**Auenbrugger** (ow-en-broog'er), **Leopold Joseph** (1722–1809). Austrian physician who was the first to use percussion of the chest as an aid in diagnosis.

**aura** (aw'ruh). Sensation which precedes an epileptic attack.

**audiology** (aw"de-ol'o-je). The science of hearing.

**audiometry** (aw"de-om'e-tre). The measurement of hearing acuity for the various frequencies of sound waves.

**Aureomycin** (aw-ree-o-migh'sin). A proprietary name for an antibiotic produced from the fungus *Streptomyces*. It is active against many bacterial and viral infections. It can clear up some staphylococcal and streptococcal infections that resist penicillin. Bad side effects are relatively rare.

**auricle** (aw'reh-kl). Means earlike; in the heart it refers to either of the two upper chambers which receive blood from the veins.

**autoimmune disease** (aw"to-i-mun'). Disease in which the body is unable to distinguish between foreign invaders and its own tissues so it produces defensive antibodies against itself, often with serious harm.

**autonomic** (aw-to-nom'ik) **nervous system.** That part of the nervous system that controls organs not consciously controlled, such as blood vessels, glands, and digestive organs.

**autopsy** (aw'tahp-si). Examination of a body after death.

**avitaminosis** (ay-vigh-tuh-min-o'sis). Disease due to lack of vitamins.

**axilla** (ak-sil'uh). Armpit.

# B

**B complex.** A group of water-soluble vitamins which occur together in nature. Some of them are essential for health, the most important being niacin, riboflavin, and thiamin.

**Babinski's** (bah-bin'skee) **reflex.** The automatic extension of the toes when the sole of the foot is stroked, a sign of a certain type of brain injury.

**bacillus** (buh-sil'uhs). One of a group of rod-shaped bacteria. Some examples are:

Typhoid bacillus. Cause of typhoid fever.

Tubercle bacillus. Cause of tuberculosis.

*Bacillus diphtheria.* Cause of diphtheria.

*Bacillus leprae.* Cause of leprosy (Hansen's disease).

*Bacillus pertussis.* Cause of whooping cough.

Shiga's bacillus. Cause of a type of dysentery and summer diarrhea of infants.

**bacitracin** (bas-eh-tray'sin). An antibiotic from Bacillus subtilis. It is active against infections of cocci and other bacteria and is used on skin infections. It is too toxic for internal use.

**bacteremia** (bak-ter-ee'mi-uh). Presence of bacteria in the blood.

**bactericidal** (bak-ter-eh-sigh'dl). Causing the death of bacteria.

**bacteriological** (bak-te-ree-o-log'ikl). Pertaining to the study of bacteria.

**bacteriolysin** (bak-te-ree-ol'is-in). Substance which dissolves bacteria.

**bacteriophage** (bak-te'ree-o-fayj). A specific type of ultramicroscopic agent which destroys bacteria.

**bacterium** (bak-te'ree-um), pl. **bacteria.** Germ; one-celled organism not visible without the aid of the microscope. Some cause diseases.

**bag of water.** Amnion; the sac in which the fetus and its surrounding fluid are held.

**baker's itch.** Irritation on the hands caused by yeast.

**baker's leg.** Knock-knee.

**BAL.** Abbreviation for British Anti-Lewisite; an antidote for metallic poisons such as arsenic and mercury.

**balm** (bahm). A soothing medicine.

**balneotherapy** (bahl-nee-o-thair'uh-pi). Treatment of disease with baths.

**bandage** (ban'dij). Gauze or other material used to wrap or cover a wound or part of the body.

**abdominal bandage.** A wide support worn around the hips for support, sometimes used in pregnancy.

**elastic bandage.** Rubber bandage used to provide constant pressure on an area; used for sprains to prevent swelling.

**bank.** Place, usually in a hospital, where reserve stocks of body fluids or parts are kept.

**eye bank.** Reserve stock of corneas used for corneal transplants.

**Banting, Frederick G.** (1891–1941) and **Charles H. Best** (b. 1899). Canadian researchers who isolated insulin from the pancreas and used it in treating diabetic patients.

**barber's itch.** Infection of the hair follicles on the face. One type which is caused by the streptococcus produces a burning, itchy area on the face, may even develop pus-filled swellings. Another type is a ringworm infection which causes itching on the lower part of the jaw.

**barbiturates** (bar-bit'yoor-ayts). A group of compounds which act as sedatives, hypnotics or sleep inducers. Phenobarbital is one of the most common.

**barium** (bair'i-um). A metallic element. It does not permit the passage of x-rays and so is often given to patients being x-rayed to make the organ being observed stand out on the film.

**barium meal.** Milk containing a barium compound which is swallowed before an x-ray of the digestive tract.

**barium enema.** Injection of fluid containing a barium compound into the anus for x-rays of the rectum or intestines.

**barley** (bahr'li) **water.** Water in which barley has been boiled. It is used in treating diarrhea in children.

**Barton, Clara** (1821–1912). American nurse who tended soldiers during the Civil War and was influential in founding the Red Cross, of which she was first president.

**basal metabolism** (bay'sl meh-tab'o-lizm) **test.** A test for thyroid activity. It depends upon the amount of energy the body uses when at rest. The oxygen intake is measured.

**base.** Alkali; a substance capable of neutralizing acid.

**base plate.** Trial plate for artificial dentures.

**basophil** (bay'so-fil). A body cell that stains with alkaline dyes.

**basophobia** (bay-so-fo'bi-uh). Fear of walking or standing erect.

**bath, alcohol.** Sponging the body with dilute alcohol, sometimes used to reduce fever.

**mustard bath.** Bath with mustard added to the water.

**bayonet** (bay'uh-net) **leg.** Condition in which the

knee joint is immovable.

**BCG.** Abbreviation for bacillus of Calmette and Guerin; an organism which is used in a vaccine for producing immunity to tuberculosis.

**Beaumont** (bo'mont), **William** (1785–1853). American army surgeon who described the digestive process. He observed the gastric fluids and food changes in Alexis St. Martin, a Canadian who had a gastric fistula from a gunshot wound.

**bedpan.** Shallow vessel of suitable shape in which a patient can urinate or defecate in bed.

**bedsore** (bed'sor). Ulcerlike sore which is caused by the pressure of the patient's body against the bed; decubitus ulcer.

**beef tea.** Water in which lean beef has soaked or in which beef extracts are dissolved.

**behaviorism** (bi-hayv'yer-izm). A theory that attempts to explain human emotional reactions.

**belching** (belch'ing). Raising gas.

**belladonna** (bel-uh-dahn'uh). A poisonous substance obtained from a plant called the deadly nightshade. Atropine is the active alkaloid in belladonna. In proper dosages, belladonna and atropine are useful medicines.

**Benadryl** (ben'uh-dril). A proprietary name for an antihistamine used in treating allergic reactions.

**bends.** Caisson disease.

**benign** (bi-nighn'). Not recurrent, harmless.

**Benzedrine** (ben'zuh-dreen). A proprietary name for a compound having stimulating properties; also used in nose sprays and inhalants.

**benzidine** (ben'zi-deen) **test.** A test used to determine whether blood is present in feces, urine, or other material.

**beriberi** (behr'i-behr'i). A disease resulting from lack of vitamin $B_1$ (thiamin) in the diet.

**Bernard** (ber-nar'), **Claude** (1813–1878). French physiologist who made many important discoveries about the liver, the pancreas, and the sympathetic nervous system.

**bicarbonate** (bigh-kar'bo-nuht). A substance which tends to neutralize the effects of both acids and bases found in the blood.

> **bicarbonate of soda.** Common compound useful for minor digestive upsets.

**biceps** (bigh'seps). Muscle of either the upper arm or thigh.

**bichloride of mercury** (bigh-klo'righd uv mer'kyoo-ri).

Germicide; highly toxic if swallowed.

**bicuspid** (bigh-kuhs'pid). A tooth having two "prongs" or cusps. There are normally eight in the mouth, two on each side of both jaws between the canines and the molars.

**bifocal** (bigh-fo'kl) **spectacles.** Spectacles which have two lenses cemented together, the lower one for reading or close vision, and the upper one for distance.

**bifurcation** (bigh-fer-kay'shun). Division into two parts.

**bile.** Bitter fluid secreted by the liver. It aids in digesting food. The yellow bile secreted by the liver is stored in the gallbladder, where it becomes dark (black bile).

**biliousness** (bil'yuhs-ness). Type of indigestion believed to be caused by an excess of bile.

**bilirubin** (bil-ee-roo'bin). Brownish substance in bile. It is found in the urine and blood in cases of jaundice.

**Binet** (bin-ay') **test.** Method of testing mental capacity.

**binocular** (bin-ahk'yuh-ler) **vision.** Seeing with the use of both eyes.

**biology** (bigh-ahl'uh-ji). The study of living things.

**biopsy** (bigh'op-si). Removal of a piece of tissue to be examined microscopically for diagnosis.

**biparous** (bip'uh-ruhs). Producing two children at one birth.

**birth control.** Prevention or regulation of conception.

**birthmark.** A colored area, a mole, or a slightly raised portion of skin which is present on the body at birth.

**bisexual** (bigh-seks'yoo-uhl). Having characteristics of both male and female.

**black death.** Bubonic plague; so called because of the dark appearance of the skin from numerous hemorrhages.

**blackhead.** A pustule formed around a skin pore plugged with fat secreted by the oil glands.

**black widow, black-widow spider.** A spider whose bite is poisonous though rarely fatal. The variety found in eastern United States has a characteristic red hourglass on its lower side.

**bladder** (blad'er). Sac which holds urine.

**blastomycosis** (blas-toh-migh-ko'sis). A disease caused by a fungus. It usually affects the lungs but may involve the whole system.

**bleb.** Raised area on the skin; blister.

**bleeding time.** Time required for bleeding from a skin prick to stop; normally 1 to 5 minutes.

**blind spot.** The spot where the optic nerve enters the retina. This area of the eye is not sensitive to light.

**blister** (blis'ter). Collection of fluid in the skin causing a raised area.

> **blood blister.** Blister containing blood.
>
> **fever blister.** Sore on the lips caused by a virus (*Herpes simplex*).

**bloat.** Puffiness, caused by accumulation of gas or fluid.

**block, nerve.** A form of local anesthetic in which nerve impulses are interrupted by injection of a drug.

**blood corpuscle** (kawr'puhsl). A blood cell, either a red cell (erythrocyte) or a white cell (leukocyte).

**blood count.** The number of red cells and white cells in a standard volume of blood. Normally there are about 4.2 to 5.5 million red cells and 5000 to 10,000 white cells per cubic millimeter.

**blood donor** (doh'ner). One who gives blood to be used for blood transfusions.

**blood plasma** (plaz'muh). The liquid part of the blood after the cells have been removed.

**blood poisoning.** Infection in the blood. It may be carried through the blood to all parts of the body.

**blood pressure.** The force of the blood in the blood vessels. It is measured by a sphygmomanometer, which consists of a cuff into which air can be pumped, and a pressure gauge. Pressure readings are made during both the systolic and diastolic phases of the heartbeat.

**blood serum** (seer'um). The fluid which separates from clotted blood.

**blood shot.** Suffused with blood.

**blood type.** Hereditary factors in the blood, e.g., A, B, AB, or O. It is important to determine the blood types of both donor and patient before a blood transfusion, as certain combinations cause agglutination of the blood cells. When blood is typed it is also tested for the Rh factor, another hereditary factor important in blood transfusion.

**blood vessel.** An artery or vein.

**blue baby.** A baby born with a malformation of the heart. The blue color results from lack of oxygen in the blood.

**boil.** Furuncle; a round, tender, pus-filled, raised area on the skin, caused by bacterial infection, usually staphylococci.

**booster shot.** Injection of a vaccine to reinforce an immunity obtained from previous vaccine injections.

**boric** (boh'rik) **acid.** A white powder which is used in skin ointments and in water solution as a mild antiseptic.

**botulism** (baht'yoo-lizm). Highly fatal food poisoning from improperly canned food. It is caused by bacteria that grow in the absence of air and produce poison. Symptoms are headache, weakness, constipation, and paralysis. The poison is easily destroyed by boiling.

**bowel** (bow'el). Intestine.

**brachial** (bray'ki-al). Relating to the arm.

**Braille** (brayl) **system.** Method of printing words by using raised dots which the blind can "read" by touching with the finger tips.

**brain waves.** Electric impulses given off by the brain. Various patterns are associated with abnormal conditions.

**breakbone** (brayk'bohn) **fever.** Dengue.

**breast, broken.** Abscess on the breast.

**breast, chicken.** Malformation in which the breastbone is very prominent. It may result from rickets. Also called pigeon breast.

**breast, funnel.** A hollow at the lower part of the breastbone.

**breast pump.** Device to empty milk from the breast.

**breech presentation.** Birth of a baby with the buttocks first.

**bridge.** A device for replacing one or more missing teeth. It is held in place by being fastened to the adjoining natural teeth.

**Bright's disease.** Nephritis; a chronic disease of the kidneys. It is named for Richard Bright (1789–1858), the English physician who described this condition.

**bromide** (bro'mighd). Compound of bromine. Some are used as sedatives and pain relievers.

**bronchiole** (brahng'ki-ohl). Small air tube in the lung, a subdivision of the bronchus.

**bronchitis** (brahn-kigh'tis). Inflammation of the bronchi.

**bronchodilator** (brong"ko-di-la'tor). Any substance that will dilate the bronchi.

**bronchopneumonia** (brahng-ko-noo-mo'ni-uh). Inflammation of the bronchioles and lung tissue caused by bacterial infection.

**bronchoscope** (brahng'kuh-skohp). Tubelike instrument containing a light which can be inserted through the mouth down into the bronchi in order to examine them.

**bronchotomy** (brahng-kaht′uh-mi). Cutting into the trachea or a bronchus.

**bronchus** (brahng′kuhs), pl. **bronchi**. One of the two main branches of the windpipe (trachea).

**brush burn**. Injury caused by friction of a rapidly moving object.

**bubo** (byoo′boh). A painful swelling in a lymphatic gland, usually one in the groin or under the arm.

**buboes** (byoo′bohs). Leishmaniasis; a disease caused by protozoa spread by flies. Found in Asia and So. America.

**bubonic** (byoo-bahn′ik) **plague**. Infectious disease caused by bacteria spread by rat fleas.

**Bufferin** (buf′er-in). A proprietary name for an aspirin preparation containing an alkaline buffer to neutralize stomach acidity.

**bulbar** (buhl′bar). Pertaining to the lower part of the brainstem.

**bulla** (boo′la). A large bleb or blister.

**bunion** (buhn′yun). A swelling at the first joint of the great toe.

**bursa** (ber′suh). Small fluid-filled sac in the joints which helps cushion the bones against friction.

**bursitis** (ber-sigh′tis). Inflammation of a bursa. Movement of the joint affected is very painful in this condition.

**Butazolidin** (byoo-tuh-zol′-i-din). A proprietary medicine sometimes used in the treatment of arthritis.

**butterfly patch**. The characteristic mark on the face in lupus erythematosus.

**butyn** (byoo′tin). A local anesthetic for the surface of the eye and mucous membranes.

## C

**caesarean** (see-zair′ri-un) **section**. Delivery of a baby by cutting through the abdominal wall.

**caffeine** (kaf′een). Stimulant found in coffee and tea.

**caisson** (kay′sn) **disease**. Paralytic disease of people who work in caissons under high air pressure. The condition occurs when workers are brought into normal pressure areas too quickly, and bubbles of nitrogen form in the blood. Also called the bends.

**calamine** (kal′uh-mighn) **lotion**. A zinc oxide compound used to treat skin diseases and irritations.

**calcaneus** (kal-kay′ni-uhs). Heel bone.

**calcareous** (kal-kair′i-uhs). Containing lime; chalky.

**calcification** (kal-si-fi-kay′shun). Hardening due to calcium deposits.

**calcium** (kal′si-um). A chemical element which is the main material in bone and teeth and is also necessary for normal functioning of heart and other muscles.

**calculus** (kal′kyuh-luhs), pl. **calculi**. A stony mass in the gallbladder, kidney, or urinary bladder.

**callus** (kal′uhs). 1. Area where the skin has thickened and become hard, often as a result of friction. 2. The substance which forms around a broken bone that is starting to heal.

**calomel** (kal′o-mel). A mercury compound which acts as a purge.

**calorie** (kal′uh-ri). Measure of heat or energy, therefore a measure of the fattening properties of a foodstuff.

**cancer** (kan′ser). Malignant tumor; uncontrolled growth of cells which are usually larger and more like embryonic cells than the normal cells of the affected tissue.

**canine** (kay′nighn) **tooth**. The sharply pointed tooth located between the incisors and the premolars.

**canker** (kang′ker). Ulcerlike sore in the mouth or on the lips.

**capillary** (kap′i-lehr-i). Very small blood vessel.

**carbohydrate** (kahr-bo-high′drayt). A class of energy foods which includes sugars and starches.

**carbolic** (kahr-bahl′ik) **acid**. Phenol; a disinfectant.

**carbuncle** (kahr′buhng-kl). A hard pus-filled painful inflammation. It is similar to a boil but it is larger and has several openings.

**carcinogen** (kahr-sin′o-jen). A substance which can cause cancer.

**carcinoma** (kahr-si-no′muh). A cancer which started from epithelial cells (skin or mucous membranes).

**cardiogram** (kahr′di-o-gram). Tracing which shows the movements of the heart.

**cardiovascular** (kahr-di-o-vas′kyoo-lar). Pertaining to the heart and blood vessels.

**cardioverter** (kahr-di-o-ver′ter). Any device that will shock the heart into action.

**carditis** (kahr-di′tis). Inflammation of the heart.

**caries** (kair′eez). Decay in teeth or bone.

**carotene** (kair′o-teen). A pigment relating to vitamin A and found in carrots.

**carotid** (kuh-raht′id) **arteries**. Arteries of the neck.

**carpal** (kahr'pl) **bones.** Bones of the wrist.

**carrier** (ka'ri-er). Person who has germs of a disease in his body but does not show symptoms of the disease.

**cartilage** (kahr'ti-lij). Gristle; white elastic tissue found around joints and forming the tip of the nose and the outer ear.

**cascara** (kas-kair'uh). A laxative or cathartic made from the dried bark of certain shrubs.

**caseous** (kay'si-uhs). Resembling cheese.

**castor** (kas'ter) **oil.** Oil obtained from a type of poisonous bean plant. It has a cathartic action.

**castration** (kas-tray'shun). Removal of the testicles or ovaries.

**casts** (kasts). Material which has hardened in body cavities and taken the shape of them. They are observed in the urine or other discharges in certain diseases.

**catalepsy** (kat'uh-lep-si). A nervous condition in which the person goes into a trance and may not change position for an indefinite time.

**cataract** (kat'uh-rakt). Cloudiness in the eye lens.

**catarrh** (kuh-tahr'). Inflammation in nose or other mucous membranes accompanied by discharge of a great deal of mucus.

**catatonic** (kat-uh-tahn'ik). Relating to a behavior disturbance characterized by catalepsy (*q.v.*), and found most commonly in schizophrenia.

**catgut** (kat'guht). Thread or string prepared from sheep's intestines, used in surgery.

**cathartic** (kuh-thahr'tik). A substance that rapidly causes the bowels to move.

**catheter** (kath'i-ter). A tubelike instrument which is used for draining fluids from body cavities, such as the bladder.

**cauliflower** (kaw'li-flau-er) **ear.** A thickened and deformed ear seen in boxers. It is caused by the accumulation of fluid and blood clots in the tissue following injury.

**cauterize** (kaw'ter-ighz). To apply burning or caustic substances or instruments.

**cecum** (see'kum). Sac of the large intestine located where the large and small intestines join.

**cell** (sel). Structural unit of life consisting of a mass of jellylike protoplasm containing a nucleus and surrounded by a membrane.

**cellulose** (sel'yoo-lohs). Starchy material in plant cells.

**cementum** (see-men'tum). The thin hard outer layer of a tooth below the gum, bony in structure.

**cerebellum** (sehr-uh-bel'um). The part of the brain which coordinates movements.

**cerebral cortex** (sehr'uh-brl kawr'teks). Outer layer of the brain.

**cerebral palsy** (sehr'uh-brl pawl'zi). Partial paralysis and lack of muscle coordination caused by brain injury.

**cerebrum** (sehr'uh-brum). The main part of the brain. It is concerned with thinking, feeling, and voluntary activities.

**cerumen** (si-roo'men). Earwax.

**cervix** (ser'viks). The narrow lower part of the uterus.

**cesarean section.** See **caesarean section.**

**chalazion** (kuh-lay'zi-un). Tumor on the eyelid caused by an infection of a sebaceous (oil) gland.

**chancre** (shang'ker). The sore that is the first sign of syphilis. It starts as a papule which breaks down into a reddish ulcer.

**chancroid** (shang'kroid). A soft nonsyphilitic sore in the genital area. It is caused by bacteria and spread by sexual contact.

**charleyhorse** (char'lee-hors). Soreness or stiffness of a muscle often resulting from athletics.

**chaulmoogra** (chaw-moo'gruh) **oil.** Oil used in treating leprosy.

**chigger** (chig'er). Larva of an insect which attaches itself to the skin causing the area to become itchy and inflamed.

**chilblain** (chil'blayn). Painful swelling of toes and feet from exposure to cold.

**chloramphenicol** (klo-ram-fen'ikl). An antibiotic from a streptomyces fungus. It is active against bacterial and viral diseases, such as typhus, undulant fever, typhoid, and viral pneumonia.

**chlorination** (klo-rin-ay'shun). Addition of chlorine to water or sewage to kill germs.

**chloroform** (klo'ruh-fawrm). Substance used as an anesthetic, a counterirritant, and an antispasmodic.

**Chloromycetin** (klo-ro-migh'suh-tin). A proprietary name of chloramphenicol.

**chlorophyll** (klo'ruh-fil). The green coloring matter in plants.

**chloroquines** (klor'oh-kwighns). A group of medicines sometimes prescribed in the treatment of rheumatoid arthritis.

**Chlor-Trimeton** (klor-trigh'muh-ton). A proprietary

antihistamine, often used to relieve the symptoms of colds and allergies.

cholera (kahl'er-uh). An epidemic disease, often fatal, spread through polluted water. The symptoms are vomiting, diarrhea, great thirst, and cramps.

cholesterol (ko-les'tuh-rohl). A fatlike substance found in all animal fats and oils as well as in the brain and blood. This substance is deposited in the walls of blood vessels in one type of hardening of the arteries, and it is also the principal material in gallstones.

chorea (ko-ree'uh). A nervous disease in which there are involuntary jerking movements of the body; St. Vitus's dance. See also **Huntington's chorea.**

chorion (ko'ree-on). The outer covering of the developing ovum. It protects and nourishes it and later becomes the placenta.

chromatin (kro'muh-tin). Substance in the cell nucleus that stains very darkly.

chromosome (kroh'muh-sohm). One of the rod-shaped bodies in the nucleus of a dividing cell which carries the hereditary factors (genes). In man there are 48 in each cell (except the spermatozoa and ova).

chronic (krahn'ik). Long continued.

chyle (kighl). Milklike fluid formed in the small intestine during digestion of fat.

chyme (kighm). Digested food in the stomach.

cilia (sil'i-uh). Fine hairs, such as the eyelashes and the hairs in the nose, which filter out dust.

ciliary (sil'i-er-i) body. A structure in the eyeball which is formed of the ciliary muscle and the ciliary processes. The ciliary muscle controls the curvature of the eyeball. The ciliary processes secrete nutrient fluids into the eye.

cinchona (sin-ko'nuh). Bark of the cinchona tree from which quinine is prepared.

circumcision (ser-km-sizh'un). Removal of the foreskin of the penis.

cirrhosis (si-ro'sis). Chronic inflammation of an organ. In the liver the disease is marked by degeneration of the liver cells and thickening of the surrounding tissue.

claustrophobia (klaws-troh-fo'bi-uh). Fear of being in a small closed place.

clavacin (klah'vuh-sin). Patulin; an antibiotic from fungi, active against many bacteria but too poisonous for medicinal purposes.

clavicle (klav'ikl). The collarbone.

cleft palate (kleft pal'it). Congenital groove in the roof of the mouth due to failure of the palate bones to unite. Harelip is often present in persons with cleft palate.

climacteric (kligh-mak-ter'ik). Menopause.

clinic (klin'ik). 1. An institution where patients not needing hospital care are treated. 2. An institution where several doctors working together study and treat patients.

clitoris (kli'to-ris). A small body at the front of the vulva. It is the female organ analogous to the penis in the male.

clonus (klo'nuhs). Spasm; muscles alternately tense and relax.

clostridium (klaws-trid'i-um). A type of bacteria. One member of the group causes tetanus (lockjaw), another causes botulism.

clot (klot). A coagulate; a soft semisolid jellylike mass formed from a liquid, such as blood or lymph.

cloves, oil of. Oily liquid used for temporary relief of toothache; also used as an antiseptic in dental work.

clubfoot. Talipes; a congenitally deformed foot. The bones are twisted causing the person to walk abnormally.

coagulation (ko-ag-yoo-lay'shun). Formation of a semisolid mass from a liquid, such as blood or lymph.

cocaine (ko-kayn'). Local anesthetic; narcotic.

coccidioidomycosis (kahk-sid-i-oi-doh-migh-ko'sis). Valley fever; fungal disease usually involving the lungs. It is found in the southwestern part of the United States.

coccus (kahk'uhs). Spherical shaped bacterium.

coccyx (kahk'siks). The bone at the lower end of the spinal column.

cochlea (kahk'li-uh). The snail-shaped tube of the ear which contains the organs of hearing.

codeine (ko'dee-in). A pain-reliever milder than morphine.

cod liver oil. An oil containing vitamin D. It is used in treating rickets.

coitus (ko'it-us). Sexual intercourse.

cold sore. Fever blister.

colic (kahl'ik). Pain and spasm in the abdomen.

colitis (ko-light'is). Inflammation of the colon.

**mucous colitis.** A condition usually associated with nervousness and worry, and marked by passage of mucus from the bowel.

**ulcerative colitis.** More serious condition, characterized by ulcers (open sores).

**colon** (ko'lon). Large intestine into which the small intestine empties. It ends in the rectum. Final stages of digestive process occur here.

**color blindness.** Inability to identify colors.

**colostomy** (ko-lahs'toh-mi). Formation of an artificial anus.

**colostrum** (ko-lahs'trum). The "first milk" which is formed in the breast.

**coma** (ko'muh). Stupor from which one cannot be aroused.

**comedo** (kom'e-do). A blackhead.

**communicable** (kuh-myoo'ni-kuh-bl) **disease.** One that can be spread from one person to another either by direct contact or by articles soiled by the sick person.

**Compazine** (kom'pa-zeen). A proprietary sedative and antinauseant. In small doses, it can control vomiting in children.

**complement-fixation** (kahm'pluh-ment fik-say'shun) **test.** A type of diagnostic blood test used to diagnose many different diseases, such as syphilis.

**complex** (kahm'pleks). In psychiatry it refers to a condition in which repressed ideas and desires influence personality.

**compound fracture** (kahm'pound frak'cher). A broken bone which has punctured the skin.

**compress** (kahm'pres). Material such as folded gauze applied as a dressing or used to produce pressure on a wound.

**concussion** (kon-kuhsh'n). Brain injury caused by a violent jar or blow.

**cone** (kohn). One of the parts of the retina that is sensitive to light.

**congenital** (kon-jen'it-l). Existing at birth.

**conjunctiva** (kon-juhngk-ti'vuh). Membrane which covers the front of the eyeball and lines the eyelid.

**conjunctivitis** (kon-juhngk-ti-vigh'tis). Inflammation of the conjunctiva.

**connective tissue** (kon-nek'tiv tish'yoo). Tissue which binds parts of the body together, such as bone, cartilage, fat, and fascia.

**constipation** (kon-sti-pay'shun). Condition in which the bowels move less often than usual and with difficulty.

**consumption** (kon-suhmp'shun). Tuberculosis of the lungs.

**contact lenses.** Corrective lenses which fit over the eyeball under the eyelid.

**contagious** (kon-tay'jus). Spread by personal contact or indirectly by articles used by a sick person.

**contraception** (kahn-truh-sep'shun). Prevention of pregnancy.

**contusion** (kon-too'zhun). Bruise.

**convalescence** (kahn-vuh-les'ns). The period of recovery after an illness.

**convulsion** (kon-vuhl'shun). An involuntary spasm.

**copulation** (kahp-yoo-lay'shun). Sexual intercourse.

**cornea** (kawr'ni-uh). Clear transparent outer layer on the front of the eyeball.

**corns.** Areas of thickened skin on the toes. They are usually caused by the pressure of ill-fitting shoes.

**coronary** (kahr'uh-nehr-i). Relating to the arteries which supply blood to the heart muscle.

**coronary thrombosis** (thrahm-bo'sis). Formation of a blood clot in the coronary artery, interfering with the blood supply to the heart muscle.

**coroner** (kahr'uh-ner). Official who examines cases of death due to unexplained causes.

**corpuscle** (kawr'puhs-l). A small mass; the red and white corpuscles are the cells in the blood.

**corpus luteum** (kawr'puhs loo'ti-um). A yellow body that forms in the ovary after an egg has been released. It secretes the hormone progesterone.

**Cort-Dome.** A proprietary medicine containing cortisone; sometimes prescribed for skin ailments.

**cortex** (kawr'teks). Outer layer.

**cortisone** (kawr'ti-zohn). Hormone produced by the adrenal cortex. It is used in treating certain diseases.

**coryza** (ko-righ'zuh). Cold in the head; a condition in which there is a large volume of mucus discharged in the nasal passages.

**counterirritant** (koun-ter-ir'i-tant). Substance applied to skin to produce inflammation which is believed to relieve underlying congestion.

**cowpox.** A viral disease of cattle which can be transmitted to humans. It is believed to be a mild form of smallpox, as immunity to both cowpox and smallpox results from an attack of cowpox or vaccination with the cowpox virus (vaccinia).

**cranial** (kray'ni-al) **nerve.** A nerve that attaches to the brain. The twelve pairs of cranial nerves are as follows:

I olfactory. Transmits the sense of smell.

II optic. Transmits the sense of sight.

III oculomotor. Moves the muscle of the eyeball in accommodation and controls the opening of the pupil.

IV trochlear. Controls movements of the eyeball.

V trigeminal. The sensory nerve of the face and the front of the scalp.

VI abducens. Controls a muscle of the eyeball.

VII facial. Moves muscles of the face, controls the salivary glands, and provides the sense of taste.

VIII acoustic. Transmits the sense of hearing and the head position.

IX glossopharyngeal. Controls muscles of the pharynx and provides sense of taste in the back part of the tongue.

X vagus. Sensory and motor nerve of the heart, esophagus, and stomach.

XI accessory. Controls muscles of larynx and pharynx and controls the muscle of the neck concerned with turning the head and raising the shoulder.

XII hypoglossal. Moves the tongue.

**cranium** (kray′ni-um). The skull.

**creosote** (kree′uh-soht). A strong antiseptic.

**curare** (koo-rah′ree). A substance obtained from poisonous plants, used to block nerve impulses and relax muscles. It is also used to prevent injury during convulsive treatments of mental patients.

**curettage** (kyoo-ret-tahzh′). Scraping out.

**Curie** (koo″ree′), **Pierre** (1859–1906) and **Marie** (1867–1934). French scientists who discovered radium.

**Cushing** (koosh′ing), **Harvey** (1869–1939). An American surgeon who greatly advanced neurosurgery and developed many important techniques of brain surgery.

**Cushing's syndrome** (sin′drohm). A group of symptoms including collection of fat in the face, abdomen, and buttocks, and caused by a tumor of the pituitary or adrenal gland.

**cuspid** (kuhs′pid). Tooth with a single point; canine tooth.

**cutaneous** (kyoo-tayn′i-uhs). Relating to the skin.

**cuticle** (kyoo′ti-kl). Outer layer of skin; dead skin, such as that at the base and sides of fingernails and toenails.

**cyanosis** (sigh-uh-no′sis). Condition in which the skin and mucous membranes are bluish from lack of oxygen in the blood.

**cyclopropane** (sigh-klo-pro′payn). An anesthetic gas especially useful when lung disease is present.

**cyst** (sist). A sac which contains gas, fluid, or a semisolid substance.

**cystine** (sis′teen). One of the amino acids.

**cystitis** (sis-tigh′tis). Inflammation of the bladder.

**cystoscopy** (sis-tahs′ko-pi). Examination of the interior of the urinary bladder.

**cytological** (sigh-toh-lahj′ikl) **smear.** A glass slide coated with material from the vagina, sputum, or other body material, in order to examine the material microscopically.

**cytoplasm** (sigh′toh-plazm). The contents of a cell not including the nucleus.

# D

**dandruff** (dan′druhf). White scales or flakes of dead skin on the scalp.

**Darvon** (dahr′vahn). A proprietary nonnarcotic pain reliever.

**Darwin** (dahr′win), **Charles Robert** (1809–1882). Originator of the theory of evolution.

**deaf-mute** (def-myoot). One who can neither hear nor speak.

**debility** (dib-il′it-i). Weakness.

**decalcification** (dee-kal-si-fi-kay′shun). Loss of calcium or calcified material in bone or teeth.

**decay** (dee-kay′). Gradual breakdown; rot.

**deciduous** (di-sij′oo-uhs) **teeth.** Temporary or baby teeth.

**decubitus** (di-kyoo′bit-uhs) **ulcer.** Bedsore.

**defecation** (def-i-kay′shun). Bowel movements.

**defibrillation** (de-fi′bri-la-shun). Stoppage of the fibrillation, or useless twitching, of the heart and the restoration of normal heart rhythm by use of drugs or an electrical current.

**defloration** (def-lo-ray′shun). Destruction of the hymen (the membrane over the vaginal opening), usually by sexual intercourse.

**dehydration** (dee-high-dray′shun). Loss or removal of water.

**delirium** (dee-leer′i-um). Mental disorder marked by excitement and illusions; may be caused by disease or drugs.

**delirium tremens** (tree′mens). Delirium in which

there is fumbling of the hands and insomnia. It is associated with alcohol poisoning, brain disease, or psychosis.

**delousing** (dee-lou'sing). Process of removing or destroying lice.

**deltoid** (del'toyd) **muscle.** The large triangular muscle over the shoulder joint.

**delusion** (di-loo'zhun). A false belief not conforming to the dictates of reason.

**dementia** (duh-men'shuh). Deterioration of the mind, especially with respect to reasoning, will power, and memory.

**dementia praecox** (pree'kahks). Schizophrenia.

**Demerol** (dem'er-ol). A proprietary medicine used as a sedative, pain reliever, and for relief from spasms.

**denatured alcohol.** Alcohol to which some substance has been added making it unfit to drink.

**dendrites** (den'drights). Threadlike parts of a nerve cell that carry impulses to the cell body.

**dengue** (deng'gay). An infectious disease found in tropical countries; symptoms are fever, severe headache, sore throat, and body pains. The disease, also known as breakbone fever and dandy fever, is caused by a virus carried by a species of mosquito.

**dental** (den'tl). Pertaining to teeth.

**dentifrice** (den'ti-fris). A substance for cleaning teeth.

**dentin** (den'tin). Calcified tissue forming major part of teeth.

**denture** (den'tyoor). Set of teeth.

**deodorant** (dee-o'dor-ant). Substance which destroys odors.

**depilatory** (dee-pil'uh-tor-i). Hair remover.

**depressant** (dee-pres'ent). A sedative; an agent which slows up a function.

**derma** (der'muh) or **dermis** (der'mis). The skin.

**dermatitis** (derm-uh-tigh'tis). Inflammation of the skin.

**dermatologist** (derm-uh-tahl'uh-jist). Physician who specializes in the treatment of diseases of the skin, hair, and scalp.

**dermatophobia** (der-mat-o-foh'bi-uh). Dread of having a skin disease.

**dermatophyte** (der-mat'o-fight). A mold or fungus that grows on the skin.

**desiccation** (des-i-kay'shun). Act of drying.

**detergent** (di-terj'nt). Cleansing agent.

**detrition** (dee-trish'un). Wearing away by rubbing or grinding.

**detritus** (dee-trigh'tus). Any broken-down material, such as tissues or tooth substance.

**Dexamyl** (dex'a-mil). A proprietary medicine used to control the appetite. It also is a stimulant for depressed moods.

**Dexedrine** (dex'i-drin). A proprietary medication used to reduce the appetite.

**dextrose** (deks'trohs). Grape sugar.

**diabetes insipidus** (digh-uh-bee'teez in-sip'id-us). A chronic disease characterized by the passing of large amounts of urine.

**diabetes mellitus** (digh-uh-bee'teez mel-light'us). A disease in which sugar is inadequately utilized by the body owing to lack of insulin.

**diagnose** (digh'ugh-nohs). To recognize a disease.

**Diamox** (die'a-mox). A proprietary diuretic medicine; used to increase the flow of urine in dropsy and other edematous conditions.

**diaphragm** (digh'uh-fram). The septum, or wall, between the chest and the abdomen.

**diarrhea** (digh-uh-ree'uh). Frequent and loose watery stools.

> **epidemic diarrhea.** An acute contagious disease of newborn infants.

**diastole** (digh-as'tuh-lee). The interval between heartbeats.

**Dick test.** Skin test for immunity to scarlet fever; redness indicates susceptibility.

**Dicumarol** (digh-koo'muh-rawl). A proprietary medicine from a substance isolated from spoiled sweet clover which interferes with blood clotting.

**diet** (digh'et). The food and drink needed for body nourishment.

**digestion** (digh-jes'chun). Process of preparing food for absorption.

**digit** (dij'it). Finger or toe.

**digitalis** (dij-i-tal'is or dij-i-tay'lis). A substance obtained from the leaves of foxglove and used as a heart stimulant.

**Dilantin** (digh-lan'tin). A proprietary medicine used to prevent epileptic seizures.

**dilation** (digh-lay'shun). Expansion of an organ, vessel, or the pupil of the eye.

**diplegia** (digh-plee'ji-uh). Paralysis of like parts on both sides of the body; bilateral paralysis.

**diplococcus** (dip-lo-kahk'us). A type of coccus

which occurs in pairs; includes the organism that causes pneumonia.

**diplopia** (dip-lo′pi-uh). Condition of seeing double.

**dipsomania** (dip-so-mayn′i-uh). Uncontrollable desire for alcoholic drink.

**disinfect** (dis-in-fekt′). Destroy disease-producing germs and substances.

**disk, vertebral** (ver′ti-brl). The pad of cartilage between the vertebrae.

**dislocation** (dis-lo-kay′shun). The separation of the parts of a joint.

**disorientation** (dis-o-ree-en-tay′shun). Mental confusion as to time, place, or identity of persons; loss of one's bearings.

**diuretic** (digh-yoo-ret′ik). Substance which increases the output of urine.

**Diuril** (dye′yoor-il). A proprietary diuretic medicine used by persons suffering from heart disease and other causes of edema. Also, used in treatment of high blood pressure.

**divergent strabismus** (digh-ver′jnt struh-biz′muhs). Eye condition in which the axes of the eyes diverge; walleye.

**diverticulum** (di-ver-tik′u-lum). A balloonlike pouch opening from an organ like the colon or esophagus.

**DNA, deoxyribonucleic acid** (dee-ox-ee-righ′boh-new-cle-ick). A chemical in the human cell that is important in controlling heredity.

**dominant trait** (dahm′in-ant trayt). Stronger of two competitive hereditary traits.

**Donnatal** (don′uh-tal). A proprietary medication to control the muscle spasms of colitis, stomach ulcers, and other ailments.

**donor** (don′er). Person who gives blood or tissue for use in another person.

**Doriden** (door′i-den). A frequently used proprietary sedative.

**dorsal** (dor′sl). Pertaining to the back.

**dose** (dohs). Measured amount of medicine to be taken at one time.

**douche** (doosh). Washing a body cavity with a stream of water.

**Down's syndrome** (downz). Mongolism, a congenital defect characterized by physical malformations and some degree of mental retardation.

**Dramamine** (dram′uh-meen). A proprietary antihistamine used to prevent motion sickness.

**dressing.** A sterile cloth to cover a wound.

**dropsy** (drahp′si). Condition in which fluid collects in the body.

**drug.** Any medicine.

**duct** (duhkt). A passage for fluids.

**ductless glands.** Endocrine glands.

**duodenum** (doo-uh-dee′nm). The part of the small intestine nearest the stomach.

**dura mater** (dyoor′uh mah′ter). Outermost layer covering the brain and spinal cord.

**dysentery** (dis′n-tehr″i). Inflammation of the large intestine resulting in diarrhea with passage of blood and mucus.

> **amebic dysentery.** Diarrhea caused by amebae. Spread by means of contaminated food and flies.

> **bacillary dysentery.** Disease marked by diarrhea and caused by bacteria (bacilli). Spread by means of contaminated food, flies, etc.

**dysmenorrhea** (dis-men-uh-ree′uh). Painful menstruation.

**dyspepsia** (dis-pep′si-uh). Indigestion.

**dysphagia** (dis-fay′juh). Difficulty in swallowing.

**dyspnea** (disp′nee-uh). Difficulty in breathing.

**dystrophy** (dis′troh-fee). Faulty nutrition.

> **progressive muscular dystrophy.** Disease in which muscles gradually weaken because of a breakdown in the muscle nerve endings (not in the spinal nerve endings).

**dysuria** (dis-yoo′ri-uh). Painful or difficult urination.

# E

**eardrum.** Tympanum; the membrane which separates the middle ear from the outer ear.

**eclampsia** (ek-lamp′si-uh). A convulsive attack during pregnancy caused by toxemia.

**ectoderm** (ek′toh-derm). Outer layer of the embryo.

**ectopic** (ek-tahp′ik). Not in the normal place; an ectopic pregnancy is one where the fetus develops outside the uterus.

**edema** (i-dee′muh). Swelling caused by collection in tissues of fluid which has escaped from the blood capillaries.

**efferent** (ef′er-ent) **nerves.** Those which carry impulses from the brain or spinal cord to other parts of the body.

**ego** (ee′goh). Self; especially the conscious mind.

**Ehrlich** (air′lik), **Paul** (1854–1915). German scientist, pioneer in immunology and in the use of chemicals in treating diseases. After 606 attempts, he obtained an arsenic compound (Salvarsan) effective against syphilis.

**ejaculation** (i-jak-yoo-lay′shun). Expulsion of semen from the penis in sexual intercourse.

**elective treatment.** Treatment helpful to the patient but not immediately necessary to save his life.

**electrocardiogram** (i-lek-troh-kahr′di-uh-gram). Graph of the electric current produced by the heart when contracting.

**electroencephalograph** (i-lek-troh-en-sef′uh-lo-graf). Instrument for recording brain waves.

**electrolysis** (i-lek-trahl′i-sis). Decomposition by means of electricity.

**electrolyte** (e-lek′tro-lite). A dissolved salt or alkali normally found in the blood and tissue fluids. Electrolytes play essential roles in the workings of cells and in maintaining fluid balance and normal acid-base balance.

**elephantiasis** (el-i-fan-tigh′uh-sis). Disease caused by the presence of a parasitic worm in the lymphatic system. It results in enlargement of parts of the body, such as a leg.

**elimination** (i-lim-in-ay′shun). Removal of wastes.

**elixir** (i-lik′ser). Sweetened and flavored medicine.

**emaciation** (i-may-shi-ay′shun). General loss of weight and wasting of the body.

**embolism** (em′buh-lizm). Obstruction of a blood vessel by a blood clot, air bubble, fat globule, or bacteria.

**embolus** (em′buh-luhs). Any material that blocks a blood vessel.

**embryo** (em′bri-oh). Fetus during its first three months of growth.

**emesis** (em′i-sis). Vomiting.

**emetic** (i-met′ik). Substance which induces vomiting.

**emetine** (em′i-tin). A medicine effective in treating acute amebic dysentery. It is injected under the skin or into a muscle.

**emission** (i-mish′n). Sudden discharge of fluid.
> **nocturnal emission.** Discharge of semen during sleep.

**emollient** (i-mahl′yent). A soothing medicine.

**empathy** (em′puh-thi). Feeling as if one were in another's place; deep understanding.

**emphysema** (em-figh-see′muh). Swelling of tissues from gas or air, particularly lung tissue.

**empyema** (em-pigh-ee′muh). Presence of pus in a body cavity, especially the lungs.

**emulsion** (i-muhl′shun). A suspension in liquid (usually water) of very fine particles such as oil droplets.

**enamel** (an-am′el). The hard shiny surface of teeth.

**encephalitis** (en-sef-uh-ligh′tis). Inflammation of the brain.
> **epidemic encephalitis.** Brain fever; a viral disease spread through domestic animals and insects. It causes languor, muscle weakness, and drowsiness.

**encephalogram** (en-sef′uh-lo-gram). X-ray of the brain.

**encephaloma** (en-sef-uh-lo′muh). Brain tumor, which may or may not be cancerous.

**encephalon** (en-sef′uh-lahn). The brain.

**endemic** (en-dem′ik). Referring to a disease which occurs fairly constantly in a locality.

**endocarditis** (en-doh-kahr-digh′tis). Inflammation of the heart lining.

**endocrine** (en′doh-krin) **gland.** One of the ductless glands which secrete directly into the bloodstream. The hormones produced by these glands stimulate and control growth, metabolism, and the digestive and reproductive systems. The endocrines include the thyroid, parathyroid, adrenal, pituitary, and thymus glands, and the ovaries and testicles.

**endoderm** (en′doh-derm′). Innermost layer of an embryo.

**endogenous** (en-dah′jen-us). Originating within an organism.

**endometrium** (en-doh-mee′tri-um). Mucous membrane lining the uterus.

**endothelium** (en-doh-thee′li-um). Membrane which lines blood vessels and body cavities.

**enema** (en′eh-muh). Liquid injected into the rectum, usually to aid bowel movement.

**enervation** (en-er-vay′shun). Lack of nervous energy.

**enteric** (en-ter′ik). Pertaining to the intestine.

**enteritis** (en-ter-igh′tis). Inflammation of the intestine.

**enuresis** (en-yoor-ees′is). Inability to control urination, especially at night; bed-wetting.

**environment** (en-vigh′rn-ment). Surroundings.

**enzyme** (en′zighm). A complex substance which causes other substances to split into simpler compounds; a catalyst.

**ephedrine** (eh-fed′rin). Substance used to dilate the pupil of the eye. It is also useful in treating asthma and hay fever.

**epidemic** (ep-i-dem'ik). A disease which affects a large number of people in a locality.

**epidemiology** (ep-i-dee-mee-ahl'o-ji). Study of epidemic disease.

**epidermis** (ep-i-der'mis). Outer layer of the skin.

**epididymis** (ep-i-did'i-mis). Small mass at the back of the testicle. It consists of a many-folded tube which opens into the vas deferens.

**epigastric** (ep"i-gas'trik). Pertaining to the region over the stomach.

**epiglottis** (ep-i-glaht'is). The flap over the larynx which closes during swallowing to prevent food from entering the windpipe.

**epilepsy** (ep'i-lep"si). Nervous disease in which there are convulsive seizures.

**epinephrine** (ep-i-nef'rin). A substance produced by the adrenal gland which affects the rate of heartbeat and blood circulation and controls muscles of the viscera. It postpones muscle fatigue, and is released in larger quantities in times of stress, permitting more activity than usual.

**epiphysis** (eh-pif'is-is). The end part of a long bone. It is separate from the shaft of the bone in young children but later unites with it.

**episiotomy** (i-piz-ee-aht'o-mi). Cutting of the vaginal lips during delivery of a baby to prevent the tissues of the mother from being torn.

**epithelium** (ep-i-thee'li-um). Type of body cells found in skin and mucous membranes.

**Epsom** (ep'sum) **salt.** Magnesium sulfate; a laxative.

**Equanil** (eck'wuh-nil). A proprietary sedative. Chemically, it is the same as Miltown, a frequently used tranquilizer.

**erection** (ee-rek'shun). State of hardness in the penis or other erectile tissues when filled with blood.

**erepsin** (ee-rep'sin). An enzyme in intestinal juice that aids in breaking down protein into amino acids.

**ergot** (er'guht). Substance obtained from a grain fungus.

**erotic** (i-raht'ik). Relating to the sex urge.

**eructation** (ee-ruhk-tay'shun). Belching.

**eruption** (i-rup'shun). Breaking out, as for example a rash.

**erysipelas** (ehr-i-sip'uh-luhs). St. Anthony's fire; a severe infectious disease in which the skin becomes swollen and inflamed. The disease is caused by a streptococcal organism which is susceptible to antibiotics.

**erythema** (ehr-i-thee'muh). Redness of the skin.

**erythroblastosis fetalis** (e-rith-roh-blas-toh'sis fee-tal'is). An anemia in newborn babies associated with the Rh factor. The anti-Rh factor in Rh-negative blood of the mother mingles with the baby's Rh-positive blood and interferes with the development of red blood cells. Treatment is replacement of the unhealthy blood by transfusion with normal blood.

**erythrocyte** (i-rith'ruh-sight). Red blood cell.

**erythromania** (i-rith-ruh-may'ni-uh). Uncontrollable blushing.

**erythromycin** (ehr-ee-throh-my'sin). An antibiotic which is unusually effective against staphylococcal germs.

**esophagus** (i-sahf'uh-guhs). Gullet; the tube which carries food from the mouth to the stomach.

**estrin** (es'trin). Estrogen; female sex hormone produced by the ovaries.

**estrogen** (es'truh-jen). A substance either natural or synthetic, which produces the changes connected with menstruation and pregnancy.

**estrone** (es'trohn). One of the female hormones.

**ether** (ee'ther). Ethyl ether; an anesthetic.

**etherize** (ee'ther-ighz). Anesthetize by inhalation of ether.

**ethmoid** (eth'moyd) **bone.** The bone that forms the roof of the nose. It contains the nasal sinuses.

**ethylene** (eth'il-een). A gas sometimes used to produce anesthesia.

**etiology** (ee-ti-ahl'uh-ji). Causes of disease or the study of the causes of disease.

**eugenics** (yoo-jen'iks). Science of improving the human race.

**eunuch** (yoo'nuhk). Man or boy whose testicles have been removed.

**euphoria** (yoo-faw'ri-uh). Sense of well-being.

**eustachian** (yoo-stay'ki-un) **tube.** The tube connecting the middle ear and the pharynx.

**euthanasia** (yoo-thn-aysh'yuh). Painless death.

**evacuation** (i-vak-yoo-ay'shun). Emptying.

**exacerbation** (eg-zas-er-bay'shun). Increase in the severity of a disease.

**excision** (ek-sizh'un). The act of cutting out.

**excoriation** (eks-kaw-ri-ay'shun). Removal of skin by scraping or scratching.

**excrescence** (eks-kres'ens). An outgrowth from the surface of an organ.

**excrete** (eks-kreet′). Give off waste products.

**exfoliation** (eks-foh-li-ay′shun). Flaking off of dead tissue.

**exhalation** (eks-huh-lay′shun). Breathing out.

**exhibitionism** (ek-si-bish′un-izm). Abnormal tendency to expose one's body to view, particularly the genitals.

**exocardia** (ek-so-kahr′di-uh). A congenital displacement of the heart.

**exophthalmos** (ek-sahf-thal′mus). Protruding eyeballs.

> **exophthalmic goiter.** Disease of the thyroid gland which causes the eyes to protrude. Loss of weight, rapid heartbeat, and enlarged thyroid are also associated with it.

**exotoxin** (ek-so-tahk′sin). A poison excreted by germs during their growth.

**expectorant** (ek-spek′tuh-rant). Substance that increases the output of sputum.

**expectoration** (eks-pek-tuh-ray′shun). The act of spitting.

**expiration** (eks-pi-ray′shun). Exhalation.

**exploratory** (eks-plawr′uh-taw-ri). Pertaining to a careful examination, as in diagnosis.

**extensor** (ek-sten′ser). A muscle used to straighten a bent limb.

**extrasystole** (ek″strah-sis′to-le). A premature heartbeat.

**extremities** (eks-trem′i-teez). The limbs.

> **lower extremities.** The legs and feet.
> **upper extremities.** The arms and hands.

**exudate** (eg′soo-dayt). Fluid given off into the tissues.

# F

**Fahrenheit** (fahr′en-hight). The temperature scale in which the boiling point of water is 212°, the freezing point 32°, and normal body temperature 98.6° (in mouth).

**faint** (faynt). Loss of consciousness because of insufficient blood in the brain.

**fallopian** (fuh-loh′pi-un) **tubes.** Oviducts; the two tubes, one on each side of the uterus, connecting the ovaries and the uterus. An egg cell released by the ovary must pass through the fallopian tube, and it is believed that a woman is most fertile during the period the ovum is in the tube.

**farsightedness.** Hyperopia; the eye is too flat, causing light rays to focus behind the retina.

**fascia** (fash′yuh). Thin tissues found beneath the skin between and around muscles and other structures.

**fauces** (faw′seez). Passage between the throat and pharynx.

**favus** (fay′vus). A contagious skin disease caused by a fungus and marked by cup-shaped yellow crusts on the hair follicles, particularly of the scalp.

**FDA.** Abbreviation for Food and Drug Administration.

**febrile** (feb′ril). Feverish.

**feces** (fee′seez). The discharge from the bowels.

**fecundity** (fi-kuhn′di-ti). Fertility.

**feeblemindedness.** Lack of intelligence caused by an underdeveloped mind. The individual may attain a mental age between 8 and 12 years.

**femoral** (fem′uh-rl). Pertaining to the thigh.

**femur** (fee′mer). The thigh bone.

**fenestrated** (fen′es-tray-ted). Pierced.

**fertile** (fer′tl). Able to produce offspring.

**fertilization** (fer-til-igh-zay′shun). Union of the egg cell with the sperm cell.

**fester** (fes′ter). To form pus.

**fetal** (fee′tl). Pertaining to the developing unborn baby.

**fetus** (fee′tuhs). The unborn baby after the third month of pregnancy.

**fever** (fee′ver). An abnormally high body temperature, above 98.6° F. (by mouth).

**fever blister.** Sore on the lips, sometimes appears when the patient has fever; cold sore, herpes labialis.

**fibril** (figh′bril). Threadlike structure, one of many that make up muscle tissue.

**fibrillation** (fib-ril-lay′shun). Tremor or twitching of muscle fibers.

> **auricular fibrillation.** Condition in which the wall of the heart auricle twitches instead of contracting normally.
> **ventricular fibrillation.** Twitching of the wall of the ventricle of the heart instead of normal contraction.

**fibrin** (figh′brin). Protein in the blood which forms into fibers when the blood clots.

**fibula** (fib′yoo-luh). The smaller of the two bones of the lower leg.

**filariasis** (fil-uh-righ′uh-sis). Chronic disease caused by parasitic worms which obstruct blood and lymph vessels. It may result in elephantiasis.

**filter** (fil′ter). To separate solid particles from a liquid by passing it through a porous substance.

**Finlay de Barres, Carlos Juan** (1833–1915). Cuban

physician who introduced the theory that yellow fever was spread by mosquitoes.

**first aid.** Immediate and temporary treatment given the sick or injured before the doctor arrives.

**fission** (fish'n). Splitting.

**fissure** (fish'er). A slit or crack.

**fistula** (fis'choo-luh). A tubelike ulcer connecting the skin to a hollow organ or abscess, or connecting two hollow organs or abscesses.

>**anal fistula.** Fistula near the anus.

>**gastric fistula.** An opening into the stomach through the abdominal wall.

>**biliary fistula.** Fistula leading into the gallbladder or bile duct.

**flaccid** (flak'sid). Flabby.

**flat foot.** Foot with a sunken arch.

**flatulence** (flah'choo-lens). A large amount of gas in the stomach or intestines.

**Fleming** (flem'ing), **Sir Alexander** (b. 1881). English scientist who discovered the antibiotic action of penicillin. He was awarded the Nobel prize (1945) together with Dr. Ernest Boris Chain and Sir Howard Walter Florey, who also worked on penicillin.

**flexor** (flek'ser). A muscle that causes bending of a joint.

**fluke** (flook). A type of parasitic worm which may infect man or other animals.

**fluorine** (floo'oh-rin). An element related to chlorine. In small amounts in water it helps prevent tooth decay.

**fluoroscope** (floo'uh-ruh-skohp). A device for projecting the x-ray image on a screen instead of on film. Used especially for observing the heart, lungs, or digestive organs.

**folic acid** (foh'lik as'id). One of the vitamin $B_2$ complex, used in treating certain types of pernicious anemia.

**follicle** (fahl'ikl). A small duct or sac.

>**hair follicle.** Small depression in the skin containing the hair root.

>**intestinal follicle.** One of the small tubular glands in the mucous membrane of the small intestine.

>**graafian follicle.** One of the many small sacs in the ovary, each of which contains an egg cell.

**fomentation** (foh-men-tay'shun). A warm application to reduce pain and inflammation; a poultice.

**fontanel** (fon-tuh-nel'). One of the "soft spots" on a baby's head where the skull bones have not yet joined.

**foramen** (foh-ray'men). An opening, especially one in a bone or other body structure where nerves or blood vessels pass through.

>**foramen ovale.** Opening in the wall between the auricles in the heart of the fetus.

>**magnum foramen.** Opening in the skull through which the spinal cord passes from the brain.

**forceps** (fawr'seps). A tonglike or tweezerlike instrument used for grasping or pinching. There are many different types and sizes, depending upon the use for which the instrument is designed.

>**obstetrical forceps.** Large tonglike instrument which fits around a baby's head and requires only gentle motion to assist birth.

**forearm** (for'arm). The part of the arm between wrist and elbow.

**forebrain** (for'brayn). The front part of the brain of an embryo.

**foreskin.** Prepuce; the fold of skin covering the head of the penis.

**formaldehyde** (fawr-mal'di-highd). A pungent gas which is used as a disinfectant. In solution it is used to harden laboratory specimens and preserve them.

**fossa** (fahs'uh). A pit or depression.

**fovea** (foh'vi-uh). A cup-shaped depression.

>**fovea centralis.** The pit in the center of the retina, which is at the point of clearest vision.

**Fracastoro** (frak-as-tor'o), **Girolamo** (1483–1553). Italian pathologist who gave syphilis its name and made many contributions to the knowledge of infectious diseases.

**Franklin, Benjamin** (1706–1790). American patriot and founder of the Pennsylvania Hospital. Among his contributions to medical science were the invention of bifocal lenses and the invention of a flexible catheter.

**freckle.** Pigmented spot on the skin. The tendency to have freckles may be hereditary, but the number is increased with exposure to the sun.

**Freud** (froyd), **Sigmund** (1856–1939). Austrian psychiatrist who emphasized the importance of the unconscious mind, particularly childhood impressions, as the cause of nervous disorders.

**Friedman** (freed'man) **test.** A pregnancy test in which urine from the woman is injected into an unmated female rabbit. If the woman is pregnant the rabbit's ovaries will show changes caused by the hormones in the urine. False results are rare.

**frigidity** (fri-jid'it-i). Inability to derive pleasure

from sexual intercourse.

**frog test.** Test for pregnancy in which urine from the woman is injected into a female frog. If the woman is pregnant the hormones in the urine will cause the frog to lay eggs.

**frontal** (fruhn'tal). Relating to the forehead.

**frostbite.** Inflammation caused by the freezing of a part of the body.

**fulminating** (fuhl'min-ay-ting). Occurring suddenly and with great severity, as a pain or disease.

**fumigation** (fyoo-mi-gay'shun). Disinfection with vapors or gas.

**fundus** (fuhn'dus). The part of an organ farthest from its opening; the base.

**fungal** (fuhng'gal). Pertaining to a fungus.

**fungicide** (fuhn'ji-sighd). Substance that destroys fungi.

**fungus** (fuhng'guhs). The fungus group includes mushrooms, molds, mildews, yeasts, and moldlike microorganisms. Some fungi cause disease.

**furuncle** (fyoo'rung-kl). A boil.

**fusiform** (fyoo'si-form). Spindle-shaped.


**G**

**Galen** (gay'len) (A.D. 131–201). Greek physician whose writings on medicine formed the basis of medical teaching until the sixteenth century.

**gall** (gawl). Bile.

**gallbladder.** Saclike organ located below the liver. It serves as a storehouse for bile.

**gallstone.** Stonelike mass which has formed in the gallbladder.

**gamma globulin** (gam'uh glahb-yoo-lin). The portion of blood plasma protein that contains antibodies, which fight infection.

**ganglion** (gang'gli-un), pl. **ganglia.** 1. Mass of nervous tissue, a nerve center. 2. A cyst in a tendon sheath.

**gangrene** (gang'green). Localized death and decay of tissues usually caused by the blood supply being cut off to one part of the body.

**Gantrisin** (gan'tri-sin). A proprietary sulfonamide medicine, used as an antibiotic.

**gastrectomy** (gas-trek'toh-mi). Cutting out of part or all of the stomach.

**gastric** (gas'trik). Pertaining to the stomach.

**gastric juice.** Digestive juice secreted by the stomach. It contains the enzymes rennin and pepsin and is acid in nature because of the presence of hydrochloric acid.

**gastric lavage** (lah-vahzh'). The washing out of the stomach.

**gastric ulcer.** See **peptic ulcer.**

**gastritis** (gas-trigh'tis). Inflammation of the stomach.

**gastrocele** (gas'troh-seel). Hernia of the stomach.

**gastrocnemius** (gas-trahk-nee'mi-us). The large muscle of the calf of the leg. It aids in bending the knee and extending the foot forward in walking.

**gastroenteritis** (gas-troh-en-ter-igh'tis). Inflammation of the stomach and intestines.

**gastroenterologist** (gas-troh-en-ter-ahl'o-jist). Physician who specializes in diseases of the stomach and intestines.

**gastrojejunostomy** (gas-troh-jeh-joo-nahs'toh-mi). Surgical formation of an opening between the stomach and the jejunum (part of the small intestine).

**gastrostomy** (gas-trahs'toh-mi). Creation of an artificial fistula in the stomach.

**gastrula** (gas'troo-lah). Early stage of an embryo.

**gene** (jeen). Basic unit which determines hereditary characteristics. It is part of the chromosome.

**genetic** (juh-net'ik). Pertaining to reproduction or the origin of a biological unit.

**genetics.** The study of heredity and transmission of characteristics.

**genitals** (jen'i-tals) or **genitalia** (jen-i-tay'li-uh). The reproductive organs.

**genitourinary** (jen-i-toh-yoo'ri-nair-i). Pertaining to both the reproductive and urinary systems.

**geriatrics** (jehr-ee-at'triks). The branch of medicine which deals with the diseases of old people.

**germ** (jerm). Microorganism, such as a bacterium, especially one which is capable of causing disease.

**German measles.** Acute contagious disease caused by a virus. It produces a red rash which lasts a couple of days.

**germicide** (jerm'uh-sighd). Substance that kills germs.

**gerontology** (jehr-un-tahl'uh-ji). Study of old age and its diseases.

**gestation** (jes-tay'shun). Pregnancy.

**giantism** (jigh'un-tizm) or **gigantism** (jigh'gan-tizm). Growth of the body or a part to an unusually large size, caused by overproduction of hormones in the pituitary.

**gingivitis** (jin-ji-vigh'tis). Inflammation of the gums.

**gland.** An organ that secretes a substance used by some other part of the body.

**glanders** (glan'ders). A disease generally of horses but communicable to man. It is characterized by fever, nodules, and a nasal discharge containing pus.

**glandular** (glan'dyoo-ler) **fever.** Infectious mononucleosis.

**glans penis** (glanz pee'nis). Head of the penis.

**glaucoma** (glaw-koh'muh). A disease of the eye in which there is increased pressure within the eye damaging the retina and the optic nerve. It may lead to blindness.

**globulin** (glahb'yoo-lin). A protein which is found in blood serum and in the placenta and helps to combat infection.

**glomerulus** (glo-mair'yoo-lus). One of the small masses of blood capillaries in the kidney which filter out waste products.

**glottis** (glah'tis). Opening between the vocal cords.

**glucose** (gloo'kohs). Dextrose; a simple sugar which is produced in the body from digestion of starchy substances and is one of the body's main sources of energy. Glucose is contained in the solution used in intravenous feeding of patients to provide nourishment.

**glucose tolerance test.** Test for diabetes.

**gluteal** (gloo'ti-al). Pertaining to the buttocks.

**gluteus maximus** and **gluteus minimus muscles.** The muscles that form the buttocks.

**glycemia** (gligh-see'mi-uh). Presence of sugar in the blood.

**glycerin** (glis'er-in). A syrupy substance used as a soothing skin lotion, and as an ingredient in suppository laxatives.

**glycine** (gligh'sin). One of the amino acids.

**glycogen** (gligh'ko-jen). Starchy substance which the body makes from carbohydrates and stores in the liver. When needed as a source of energy it is converted into glucose and released into the blood.

**glycopenia** (gligh-ko-pee'ni-uh). Unusually low amount of sugar in the blood.

**glycoprotein** (gligh-ko-pro'ti-in). Compound of a protein and a carbohydrate.

**glycosuria** (gligh-ko-shoo'ri-uh). Abnormal increase in the amount of sugar in urine.

**gnathoplasty** (nay'thoh-plas-ti). Plastic surgery of the lower part of the face.

**goblet cell.** A secreting cell in the mucous membrane lining the intestine.

**goiter** (goy'ter). Enlargement of the thyroid gland, which appears as a swelling on the front of the neck.

**gonad** (goh'nad). A sex gland, either the ovary of the female or the testis of the male.

**gonococci** (gahn-o-kahk'igh). The round bacteria which cause gonorrhea.

**Gorgas** (gawr'guhs), **William C.** (1854–1920). Surgeon General of the army who directed the eradication of the mosquito of yellow fever in Panama.

**graafian** (graf'i-en) **follicle.** See **follicle.**

**graft.** Transplantation of skin or tissue from one part of the body to another.

**gram-negative** or **gram-positive.** Referring to the reaction of bacteria to the Gram stain. Those that can be decolorized with alcohol after being stained are gram-negative, such as gonococci, *B. coli,* and typhoid bacilli. Those that cannot be decolorized are gram-positive, such as streptococci, staphylococci, and pneumococci.

**gramicidin** (gram-i-sigh'din). An antibiotic from soil bacteria, one of the two substances which make up tyrothricin.

**grand mal** (grahn mahl). An epileptic attack in which the patient loses consciousness.

**granulation** (gran-yoo-lay'shun). The formation of flesh on the surface of a wound.

**granuloma** (gran-yoo-lo'muh). A tumor composed of granulation tissue.

**granuloma inguinale** (in'gwigh-nl). A chronic infection marked by ulcer on the moist surfaces of the external genital region and caused by bacteria.

**gray matter.** The inner portion of the brain and spinal cord. It is gray in color and is composed of nerve cell bodies and nerve fibers.

**grippe** (grip). Influenza.

**groin** (groyn). The region where the thigh and the trunk join.

**gullet.** The esophagus and pharynx.

**gumma** (gum'uh). Small tumor of late syphilis, usually in the brain, liver, or heart. It consists of a fibrous capsule filled with a rubberlike substance.

**gustatory** (guhs'tuh-taw''ri). Relating to the sense of taste.

**gynecology** (jin-uh-kahl'uh-ji). The branch of medicine that deals with diseases of women.

**gynecomastia** (jin''eh-ko-mas'ti-uh). Unusual development of the breasts in the male.

# H

**Hahnemann** (hah′ni-man), **Christian Friedrich Samuel** (1755–1843). German who founded the homeopathic system of treatment.

**halibut liver oil.** An oil containing vitamins A and D and requiring a smaller dosage than cod liver oil.

**halitosis** (hal-i-toh′sis). Offensive breath.

**hallucination** (huh-loo″si-nay′shun). Imaginary experience thought to be real.

**hallux** (hal′uks). The great toe.

**Halsted** (hal′sted), **William Stewart** (1852–1922). Baltimore surgeon who made many contributions to surgical technique, including the use of sterile rubber gloves during operations.

**hammer.** One of the three small bones of the inner ear; malleus.

**hamstring.** Either of the groups of tendons at the back of the knee.

**hand, claw.** Paralysis of the hand in a clawlike position.

**hand, dead.** Condition in which the hand becomes blue and painful, caused by use of vibratory tools.

**hangnail.** Inflammation around a partly detached piece of skin at the side of the nail.

**Hansen's** (han′senz) **disease.** Leprosy; named after the Norwegian physician who discovered the bacillus that causes leprosy.

**harelip.** Congenital cleft in the upper lip due to a failure of the bones to unite.

**Harvey, William** (1578–1657). English physician who investigated heart action and was the first to describe the circulation of the blood.

**hashish** or **hasheesh** (hash-eesh′). Marijuana; a narcotic with no medicinal value.

**health** (helth). Normal condition of the body and mind.

**healthful.** Aiding health.

**healthy.** In a normal condition; free from disease.

**hearing aid.** An instrument to amplify sounds for the hard of hearing. There are two types of electric hearing aids: the air-conduction type, which is worn in the ear canal; and the bone-conduction type, which is worn in back of the ear over the mastoid bone.

**heart.** Muscular organ that pumps blood. It consists of two symmetrical halves each containing two chambers separated by a valve. The upper chambers, called auricles or atria (sing. atrium), receive blood from the veins and pump it into the lower chambers, called ventricles, which then pump it into the arteries.

**heart block.** Condition in which the auricles and ventricles contract independently, resulting in a beat of varying intensity. It is caused by some abnormality in the tissue connecting auricles and ventricles.

**heartburn.** Burning sensation in the esophagus or below the breastbone.

**heart failure.** Weakening of the heart so that it cannot pump blood sufficient for normal circulation.

**heart murmur.** Any sound heard in the heart region in addition to the regular beat.

**heat prostration** or **exhaustion.** Collapse caused by overexposure to heat; characterized by moist, cold skin, weak pulse, restlessness, and anxiety.

**hemacytometer** (heem-uh-sigh-tah′mi-ter) or **hematocytometer** (heem-uh-toh-sigh-tah′mi-ter). Device used in counting blood cells.

**hemangioma** (hee-man-ji-oh′muh). Tumor composed of blood vessels.

**hematology** (he″mah-tol′o-je). The science dealing with the study of the blood.

**hematoma** (heem-uh-toh′muh). A swelling or tumor filled with blood. It may result from hemorrhage under the skin, as in a "black" eye.

**hematuria** (heem-uh-tyoo′ri-uh). Presence of blood in the urine.

**hemiplegia** (hem-i-plee′ji-uh). Paralysis of one side of the body.

**hemoglobin** (hee-moh-gloh′bin). The coloring matter in red blood cells. It is a compound of protein and oxygen. Normally 100 milliliters of blood contain 13 to 16 grams of hemoglobin.

**hemolysis** (hee-mahl′is-is). The breaking down of red blood cells.

**hemophilia** (hee-moh-feel′ee-uh). A hereditary condition in which the blood cannot coagulate, resulting in severe bleeding from any wound. The condition affects only males but is passed from mother to son.

**hemoptysis** (hee-mahp′tis-is). Spitting up blood.

**hemorrhage** (hem′or-ij). Abnormal bleeding.

**hemorrhoid** (hem′o-royd). Pile; enlargement of the veins of the anal region, causing pain, bleeding, and constipation.

**hemostat** (hee′mo-stat). Instrument which pinches a blood vessel to prevent bleeding.

**Henle's** (hen'leez) **loop.** Part of the small tubules in the kidney where fluid is reabsorbed from the urine.

**heparin** (hep'uh-rin). Substance found in the liver and other tissues which prevents the clotting of blood. It is sometimes given following an operation in order to prevent blood clots from forming within blood vessels.

**hepatic** (hep-at'ik). Pertaining to the liver.

**hepatitis** (hep-uh-tigh'tus). Inflammation of the liver.

>**infectious hepatitis.** A viral disease of the liver producing jaundice, nausea, and vomiting.

**hereditary** (hi-red'i-tair-i). Inherited; passed from parents to offspring.

**heredity** (hi-red'i-ti). The characteristics transmitted from parent to offspring and determined by the genes and chromosomes of the cells.

**hermaphrodite** (her-maf'ro-dight). Person having characteristics of both sexes.

**hernia** (her'ni-uh). Rupture; abnormal condition in which part of an organ pushes through the wall around it. Usually refers to a rupture of the abdominal wall by the intestine but is also used to describe similar ruptures by other organs.

**heroin** (hehr'o-in). A narcotic banned by federal law because of the danger of addiction.

**herpes** (her'peez). Blisterlike skin eruption.

>**herpes simplex** (sim'pleks). Blisterlike sores on the edge of the lips, the nostrils, or the genitals; caused by a virus.

>**herpes zoster** (zahs'ter). Shingles; groups of small blisters following the path of a nerve, usually on one side of the body, accompanied by a burning or tingling sensation and neuralgic pains; caused by a virus.

**hesperidin** (hes-pehr'i-din). Vitamin P.

**Hetrazan** (het'ruh-zan). A proprietary substance believed helpful for treating filariasis.

**hiccup** or **hiccough** (hik'up). Involuntary spasm of the glottis and diaphragm.

**hilum** (high'lum). The depression in a gland at the point where nerves or vessels enter.

**Hippocrates** (hi-pahk'ruh-teez) (460–370 B.C.). Famous Greek physician, often called the "Father of Medicine." He taught high ethical standards and the importance of clinical experience.

**histamine** (his'tuh-meen). A substance produced in the body from the breakdown of histidine. It dilates blood vessels and stimulates secretions. It is produced in excess in allergy and is believed to be the cause of most of the allergic reactions.

**histidine** (his'tid-in). One of the essential amino acids.

**histology** (his-tahl'uh-ji). Study of microscopic structure of tissues.

**histoplasmosis** (his-toh-plaz-mo'sis). A disease caused by a yeastlike organism.

**hives.** Urticaria; itchy swellings which suddenly appear on the skin. They are caused by an allergic reaction.

**Hodgkin's** (hahj'kinz) **disease.** A serious disease of the lymph nodes. The cause is not known. It is named after Thomas Hodgkin (1798–1866), who described this disease of lymph nodes and also aortic insufficiency.

**Holmes** (holmz), **Oliver Wendell** (1809–1894). Professor at Harvard Medical School who coined the word "anesthesia" and was largely responsible for reducing puerperal fever among American mothers.

**homeopathy** (ho-mi-ahp'uh-thi). System of treatment founded by Hahnemann in which drugs able to produce certain symptoms in healthy persons are used in minute quantities to treat the same symptoms in diseased persons.

**homosexuality** (ho-mo-seks-yoo-al'i-ti). Sexual desire for a person of the same sex.

**hookworm.** A worm which lives as a parasite in the intestines and causes hookworm disease (ancylostomiasis or uncinariasis). It enters through the feet or in drinking water. The disease is characterized by anemia, emaciation, and listlessness.

**hormone** (hor'mohn). A glandular secretion carried by the bloodstream to the organs which it regulates.

**housemaid's knee.** Bursitis in the joint behind the kneecap; caused by the pressure from kneeling a great deal.

**humerus** (hyoo'mer-us). The bone of the upper arm.

**Hunter, John** (1728–1793). Scottish surgeon who contributed greatly to knowledge of pathology and gave a classic description of inflammation.

**Huntington's chorea** (hunt'ing-tunz koh-ree'uh). A hereditary mental affliction characterized by irregular movements, disturbance in speech, and progressive muscular weakness.

**hyalin** (high'uh-lin). A glassy substance which occurs normally in cartilage, the inside of the eyeball, and other structures.

**hydrocele** (high′droh-seel). An abnormal collection of fluid, usually in the covering of the testicle.

**hydrocephaly** (high-dro-sef′uh-li). A condition usually congenital in which the head and forehead are enlarged because of an abnormal increase in the cerebral fluid.

**hydrochloric** (high-dro-klor′ik) **acid.** An acid composed of hydrogen and chlorine. It is normally secreted in the stomach to aid digestion.

**hydrogen peroxide** (high′dro-jen per-ahk′sighd). A disinfectant.

**hydrolysis** (high-drahl′is-is). Decomposition due to water.

**hydrophobia** (high-dro-foh′bi-uh). See **rabies.**

**hydrotherapy** (high-dro-thehr′uh-pi). Treatment of disease with water by means of wet packs or baths.

**hygiene** (high′jeen). The science dealing with the maintenance of health.

**hymen** (high′men). Membrane partially covering the vaginal opening.

**hyoid** (high′oyd) **bone.** The U-shaped bone which supports the tongue.

**hyperacidity** (high-per-uh-sid′it-i). Excessive acidity.

**hyperchlorhydria** (high-per-klor-high′dri-uh). Excess of hydrochloric acid in gastric juice.

**hyperemia** (high-per-eem′i-uh). An excess of blood in any part of the body; plethora.

**hyperesthesia** (high-per-es-thee′zhi-uh). Unusual sensitivity to touch, pain, or other sensations.

**hyperinsulinism** (high-per-in′soo-lin-izm). Condition of excessive insulin secretion in the body, resulting in a low level of sugar in the blood.

**hyperkinesis** (high″per-ki-nee′sis). Abnormally increased motor function or activity.

**hyperlipemia** (high″per-li-pee′me-ah). Excessive amounts of fats in the blood.

**hyperopia** (high-per-o′pi-uh). Farsightedness; a condition in which only distant objects are seen clearly because the eye cannot accommodate properly. The eyeball is too flat, causing images to be focused behind the retina.

**hyperplasia** (high-per-play′zhi-uh). Enlarged size of an organ caused by increase in the number of cells.

**hypertension** (high-per-ten′shun). High blood pressure.

**hyperthyroidism** (high-per-thigh′royd-izm). Overactivity of the thyroid.

**hypertrophy** (high-per′truh-fi). Abnormal enlarge-ment of a part due to its excessive activity.

**hypnosis** (hip-no′sis). An induced trance in which the person is susceptible to suggestion.

**hypnotic** (hip-naht′ik). 1. A substance which induces sleep. 2. Pertaining to hypnosis.

**hypoacidity** (high-po-as-id′i-ti). Decreased acid content of the stomach juices.

**hypocalcemia** (high-po-kal-see′mi-uh). Abnormally small amount of calcium in the blood.

**hypochondriac** (high-puh-kahn′dri-ak). A person abnormally worried about his health.

**hypodermic** (high-puh-derm′ik). Injected under the skin.

**hypoglossal** (high-puh-glahs′ul). Situated under the tongue.

**hypoglycemia** (high-po-gligh-see′mi-uh). Deficiency of sugar in the blood.

**hypoinsulinism** (high-po-in′soo-lin-izm). Insufficient insulin secretion by the pancreas; diabetes mellitus.

**hypophysis** (high-pahf′is-is). The pituitary gland.

**hypoplasia** (high-po-play′zhi-uh). Defective or incomplete development of a tissue or organ.

**hypotension** (high-poh-ten′shun). Low blood pressure.

**hypothalamus** (high-po-thal′uh-mus). The part of the brain which plays a part in controlling internal organs and in maintaining uniform body temperature.

**hypothyroidism** (high-po-thigh′royd-izm). Abnormal condition caused by a decrease in the activity of the thyroid.

**hysterectomy** (his-ter-ek′tuh-mi). Surgical removal of the uterus; uterectomy.

**hysteria** (his-tier′i-uh). A psychoneurosis in which there is a loss of control over the will, resulting in any of a variety of symptoms such as causeless laughing or crying, emotional excitement, or even convulsions or paralysis.

# I

**iatrogenic** (i-at″ro-jen′ik). Resulting from an attitude or activity of a physician. An iatrogenic disorder is one produced unintentionally as a result of treatment for some other disorder.

**icterus** (ik′ter-us). Jaundice.

**ictus** (ik′tus). 1. A sudden attack. 2. Heartbeat.

**id.** In psychiatry it refers to the unconscious part of one's self; the part that has to do with instincts, such as those of sex and self-preservation.

**idiocy** (id'i-o-si). Extreme mental deficiency, usually congenital. The individual is absolutely helpless and has a mental age of less than 3 years.

**idiomuscular** (id-i-o-mus'kyoo-lar) **contraction.** Motion of muscle not caused by nerve stimulus; seen in degenerative or fatigued muscle.

**idiopathic** (id-i-o-path'ik). Of unknown origin.

**ileitis** (il-i-igh'tis). Inflammation of the ileum. A special chronic form is called regional ileitis or Crohn's disease and is also known as terminal ileitis.

**ileocolostomy** (il-i-o-ko-lahs'tuh-mi). An operation connecting the ileum with the large intestine.

**ileum** (il'i-um). The lower portion of the small intestine between the jejunum and the large intestine.

**ilium** (il'i-um). Wide upper part of the hipbone.

**imbecility** (im-bi-sil'i-ti). A condition of mental deficiency in which the individual has a mental age between 3 and 7.

**immobilization** (im-o-bil-uh-zay'shun). Making a part immovable to aid healing.

**immunity** (i-myoo'ni-ti). Condition of being resistant to a disease.

    **active immunity.** Immunity acquired as a result of having had the disease or as a result of an inoculation against it.

    **passive immunity.** Immunity acquired by injection of serum from an animal which has active immunity to the disease.

**impacted** (im-pak'ted). Wedged in so tightly as to be immovable.

    **impacted tooth.** One placed in such a way in the gum that it cannot break through.

**imperforate** (im-per'fuh-rayt). Without the normal opening.

**impetigo** (im-pee-tigh'go). A contagious skin disease characterized by blisterlike pustules; probably caused by staphylococci or streptococci. It is spread by direct contact with the moist discharges of the sores.

**implantation** (im-plan-tay'shun). Embedding of the embryo into the wall of the uterus. This takes place about ten days after the egg is fertilized.

**impotence** (im'puh-tns). Inability of a male to perform the sexual act.

**impregnation** (im-preg-nay'shun). Fertilization of the ovum by a sperm.

**inactivation** (in-ak-ti-vay'shun). Process of destroying the activity of a substance.

**incipient** (in-sip'i-ent). Just beginning.

**incised** (in-sigh'zd) **wound.** A wound made by cutting.

**incisor** (in-sigh'zer). One of the sharp cutting teeth. There are eight, four in each jaw.

**incompetence** (in-kahm'pi-tens). Inadequacy; being unable to perform the normal function.

**incontinence** (in-kahn'ti-nens). 1. Inability to control urination or bowel movements. 2. Lack of self-restraint sexually.

**incoordination** (in-ko-or-di-nay'shun). Inability to use muscles harmoniously in performing a voluntary action.

**incrustation** (in-krus-tay'shun). Formation of a scab or hard coating.

**incubation** (in-kyoo-bay'shun) **period.** The time between the entrance of germs into the body and the appearance of symptoms.

**incubator** (in'kyoo-bay-ter). A container in which the temperature and atmosphere are controlled; used for premature babies.

**incus** (ing'kus). Anvil; one of the small bones of the inner ear.

**Indocin** (in'doh-sin). A proprietary medicine sometimes used in the treatment of arthritis. Its action is to reduce inflammation.

**induration** (in-dyoo-ray'shun). Process of becoming hard.

**infantile paralysis** (in'fun-tighl puh-ral'i-sis). Poliomyelitis; see text.

**infarct** (in'farkt). Area in which the tissue has broken down because of some obstruction in the blood supply to the area.

**infection** (in-fek'shun). Invasion of body tissue by disease germs; or the disease itself.

**inferiority** (in-feer-i-or'i-ti) **complex.** A group of symptoms associated with a feeling of inadequacy usually based on imagined defects.

**inflammation** (in-fluh-may'shun). Condition of redness and swelling accompanied by heat and pain; caused by irritation from bacteria or other agents.

**infrared** (in-fruh-red'). The invisible long-wave heat rays.

**inguinal** (ing'gwigh-nl). Pertaining to the groin.

**INH.** Abbreviation of isonicotinic acid hydrazide, a substance used in the treatment of tuberculosis.

**inhalation** (in-huh-lay'shun). Intake of breath.

**inheritance** (in-hair'i-tns). Characteristics transmitted from parent to offspring.

**inhibition** (in-hi-bish'un). Interference with or impediment to an action.

**injection** (in-jek'shun). Forcing a substance into an area, usually by means of a syringe with a hollow needle.

**innocuous** (in-ahk'yoo-uhs). Harmless.

**innominate** (in-ahm'uh-nayt) **bone.** Hipbone.

**inoculation** (in-ahk-yoo-lay'shun). The intentional planting in the body of germs or extracts to protect against disease.

**inoperable** (in-ahp'er-uh-bl). Not able to be cured by operation.

**inorganic** (in-or-gan'ik). Not of organic origin.

**insanity** (in-san'i-ti). Unsoundness of mind; mental disorder, usually chronic, in which the individual is not capable of reasoning, is irresponsible, and may suffer from delusions.

**insemination** (in-sem-uh-nay'shun). Depositing semen in the vagina.

> **artificial insemination.** Introduction of semen into the vagina by artificial means.

**insomnia** (in-sahm'ni-uh). Inability to sleep.

**inspiration** (in-spi-ray'shun). Breathing in.

**insufficiency** (in-suh-fish'en-si). Weakness of an organ or a condition in which it is unable to perform its function.

**insulin** (in'suh-lin). Hormone produced in the pancreas and used by the tissues to get energy from blood sugar. This substance can be isolated from the pancreas of slaughterhouse animals and is used in treating diabetes.

**insulin shock.** Loss of consciousness caused by an overdose of insulin.

**integument** (in-teg'yoo-ment). The skin.

**intelligence** (in-tel'i-jens). Mental development.

**intention tremor.** Involuntary trembling when movement is attempted.

**intercellular** (in-ter-sel'yoo-lar). Between the cells.

**intercostal** (in-ter-kahs'tl). Between the ribs.

**intercurrent infection.** An infection occurring while another disease is present.

**intern** or **interne** (in-tern'). A hospital physician who lives within the institution and is in his first year of service.

**internist** (in-ter'nist). A physician who specializes in diseases of the internal organs.

**intervertebral disk.** See **Disk.**

**intestine** (in-tes'tin). The long coiled tube of the digestive system. It extends from the stomach to the anus.

**intima** (in'ti-muh). The innermost of the three layers of an artery.

**intoxication** (in-tahk-si-kay'shun). 1. Poisoning. 2. Drunkenness.

**intradermal** (in-truh-der'ml). Within or into the skin.

**intramuscular** (in-truh-mus'kyoo-lar). Within or into a muscle.

**intravenous** (in-truh-vee'nus). Within or into a vein.

**intravenous feeding.** Giving nourishment by allowing a solution of glucose to flow through a tube directly into a vein.

**introvert** (in'troh-vert). One whose attention is focused on his inner self and has no interest in others or in things around him.

**intubation** (in-too-bay'shun). Insertion of a tube into the body or into an organ.

**intumescence** (in-too-mes'ens). Swelling.

**in utero** (in yoo'ter-o). Within the uterus.

**invertase** (in-ver'tays). An enzyme from the pancreas which aids in converting cane sugar to invert sugar.

**involution of the uterus.** Shrinking of the uterus to normal size after childbirth.

**iodine** (igh'uh-dighn). A nonmetallic element which is necessary for the normal function of the thyroid gland. Medicinally, an alcoholic solution used as an antiseptic on the skin.

> **radioactive iodine.** Used in treating goiter and cancers originating in thyroid tissue.

**iodoform** (igh-o'doh-form). A yellow powder with a penetrating odor used as an anesthetic and antiseptic, particularly on wounds.

**ipecac** (ip'i-kak). An emetic obtained from the root of a tropical plant.

**IQ.** Abbreviation of intelligence quotient; 100 multiplied by the ratio of mental age to age in years.

**iris** (igh'ris). The colored part of the eye, located between the lens and the cornea with an opening in the middle (the pupil).

**iritis** (igh-righ'tis). Inflammation of the iris.

**iron lung** (igh'ern luhng'). A respirator; a device which artificially expands and contracts the chest of a patient whose respiratory muscles are paralyzed.

**irradiation** (ir-ray-di-ay'shun). Treatment of disease with x-ray, radioactive material, ultraviolet rays, or infrared rays.

**ischemia** (is-kee'me-ah). Deficiency of blood in a part.

**ischium** (is'ki-um). The lower hind part of the hip-bone.

**islands** or **islets of Langerhans** (lahng'er-hans). Masses of very small cells in the pancreas which secrete insulin.

**isolation** (igh-suh-lay'shun). Placing a person having a communicable disease separate from others to prevent the disease from being spread to other people.

**isoleucine** (igh-so-loo'sin). An essential amino acid.

**isonicotinic** (igh'so-nik'o-tin-ik) **acid.** See INH.

**isotope** (igh'suh-tohp). A chemical element like another in structure and chemical properties but differing slightly in atomic weight or in radioactivity.

# J

**jaundice** (jawn'dis). Yellowness of skin and eyes caused by an excess of bile pigment in the blood.

**jaw, lumpy.** A fungal disease of cattle transmissible to man.

**jejunum** (ji-joo'num). The part of the small intestine between the duodenum and the ileum.

**Jenner** (jen'er), **Edward** (1749–1823). English physician who introduced vaccination with cowpox virus to immunize against smallpox.

**joint.** Connection of two bones.

**jugular** (jug'yoo-ler). Pertaining to the neck or throat.

> **jugular veins.** The large veins in the neck which carry blood from the head.

**Jung** (yoong), **Carl Gustav** (1875–1961). Swiss psychiatrist who carried on the work of Freud and has added many contributions of his own.

**jungle rot.** Common term for any fungal infection of the skin occurring in tropical regions.

# K

**Kahn test.** A blood test for syphilis.

**kala azar** (kah'lah ah'zar). A chronic, often fatal disease found mainly in Asia. It is caused by a protozoan which is carried by sand flies that have bitten an infected person.

**kaolin** (kay'o-lin). A fine clay sometimes used in treating skin diseases.

**Kenalog** (ken'uh-log). A proprietary preparation containing a derivative of cortisone, used in treatment of skin ailments.

**Kenny** (ken'ee) **method.** Treatment of muscles affected by poliomyelitis developed by Sister Elizabeth Kenny, an Australian nurse. It is based on the use of hot packs to prevent muscle spasms and exercises to reeducate the muscles.

**keratin** (kehr'uh-tin). Substance which forms the principal part of horny tissues, such as fingernails and toenails, and is also found in the skin and hair. It is not dissolved by gastric juice and so is used to coat pills that are meant to be dissolved in the intestines.

**keratitis** (kehr-uh-tigh'tis). Inflammation of the cornea.

> **infectious keratitis.** A viral infection of the eye causing swelling, a watery discharge, and opaque spots on the cornea. It is spread by the handling of articles soiled by an infected person.

**kidney** (kid'ni). One of the two bean-shaped glands in the back of the abdomen. It acts as a purifying system for the blood and excretes urine.

**kineplasty** (kin'i-plas-ti). Method of amputation which permits the use of the voluntary muscles in regulating an artificial limb.

**kinesia** (kuh-nee'zhuh). Motion sickness.

**kinesthesia** (kin-es-thee'zhuh). The sense of position, weight, and motion.

**kleptomania** (klep-tuh-may'ni-uh). Abnormal desire to steal.

**kneecap.** Patella.

**knee jerk.** Reflex that causes the foot to kick forward when the ligament below the kneecap is tapped.

**Koch** (kohk), **Robert** (1843–1910). German physician who isolated and described the organisms causing tuberculosis, cholera, and anthrax.

**kyphosis** (kigh-foh'sis). Body deformity resulting in round shoulders or humpback.

# L

**labia** (lay'bi-uh). Liplike structures.

> **labia majora** and **minora.** Vaginal lips.

**labor.** The process of childbirth.

**lacerated** (las'er-ay-ted). Torn.

**laceration** (las-er-ay'shun). A wound caused by the cutting or tearing of tissue.

**lacrimal** (lak'ri-mul). 1. Pertaining to tears. 2. The gland which secretes tears.

**lactase** (lak'tays). An enzyme found in the intestinal juice to digest milk sugar.

**lactation** (lak-tay'shun). The secretion of milk.

**lacteal** (lak'ti-ul). One of the lymphatic ducts in the intestines which takes up digested fat (chyle).

**lactic** (lak'tik) **acid.** A waste product from muscles.

**Laënnec** (lan-ek, or lay-uh-nek'), **René Théophile Hyacinthe** (1781–1826). French physician who invented the stethoscope.

**lance** (lans). To cut open with a knife.

**lancet** (lan'set). A small two-edged surgical knife.

**Landsteiner** (land'stigh-ner), **Karl** (1868–1943). Scientist who developed a method of blood typing and helped show the significance of the Rh factor.

**lanolin** (lan'o-lin). A fat obtained from wool and used as a base for ointments and skin lotions.

**Lanoxin** (lan-ox'in). A proprietary digitalis compound, used in treatment of heart disease.

**laryngectomy** (lar-in-jek'tuh-mi). Surgical removal of the larynx.

**laryngitis** (lar-in-jigh'tis). Inflammation of the larynx.

**larynx** (lar'ingks). The voicebox; a cartilaginous structure which contains the vocal cords and produces most of the sounds made by the voice.

**latent** (lay'tent). Hidden.

**laudanum** (law'duh-nm). Tincture of opium.

**laxative** (laks'uh-tiv). An agent that loosens the bowels; a mild cathartic.

**lecithin** (les'i-thin). A waxy compound containing fatty acids and found normally in plant and animal tissues, especially nervous tissue.

**Leeuwenhoek** (lay'ven-hook), **Antony van** (1632–1723). Dutch maker of microscopes who described many microorganisms and microscopic structures.

**Leishmania** (lighsh-may'ni-uh). A genus of protozoa which includes some disease producers. They are generally spread by a certain type of fly found mainly in Asia and South America.

**leishmaniasis** (lighsh-muh-nigh'uh-sis). Buboes; any infection caused by Leishmania.

**lens, crystalline.** The colorless capsule behind the pupil of the eye. It focuses light rays on the retina.

**leprosy** (lep'ruh-si). Hansen's disease; a chronic infectious disease caused by bacteria and found mainly in tropical and semitropical regions. It affects the nerves or the skin with its subcutaneous tissues causing ulcers and mutilation. It is not easily communicable to others.

**leptospirosis** (lep-toh-spigh-ro'sis). A disease caused by spirochetes and seen mainly in dogs and rats but communicable to man. It may be manifest by the appearance of jaundice.

**lesion** (lee'zhn). Any wound, sore, tumor, or area of tissue breakdown.

**leukocyte** (loo'kuh-sight). One of the white blood cells. The leukocytes are larger than the red blood cells and have large irregularly shaped nuclei. One of the functions of these cells is to engulf any germs or foreign particles in the blood, thus helping the body to resist infection.

**leukopenia** (loo-ko-pee'ni-uh). Condition in which there are fewer leukocytes present in the blood than normally.

**leukorrhea** (loo-ko-ree'uh). A whitish mucus discharged from the vagina. A small amount of discharge is not abnormal but an increase in the amount may be an indication of infection.

**leukotomy** (loo-kaht'uh-mi). See **lobotomy.**

**libido** (li-bee'do). Conscious or unconscious sexual desire.

**Librium** (lib'ree-um). A proprietary tranquilizer.

**ligament** (lig'uh-ment). A tough band of tissue which connects bones or supports organs.

**ligature** (lig'uh-tyoor). The thread used in surgery for tying off blood vessels to prevent bleeding or for constricting any other structures.

**liniment** (lin'i-ment). A liquid to be rubbed on the skin.

**lipase** (lip'ays). An enzyme which digests fats. It is produced in most of the digestive organs.

**lipid** (lip'id). A fat or fatlike substance, such as fatty acids or soap.

**Lister** (lis'ter), **Joseph** (1827–1912). English Quaker surgeon who introduced the idea of antiseptic surgery by using carbolic acid on the wound, to clean instruments and to spray the air of the operating room.

**litholapaxy** (lith-ahl'uh-pak-si). Crushing of a stone in the bladder and removal of the fragments by washing out the bladder through a catheter.

**lithotomy** (lith-aht'uh-mi). Removing a stone by cutting through the bladder.

**liver** (liv'er). The large four-lobed red organ situated in the upper right portion of the abdomen. It has many functions, including the manufacture of bile and storage of excess carbohydrates.

**liver injection.** Extract from livers of slaughterhouse animals, used to treat pernicious anemia.

**lobotomy** (lo-baht'uh-mi). An operation performed on violent uncontrollable mental patients to calm them. The nerve fibers leading to the frontal lobes of the brain are cut.

**lochia** (lo'ki-uh). Vaginal discharge which follows childbirth. It consists of blood, mucus, and tissue, and lasts for several weeks.

**lockjaw.** See **tetany.**

**lordosis** (lor-doh'sis). Swayback; abnormal posture in which the inward curve of the back is exaggerated.

**louse** (lous). A small parasitic animal which infects the hairy parts of the body and may carry disease germs.

**lozenge** (lahz'inj). A medicated tablet meant to be dissolved slowly in the mouth.

**lues** (loo'eez). Syphilis.

**lumbago** (lum-bay'go). An ache in the lower part of the back.

**lumbar** (lum'ber). Pertaining to the lower back just between the pelvis and the ribs.

**lung.** One of the two organs of breathing which are situated in the chest beneath the ribs. Each consists of spongy red tissue surrounding treelike branches of the bronchus. In the lungs the blood receives oxygen from the air and gives up carbon dioxide.

**lupus** (loo'pus), or **lupus vulgaris.** Tuberculosis of the skin.

**lupus erythematosus** (ehr-i-thee-muh-toh'sus). A disease, inflammatory in nature, that takes two forms. One, the *systemic,* causes deterioration of connective tissues in various parts of the body. The other, *discoid,* is a fairly mild skin disorder.

**lymph** (limf). The clear yellowish watery fluid which is contained in the lymph vessels and around body cells.

**lymph node.** One of the many oval-shaped nodules along a lymph vessel. These nodes filter out germs and foreign bodies from the lymph.

**lymphocyte** (lim'foh-sight). A type of leukocyte found in the lymph and the blood. It contains few granules and has a single nucleus.

**lymphocytic choriomeningitis** (lim-foh-si'tik koh-ri-o-men-in-jigh'tis). A type of meningitis caused by a virus carried by the house mouse and spread to man by objects contaminated with mouse secretions or feces.

**lymphogranuloma venereum** (veh-neer'i-um). A viral disease which causes sores in the genital region and, in the male, enlargement of the lymph nodes in the groin.

**Lysol** (ligh'sawl). A proprietary disinfectant and antiseptic which contains a substance related to cresol.

**lytic** (lit'ik). 1. Pertaining to breakdown of cells by a lysin. 2. Pertaining to the subsiding of symptoms of a disease.

## M

**maceration** (mas-er-ay'shun). The softening and deterioration of tissue.

**macroscopic** (mak-ro-skahp'ik). Seen with the naked eye.

**macula** (mak'yuh-luh). Discolored area on the skin; spot.

**madarosis** (mad-uh-ro'sis). Loss of eyelashes and eyebrows.

**Madura** (mad-yoo'ruh) **foot.** Mycetoma; a fungal infection of the foot found in India.

**Magendie** (maj-jen'dee), **Francois** (1783–1855). French physiologist who investigated the action of nerves and the effects of drugs. He showed that some nerves transmit sensation and others stimulate muscles.

**maidenhead.** Hymen; the membrane that partly covers the vaginal opening.

**malacotic** (mal-uh-kaht'ik) **teeth.** Teeth of a rather soft texture which decay more easily than normal teeth.

**malaise** (mal-ayz'). Discomfort; a feeling of being sick.

**malaria** (muh-lair'i-uh). A disease found mainly in tropical and subtropical areas and marked by intermittent attacks of fever, chills, and sweating. It is caused by a protozoan parasite carried by the anopheles mosquito.

**mal de mer** (mal"duh-mair'). Seasickness.

**malignant** (muh-lig'nent). Harmful; the opposite of benign.

**malingerer** (muh-ling'ger-er). One who pretends to be ill.

**malleolus** (mal-ee'o-lus). The round protruding bone

on either side of the ankle.

**malleus** (mal′i-us). The hammer-shaped bone of the inner ear. It is the largest of the three small bones.

**malnutrition** (mal-noo-trish′un). Improper nourishment resulting either from some defect in the body's assimilation or from poor diet.

**malocclusion** (mal-ahk-kloo′zhun). Abnormal position of the teeth in such a way that the teeth of the upper jaw do not mesh perfectly with those of the lower jaw, thus decreasing efficiency in chewing.

**Malta** (mawl′tuh) **fever.** Undulant fever; brucellosis.

**mammary** (mam′uh-ri) **gland.** The gland in the breast of a female which secretes milk.

**mandible** (man′di-bl). The lower jaw.

**mandrake** (man′drayk). A plant with properties like belladonna.

**mania** (may′ni-uh). 1. A type of insanity marked by great excitement, exaggerated feelings of happiness, hallucinations, and violent action. 2. Strong desire or enthusiasm.

**manic-depressive psychosis.** A type of mental illness in which periods of melancholy and depression alternate with periods of great excitement.

**manubrium** (man-oo′bri-um). The upper part of the breast bone or the "handle" of the malleus bone.

**marijuana** or **marihuana** (mah-ri-hwah′-nah). The hemp or cannabis plant.

**marrow** (mar′oh). The soft material in the cavities of bones.

> **red marrow.** Marrow in which red blood cells are formed. In adults only a few areas have red marrow but in children most marrow is red.
>
> **yellow marrow.** Marrow which no longer makes red blood cells. It contains mostly fat cells.

**masochism** (mas′uh-kizm). A perversion, usually sexual, in which an individual gets pleasure from being hurt.

**massage** (muh-sahzh′). Rubbing and kneading the muscles.

**mastectomy** (mas-tek′tuh-mi). Surgical removal of the breast.

**mastication** (mas-ti-kay′shun). Act of chewing.

**mastitis** (mas-tigh′tis). Inflammation of the breast.

**mastoid** (mas′toyd) **bone.** The part of the skull which forms the hump behind the ear. It contains several hollow areas (cells) which connect with the middle ear.

**mastoidectomy** (mas-toyd-ek′tuh-mi). Operation of scraping out the mastoid bone and removing the bony partitions between the cells.

**mastoiditis** (mas-toyd-igh′tis). Inflammation in the mastoid bone.

**masturbation** (mas-ter-bay′shun). Handling one's own genitals to produce sexual excitement.

**materia medica** (muh-tir′i-uh med′i-kuh). Branch of medical study which deals with medicines, their preparation and use.

**maxilla** (mak-sil′uh). The upper jaw.

**Mayo** (may′o), **William James** (1861–1939) and **Charles Horace** (1865–1939). American surgeons who started a famous clinic.

**McDowell, Ephraim** (1771–1830). Backwoods Kentucky doctor who successfully removed a large ovarian cyst.

**meatus** (mee-ay′tus). Passage or opening.

**meconium** (mi-ko′ni-um). The pasty greenish feces passed by newborn babies.

**mediastinum** (mee-di-as-tee′num). 1. A partition in an organ or cavity. 2. The space in the middle of the chest which separates the lungs. The mediastinum contains the heart, trachea, esophagus, and thymus.

**medicine** (med′i-sin). 1. A substance used to treat disease. 2. Science of healing.

> **internal medicine.** The study of those diseases which are not treated by surgery.
>
> **patent medicine.** A manufactured medicine whose composition is patented.
>
> **preventive medicine.** A branch of medicine which aims at preventing disease.
>
> **proprietary medicine.** A trademarked medicine whose formula or method of preparation belongs to the manufacturer.

**medicolegal** (med-i-ko-lee′gl). Aspects of medicine which also relate to law.

**medulla** (mi-dul′uh). Central portion of an organ.

**medulla oblongata** (ahb′lawng-gah′tuh). The lower portion of the brain which connects with the spinal cord.

**megalomania** (meg-uh-lo-mayn′i-uh). Insanity in which the patient thinks himself great or powerful.

**melancholia** (mel-en-ko′li-uh). Depressed mental state in which the patient is indifferent to his surroundings and shows lessened mental and physical activity.

**melanin** (mel′uh-nin). The dark pigment in hair, tanned skin, and other dark-colored tissues.

**melanoma** (mel-uh-no'muh). A tumor made up of cells containing melanin.

**membrane** (mem'brayn). A thin layer of tissue which covers, lines, or partitions an organ.

**menarche** (men-ar'ki). The first menstrual period.

**meninges** (mi-nin'jeez). The membranes covering the brain and spinal cord.

**meningitis** (men-in-jigh'tis). Inflammation of the meninges.

> **epidemic cerebrospinal meningitis.** An acute infectious disease especially of children, marked by vomiting, convulsions, and headache. It is caused by bacteria (meningococcus).

**menopause** (men'o-pawz). Period when the menstrual cycle stops; the change of life.

**menorrhagia** (men-o-ray'ji-uh). Unusually long or profuse menstrual flow.

**menorrhalgia** (men-o-ral'ji-uh). Pain in menstruation.

**menorrhea** (men-o-ree'uh). Normal menstruation.

**menstruation** (men-stroo-ay'shun). The periodic discharge of blood from the vagina (usually monthly) in women.

**menthol** (men'thol). A pleasant-smelling substance which has anesthetic and antiseptic properties. It increases the ability to feel cold and so seems to produce a cooling effect.

**Mercurochrome** (mer-kyoo'ro-krohm). Trademark for a red antiseptic containing mercury.

**Merthiolate** (mer-thigh'o-layt). Trademark for a disinfectant and antiseptic substance which contains mercury.

**mesencephalon** (mes-en-sef'uh-lon). Midbrain; the part of the brain between the cerebrum and the cerebellum.

**mesentery** (mes'en-ter-i). The folds in the abdominal lining (peritoneum) that support the abdominal organs and attach the intestines to the abdominal wall. It carries the nerves and blood vessels to the abdominal organs.

**Mesmer** (mes'mer), **Franz A.** (1733–1815). Used "animal magnetism" or hypnotism to treat mental patients.

**metabolism** (meh-tab'o-lizm). The sum total of all the chemical and physical changes in the body, including tissue construction, destruction, and maintenance. See also **basal metabolism.**

**metacarpus** (met-uh-kar'pus). The part of the hand between the wrist and the fingers.

**metastasis** (meh-tas'tuh-sis). The spread of a disease from one part of the body to another usually by means of germs or cells carried from the diseased part by the blood or lymph.

**Metchnikoff** (mech'ni-kahf), **Elie** (1845–1916). Investigated the mechanism of immunity to disease and discovered that white blood cells engulf and ingest bacteria. He received the Nobel prize together with Ehrlich in 1908.

**metencephalon** (met-en-sef'uh-lon). 1. The cerebellum. 2. The hindbrain of the embryo.

**methemoglobin** (met-hee-mo-glo'bin). Hemoglobin which has decomposed or been deoxidized and changed by poisons, causing it to become chocolate brown in color.

**metritis** (mi-trigh'tis). Inflammation of the uterus.

**microbe** (migh'krohb). 1. Germ. 2. Microorganism; an organism which cannot be seen with the unaided eye, such as bacteria and protozoa.

**microcardia** (migh-kro-kar'di-uh). Abnormally small heart.

**microcephalic** (migh-kro-seh-fal'ik). Having a small head.

**microscope** (migh'kro-skohp). An instrument to magnify very small objects.

> **electron microscope.** An instrument that magnifies by means of electric and magnetic fields instead of lenses.

> **light microscope.** One which contains lenses arranged in such a way as to magnify objects.

**microtome** (migh'kro-tohm). Instrument for making extremely thin slices of tissue for microscopic study.

**micturition** (mik-tyoo-rish'un). Urination.

**migraine** (migh'grayn). Periodic sick-headache; pain in the head usually only on one side, accompanied by nausea, vomiting, and interferences in vision.

**milk of magnesia** (mag-nee'zhi-uh). A suspension of magnesium hydroxide that has laxative action.

**milligram.** A thousandth of a gram.

**Miltown** (mil'town). A proprietary tranquilizer, chemically the same as Equanil.

**mineral oil.** An oil obtained from petroleum and used as a laxative.

**Minot, George Richards** (1885–1950). American physician who developed dietary use of liver in treating pernicious anemia. He received the Nobel prize in 1934 together with W. P. Murphy and G. H. Whipple.

**miosis** (migh-o′sis). 1. Contraction of the pupil of the eye. 2. The last phase in the development of an egg or sperm.

**miscarriage** (mis-ka′rij). Expulsion of the fetus from the uterus before it is able to live, between the fourth and seventh months of pregnancy.

**mite** (might). A small parasitic insect which may infest man and cause skin irritations and spread disease germs.

**mitosis** (migh-toh′sis). Cell division.

**mitral** (migh′tral) **valve.** The valve between the upper and lower chambers in the left side of the heart.

**molar** (mo′ler). One of the grinding teeth in the back of both jaws.

**mole** (mohl). A brownish spot on the skin; a nevus.

**mongolism** (mahn′go-lizm). See **Down's syndrome.**

**moniliasis** (mahn-il-igh′uh-sis). Any infection caused by fungus of the Monilia group. Thrush is one type.

**monocyte** (mahn′o-sight). The largest type of leukocyte. It contains a single nucleus and faint granules. Two to 6 percent of all leukocytes are monocytes.

**mononucleosis** (mahn-o-noo-klee-o′sis). Condition in which there is a large number of monocytes in the blood; glandular fever.

> **infectious mononucleosis.** A communicable disease of unknown origin which is marked by fever, swollen lymph nodes, and an increase in monocytes in the blood.

**mons pubis** (monz pyoo′bis) or **mons veneris.** The elevated area in the front of the body of the female, formed by a pad of fatty tissue over the pubic symphysis.

**monster** (mon′ster). A malformed fetus.

**morbid** (mor′bid). Unhealthy.

**morbidity rate.** Sick rate; the number of cases per year of a specific disease per 100,000 people.

**morgue** (morg). Place where dead bodies are stored temporarily.

**moribund** (mawr′uh-buhnd). Near death.

**morning sickness.** Feeling of nausea in the first few months of pregnancy. It occurs chiefly in the morning.

**moron** (mo′rahn). Feebleminded person with a mental age between 7 and 12.

**morphine** (mawr′feen). A narcotic obtained from opium and used to relieve pain.

**mortality** (mor-tal′i-ti). Death rate.

**Morton, William T. G.** (1819–1868). American physician who pioneered in the use of ether for painless surgery.

**motor** (mo′ter). Affecting movement.

**mountain fever.** Tick fever.

**mountain sickness.** Sickness caused by low atmospheric pressure such as is found on mountains and in airplanes. It is marked by nausea, headache, thirst, and difficulty in breathing.

**mucin** (myoo′sin). A glycoprotein which is the main part of mucus.

**mucopurulent** (myoo-ko-pyoo′roo-lent). Containing mucus and pus.

**mucosa** (myoo-ko′suh). Mucous membrane; tissues that secrete mucus.

**mucous** (myoo′kus). Pertaining to mucus.

**mucus** (myoo′kus). The slimy secretion of the mucous glands which moistens body linings.

**multicellular** (mul-ti-sel′yoo-ler). Composed of many cells.

**murmur** (mer′mer). See **heart murmur.**

**muscle** (muhs′l). An organ which causes movement of some part of the body by means of its ability to shorten.

**musculature** (mus′kyoo-luh-tyoor). The muscles of the body or of any part.

**mute** (myoot). Unable to speak.

**myalgia** (migh-al′ji-uh). Pain in a muscle.

**myasthenia** (migh-as-thee′ni-uh). Muscle weakness; fatigue.

**mycetoma** (migh-si-toh′muh). Madura foot; a fungal infection of the foot which produces large pus-filled nodules. Found in India.

**mydriasis** (mid-righ′uh-sis). Dilatation of the pupil of the eye.

**myelin** (migh′el-in). The fatlike substance which forms a sheath around some nerves.

**myelitis** (migh-uh-ligh′tis). 1. Inflammation of the spinal cord. 2. Inflammation of marrow.

**myeloma** (migh-el-o′muh). A malignant tumor composed of cells of the same type as those in bone marrow.

**myoma** (migh-o′muh). Tumor formed of muscular tissue; may or may not be cancerous.

**myopia** (migh-o′pi-uh). Nearsightedness; condition in which the eyeball is too convex, causing light rays to focus in front of the retina.

**myxadenoma** (miks-ad-en-o′muh). A tumor that contains structures like those of a mucous gland.

## N

**nail bed.** The part of the finger covered by the nail.

**narcosis** (nar-ko′sis). A condition of stupor and loss of feeling produced by a narcotic.

**narcosynthesis** (nar-ko-sin′thi-sis). A method of treating psychoneurosis in which the patient is put into a hypnotic state to bring out his hidden emotions.

**narcotic** (nahr-kaht′ik). A medicine which produces sleep or stupor and relieves pain.

**nares** (nay′reez). Nostrils; the openings of the nose.

**nasal feeding.** Giving nourishing fluids through a rubber tube which has been passed through the nose down into the stomach.

**nasopharyngeal** (nay-zo-fuh-rin′ji-ul). Pertaining to the part of the pharynx directly over the roof of the mouth.

**nausea** (naw′se-uh). State of feeling sick at the stomach; a tendency to vomit.

**navel** (nay′vl). Umbilicus; the depression in the belly which marks the point where the umbilical cord had been attached during fetal life.

**nearsightedness.** See myopia.

**nebula** (neb′yoo-luh). Faint cloudiness on the cornea of the eye.

**necatoriasis** (ni-ka-tuh-righ′uh-sis). Hookworm disease.

**necropsy** (nek′rahp-si). Examination after death.

**necrosis** (ni-kro′sis). The death and breakdown of tissues which are surrounded by healthy tissues.

**Nembutal** (nem′byoo-tal). A proprietary barbiturate used as a sedative, and for relief from convulsions; pentobarbital sodium.

**neomycin** (nee-o-migh′sin). An antibiotic from a mold. It is used against infections which have become resistant to other antibiotics, but must be used with caution to avoid kidney damage.

**neoplasm** (nee′o-plazm). New and abnormal growth; tumor.

**Neo-Synephrine** (nee-o-sin-ef′rin) **hydrochloride.** A proprietary name for phenylephrine hydrochloride, which is used in nosedrops and eyedrops to relieve congestion.

**nephrectomy** (nef-rek′tuh-mi). Surgical removal of a kidney.

**nephritis** (ni-frigh′tis). Inflammation of a kidney.

**nephron** (nef′ron). One of the many units of a kidney in which waste is removed from the blood and carried to the kidney pelvis.

**nephrosis** (ni-fro′sis). A disease of the kidney in which there is degeneration of tissue without any apparent inflammation.

**nephrostomy** (ni-frahs′tuh-mi). Surgical formation of an artificial outlet from the kidney to the outside of the body.

**nerve** (nerv). A white cordlike tissue composed of fibers that can carry nerve impulses. It connects the brain and spinal cord with other parts of the body.

    **cranial nerve.** A nerve that connects with the brain. See **cranial** for the list of cranial nerves.

    **mixed nerve.** One which contains both sensory and motor fibers.

    **motor nerve.** One which carries impulses from the brain or spinal cord to muscles of the body and causes them to contract.

    **sensory nerve.** One which carries impulses to the brain or spinal cord from another part of the body.

    **spinal nerve.** A nerve which connects with the spinal cord. There are 31 pairs of spinal nerves.

**nervous system.** The entire apparatus of the body concerned with carrying impulses throughout the body. It includes the brain, spinal cord, nerves, and ganglions.

    **autonomic nervous system.** The system of nerves which regulate involuntary actions, such as those of the digestive organs, blood vessels, heart, kidneys, glands, etc. It is divided into the sympathetic and the parasympathetic nervous systems.

    **parasympathetic nervous system.** Nerves that dilate blood vessels, slow the heartbeat, and stimulate secretions.

    **sympathetic nervous system.** Spinal nerves that act in opposition to the parasympathetic nerves. They contract blood vessels, increase the heart rate, and inhibit stomach and glandular secretion.

**neuralgia** (noo-ral′ji-uh). Pain in a nerve or along the course of a nerve. The sharp stabbing pain usually lasts only a short time but recurs suddenly.

**neurasthenia** (noo-ras-thee′ni-uh). Nervous prostration; a condition in which one tires easily and suffers from weakness and various aches and pains.

**neuritis** (noo-righ′tis). Inflammation of a nerve. There are many different forms with different effects. Some increase the sensitivity in the affected part; others produce paralysis or numbness; some cause pain and inflammation.

**neurofibroma** (noo-ro-figh-bro′muh). A tumor made up of both nervous and connective tissues, caused by the overgrowth of the tissues surrounding the nerve fibers.

**neurofibromatosis** (noo-ro-figh-bro-muh-toh′sis). Condition in which there are many painless neurofibromas under the skin or along the course of a nerve. The tendency to this condition seems to be inherited.

**neuroglia** (noo-rahg′li-uh). The structure which supports the nervous tissue in the brain, spinal cord, and nerves. It consists of a fibrous network in which there are "spider cells," cells which have thin extensions in every direction.

**neurology** (noo-rahl′uh-ji). The study of nerves.

**neuron** (noo′rahn). A nerve cell.

**neurosis** (noo-ro′sis). A nervous disorder with no changes in tissue structure.

**neurotic** (noo-raht′ik). Pertaining to or affected by neurosis.

**neutralize** (nyoo′truh-lighz). To counteract the effect of a substance such as a toxin, an acid, or an alkali with another substance of equal strength but producing the opposite effect.

**nevus** (nee′vus). A congenital mark on the skin, either a pigmented area or a collection of tiny blood vessels; birthmark or mole.

**niacin** (nigh′uh-sin) or **nicotinic** (nik′o-tin-ik) **acid.** One of the vitamins in the vitamin B complex. It is found in lean meat, liver, milk, and rice. Medicinally it is used to treat pellagra.

**nictation** (nik-tay′shun) or **nictitation** (nik-tuh-tay′-shun). The act of winking or an abnormal spasm in the eyelid.

**Nightingale, Florence** (1820–1910). English nurse who organized a nursing corps during the Crimean War and founded the modern form of nursing.

**nit.** Egg of a louse.

**nitrogen mustard.** A gas used medicinally to destroy diseased tissue in Hodgkin's disease, lymphosarcoma, and chronic leukemia.

**nitroglycerin** (nigh-tro-glis′er-in). An oily explosive liquid used medicinally to prevent attacks of asthma, angina pectoris, and apoplexy.

**nitrous oxide.** Laughing gas; a gas which produces general anesthesia when inhaled.

**nocturia** (nok-tu′re-ah). Excessive urination at night.

**node** (nohd). A knoblike structure.

**Noludar** (nohl′oo-dahr). A proprietary medicine used for sedation.

**Novocain** (no′vuh-kayn). Proprietary name of procaine hydrochloride, an anesthetic.

**nucleus** (noo′kli-us). The central body and most essential part of a cell. All human body cells except mature red blood cells have nuclei.

**nurse.** A person who takes care of the sick, injured, or helpless.

> **graduate nurse.** One who has graduated from an accredited training school.
>
> **practical nurse.** One trained in the less technical duties of nursing.
>
> **private nurse.** One who takes care of only one patient.
>
> **public health nurse.** A graduate nurse employed by the community board of health to promote health by teaching good health practices, by aiding in disease prevention, and by visiting sick persons.
>
> **registered nurse.** A graduate nurse who has been licensed and registered by a state authority.
>
> **visiting nurse.** A graduate nurse employed by an agency to visit and care for patients in their homes, if they cannot afford a full-time private nurse.

**nutrient** (noo′tri-ent). 1. A food which provides material needed by the body. 2. Providing nourishment.

**nutrition** (noo-trish′un). The process of supplying food and necessary material to the body or any of its parts so that it may grow or maintain itself in a healthy condition.

**nycturia** (nik-tyoo′ri-uh) or **nocturia** (nahk-tyoo′ri-uh). Excessive urination at night.

**nymphomania** (nim-foh-mayn′i-uh). Abnormally great sexual desire in a woman.

**nystagmus** (nis-tag′mus). Continuous involuntary movements of the eyeball. The condition may be congenital or the result of a disease.

# O

**obesity** (oh-bees'i-ti). Excessive fatness; corpulence.

**obstetrics** (ahb-stet'riks). The branch of medicine which deals with care of women during pregnancy, childbirth, and the period immediately following childbirth.

**occipital** (ahk-sip'uh-tl). Pertaining to the back part of the head or to the part of the brain in this part of the skull.

**occlusion** (ahk-kloo'zhun). The act of closing; in reference to teeth it means the fitting together of the upper and lower teeth in chewing.

    **coronary occlusion.** Blocking of an artery that supplies blood to the heart muscle.

**occult** (uh-kuhlt') **blood.** Blood present in feces or other material in such small amount that it can be detected only by chemical tests.

**occupational therapy.** The teaching of some useful trade or handicraft to sick or handicapped persons to give them something to do while recovering or to help them to earn a living.

**ocular** (ahk'yuh-ler). Pertaining to the eye.

**oculist** (ahk'yuh-list). A physician who specializes in treating eye diseases.

**odontitis** (o-dahn-tigh'tis). Inflammation of a tooth.

**odontoscope** (o-dahn'tuh-skohp). A dental mirror for examining teeth.

**odynophagia** (od-in-o-fay'ji-uh). Pain in swallowing food.

**Oedipus** (ed'i-pus) **complex.** A series of reactions thought to be caused by a son's suppressed sexual desire for his mother.

**ointment** (oynt'ment). A medicine for the skin prepared with a fatty base.

**olfactory** (ahl-fak'tuh-ri). Pertaining to the sense of smell.

**oliguria** (ahl-i-gyoo'ri-uh). Abnormally scanty urine.

**omentum** (o-men'tum). The fold of peritoneum which covers and connects the stomach and other abdominal organs.

    **greater omentum.** The fold which covers the large curve of the stomach and the intestines and attaches to the large intestine.

    **lesser omentum.** The fold which joins the small curve of the stomach and the liver.

**omphalitis** (ahm-ful-ligh'tis). Inflammation of the navel.

**oncology** (ahng-kahl'uh-ji). Study of tumors.

**onychia** (o-nik'i-uh). Inflammation of the tissue from which the nail grows.

**onycholysis** (ahn-i-kahl'is-is). Loosening of the nail.

**onychophagy** (ahn-i-kahf'uh-ji). Nail-biting.

**oophoroma** (o-ahf-o-ro'muh). Cancer of the ovary.

**ophthalmia** (ahf-thal'mi-uh). Inflammation of the eye or of the mucous lining of the eyelid.

**ophthalmitis** (ahf-thal-migh'tis). Inflammation of the eye.

**ophthalmology** (ahf-thal-mahl'uh-ji). The branch of medicine dealing with the eye, its defects and diseases.

**ophthalmoscope** (ahf-thal'muh-skohp). An instrument for examining the interior of the eye.

**opiate** (o'pi-ayt). 1. A substance containing opium. 2. A substance which produces sleep.

**opium** (o'pi-um). Narcotic obtained from the juice of the opium poppy. It is habit-forming and poisonous. Used medicinally as a pain reliever, hypnotic, and treatment for some types of diarrhea and other conditions.

**optician** (ahp-tish'n). One trained to grind lenses or glasses from a prescription.

**optometrist** (ahp-tahm'i-trist). One trained in examining eyes for the purpose of prescribing glasses.

**oral** (oh'rul). Pertaining to the mouth.

**orbit** (or'bit). Eye socket.

**orchiectomy** (or-ki-ek'tuh-mi) or **orchectomy** or **orchotomy.** Surgical removal of a testicle.

**orchiorrhaphy** (or-ki-or'uh-fi). Surgical correction of an undescended testis.

**orchitis** (or-kigh'tis). Inflammation of the testicle.

**organ** (or'gan). Any part of the body with a special function.

**orgasm** (or'gazm). Climax of sexual intercourse.

**origin of a muscle.** The more fixed end of a muscle.

**orthodontics.** Straightening of teeth.

**orthopedics** (or-tho-pee'diks). The branch of surgery concerned with correcting deformities and treating diseases of the bones, joints, muscles, and spine. Treatment may be by use of apparatus, manipulation, or operation.

**orthopedic surgeon.** Orthopedist; one who practices orthopedics.

**orthopnea** (or-thahp-nee'uh). Condition in which the person must stand or sit up in order to breathe easily.

**orthostatic** (or-tho-stat'ik). Standing erect.

**orthotonus** (or-thaht'o-nus). A spasm in which the body becomes straight and rigid. Seen in tetanus.

**os** (ahs), pl. **ora.** Mouth.

**os** (ahs), pl. **ossa.** Bone.

**oschitis** (ahs-kigh'tis). Inflammation of the scrotum.

**Osler** (ohs'ler), **Sir William** (1849–1919). Famous professor of medicine at Johns Hopkins and Oxford.

**osmosis** (ahs-mo'sis). Passage of a substance from one solution to another through a porous membrane. This is the method by which substances in tissues and blood are exchanged.

**ossicle** (ahs'i-kl). A very small bone, such as the three bones of the inner ear.

**ossification** (ahs-i-fi-kay'shun). Formation of bone or the process of changing cartilage into bone.

**osteitis** (ahs-ti-igh'tis). Inflammation of bone.

**osteochondritis** (ahs-ti-o-kahn-drigh'tis). Inflammation of bone and cartilage.

**osteoclasia** (ahs-ti-o-klay'zhi-uh). Surgical breaking of a bone to correct a deformity.

**osteoma** (ahs-ti-o'muh). Tumor composed of bone tissue. It may be an outgrowth of bone or may occur in the tissues.

**osteomalacia** (ahs-ti-o-muh-lay'shi-uh). Softening of the bones due to calcium deficiency and lack of vitamin D, and some hormonal disturbances. The bones become more flexible and brittle and cause pain. Similar to rickets in children.

**osteomyelitis** (ahs-ti-o-migh-eh-ligh'tis). Inflammation of bone.

**osteopathy** (ahs-ti-ahp'uh-thi). A system of treating diseases that uses generally accepted physical, medicinal, and surgical methods with emphasis on manipulation.

**otitis** (o-tigh'tis). Inflammation of the ear.

**otitis media.** Inflammation of the middle ear.

**otomycosis** (o-toh-migh-ko'sis). A disease of the ear caused by a fungus.

**otorhinolaryngology** (o-toh-rine'-o-lar-in-gahl'uh-ji). Branch of medicine dealing with the ear, nose, and throat.

**otoscope** (o'toh-skohp). Instrument for examining the ear.

**outpatient department.** Dispensary; part of the hospital where persons are treated who do not need to be kept at the hospital. In many hospitals such care is given at low cost or free to those who can prove their need.

**ovariectomy** (o-va-ri-ek'tuh-mi). Surgical removal of an ovary.

**ovariostomy** (o-va-ri-ahs'tuh-mi). Cutting into the ovary to drain an ovarian cyst.

**ovaritis** (o-va-righ'tis). Inflammation of an ovary.

**ovary** (o'vuh-ri). Either of the two female reproductive glands which produce the eggs (ova) and female hormones.

**overbite.** A condition in which the upper front teeth overlap the lower teeth when biting.

**oviduct** (o'vuh-dukt). The tube connecting the ovary and the uterus through which the egg cell must pass; also called the fallopian tube.

**ovulation** (o-vyoo-lay'shun). The maturing of an egg cell and its release from the ovary. This takes place approximately every 28 days, midway during the menstrual cycle.

**ovum** (o'vum). An egg cell; the sex cell from the woman. When fertilized the cell develops from a size of 1/125 inch diameter into a human baby.

**oxygen** (ahk'si-jen). A colorless gas found in air and necessary for life.

**oxygenation** (ahk-si-jen-ay'shun). Saturation of a substance with oxygen.

**oxyhemoglobin** (ahk'si-hee'mo-glo-bin). Hemoglobin which has combined with oxygen. It gives blood a bright red color.

**oxyhydrocephalus** (ahk-si-high-dro-sef'uh-lus). A condition in which there is an excess of fluid in the head, causing the head to assume a pointed shape.

**oxytocic** (ahk-si-toh'sik). 1. A substance which hastens the process of childbirth. 2. Hastening childbirth.

**oxytocin** (akh-si-toh'sin). A substance produced by the pituitary gland which stimulates the uterus to contract in childbirth.

**ozone** (o'zohn). A form of oxygen. It is used as an antiseptic and as a disinfectant, particularly for swimming pools.

# P

**PABA.** Abbreviation for para-aminobenzoic acid; an agent believed to be a member of the vitamin B complex. It is used in treatment for rickettsial diseases such as Rocky Mountain spotted fever.

**pabulum** (pab'yoo-lum). A cooked cereal for babies.

**pachycephaly** (pak-i-sef'uh-li). Condition of having

an abnormally thick skull.

**pachydermia** (pak-i-der′mi-uh). Condition in which the skin thickens abnormally.

**pack treatment.** Treatment by wrapping the patient in a blanket.

    **cold pack.** Wrapping in a covering wrung out of cold water.

    **dry pack.** Wrapping in dry hot blankets.

    **half pack.** Wrapping the body from the armpits to the knees.

    **hot pack.** Wrapping in hot blankets, wet or dry.

    **ice pack.** A substitute for an ice bag made by wrapping ice in a towel.

    **wet pack.** Wrapping in wet blankets, hot or cold.

**Paget's** (paj′ets) **disease.** 1. A disease of the nipple associated with breast cancer. 2. Also a disease of the bones and skull, called *osteitis deformans*.

**palate** (pal′it). The roof of the mouth.

    **artificial palate.** A plate inserted to close the gap of a cleft palate.

    **cleft palate.** Congenital condition in which the bones of the roof of the mouth fail to unite, leaving a cleft.

    **hard palate.** The bony front portion of the roof of the mouth.

    **soft palate.** The fleshy part of the roof of the mouth near the throat.

**palliative** (pal′i-uh-tiv). A medicine which relieves symptoms of a disease but does not cure it.

**pallor** (pal′or). Paleness.

**palpation** (pal-pay′shun). Examination by feeling with the hand.

**palpitation** (pal-pi-tay′shun). Rapid beating of the heart.

**palsy** (pawl′zi). Paralysis.

    **birth palsy.** 1. Paralysis from an injury received at birth. 2. Spastic diplegia.

    **cerebral palsy.** 1. Paralysis caused by brain injury. 2. Spastic diplegia.

    **crutch palsy.** Paralysis caused by the pressure of a crutch against the armpit.

    **lead palsy.** Paralysis of arm muscles from lead poisoning.

    **shaking palsy.** Parkinson's disease; paralysis agitans.

**panacea** (pan-uh-see′uh). A cure-all.

**pancreas** (pan′kri-uhs). The gland (6 to 8 inches long) located behind the stomach. It secretes a juice that aids in digesting food and also secretes insulin which regulates the blood-sugar level.

**pancreatin** (pan′kri-uh-tin). An extract from ox or hog pancreas which contains a mixture of digestive enzymes. Used in treating certain types of digestive failures and also used in preparing predigested foods.

**pancreatitis** (pan-kri-uh-tigh′tis). Inflammation of the pancreas.

**pandemic** (pan-dem′ik). Epidemic which covers a very large area.

**pantothenic** (pan-toh-then′ik) **acid.** One of the vitamin B complex. It is important in the nutrition of certain animals, but its importance for human beings has not yet been established.

**pap.** Any soft food.

**Papanicolaou's** (pap-uh-nik-o-lay′ooz) (**Pap**) **smear.** A test made with body excretions, secretions, or tissue scrapings used in detection mainly of cancer of the uterus and cervix but also of the lung, stomach, and bladder.

**papilla** (puh-pil′uh). A nipple-shaped elevation.

    **gustatory** or **lingual papilla.** One of the small elevations on the tongue which contains taste buds.

**papilloma** (pap-i-lo′muh). An overgrown papilla of the skin or mucous membranes. Such tumors are usually benign and may be due to a virus or a chemical factor.

**papule** (pap′yool). Small abnormal elevation on the skin; a pimple.

**para-anesthesia** (par-uh-an-es-thee′zi-uh). Anesthesia of the body below the waist.

**Paracelsus** (par-uh-sel′sus) (1493–1541). Swiss physician who contributed to the advance of medicine, particularly in the use of chemicals to treat disease.

**paraldehyde** (par-al′duh-highd). A liquid with a characteristic odor and unpleasant taste used as a hypnotic, a pain reliever, and a sleep inducer for patients with delirium tremens or other cases where fast action is desirable.

**paralysis** (puh-ral′i-sis). Loss of sensation or movement in a part.

    **paralysis agitans.** A nervous disease of the aged marked by tremor of the hands.

**paranoia** (par-uh-noy′uh). A chronic mental disorder in which there are delusions, usually of persecution.

**paraplegia** (par-uh-plee′ji-uh). Paralysis of the legs and lower part of the body.

> **ataxic paraplegia.** A form caused by sclerosis of the spinal cord in which paralysis progresses slowly.

**parasite** (par′uh-sight). A plant or animal that lives in or on another organism and gets nourishment from it.

**parasympathetic nervous system.** Part of the autonomic nervous system. It dilates blood vessels, slows the heart beat, and stimulates secretions.

**parathyroid** (par-uh-thigh′royd). Any one of four small glands located behind or imbedded in the thyroid gland. They control the calcium-phosphorus levels in the body.

**paratyphoid** (par-uh-tigh′foyd) **fever.** A disease with symptoms similar to typhoid fever but caused by different bacteria. It is spread through polluted water or milk.

**Paré** (par-ay′), **Ambroise** (1510–1590). French surgeon who substituted the use of ligatures to tie off arteries for cauterization as a means of preventing bleeding.

**paregoric** (par-eh-gor′ik). An opium compound used to relieve cramps.

**parenchyma** (par-eng′kigh-muh). The parts of an organ that are especially adapted for its function rather than the supporting or protective tissues of the organ.

**parenteral** (par-en′ter-ul). Not into the intestine; designates substances introduced or injected through the mucous membranes, skin, blood, or other means than the intestine.

**paresis** (puh-ree′sis). 1. A slight paralysis. 2. A chronic disease of the brain resulting from syphilis and causing progressive mental and physical deterioration.

**parietal** (puh-righ′i-tal) **bones.** Bones at the sides of the skull.

**parietal lobe.** A cerebral lobe of the brain located at the side of the head, composed of gray matter.

**paronychia** (par-o-nik′i-uh). Inflammation around a finger or toe nail.

**parotid** (puh-rot′id) **gland.** The largest of the salivary glands, located near the ear.

**parotitis** (par-o-tigh′tis). Mumps; a viral disease marked by the swelling of one or both parotid glands.

**paroxysm** (par′uhk-sizm). 1. The sudden appearance of symptoms or sudden increase in intensity of symptoms of a disease. 2. Fit; convulsions; spasm.

**parrot fever.** See **psittacosis.**

**parturition** (par-tyoo-rish′un). The act of giving birth to a child.

**PAS.** Abbreviation for para-aminosalicylic acid; a substance which stops the growth of tubercle bacilli and is used in association with streptomycin in tuberculosis treatment.

**Pasteur** (pahs″ter′), **Louis** (1822–1895). French scientist who discovered that many diseases are caused by germs. His contributions include the pasteurization of milk and wine and the development of a vaccine against rabies.

**Pasteur treatment.** Prevention of rabies by a series of inoculations with vaccine containing a milder form of the rabies virus obtained from rabbits.

**pasteurization** (pas-tyoor-uh-zay′shun). A method of destroying harmful bacteria in milk or other liquids by heating for 30 minutes at 60 C. (140 F.).

**patch test.** Test for allergy to a substance by applying to the skin a piece of cloth containing the substance.

**patella** (puh-tel′uh). Kneecap.

**pathogen** (path′o-jen). Any substance or organism that can cause disease.

**pathogenic** (path-o-jen′ik). Capable of causing disease.

**pathological** (path-o-lahj′i-kal). Diseased.

**pathology** (puh-thahl′uh-ji). 1. The branch of medicine which deals with the changes in the body produced by disease. 2. Effects produced by a disease.

**patient** (pay′shent). Person who is ill or is undergoing treatment.

**Pavlov** (Pahf′lohf), **Ivan Petrovich** (1849–1936). Russian physiologist who described and demonstrated the conditioned reflex.

**pectoral** (pek′tuh-ral). Relating to the chest.

**pediatrics** (pee-di-at′riks). The branch of medicine that deals with the development and the diseases of children.

**pedicle** (ped′i-kl). The stem of a tumor.

**pediculosis** (pee-dik′yoo-lo′sis). Condition of being infested with lice.

**pellagra** (pel-lag′ruh or puh-lay′gruh). A disease caused by lack of vitamin $B_2$ (nicotinic acid) in the diet. It is marked by weakness, redness on parts of the body, diarrhea, etc.

**pelvic girdle.** The bony cup formed by the hip-bone and the lower bones of the back.

**pelvis** (pel'vis). 1. A basin-shaped cavity, such as the cavity in the kidney. 2. The pelvic girdle.

**pemphigus** (pem'fi-gus). A skin disease marked by the appearance of watery blisters.

**penicillin** (pen-i-sil'in). An antibiotic obtained from the *Penicillium* mold and active against many bacteria such as those that cause gonorrhea, syphilis, lobar pneumonia, etc.

**penis** (pee'nis). The external male sex organ from which semen is discharged in sexual intercourse. It also contains the passage for urine.

**Pentothal** (pen'toh-thal) **sodium.** A proprietary hypnotic given intravenously.

**pepsin** (pep'sin). An enzyme secreted in the stomach to aid in digesting proteins.

**peptic ulcer** (pep'tik ul'ser). An ulcer in the stomach or intestine caused by the abnormal action of digestive juices on the tissues. This condition causes burning pains in the stomach and seems to be related to the mental stress of the patient.

**percaine** (per'kayn). Local or spinal anesthetic; nupercaine hydrochloride.

**percomorph** (per'ko-morf) **oil.** Oil from the liver of a certain type of fish. It contains vitamin D.

**percussion** (per-kush'un). The act of tapping or thumping a part, particularly the chest and back, as an aid to diagnosis. The sounds indicate the size, position, and density of the organs underneath.

**pericardium** (pehr-i-kar'di-um). The membrane which surrounds the heart.

**perineum** (pehr-i-nee'um). The region between the anus and the genitals.

**periodontal** (pehr-i-o-dahn'tal) **membrane.** A tough tissue covering the roots of the teeth and connecting them to the jaw.

**periodontitis** (pehr"e-o-don-tigh'tis). Inflammation of the tissues around a tooth. If unchecked, it is a major cause of tooth loss.

**periosteum** (pehr-i-ahs'ti-um). The fibrous membrane which covers bones.

**peristalsis** (pehr-i-stahl'sis). The progressive wave of muscular contraction which pushes food along in the esophagus and the intestines. The motion appears wormlike.

**peritoneum** (pehr-i-tuh-nee'um). The membrane which forms the lining of the abdominal cavity and covers the stomach, intestines, and other organs.

**peritonitis** (pehr-i-toh-nigh'tis). Inflammation of the peritoneum.

**perlèche** (per-lesh'). A contagious disease in which the corners of the mouth become raw and thickened.

**pernicious** (per-nish'us). Tending to cause death.

**personality** (per-sun-al'i-ti). The characteristics and behavior that are seen in an individual.

    **dual** or **alternating personality.** Existence in an individual of two distinct personalities.

**perspiration** (per-spi-ray'shun). 1. Sweat; the substance excreted through the sweat glands of the skin and consisting of water, salts, urea, ammonia, and other substances. 2. The act of sweating.

**pertussis** (per-tus'is). Whooping cough.

**perversion** (per-ver'zhun). A turning away from the normal or correct.

    **sexual pervert.** One who indulges in unnatural sexual practices.

**pessary** (pes'uh-ri). 1. A device placed in the vagina to support the uterus or rectum. 2. A vaginal suppository.

**petit mal** (pet-i-mahl'). A mild epileptic attack.

**petrolatum** (pet-ruh-lay'tum). A jellylike substance obtained from petroleum. It is used as an ointment base and for treatment of burns and minor skin irritations.

**phacolysis** (fu-kahl'is-is). 1. Disintegration of the lens of the eye. 2. Removal of the lens of the eye to relieve high myopia.

**phacomalacia** (fak-o-muh-lay'shi-uh). Abnormal softening of the lens of the eye.

**phagocyte** (fag'uh-sight). Any cell that is able to engulf bacteria or foreign particles. Many of the white blood cells are phagocytes.

**phalanx** (fay'langks), pl. **phalanges** (fuh-lan'jeez). Bone of the finger or toe, three in each digit.

**phallitis** (fal-igh'tis). Inflammation of the penis.

**phallus** (fal'us). The penis.

**phantasm** (fan'tazm). An optical illusion.

**pharmaceutical** (far-muh-soo'ti-kal). A medicine.

**pharmacist** (far'muh-sist). A druggist who is trained to fill prescriptions.

**pharyngeal** (fuh-rin'ji-ul). Pertaining to the tube which connects the mouth, nose, and esophagus.

**pharyngectomy** (far-in-jek'tuh-mi). Surgical removal of part of the pharynx.

**pharyngitis** (far-in-jigh'tis). Inflammation of the pharynx; sore throat.

**pharynx** (far'ingks). The throat. The tube composed of muscle and membranes, which extends from the back of the nose and mouth to the esophagus. It is a passage for both food and air and also plays a part in voice resonance.

**phenacetin** (fee-nas'i-tin). A brand of acetopheneti-din used to relieve pain and fever.

**phenobarbital** (feen-o-bar'bi-tal). A barbiturate. It is a sedative and is also used to control epileptic convulsions.

**phenol** (fee'nohl). Carbolic acid; a disinfectant.

**phenolphthalein** (fee-nohl-thal'i-in). A cathartic and a dye. It is the active agent in most "candy" laxatives.

**phimosis** (figh-mo'sis). Condition in which the foreskin is too tight to be drawn back over the glans penis.

**phlebitis** (fli-bigh'tis). Inflammation of a vein.

**phlegm** (flem). Mucus.

**phobia** (fo'bi-uh). Any abnormal and persistent fear.
> **acrophobia.** Fear of high places.
> **algophobia.** Fear of pain.
> **androphobia.** Fear of men.
> **apiphobia.** Fear of bees.
> **astrapophobia.** Fear of lightning.
> **claustrophobia.** Fear of closed places.
> **cynophobia.** Fear of dogs.
> **gephyrophobia.** Fear of crossing a bridge.
> **haphephobia.** Fear of touching or being touched by others.
> **hematophobia** or **hemophobia.** Fear of blood.
> **lalophobia.** Fear of speaking.
> **necrophobia.** Fear of a corpse.
> **ophidiophobia.** Fear of snakes.
> **pyrophobia.** Fear of fire.
> **thanatophobia.** Fear of death.
> **triskaidekaphobia.** Fear of the number thirteen.
> **zoophobia.** Fear of animals.

**phosphate** (fahs'fayt). A type of phosphorus compound which is an important part of bone.

**photophobia** (fo-toh-fo'bi-uh). A condition in which light causes pain in the eyes.

**phthisis** (thigh'sis). 1. Tuberculosis. 2. Wasting of the body.

**physic** (fiz'ik). A medicine, especially one which loosens the bowels.

**physician** (fi-zish'un). One who is licensed to practice medicine.

**physiology** (fiz-i-ahl'uh-ji). The study of the functions and activities of cells, tissues, and organs.

**pia, pia mater** (pi'uh may'ter). The delicate membrane which is the innermost of three layers covering the brain and spinal cord.

**pigeon breast.** Chicken breast; condition of prominent sternum.

**pigeon-toed.** Walking or standing with the toes turned in.

**pigment** (pig'ment). Coloring matter; dye.

**piles.** See **hemorrhoid.**

**pimple** (pim'pl). Pustule or papule; a nipple-shaped growth on the skin caused by inflammation of a skin pore.

**pineal** (pin'i-ul) **body.** A small gland located in the back of the brain. Its function is not known.

**pink-eye.** A contagious inflammation of the eye caused by bacteria. Also called acute contagious conjunctivitis.

**pinworm.** A parasitic worm which is the cause of enterobiasis, a disease marked by loss of appetite, insomnia, and itching at the anus.

**Pitocin.** Proprietary name for oxytocin.

**Pitressin.** Proprietary name for vasopressin.

**pituitary** (pi-too'i-tehr-i) **gland.** A small bean-shaped gland lying at the base of the brain. It has many functions including growth and sexual development.

**Pituitrin** (pi-too'i-trin). A proprietary name for a substance obtained from dried pituitary glands of slaughterhouse animals.

**pityriasis** (pit-i-righ'uh-sis). A skin disease in which colored flaky patches appear.

**placebo** (pluh-see'bo). An inert substance given to a patient like medicine. It may be given for the mental effect on the patient, or it may be a control in tests of a new medicine.

**placenta** (pluh-sen'tuh). The structure on the wall of the uterus through which nourishment passes to the umbilical cord from the mother to the fetus in pregnancy; the afterbirth.

**Placidyl** (plass'i-dil). A proprietary sedative, taken orally.

**plague** (playg). 1. Any contagious fatal epidemic disease. 2. Bubonic plague; a highly contagious fatal fever caused by bacteria carried in infected rats and transmitted to man by rat fleas.
> **black plague.** The fourteenth-century epidemic disease which killed many people and caused

them to appear black because of severe hemorrhages.

**plantar** (plan'tar). Pertaining to the sole of the foot.

**plaque** (plak). 1. Patch or film. 2. A blood platelet.

**plasma** (plaz'muh). The fluid part of the circulating blood. It differs from blood serum in that it contains fibrin while serum does not.

**plastic** (plas'tik). Concerned with building up or repairing tissues.

**plastic surgery.** Surgery to restore lost parts or repair defects, often by grafting tissue from another part.

**platelet** (playt'let). Thrombocyte; one of the small colorless round bodies found in blood and believed to play a part in blood clotting.

**pledget** (plej'et). A small compress or wad of cotton, gauze, etc.

**plethora** (pleth'uh-ruh). A condition in which there is an excess of blood in the blood vessels causing redness of the face and a tendency to nosebleed.

**pleura** (ploor'uh). The membrane which lines the chest cavity and covers the lungs.

**pleurisy** (ploor'i-si). Inflammation of the pleura.

**pleuropneumonia** (ploor-o-noo-mo'ni-uh). Inflammation of the pleura and the lung.

**plexus** (plek'sus). A network or tangle of veins, lymphatic vessels, or nerves.

>   **solar plexus.** A large ganglion or network of nerves located behind the stomach.

**plumbism** (plum'bizm). Lead poisoning.

**pneumococcus** (noo-mo-kahk'us). A type of bacterium which is seen in pairs, and can cause lobar pneumonia.

**pneumonitis** (noo-mo-nigh'tis). Inflammation of the lung.

**pneumoresection** (noo-mo-ree-sek'shun). Surgical removal of a part of the lung.

**pneumothorax** (noo-mo-tho'raks). A collection of air or gas in the chest cavity causing the lung to collapse. It can result from injury to the chest or may occur spontaneously.

>   **artificial pneumothorax.** Collapse of the lung induced by injection of air or gas into the pleural cavity in order to rest the lung.

**pock.** A pustule, particularly of smallpox.

**pock-marked.** Having small pits or scars on the skin resulting from smallpox.

**podiatrist** (po-digh'uh-trist). One who treats foot ailments; a chiropodist.

**polioencephalitis** (pahl-i-o-en-sef-uh-ligh'tis). Inflammation of the gray matter of the brain.

**polluted** (po-loo'ted). Impure.

**polycythemia** (pahl-i-sigh-thee'mi-uh). An abnormal increase in the number of red blood cells.

**polydactylism** (pahl-i-dak'til-izm). Having more than five fingers on a hand.

**polymyxin** (pahl-i-mik'sin). Antibiotic from bacteria; active against gram-negative bacteria, such as those causing urinary infections. It is very toxic when injected but can safely be taken by mouth.

**polyp** (pahl'ip). A nodular tumor growing from mucous tissues, such as the linings of the nose, bladder, stomach, intestine, or uterus.

**polyphagia** (pahl-i-fay'ji-uh). Excessive eating.

**portal vein.** Blood vessel which carries blood through the liver.

**postpartum** (pohst-par'tum). After childbirth.

**PPD.** Abbreviation for purified protein derivative, a substance obtained by purifying tuberculin and used like tuberculin in skin tests for tuberculosis.

**precancerous** (pree-kan'ser-us). Likely to develop into cancer.

**pregnancy** (preg'nen-si). Being with child; the period between conception and childbirth (approximately 280 days).

**Preludin** (pray-lude'in). A proprietary appetite depressant.

**Presate** (pree'sate). A proprietary appetite-reducing medication.

**prescription** (pree-skrip'shun). Written directions for preparing a medicine.

**pressor** (pres'or). Tending to raise the blood pressure.

**prickly heat.** Miliaria; a rash caused by the skin being irritated by perspiration. Occurs particularly where the skin is folded or rubbed by clothing.

**primaquine** (prigh'muh-kwin). A medicine used against malaria.

**Pro-Banthine** (pro-bann'theen). A proprietary antispasmodic preparation, used to treat stomach ulcers, colitis, and other diseases that involve the involuntary muscles.

**probe** (prohb). A slender flexible instrument used for exploring wounds or body passages.

**procaine** (pro'kayn). A local anesthetic; also a spinal anesthetic used when it is desired to anesthetize for only a short time.

**process** (prahs'ses). In reference to a cell, bone, or

organ it means a projecting part or thin extension.

**procreation** (pro-kree-ay'shun). The act of producing offspring.

**proctitis** (prahk-tigh'tis). Inflammation of the rectum or anus.

**proctocele** (prahk'toh-seel). A hernia of part of the rectum.

**progesterone** (pro-jes'ter-ohn). The female sex hormone produced by the corpus luteum and causing the lining of the uterus to thicken and other body changes necessary before conception can occur.

**prognosis** (prahg-no'sis). Prediction of the probable results of a disease.

**projection** (pro-jek'shun). In psychiatry it refers to a tendency to see in other people one's own repressed feelings.

**prolapse** (pro-laps'). Downward displacement of an organ or the falling down of an organ from its usual place.

**proliferation** (pro-lif-er-ay'shun). Multiplication of cells.

**prophylactic** (pro-figh-lak'tik). An agent that prevents the development of a disease.

**prophylaxis** (pro-figh-lak'sis). Disease prevention.

**proprietary medicine.** See **medicine, proprietary.**

**proprioceptor** (pro-pree-o-sep'tor). A nerve that is stimulated from within the body, giving information concerning movement or position.

**propylthiouracil** (pro-pil-thigh-o-yoor'uh-sil). Medicine which is used in treating overactive thyroid.

**prostate** (prahs'tayt) **gland.** A male sex gland located at the neck of the bladder. It secretes prostatic fluid, which is part of the seminal fluid.

**prostatectomy** (prahs-tuh-tek'tuh-mi). Surgical removal of part of the prostate gland.

**prosthetic** (prahs-thet'ik) **device.** An artificial substitute for a missing part, such as a hand, leg, or eye. It may be used to improve the appearance or it may be functional as well.

**prostration** (prahs-tray-shun). Extreme exhaustion.

**protein** (pro'tee-in). A type of nitrogen compound which forms most of the tissues of the body, especially muscles.

**prothrombin** (pro-thrahm'bin). One of the substances in blood which combines to form thrombin, the enzyme which clots blood.

**protoplasm** (pro'toh-plazm). The jellylike substance which composes all living cells and is the essential material of life.

**protozoa** (pro-toh-zo'uh). The lowest division of the animal kingdom. It includes one-celled organisms such as amebae and paramecia, some of which cause disease.

**prurigo** (proo-righ'go). A chronic skin disease marked by intense itching and the development of small pale papules.

**pruritus** (proo-righ'tis). Intense itching.

**psittacosis** (sit-uh-ko'sis). Parrot fever; a contagious disease of birds, such as pigeons and parakeets, which can be transmitted to man. In man it causes inflammation of the lung accompanied by fever.

**psyche** (sigh'ki). The mind, including both conscious and unconscious processes.

**psychiatry** (sigh-kigh'uh-tri). The branch of medicine that deals with mental disorders.

**psychoanalysis** (sigh-ko-uh-nal'is-is). A technique used for treating various mental disorders. By means of free association the patient brings up past experiences and ideas which give insight into the unconscious mind.

**psychology** (sigh-kahl'uh-ji). The branch of science that deals with the mind and behavior.

**psychomotor** (sigh-ko-mo'ter). Pertaining to voluntary movement.

**psychoneurosis** (sigh-ko-noo-ro'sis). A disorder of the mind not caused by any damage or change in brain tissue. The personality is only partially disorganized but marked by anxiety, preoccupation, and tension.

**psychopath** (sigh'ko-path). A person mentally ill yet apparently of sound mind except for an abnormal criminal or sexual drive.

**psychosis** (sigh-ko'sis). A disorder of the mind; insanity.

**psychosomatic** (sigh-ko-so-mat'ik). Pertaining to both the mind and the body, such as diseases which are traced to emotional causes.

**ptomaine** (toh'mayn). An indefinite term for poisonous substances produced by decomposition of protein by bacteria.

**ptyalin** (tigh'uh-lin). An enzyme in saliva which changes starch to sugar.

**puberty** (pyoo'ber-ti). The period of life in which the reproductive organs become capable of functioning. In boys it is marked by the change in voice and discharge of semen. In girls it is marked by the start of menstruation.

**pubic bone** (pyoo'bik). The lower front part of the

hipbone.

**pubic symphisis** (sim'fi-sis). The place where the two pubic bones join.

**puerperium** (pyoo-er-pee'ri-um). The period after childbirth during which the uterus returns to normal. Usually considered to last about six weeks.

**pulmonary** (puhl'muh-nehr-i). Pertaining to the lungs.

**pulmotor** (puhl'mo-ter). An apparatus for automatically giving artificial respiration.

**pulse** (puhls). The expansion and contraction of an artery. The contractions of the arterial walls correspond to the contractions of the heart and so are indications of the rate of heartbeat. Normal rate in men: 65 to 72 beats per minute; in women: 70 to 80 beats per minute; more rapid in children.

**pump, breast.** Pump for removing milk from the breasts.

> **stomach pump.** Pump for removing poisons from the stomach.

**puncture, lumbar** or **spinal.** Making a hole through the membranes of the spinal cord in the lower back region in order to withdraw fluid from the spine.

**pupil** (pyoo'pil). The opening in the center of the iris through which light passes.

**purge** (perj). 1. To evacuate the bowels by means of a medicine. 2. Also a medicine which causes a very active bowel movement; a cathartic.

**purpura** (per'pyoo-ruh). A condition in which purple patches appear on the skin or other membranes as a result of hemorrhages of the tiny blood vessels.

**purulent** (pyoo'roo-lent). Containing or forming pus.

**pus.** A thick yellowish fluid containing cells, serum, and the products of inflammation.

**pustule** (pus'tyool). A pus-filled pimple or papule.

**pyelitis** (pigh-eh-ligh'tis). Inflammation of the kidney pelvis.

**pyemia** (pigh-ee'mi-uh). Presence of pus in the blood. Pus-forming germs invade the whole system through the bloodstream and may produce abscesses in many different parts of the body.

**pyloric** (pigh-lor'ik). Pertaining to the opening between the stomach and the small intestine.

**pylorus** (pigh-lor'us). The opening of the stomach into the small intestine.

**pyogenic** (pigh-o-jen'ik). Producing pus.

**pyorrhea** (pigh-o-ree'uh). Discharge of pus.

> **pyorrhea alveolaris.** A pus-producing inflam-

mation around the roots of teeth, marked by shrinking of gums and loosening of teeth. See also **periodontitis.**

**pyretic** (pigh-ret'ik). Pertaining to or characterized by fever.

**pyrexia** (pigh-rek'si-uh). Fever.

**Pyribenzamine** (peer-i-ben'zuh-meen). A proprietary antihistamine used in allergic conditions.

**pyrogen** (pigh'ro-jen). A substance which causes a rise in temperature. It is believed to come from bacteria but is not destroyed by sterilization and is frequently found in sterile solutions prepared for injections.

**pyromania** (pigh-ro-mayn'i-uh). An abnormal impulse to set fires.

## Q

**Q fever.** A mild typhuslike disease characterized chiefly by headache. It is caused by a rickettsia germ and seems to be spread through livestock and milk from infected cows.

**quack.** One who pretends to have medical knowledge and skill which he does not possess.

**quarantine** (kwor'an-teen). 1. To isolate persons exposed to or sick with communicable diseases. 2. To detain ships and their passengers coming from places where they were exposed to some communicable disease.

**quickening.** The first fetal movements felt by a pregnant woman. They usually occur in the fourth or fifth month.

**quinine** (kwigh'nighn). A bitter substance obtained from bark of the cinchona tree. It is most important as the oldest treatment for malaria, although it has other medicinal uses.

**quinsy** (kwin'zi). An acute inflammation of the tonsil with formation of pus.

## R

**rabbit fever.** See **tularemia.**

**rabies** (ray'beez). An acute infectious disease caused by a virus and marked by fever, muscle spasm, and delirium. It is communicated to man by the bite of infected animals, usually dogs. Also called hydrophobia.

**rachitic** (ray-kit′ik). Pertaining to rickets.

**radiation sickness.** A disease marked by nausea and diarrhea and caused by overabsorption of radiation products.

**radioactive** (ray-di-o-ak′tiv). Emitting energy rays which can pass through substances opaque to light and produce electrical or chemical effects.

**radium** (ray′di-um). A highly radioactive element used in treating cancer.

**radius** (ray′di-us). The bone of the forearm on the thumb side.

**ranula** (ran′yoo-luh). Cystic tumor under the tongue due to obstruction of one of the glandular ducts.

**rash.** A temporary eruption on the skin.

**rat-bite fever.** A disease caused by bacteria transmitted to man by the bite of a rat.

**Rauwolfia** (raw′wolf-i-a). An ancient Hindu medicine used in the treatment of high blood pressure. It also produces a tranquil mood. Some of its purified components are called Serpasil, Reserpine, etc., and have similar medical properties.

**receptors** (ree-sep′ters). Nerve endings in the skin which are sensitive to heat, touch, pain, etc., and carry impulses to the brain.

**recessive characteristic.** The weaker of two competitive hereditary traits.

**recrudescence** (ree-kroo-des′ens). An increase in the symptoms of a disease after a period of improvement.

**rectal** (rek′tl). Pertaining to the rectum.

**rectum** (rek′tum). The part of the large intestine nearest the anus.

**red blood cell.** See **erythrocyte.**

**Reed, Walter** (1851–1902). Leader of the army medical commission which eliminated the danger of yellow fever in Panama, permitting construction of the Panama Canal.

**reflex** (ree′fleks). Automatic reaction; action done unconsciously in response to a stimulus.

**refractory** (ree-frak′tuh-ri). Not being cured by treatment.

**regeneration** (ree-jen-er-ay′shun). Repair of injured tissue.

**regressive** (ree-gres′iv). In psychology it refers to a return to a more childish state that had been more satisfying to the individual but is no longer in keeping with the age or social status.

**regurgitation** (ri-ger-ji-tay′shun). 1. Throwing up undigested food from the stomach. 2. Backward flow of blood through a leaky heart valve.

**rehabilitation** (ree-huh-bil-i-tay′shun). Restoring a handicapped person to useful activity.

**relapse** (re-laps′). The return of a disease after the patient has started to recuperate.

**relapsing fever.** Any one of several infectious diseases caused by bacteria carried in lice or ticks. It is marked by alternating periods of fever and normal temperature. Includes tick fever, louse fever, famine fever.

**relaxation** (ree-lak-say′shun). Release of tension.

**remedial** (ri-mee′di-ul). Curative; acting as a remedy.

**remission** (ree-mish′un). A lessening of symptoms.

**renal** (ree′nal). Pertaining to the kidney.

**rennin** (ren′in). An enzyme in the stomach which digests milk.

**repression** (ree-presh′un). Rejection of an unpleasant matter from the conscious mind. It remains in the unconscious mind and may be expressed in a different form.

**resection** (ree-sek′shun). Surgical removal of a part of an organ.

**reserpine** (res′er-peen). See **Rauwolfia.**

**residual** (ree-zid′yoo-ul). Remaining.

    **residual air.** Air that still remains in the lungs after breathing out forcibly.

**resorcin** (ree-zor′sin) or **resorcinol** (ree-zor′si-nul). An antiseptic used especially for skin diseases.

**respiration** (res-pi-ray′shun). The act of breathing; also the taking in of oxygen and throwing off of carbon dioxide by any part of the body.

**rest cure.** Treatment of disease by prolonged rest, usually in bed.

**restraint** (ree-straynt′). Controlling the actions of mental patients by means of force.

**resuscitation** (ree-sus-i-tay′shun). Revival of one apparently dead.

**retching** (rech′ing). A strong involuntary effort to vomit.

**retention** (ree-ten′shun). Keeping within the body substances normally excreted.

**reticular** (ree-tik′yoo-lar). Like a network.

**reticuloendothelial** (ree-tik-yoo-lo-en-doh-thee′li-ul) **system.** Tissue network containing phagocytes and found in the spleen, liver, lymph glands, and bone marrow.

**retina** (ret′i-nuh). The inner coat of the eye on which light rays are focused. It is sensitive to light and transmits impulses to the brain through the optic nerve.

**retractor** (ree-trak'ter). An instrument for drawing back the edges of a wound.

**retrograde** (ret'ro-grayd). Going backward.

**Rh factor.** Hereditary factor in blood which can cause complications if an Rh-negative mother carries a fetus with Rh-positive blood.

**rheum** (room). Watery discharge.

**rhinitis** (righ-nigh'tis). Inflammation of the mucous membrane of the nose.

    **acute rhinitis.** Cold in the head.

**rhinoplasty** (righ'no-plas-ti). Plastic surgery of the nose.

**rhodopsin** (ro-dahp'sin). Visual purple; the purplish pigment in the rods of the retina which is bleached on exposure to light.

**Rhus** (rus). A genus of trees and shrubs which includes several poisonous plants.

    *Rhus diversiloba.* Poison oak.

    *Rhus toxicodendron.* Poison ivy.

    *Rhus venenata.* Poison sumac.

**rib.** Any one of the twenty-four bones of the chest, attached to the vertebrae in the back, and, except for the last five pairs, to the sternum in the front.

    **false ribs.** The ribs not attached to the sternum.

    **floating ribs.** The last two pairs of ribs.

**riboflavin** (righ-bo-flay'vin). Vitamin $B_2$. It is found in eggs, milk, liver, and other foods. A deficiency of riboflavin results in soreness around the corners of the mouth, redness of eyes, and changes in the skin and tongue.

**rice-water stools.** Bowel discharge which looks like water in which rice has been boiled. It is a characteristic of cholera.

**ricin** (righ'sin). Poison from the seeds of the castor-oil plant.

**rickets** (rik'its). A disease of infants and children caused by lack of vitamin D. It is marked by improper development of bones and teeth; the bones may become crooked and deformed and the fontanels are delayed in closing.

**Rickettsia** (rik-et'si-uh). A group of microorganisms some of which cause disease. They are smaller than most bacteria but larger than the viruses.

**rickettsialpox.** A rickettsial disease characterized by the appearance of a firm red papule on covered parts of the body, later followed by fever and rash.

**rigor mortis** (rig'er mor'tis). Stiffening after death.

**ringworm.** A general term for skin disease caused by fungus and marked by ring-shaped patches. Includes tinea capitis, athlete's foot, dermatomycosis.

**RN.** An abbreviation for registered nurse.

**RNA, ribonucleic** (righ'boh-new-clee-ick) **acid.** One of the chemicals that make up the chromosomes and control the mechanism of heredity.

**Rocky Mountain spotted fever.** A rickettsial disease marked by fever, headache, muscle and point pains, and rash. It is spread by ticks.

**rod.** Stick-shaped structure in the retina which contains rhodopsin, a substance affected by light.

**roentgen** (rent'gen) **rays.** X-rays. Named for Wilhelm Konrad von Röntgen (1845–1923), German physicist who discovered them.

**Rorschach** (ror'shahk) **test.** Inkblot test; a test for personality traits based on the interpretation of ten inkblots of different shapes and colors. Named for Herman Rorschach (1884–1922), Swiss psychiatrist who developed the test.

**rose fever.** An allergic reaction to roses, similar to hay fever.

**roseola** (ro-zee-o'luh). 1. A rose-colored skin rash. 2. Epidemic roseola; German measles.

**roughage** (ruf'ij). Any undigestible matter in food which helps to stimulate bowel movements.

**roundworms.** Parasites which can infect man causing ascariasis, a condition marked by digestive disturbance and abdominal pain. The worms are spread through material contaminated with feces.

**rubella** (roo-bel'uh). German measles.

**rubeola** (roo-bee'o-luh). Measles.

**rudimentary** (roo-di-men'tuh-ri). Undeveloped.

**rupture** (rup'cher). 1. A tearing or breaking apart. 2. Hernia.

**Rush, Benjamin** (1745–1813). American physician, a signer of the Declaration of Independence, who described dengue fever.

## S

**Sabin, Albert B.** (b. 1906). American physician and scientist. Dr. Sabin developed an effective antipolio vaccine containing live viruses. It was first licensed for public use in 1961.

**saccharin** (sak'uh-rin). A crystalline substance obtained from coal tar and used as a substitute for sugar. It is many times sweeter than sugar.

**sacroiliac** (say-kro-il'i-ak). The joint of the upper

portion of the hipbone and the large bone in the lower part of the spine.

**sacrum** (say'krum). The large bone near the lower end of the spine just above the coccyx. It is formed by the fusion of segments which are separate in infancy.

**sadism** (sad'izm). A perversion, usually sexual, in which one gets pleasure from inflicting cruelty on others.

**Saint Anthony's fire.** Erysipelas; a disease marked by fever and redness of skin. It is caused by bacteria (streptococcus).

**St. Vitus's dance.** Chorea; a nervous condition in which the muscles twitch involuntarily.

**saline** (say'lighn). Salty.

**saliva** (suh-ligh'vuh). The fluid secreted into the mouth by the salivary glands. It mixes with the food, lubricating it and aiding in the digestion of starch.

**salivary** (sal'i-vehr-i) **glands.** The glands of the mouth that secrete saliva. The principal ones are the parotid, submaxillary, and sublingual.

**Salk, Jonas E.** (b. 1914). Dr. Salk, American physician and scientist, and co-workers developed an effective antipolio vaccine consisting of chemically killed viruses. It was approved for general use in 1955.

**salpingectomy** (sal-pin-jek'tuh-mi). Surgical removal of a fallopian tube.

**Salvarsan** (sal'var-san). A proprietary name for arsphenamine, an arsenic compound used in treating syphilis and other infections.

**salve** (sav). Ointment.

**sanatorium** (san-uh-taw'ri-um). An institution for treatment of certain diseases, especially tuberculosis, chronic diseases, and mental disorders.

**sanitary** (san'uh-tehr-i). Promoting health.

**sanity** (san'i-ti). Soundness of mind.

**sarcoma** (sar-ko'muh). A cancerous tumor from connective tissue.

**satyriasis** (sat-ir-igh'uh-sis). Excessive sexual desire in a man.

**scab.** A crust formed over a sore or wound.

**scapula** (skap'yoo-luh). Shoulder blade.

**scarification** (skar-i-fi-kay'shun). Operation of making many small scratches or pricks in the skin.

**Schick** (shik) **test.** Skin test for diphtheria immunity. A small amount of diphtheria toxin is injected into the skin.

**schizoid** (skiz'oyd). An individual who is unusually unsocial and introverted.

**schizophrenia** (skiz-o-free'ni-uh). Dementia praecox; a mental disorder in which the person withdraws from reality into a mental world of his own.

**Schleiden, Matthias Jakob** (1804–1881) and **Theodor Schwann** (1810–1882). Two German scientists who collaborated on the theory that living tissue is composed of units or cells.

**sciatic** (sigh-at'ik) **nerve.** The largest nerve of the body. It is attached to the lower part of the spinal cord, and branches to form the sensory and motor nerves of the legs and feet.

**sciatica** (sigh-at'i-kuh). Inflammation of the sciatic nerve with pain at the back of the thigh.

**scirrhus** (skeer'us). A hard carcinoma.

**sclera** (sklee'ruh). The tough outer coat which covers all of the eyeball except the portion covered by the cornea.

**sclerosis** (skli-ro'sis). Hardening of connective tissue, particularly the thickening of the walls of blood vessels.

**scoliosis** (sko-li-o'sis). Sideward curvature of the spine.

**scopolamine** (sko-pahl'uh-min). A compound used as a sedative and sleep inducer.

**scorbutic** (skor-byoo'tik). Affected with scurvy.

**scrofula** (skrahf'yoo-luh). Tuberculosis of the lymph nodes, a disease causing pus-filled abscesses and tissue breakdown in the affected areas.

**scrotum** (skro'tum). The pouchlike structure that holds the testicles.

**scrubbing.** The thorough washing of hands and arms with soap, water, and a nail brush which is carried out by surgeons and others before assisting with an operation.

**scurvy** (sker'vi). A disease caused by lack of vitamin C in the diet. It is marked by anemia, weakness, and bleeding gums.

**sebaceous** (see-bay'shus) **glands.** The oil glands of the skin, which secrete a fatty substance to lubricate the skin.

**seborrhea** (seb-o-ree'uh). A disease of the sebaceous glands in which they secrete abnormally. The secretion may collect on the skin as an oily coating or in crusts.

**sebum** (see'bum). The secretion of the sebaceous glands, a fatty substance.

**Seconal** (sek'uh-nal). A proprietary name for a barbiturate used as a sedative.

**secretion** (see-kree'shun). Substance given off by glands or tissues to be used in the body. It differs from an excretion, which is a waste product, not usable by the body.

**section** (sek'shun). In surgery it means to cut or divide.

**sedation** (si-day'shun). Act of calming the nerves by use of a sedative.

**sedative** (sed'uh-tiv). A substance that calms and quiets nervous excitement.

**sedimentation** (sed-i-men-tay'shun) **rate**. The time required for blood cells to settle out of a standard volume of unclotted blood. The rate changes in certain diseases.

**semen** (see'men). Thick whitish liquid containing spermatozoa secreted by the testes and released in sexual intercourse.

**semicircular canal.** The passage of the inner ear that controls the sense of balance.

**seminal vesicle** (sem'uh-nal ves'i-kl). The sac in which semen is stored.

**Semmelweis** (sem'el-vighs), **Ignaz Philipp** (1818–1865). Viennese physician who showed that infection following childbirth was caused by germs carried on the unwashed hands of physicians. He stressed the importance of cleanliness of doctors and hospitals.

**senescence** (si-nes'ens). Aging; growing old.

**senility** (suh-nil'i-ti). 1. Old age. 2. Feebleness of mind and body associated with old age.

**senna** (sen'uh). Dried leaves which produce a laxative action.

**sensation** (sen-say'shun). Feeling or mental impression produced when nerves are stimulated.

**sensitized** (sen'si-tighzd). Made more sensitive or susceptible to a particular substance; allergic.

**sepsis** (sep'sis). Presence of germs in blood or tissues.

**septicemia** (sep-ti-see'mi-uh). Presence in the blood of germs or poisons from them.

**septum** (sep'tum). A partition or dividing wall in an organ.

**Serpasil** (serp'a-sill). See **Rauwolfia**.

**serum** (seer'um). Clear liquid separated from a blood clot.

    **pooled serum.** Mixture of serum from several different people.

    **serum albumin.** Albumin found in blood.

**serum sickness.** An allergic reaction from injection of serum. It may be marked by hives, fever, and enlarged glands.

**shin.** The front of the leg below the knee.

**shingles.** Herpes zoster; inflammation of a nerve with pain and blisters along the path of the nerve.

**shock.** Condition in which the body processes are slowed down considerably. It is brought on as a result of bodily injury or extreme emotion, and is marked by weakness, paleness, and rapid pulse.

    **anaphylactic shock.** Shock caused by injection of a substance to which the patient is sensitized.

    **electric shock.** Shock caused by electric current passing through the body. Electric shock from current through the brain is used in treating certain mental illnesses.

    **insulin shock.** Coma caused by overdose of insulin. Used in treating certain mental illnesses.

    **shell shock.** A general term for serious mental disorders resulting from war service; battle fatigue.

**sickle-cell anemia.** Type of anemia caused by malformed blood cells.

**siderosis** (sid-er-o'sis). Inflammation of the lungs caused by inhaling iron dust. Found particularly among miners and welders who are exposed to the dust in their work.

**silicosis** (sil-i-ko'sis). A disease in which the lung is damaged by silicon dioxide. It is associated with occupations such as sand blasting, stone cutting, and others in which there is sand in the air.

**silver nitrate.** Compound used in solution as an antiseptic and germicide, especially for mucous membranes.

**Simpson, James Young** (1811–1870). Edinburgh obstetrician who first used anesthetics in childbirth.

**sinus** (sigh'nus). A cavity or hollow space, particularly those in the bones of the nose.

**sinusitis** (sigh-nus-igh'tis). Inflammation of a sinus, especially the maxillary sinus.

**skeleton** (skel'i-tun). Bony framework of the body.

**sleeping sickness.** Disease found in Africa in which the patient shows increasing drowsiness. It is caused by a protozoan parasite transmitted to man by the bite of a tsetse fly.

**slide.** A thin rectangle of glass on which objects are placed for microscopic study.

**smallpox.** An acute contagious disease caused by a

virus and characterized by fever and pustules.

**smegma** (smeg'muh). The thick secretion of the sebaceous glands of the external genitalia.

**soap, tincture of green.** A liniment made from a medicinal potassium soap. Useful against some skin diseases.

**sodium amytal** (am'i-tal). Substance used for sedation.

**sodium benzoate.** Food preservative; also used to test liver function.

**sodium bicarbonate.** Baking soda; used to counteract stomach acidity.

**sodium chloride.** Table salt.

**sodium citrate** (sit'rayt). White powder which can alkalinize urine. Also used by blood banks to keep collected blood from clotting.

**sodium salicylate** (sal'i-sil-ayt). Substance used in treating acute rheumatic fever.

**sodium thiosulfate.** An antidote for certain metallic poisons; also the hypo of photography.

**soft palate.** The roof of the mouth near the throat.

**solar plexus** (so-ler plek'sus). Celiac plexus; a large knot of nerves in the abdomen.

**somnambulism** (sahm-nam'byoo-lizm). Sleepwalking.

**soporific** (so-puh-rif'ik). 1. Producing sleep. 2. A substance capable of producing sleep.

**spansule** (span'syul). A form of medication in special capsules designed to release the medicine inside the body over many hours.

**spasm** (spazm). A sudden violent involuntary contraction, usually of muscles.

> **clonic spasm.** One in which the muscles relax quickly.

> **tonic spasm.** One in which the muscles remain rigid for a long time.

**spastic** (spas'tik). Convulsive or resembling a spasm.

> **spastic hemiplegia.** Partial paralysis of one side in which spasms are induced by movement of the affected muscles.

> **spastic paraplegia.** Paralysis of the lower legs with muscle spasms when the affected parts are moved.

**speculum** (spek'yoo-lum). An instrument for stretching a passageway or opening in order that it may be examined more easily.

**spermatocele** (sper'muh-toh-seel). Cystic enlargement of the epididymis.

**spermatocystitis** (sper-muh-toh-sis-tigh'tis). Inflammation of the seminal vesicles.

**sphincter** (sfingk'ter). A ring of muscle which contracts to close an opening.

> **anal sphincter.** One of the two muscles that close the anus.

> **pyloric sphincter.** The circular muscle at the opening between the stomach and small intestine.

**sphygmomanometer** (sfig-mo-muh-nahm'i-ter). Instrument used to determine blood pressure.

**spinal** (spigh'nal) **canal.** The passage formed by the arches of the vertebrae and containing the spinal cord.

**spinal column.** The backbone; the vertebral column.

**spinal cord.** The long cordlike structure of nerves and nervous tissue which extends down from the brain and serves as the main center for reflex actions and other involuntary actions.

**spinal nerves.** Nerves which attach to the spinal cord.

**spirochete** (spigh'ro-keet). A spiral-shaped bacterium. One type causes syphilis.

**splanchnic** (splangk-'nik) **nerves.** Nerves of the internal organs.

**spleen.** A large reddish brown gland lying between the stomach and the diaphragm in the upper portion of the abdomen. Its functions are not yet understood, but it is believed to aid blood cell and antibody formation.

**splint.** A support for a broken bone or other injured part.

> **Stader splint.** A splint consisting of a metal bar fastened to the bone with steel pins.

**spondylitis** (spahn-duh-ligh'tis). Inflammation of the vertebrae.

**spondylosis** (spahn-duh-lo'sis). Abnormal stiffening of a vertebral joint.

**sport.** An organism that is unusually different from its parents; a mutation.

**spotted fever.** 1. Typhus fever. 2. Epidemic cerebrospinal meningitis. 3. Tick fever.

**sprain.** Wrenching of a joint, producing stretching or tearing of ligaments or tendons.

**sprue** (sproo). A disease in which the body is unable to absorb fats and there is difficulty in blood formation. Symptoms are diarrhea, indigestion, soreness of mouth and tongue, and loss of weight. Administration of vitamin $B_{12}$ is usually effective in relieving symptoms.

**sputum** (spyoo'tum). Discharge from lungs and

throat expelled by spitting. It is composed of saliva and mucus.

**stapes** (stay'peez). The small stirrup-shaped bone of the inner ear; stirrup.

**staphyledema** (staf-il-i-dee'muh). Swelling of the uvula.

**staphylococcus** (staf-i-lo-kahk'us). A spherical bacterium usually found in clusters. Bacteria of this type cause boils and pus-forming infections of wounds.

**steapsin** (stee-ap'sin). An enzyme which aids in digesting fat. It is produced in the pancreas.

**stenosis** (stuh-no'sis). Narrowing of a body tube or opening.

**sterile** (stehr'il). 1. Free from germs. 2. Not able to produce offspring.

**sternum** (ster'num). Breastbone; the bone in the middle of the front of the chest to which the ribs attach.

**stethoscope** (steth'uh-skohp). An instrument used to discover and amplify the sounds of the heart, lungs, and other organs.

**stigma** (stig'muh). A spot or mark on the skin.

**stillborn.** Dead at birth.

**stimulus** (stim'yoo-lus). Anything which arouses action in a body organ, such as muscle contraction, gland secretion, or nerve impulse.

**stirrup** (stir'up). See **stapes.**

**stomach** (stum'uk). The saclike organ just below the diaphragm between the esophagus and the intestine. It can hold about one quart of food, which it digests by the action of enzymes and hydrochloric acid.

**stomatitis** (sto-muh-tigh'tis). Inflammation of the inside of the mouth; sore mouth.

**stool.** Feces; waste from the bowels.

**strabismus** (struh-biz'mus). A squint; an eye condition in which both eyes cannot be focused at the same time.

**strain, muscle.** An injury from overuse or misuse which caused unusual tension in the muscle.

**strait jacket.** A device preventing movement of the arms; used to restrain a violent mental patient.

**strawberry tongue.** One with enlarged papillae that project as bright red points; seen in scarlet fever.

**streptococcus** (strep-toh-kahk'us). A spherical-shaped bacterium found in chain arrangement, when observed microscopically. Some types cause disease, such as scarlet fever and sore throat.

**streptomycin** (strep-toh-migh'sin). An antibiotic from a fungus, effective against tuberculosis and other infections.

**striated** (strigh'ayt-id). Having streaks or stripes.

**stroke.** A sudden severe attack as of paralysis, apoplexy, or sunstroke.

**stroma** (stro'muh). The tissue, usually connective tissue, which forms the framework of an organ, as distinguished from parenchyma, the tissue which carries out the specialized function.

**stupe** (stoop). A cloth wrung out of hot water and applied to the skin as a counterirritant. Sometimes used with turpentine or other irritants.

**stupor** (stoo'per). A state of partial unconsciousness in which the individual seems hardly to feel or notice anything.

**sty** or **stye.** Inflammation caused by the infection or blocking of one of the sebaceous glands of the eyelid.

**styptic** (stip'tik). Stopping bleeding with an astringent.

**subconscious** (sub-kahn'shus). The contents of the mind not on the conscious level.

**subcutaneous** (sub-kyoo-tay'ni-us). Under the skin.

**Sucaryl** (soo'kuh-ril). A proprietary name of a sweet substance used instead of sugar in diabetic diets.

**sulfadiazine** (sul-fuh-digh'uh-zeen). One of the sulfa drugs active against many infections; used in treating meningococcal meningitis, urinary tract infections, and some fungal diseases. In powder form it has been used in surgery and on wounds to prevent infection.

**sulfonamides** (sul-fo'nuh-mighds). The sulfa drugs; a group of medicines which stop growth of bacteria. Some of the most important are sulfadiazine, sulfaguanidine, sulfamerazine, and sulfasuxidine.

**sulfones** (sul'fohns). A group of compounds related to the sulfonamides and also active against many bacterial infections. They are used in the treatment of Hansen's disease (leprosy).

**sunstroke.** A form of heatstroke caused by overexposure to the sun. There may be headache or collapse.

**superego** (soo'per-ee-go). The part of the unconscious mind that opposes and criticizes.

**supine** (soo-pighn'). Lying on the back.

**suppository** (suh-pahz'i-taw"ri). A medicated mass shaped to fit into one of the body openings. It is solid at room temperature but melts when in the body. Suppositories are used especially for diseases of the rectum or to treat constipation.

**suppuration** (sup-yoo-ray'shun). Formation of pus.

**suprarenal** (soo-pruh-ree'nul). Above the kidney; adrenal.

**suprarenal body.** See **adrenal gland.**

**surgery** (ser'jer-i). Branch of medicine dealing with wounds, deformities, and diseases treated by operation or manipulation.

**susceptible** (sus-sep'ti-bl). Not immune; capable of being affected by a substance or by disease germs.

**suture** (soo'cher). 1. Uniting of two surfaces, particularly by stitching. 2. The thread, catgut, or other material used in uniting tissues.

**swab** (swahb). A stick with a tuft of absorbent cotton at the end. It is used to cleanse wounds, apply medicines, or obtain samples of secretions.

**Sydenham** (sid'en-ham), **Thomas** (1624–1689). Englishman who was an outstanding physician of the seventeenth-century. He used practical methods of treatment and observed and described various diseases.

**sympathectomy** (sim-puh-thek'tuh-mi). Surgical removal of a part of the sympathetic nervous system.

**sympathetic nervous system.** The spinal nerves which cause contraction of blood vessels, increase in heart rate, and inhibition of stomach and glandular secretions.

**symphysis** (sim'fi-sis). 1. Growing together of bones. 2. The line of union between bones which were originally separate but have grown together.

**symptom** (simp'tum). Any change from the normal which indicates disease.

**synapse** (sin'aps). The point of contact between nerve endings.

**syncope** (sin'ko-pi). A swoon or faint; temporary unconsciousness caused by lack of oxygen or blood in the brain.

**syndrome** (sin'drohm). A group of symptoms which occur together and seem to have the same cause.

**synergy** (sin'er-ji). Cooperation in action, such as among muscles carrying out a task, or among medicines used together in treating a disease.

**synovia** (sigh-no'vi-uh). The lubricating fluid of the joints. It is secreted by membranes lining the joint capsules and surrounding the tendons.

**syringe** (seer'inj). A device used to inject fluids into the body.

**systemic** (sis-tem'ik). Affecting the entire body.

**systole** (sis'toh-li). Contraction of the heart.

**systolic** (sis-tahl'ik) **murmur.** A murmur of the heart heard during the contraction.

**Szent-Györgyi, Albert** (b. 1893). Hungarian-born biochemist who isolated vitamin C. Winner of the Nobel prize in 1937.

**T**

**tabes** (tay'beez). 1. A gradual wasting away of the body or of a part of the body; emaciation. 2. Tabes dorsalis; a form of late syphilis characterized by degeneration of part of the spinal cord.

**tachycardia** (tak-i-kar'di-uh). Abnormally rapid heartbeat.

**talipes** (tal'i-peez). Clubfoot; a deformity of the foot in which it is twisted out of normal position, occurring congenitally or from paralysis.

**tampon** (tam'pun). A cotton plug.

**tannic acid.** Substance obtained from trees and used as a dressing for burns, as an astringent, and as an antidote for metallic poisons.

**tantalum** (tan'tuh-lum). A metal used to repair defects of the skull.

**tarsus** (tahr'sus). The instep.

**tartar** (tahr'tahr). A calcium compound deposited on the teeth by the saliva.

**taste buds.** The tiny structures on the tongue which are sensitive to taste.

**tattooing** (tat-too'ing). Coloring the skin permanently by injecting pigment into the skin. It is used to hide white spots on the eye which may result from infections and is also used to cover up unsightly birthmarks.

**telangioma** (tel-an-ji-o'muh). A tumor made up of tiny blood vessels which have become dilated.

**telangiosis** (tel-an-ji-o'sis). Any disease of the capillary blood vessels.

**temperature** (tem'per-uh-choor). The degree of heat or cold. Normal body temperature is 98.6 F.

**temple** (tem'pl). The region of the head above the eye socket and between the eye and the ear.

**temporal** (tem'puh-ral) **bone.** One of the bones of the skull covering the inner ear.

**tendinitis** (ten-di-nigh'tis). Inflammation of a tendon.

**tendon** (ten'dun). A white fibrous cord which connects muscle to bone.

**tenesmus** (ti-nez'mus). Straining, especially during urination or bowel movement.

**tenia** (tee'ni-uh) or **teniasis** (tee-nigh'uh-sis). Condition of infection with a tapeworm.

**teniafuge** (tee'ni-uh-fyooj). A medicine that causes tapeworms to be expelled.

**tenositis** (ten-o-sigh'tis). Inflammation of a tendon.

**tension** (ten'shun). Condition of being tense or stretched.

**tensor** (ten'ser). A muscle which makes a part firm or tense.

**Tepanil** (tepp'uh-nil). A proprietary preparation prescribed to help overweight persons by reducing the appetite.

**Terramycin** (tehr-uh-migh'sin). A proprietary antibiotic from a fungus. It is very similar to Aureomycin.

**testicle** (tes'ti-kl) or **testis** (tes'tis). One of the two male sex glands located in the scrotum which produce spermatozoa and semen.

**test meal.** A meal given and later withdrawn from the stomach to show the digestive power of the stomach.

**testosterone** (tes-tahs'ter-ohn). Male sex hormone which induces development of male characteristics. It is prepared commercially from the testes of bulls and is used in treating certain conditions.

**tetany** (tet'uh-ni). A nervous disorder in which there are muscular spasms, cramps, and convulsions. It may accompany certain gastric or intestinal disorders or result from a calcium deficiency such as might occur after removal of parathyroids.

**tetracycline** (tet-ra-cy'clean). An antibiotic administered by mouth. It is active against many diseases caused by microorganisms.

**thalamus** (thal'uh-mus). An egg-shaped structure of the brain.

**theca** (thee'kuh). A sheath such as the one enclosing a tendon.

**therapeutics** (thehr-uh-pyoo'tiks). Science of healing.

**therapy** (thehr'uh-pi). Treatment of disease.

    **shock therapy.** Treatment of mental disease by producing convulsions with electric current or insulin. It is believed that the brain waves are altered or interrupted.

**thermolabile** (ther-mo-lay'bil). Changed or destroyed by heat.

**thermometer** (ther-mahm'i-ter). Instrument to measure temperature.

    **oral thermometer.** One for taking temperature by mouth.

    **rectal thermometer.** One for taking the temperature through the anus.

**thiamine** (thigh'uh-min). Thiamine hydrochloride; vitamin B₁; a vitamin found in yeast and other foods and necessary to prevent beriberi.

**thiouracil** (thigh-o-yoo'ruh-sil). A compound used to treat conditions of overactive thyroid. It interferes with the utilization of iodine by the thyroid gland.

**thoracic** (tho-ras'ik). Pertaining to the chest.

**thoracolysis** (tho-ruh-kahl'is-is). The process of breaking up lung adhesions. This operation requires removal of part of the ribs.

**thorax** (tho'raks). The chest.

**Thorazine** (thor'a-zeen). A proprietary medicine with powerful antinauseant and antivomiting properties. It is also used in some types of emotional illness.

**threshold** (thresh'old). The point at which a sensation can just barely be felt or sensed.

**thrombin** (thrahm'bin). An enzyme which is necessary for blood to clot. It forms from other substances in the blood after blood is shed.

**thromboclasis** (thrahm-bahk'luh-sis). Breaking up of a blood clot.

**thrombocyte** (thrahm'bo-sight). A blood platelet.

**thrombosis** (thrahm-bo'sis). Formation of a blood clot blocking a blood vessel.

**thrombostasis** (thrahm-bahs'tuh-sis). Collecting of blood in a part, leading to formation of a thrombus.

**thrombus** (thrahm'bus). A blood clot formed in a blood vessel.

**thrush.** A disease of infants caused by a fungus and marked by the appearance of small white spots or sores in the mouth and on the tongue.

**thymus** (thigh'mus). Gland of children located in the mediastinum.

**thyroid** (thigh'royd) **gland.** A large ductless gland located in the neck. Its secretions regulate body metabolism.

**thyroidectomy** (thigh-royd-ek'tuh-mi). Surgical removal of the thyroid.

**thyroxin** (thigh-rahk'sin). A chemical compound produced by the thyroid gland.

**tibia** (tib'i-uh). The bone on the inner side of the lower leg.

**tic.** Twitching.

**tick.** A blood-sucking insect related to the mites but larger.

**tick fever.** Any disease which is transmitted by ticks, such as Rocky Mountain spotted fever, Colorado tick fever, or Texas cattle fever.

**tincture** (tingh-cher). A medicinal alcoholic solution weaker than an extract.

**tinea** (tin'i-uh). Ringworm.

**tissue** (tish'yoo). A collection of cells of the same type forming a definite structure.

**tone.** Normal strength and tension of the body or of muscles.

**tonic** (tahn'ik). A medicine that helps restore normal tone.

**tonsil** (tahn'sil). A mass of lymphoid tissue, especially one of the two located at the back of the tongue.

**tonsillectomy** (tahn-si-lek'tuh-mi). Surgical removal of the tonsils.

**tonsillitis** (tahn-si-ligh'tis). Inflammation of a tonsil.

**topical** (tahp'i-kal). Local; in a definite area.

**torpor** (tor'per). Numbness; apathy.

**torticollis** (tor-ti-kahl'is). Stiff neck in which the head is turned to one side.

**tourniquet** (toor'ni-ket). Device to press on blood vessels to stop bleeding.

**toxemia** (tahk-see'mi-uh). Blood poisoning.

**toxic** (tahk'sik). Poisonous.

**toxin** (tahk'sin). A poison produced by germs.

**toxin-antitoxin.** A mixture of diphtheria toxin and its antitoxin used for vaccination against diphtheria.

**toxoid** (tahk'soyd). A toxin changed so that it is no longer poisonous.

**trachea** (tray'ki-uh). Windpipe; the tube which extends from the voicebox to the bronchi.

**tracheitis** (tray-ki-igh'tis). Inflammation of the trachea.

**tracheostenosis** (tray-ki-o-sti-no'sis). Narrowing of the trachea.

**tracheotomy** (tray-ki-aht'uh-mi). A surgical operation to produce an artificial opening in the trachea through the tissues of the neck.

**trachoma** (truh-ko'muh). A chronic communicable disease of the eye caused by a virus. It is characterized by inflammation of the conjunctiva and may lead to blindness.

**traction** (trak'shun). The act of pulling, such as is used in correcting dislocations.

**trance** (trans). An abnormal sleep.

**transference** (trans-fer'ens). Shifting of a mental attitude from one person or thing to another.

**transfusion** (trans-fyoo'zhun). Injection of fluid, especially blood or plasma, into a vein.

**transpiration** (tran-spuh-ray'shun). Excretion through the skin of air, sweat, or vapor.

**transplantation** (trans-plan-tay'shun). Grafting of tissues from one part of the body to another part, or to another body.

**transvestitism** (trans-ves'ti-tizm). A perversion in which the individual prefers to wear the clothing worn by the opposite sex.

**trauma** (traw'muh). Injury.

    **psychic trauma.** A painful emotional experience.

**tremor** (trem'er). An involuntary quiver.

**trench mouth.** Vincent's angina.

**trephine** (tree-fighn'). 1. To cut a circular piece of bone out of the skull to relieve pressure on the brain. 2. The saw used in the operation, an improvement over the trepan.

**triceps** (trigh'seps) **muscle.** The muscle which extends the forearm.

**trichiasis** (trigh-kigh'uh-sis). Ingrown hair.

**trichinella** (trik-uh-nel'uh). The parasites of the type that cause trichinosis.

**trichinosis** (trik-i-no'sis). Disease caused by eating insufficiently cooked pork or other meat infected with a parasitic worm. The disease is marked by nausea, diarrhea, muscle soreness, edema, difficulty in breathing, and fever.

**tricuspid** (trigh-kus'pid). See **valve.**

**trigeminal** (trigh-jem'i-nal) **nerve.** The fifth cranial nerve. It serves the forehead, cheek, teeth, tongue, and interior of the mouth.

**troche** (tro'kee). A medicated tablet.

**trochlear** (trahk'li-er) **nerve.** The fourth cranial nerve. It controls eye movements.

**Trudeau** (troo-doh'), **Edward Livingston** (1848–1915). American physician who established a tuberculosis sanatorium at Saranac Lake and advocated open-air treatment of tuberculosis.

**truss** (trus). Device to hold a hernia in place.

**trypsin** (trip'sin). An enzyme produced by the pancreas to digest proteins.

**tsetse** (tset'see) **fly.** The fly that spreads African sleeping sickness.

**tsutsugamushi** (soot-soo-guh-moosh'i) **disease.** Japanese river fever; scrub typhus; disease found in southwest Asia and Japan and caused by rickettsia spread through mites of mice and rats.

**tubercle** (too′ber-kl). A nodule.

**tuberculin** (too-ber′kyoo-lin). An extract from tubercle bacilli used in diagnostic tests for tuberculosis.

**tuberculin test.** A skin test for tuberculosis sensitivity. A small amount of tuberculin is injected into the skin. If there is no marked inflammation or tissue breakdown after two days, the test is negative, indicating absence of tuberculosis infection. A change from a negative to a positive skin reaction is suggestive of tuberculosis.

**tubule** (too′byool). Any small tube.

**Tuinal** (too′in-all). A trade name for a barbiturate prescribed as a medicine to induce sleep.

**tularemia** (too-luh-ree′mi-uh). Rabbit fever; a disease caused by bacteria from small wild animals, particularly rabbits. It is marked by a sudden attack of chills and fever accompanied by swollen lymph nodes. It is transmitted by bites of flies or ticks which have previously bitten infected animals, or it may be transmitted through handling infected animals or eating the insufficiently cooked meat of infected animals.

**tumefaction** (too-mi-fak′shun). Swelling or puffiness.

**tumor** (too′mer). 1. Swelling. 2. New and abnormal growth; neoplasm.

**turgid** (ter′jid). Swollen.

**twilight sleep.** A state of consciousness in which one reacts to pain and other sensations but has no memory of them afterward. It is used in childbirth and is usually produced by scopolamine.

**twins, fraternal.** Two children developed from different ova but born at the same time. May be of the same or different sex.

**twins, identical.** Two children developed from the same ovum. They are of the same sex and of very similar appearance.

**tympanic** (tim-pan′ik) **membrane.** Eardrum.

**tympanum** (tim′puh-num). The middle ear.

**typhlitis** (tif-ligh′tis). Inflammation of the cecum.

**typhoid** (tigh′foyd) **fever.** A bacterial infection marked by fever and diarrhea. Spread by contaminated water, milk, or food, especially shellfish.

**typhus** (tigh′fus). Disease marked by headache, chills, fever, and general pains. It is caused by rickettsia carried by lice. It cannot be spread from man to man.

**murine typhus.** A disease similar to but milder than the louse-borne typhus. It is carried by rodents and spread to man through fleas.

**scrub typhus.** See **tsutsugamushi disease.**

## U

**ulcer** (ul′ser). An open sore other than a wound.

**ulceration** (ul-ser-ay′shun). Formation of an ulcer.

**ulna** (ul′nuh). The larger bone of the forearm located on the side opposite the thumb.

**ulotomy** (yoo-laht′uh-mi). 1. Cutting into the gum. 2. Cutting into scar tissue to relieve or correct deformity.

**ultramicroscopical** (ul-truh-migh-kro-skahp′i-kl). Too small to be seen with a microscope.

**ultraviolet** (ul-truh-vigh′uh-lit). Invisible rays of light shorter than the violet rays of the visible spectrum.

**umbilical** (um-bil′i-kal) **cord.** The cord which connects the fetus to the placenta. It contains the blood vessels which provide nourishment to the developing child.

**umbilicus** (um-bil′i-kus). The navel; the round depression on the skin of the abdomen marking the point of attachment of the umbilical cord during fetal life.

**unconscious** (un-kahn′shus). 1. In psychiatry it refers to behavior not controlled by the conscious mind. 2. Insensible.

**undulant** (un′dyoo-lent) **fever.** Brucellosis; see text.

**unguent** (ung′gwent). Ointment or salve.

**urea** (yoo-ree′uh). A nitrogen compound which is the chief product of protein breakdown in the body and is excreted in urine.

**uremia** (yoo-ree′mi-uh). Condition in which waste products normally excreted in urine remain in the blood.

**ureter** (yoo-ree′ter). The tube through which urine passes from the kidney to the bladder.

**urethra** (yoo-ree′thruh). The canal through which urine is discharged from the bladder.

**urethritis** (yoo-ri-thrigh′tis). Inflammation of the urethra.

**uric** (yoo′rik) **acid.** One of the waste products of metabolism found in blood and urine.

**urinalysis** (yoo-ri-nal′i-sis). Examination of the urine for chemical and microscopic contents.

**urination** (yoo-ri-nay′shun). Act of discharging urine from the bladder; micturition.

**urine** (yoo′rin). Liquid waste of the body which is collected by the kidneys and stored temporarily in the bladder for excretion. It is normally a clear pale amber fluid with a faint odor.

**uriniferous** (yoo-ri-nif′er-us) **tubule.** One of the many tubes in the kidney which carry urine from the capsules to the kidney pelvis.

**urology** (yoo-rahl′uh-gy). The branch of medicine dealing with the diseases of the male urogenital system and the female urinary system.

**urticaria** (er-ti-kay′ri-uh). Hives; a condition in which itchy elevations (wheals) appear on the skin. They usually are not accompanied by any other symptoms and disappear in a day or two. They are caused by an allergic reaction.

**USP.** Abbreviation for United States Pharmacopoeia. On medicines it indicates that they comply with standards of strength and purity set by the U. S. Pharmacopoeia.

**uterectomy** (yoo-ter-ek′tuh-mi). Hysterectomy; surgical removal of the uterus.

**uterotomy** (yoo-ter-aht′uh-mi). Cutting into the uterus.

**uterus** (yoo′ter-us). The womb; the hollow pear-shaped organ in the pelvis which holds the developing fetus.

**uvula** (yoo′vyoo-luh). The small conical structure which hangs down from the roof of the mouth near the throat.

# V

**vaccination** (vak-si-nay′shun). Inoculation with weakened or dead germs to develop immunity to a specific disease.

**vaccine** (vak′seen). A substance containing weakened or dead germs prepared for vaccination.

**vaccinia** (vak-sin′i-uh). See **cowpox.**

**vagina** (vuh-jigh′nuh). The passageway in the female between the uterus and the external genitalia.

**vaginismus** (vaj-uh-niz′mus). A painful spasm of the vagina.

**vaginitis** (vaj-uh-nigh′tis). Inflammation of the vagina.

**vagotonia** (vay-go-toh′ni-uh). Increase in the excit-ability of the vagus nerve, slowing the heart, etc.

**vagus** (vay′gus) **nerve.** The tenth cranial nerve, which has both motor and sensory functions and serves the stomach, intestines, heart, lungs, larynx, esophagus.

**valve, aortic.** The valve between the aorta and the left ventricle of the heart.

> **bicuspid** or **mitral valve.** The valve between the left auricle and the left ventricle of the heart.
>
> **pulmonary valve.** The valve at the junction of the pulmonary artery and the right ventricle.
>
> **pyloric valve.** The valve between the stomach and the small intestine.
>
> **tricuspid valve.** The valve between the right auricle and the right ventricle of the heart.

**varicella** (var-uh-sel′uh). Chickenpox; see text.

**varicocele** (var′i-ko-seel). Swollen veins in the spermatic cord.

**varicose** (var′i-kohs) **vein.** An unnaturally swollen vein.

**varicotomy** (var-i-kaht′uh-mi). Surgical cutting out of a varicose vein.

**variola** (vuh-righ′uh-luh). See **smallpox.**

**vas deferens** (vas def′er-ens). The tube which extends from the epididymus to the ejaculatory duct.

**vascular** (vas′kyoo-ler). Pertaining to or containing blood vessels or other vessels.

**vasectomy** (vas-ek′tuh-mi). Surgical removal of the vas deferens.

**Vaseline** (vas′uh-leen). A proprietary name of petroleum jelly.

**vasoconstrictor** (vas-o-kahn-strick′ter). A substance which causes blood vessels to contract or narrow.

**vasodepressor** (vas-o-dee-pres′er). A substance that lowers the blood pressure.

**vasodilator** (vas-o-digh-lay′ter). A substance that causes blood vessels to enlarge.

**vasomotor** (vas-o-mo′ter). Any substance that causes contraction or enlargement of blood vessels.

**vasopressin** (vas-o-pres′in). A hormone produced by the pituitary gland that raises blood pressure.

**vector** (vek′ter). A person or animal that carries disease germs.

**vein** (vayn). A blood vessel which carries blood to the heart from other parts of the body.

> **jugular vein.** The vein in the neck which carries blood from the brain.

**vena cava** (vee′nuh kay′vuh). One of the two large

veins which empty into the right auricle.

**venereal** (vi-neer′i-ul) **disease.** A disease spread by sexual intercourse. Syphilis, gonorrhea, and chancroid are the principal ones.

**venesection** (ven-i-sek′shun). Cutting open a vein for withdrawal of blood.

**venipuncture** (ven′i-punk-tyoor). Puncture of a vein for injection of fluid or withdrawal of blood.

**venom** (ven′um). Poison produced by a snake or other animal.

**venous** (vee′nus). Pertaining to the veins.

**ventral** (ven′trul). Pertaining to the front of the body.

**ventricle** (ven′tri-kul). 1. Either of the lower chambers of the heart from which blood is pumped to the arteries. 2. A small cavity.

**venule** (ven′yool). A little vein.

**vermiform** (ver′mi-form) **appendix.** See text.

**vermin** (ver′min). Harmful animals or insects such as lice, mice, worms that are parasitic, and flies.

**verruca** (vee-roo′kuh). A wart.

**vertebra** (ver′ti-bruh). Any one of the thirty-three bones of the spinal column.

**vertigo** (ver′ti-go). Dizziness.

**Vesalius** (vi-say′li-us), **Andreas** (1514–1564). Belgian physician who prepared a treatise on body structure and laid the basis for the modern study of anatomy.

**vesicle** (ves′i-kl). A saclike structure either normal or abnormal.

**vesicotomy** (ves-i-kaht′uh-mi). Cutting into the bladder.

**vestigial** (ves-tij′i-ul). Rudimentary.

**viable** (vigh′uh-bl). Able to live.

**vibrio** (vib′ri-o). A type of bacteria such as the one that causes cholera.

**villus** (vil′us), pl. **villi.** One of the tiny projections on the lining of the intestine.

**Vincent's angina.** Trench mouth; a contagious infection of the mouth which causes bleeding gums and bad breath. It is caused by the combined action of a spirochete and a bacillus.

**viosterol** (vigh-ahs′ter-ol). A vitamin D preparation made by irradiating ergosterol, a substance found in plant and animal tissues.

**viral** (vigh′ral). Pertaining to a virus.

**Virchow** (feer′ko), **Rudolf** (1821–1902). German pathologist who applied the cellular theory to disease and showed how disease could be identified through observation of cells and tissues.

**virulent** (veer′yoo-lent). Extremely poisonous or harmful.

**virus** (vigh′rus). A small organism too small to be seen with the ordinary microscope.

**viscera** (vis′er-uh). The internal organs.

**viscid** (vis′id). Sticky.

**visual purple.** The purple pigment in the rods of the retina of the eye; rhodopsin.

**vital statistics.** Death rates, birth rates, sickness rates, etc.

**vitamin** (vigh′tuh-min). A substance present in small amounts in food and necessary for normal functioning of the body. The following are known vitamins:

    **vitamin A**
    **vitamin $B_1$**   Thiamine
    **vitamin $B_2$**   Riboflavin
    **vitamin $B_3$**   Niacin (nicotinic acid)
    **vitamin $B_6$**   Pyridoxine
    **vitamin $B_{12}$**   Cyanocobalamin
    **vitamin C**   Ascorbic acid
    **vitamin D**
    **vitamin E**
    **vitamin K**
    **folic acid**
    **pantothenic acid**

**vitreous** (vit′ri-us) **body** or **vitreous humor.** Transparent semifluid mass between the lens and the retina of the eye.

**vocal cords.** The ligaments in the larynx which vibrate in speech.

**voice box.** The larynx.

**void** (voyd). To release waste matter.

**volvulus** (vahl′vyoo-lus). A twisting of the intestine causing blockage.

**vomit** (vahm′it). 1. To throw up matter from the stomach. 2. The material from the stomach ejected through the mouth.

**voyeurism** (voy′er-izm). Sexual excitement from seeing suggestive pictures or sights.

**vulva** (vul′vuh). The external genital organs of the female including the vaginal lips, clitoris, and other structures.

**vulvitis** (vul-vigh′tis). Inflammation of the vulva.

**vulvovaginitis** (vul-vo-vaj-uh-nigh′tis). Inflammation of the vulva and the vagina, particularly an infection seen in children. This infection is caused by bacteria and produces redness, swelling, and a copious discharge.

**W**

**walleye** (wawl′igh). 1. A condition in which the cornea is white and opaque; leukoma. 2. A condition in which the images seen by the eyes are slanted in different directions; divergent strabismus.

**ward.** A large room in a hospital where there are several patients.

  **isolation ward.** One where persons having contagious diseases are kept safely apart from other patients.

  **probationary ward.** One where patients are kept until it is determined whether they have a contagious disease.

  **psychopathic ward.** One where patients with mental disease are kept temporarily.

**wart.** A small overgrowth on the skin.

**Wassermann** (wahs′er-mun) **test.** A blood test for syphilis; named for August Paul von Wassermann, (1866–1925), German bacteriologist who developed the test.

**Wells, Horace** (1815–1848). An American dentist who led the way for general anesthesia in surgery by using nitrous oxide (laughing gas) during tooth extractions.

**wen.** A cyst of an oil gland of the skin, particularly on the scalp.

**wet nurse.** A woman who breast-feeds another's baby.

**wheal** (hweel). A smooth elevation on the skin, such as hives.

**whelk** (hwelk). A wheal on the face.

**white cell.** See **leukocyte.**

**white matter.** The white portion of the brain and spinal cord. It contains only fibers, no nerve cell bodies.

**whites.** Leukorrhea.

**Widal** (vee′dal) **test.** A blood test for typhoid diagnosis.

**windpipe.** Trachea.

**wintergreen oil.** Methyl salicylate; gaultheria oil; an oily liquid used as a liniment for rheumatic pains, as a local antiseptic, or as a flavoring agent.

**wisdom tooth.** The last molar on either side of each jaw.

**witch hazel.** An astringent.

**writer's cramp.** Pain in the arm, hand, and fingers caused by writing.

**X**

**xanthoma** (zan-tho′muh). Condition in which fatty tumors form in the skin especially in the eyelids.

**xerophthalmia** (zee-rahf-thal′mi-uh). Drying of the eyes; often associated with lack of vitamin A.

**xerosis** (zi-ro′sis). Abnormal dryness of skin or eyes.

**xiphoid** (zif′oyd) **process.** The cartilage projecting from the lower edge of the breastbone.

**x-ray dermatitis.** A skin eruption caused by overexposure to x-rays.

**Y**

**yaws.** Frambesia; a chronic disease caused by a spirochete and characterized by sores which first appear in the genital area. It is found in tropical countries.

**yellow fever.** A viral disease spread from infected persons or monkeys by mosquitoes. Symptoms are fever, headache, weakness, backache, and nasal congestion. Found in South America and Africa.

**yogurt** (yo′goort). Cultured milk; milk fermented by certain bacteria.

**yolk sac** or **yolk** (yohk). The part of the egg that nourishes the embryo; the yellow portion in birds' eggs.

**Z**

**zinc acetate** (zink as′i-tayt). An astringent; an antiseptic for treating eye inflammations.

**zinc oxide.** A white powder or ointment used in treating skin disorders and burns.

**zona** (zo′nuh). 1. A beltlike structure or band. 2. Herpes zoster.

**zoonosis** (zoh-oh-noh′sis). A disease transmitted by an animal to a human.

**zoster** (zahs′ter). See **herpes zoster.**

**zwieback** (zwee′bak). Pieces of rich bread which have been heated in the oven until they turned yellow.

**zygote** (zigh′goht). The cell formed by the union of an egg and a sperm; a fertilized egg.

# ABOUT THE AUTHORS

Dr. Benjamin F. Miller received his undergraduate training at the Massachusetts Institute of Technology and his medical training at the Harvard Medical School, the Cornell Medical Center, and the Rockefeller Institute for Medical Research. During World War II he attained the rank of major in the Public Health Service. Falling ill, and spending more months in hospitals than anyone could ever expect to endure, he busied himself writing pamphlets for the U.S. Public Health Service. It was at that time that the idea for this book first developed.

Other books written or edited by Dr. Miller include *You and Your Doctor, When Doctors Are Patients* (with Max Pinner, M.D.), *Man and His Body* (with Ruth Goode), *Good Health* (with J. Burt), *Family Health Guide and Medical Encyclopedia, Investigating Your Health, The Family Book of Preventive Medicine* and *Freedom From Heart Attacks* (both with Lawrence Galton), and *The Encyclopedia and Dictionary of Medicine and Nursing.* He was editor-in-chief of *The Modern Medical Encyclopedia* and *The Modern Encyclopedia of Baby and Child Care.* He also contributed 125 scientific papers and many articles to major magazines.

Dr. Miller was on the faculty of Harvard Medical School and professor at the University of Pennsylvania School of Medicine. He engaged in research on diseases of the heart, arteries and kidneys and was awarded the Francis Amory Prize of the American Academy of Arts and Sciences in 1962 for his pioneer work in kidney transplantation at the Peter Bent Brigham Hospital.

His wife, Judith, was formerly director of the early childhood division at the Walden School.

Lawrence Galton is a noted medical writer and editor and a former visiting professor at Purdue University. He is a columnist for the Washington Star Syndicate and *Family Circle,* and his articles frequently appear in *The New York Times Magazine, Reader's Digest, Parade,* and other national publications. He is the author of more than a dozen other books.